Cochlear Implants: Audiologic Management

Cochlear Implants: Audiologic Management

Editor: Rowland Halsey

AMERICAN
MEDICAL PUBLISHERS
www.americanmedicalpublishers.com

AMERICAN
MEDICAL PUBLISHERS
www.americanmedicalpublishers.com

Cataloging-in-Publication Data

Cochlear implants : audiologic management / edited by Rowland Halsey.
p. cm.
Includes bibliographical references and index.
ISBN 979-8-88740-015-0
1. Cochlear implants. 2. Hearing aids. 3. Audiology. 4. Hearing disorders--Treatment. I. Halsey, Rowland.
RF305 .C63 2023
617.89--dc23

American Medical Publishers,
41 Flatbush Avenue,
1st Floor, New York,
NY 11217, USA

ISBN 979-8-88740-015-0 (Hardback)

Contents

Preface

Cochlea is a coiled sensory structure that is present in the inner ear and plays a significant role in hearing. This sensory structure is stimulated by the cochlear nerve, which bifurcates from the larger vestibulocochlear nerve and serves as the primary fiber for the relay of electrical impulses transferring information about sound from the external environment to the auditory nucleus, or sound-processing centre of the brain. An electrical device inserted surgically into the human ear that enables hearing impaired people to detect sound is called a cochlear implant. Adults affected by extreme sensorineural hearing loss often use these implants. There are certain drawbacks associated with the implantation procedure such as a person may experience complete hearing loss in the affected ear. Infection, numbness around the ear, tinnitus, and implant failure are some other side effects related with cochlear implant. Improvements in electrode technologies and device materials have lowered the risk of infection caused by these implants. This book is compiled in such a manner, that it will provide in-depth knowledge about cochlear implants. It aims to equip students and experts with the advanced topics and upcoming concepts on these implants.

This book is the end result of constructive efforts and intensive research done by experts in this field. The aim of this book is to enlighten the readers with recent information in this area of research. The information provided in this profound book would serve as a valuable reference to students and researchers in this field.

At the end, I would like to thank all the authors for devoting their precious time and providing their valuable contribution to this book. I would also like to express my gratitude to my fellow colleagues who encouraged me throughout the process.

Editor

1

Music Perception Testing Reveals Advantages and Continued Challenges for Children Using Bilateral Cochlear Implants

Morrison M. Steel[1], Melissa J. Polonenko[1], Sara Giannantonio[1], Talar Hopyan[1], Blake C. Papsin[1,2] and Karen A. Gordon[1,2]*

[1] *Archie's Cochlear Implant Laboratory, The Hospital for Sick Children, Toronto, ON, Canada,* [2] *Department of Otolaryngology-Head and Neck Surgery, University of Toronto, Toronto, ON, Canada*

***Correspondence:**
Karen A. Gordon
karen.gordon@utoronto.ca

A modified version of the child's *Montreal Battery of Evaluation of Amusia* (cMBEA) was used to assess music perception in children using bilateral cochlear implants. Our overall aim was to promote better performance by children with CIs on the cMBEA by modifying the complement of instruments used in the test and adding pieces transposed in frequency. The 10 test trials played by piano were removed and two high and two low frequency trials added to each of five subtests (20 additional). The modified cMBEA was completed by 14 children using bilateral cochlear implants and 23 peers with normal hearing. Results were compared with performance on the original version of the cMBEA previously reported in groups of similar aged children: 2 groups with normal hearing (n = 23: Hopyan et al., 2012; n = 16: Polonenko et al., 2017), 1 group using bilateral cochlear implants (CIs) (n = 26: Polonenko et al., 2017), 1 group using bimodal (hearing aid and CI) devices (n = 8: Polonenko et al., 2017), and 1 group using unilateral CI (n = 23: Hopyan et al., 2012). Children with normal hearing had high scores on the modified version of the cMBEA and there were no significant score differences from children with normal hearing who completed the original cMBEA. Children with CIs showed no significant improvement in scores on the modified cMBEA compared to peers with CIs who completed the original version of the test. The group with bilateral CIs who completed the modified cMBEA showed a trend toward better abilities to remember music compared to children listening through a unilateral CI but effects were smaller than in previous cohorts of children with bilateral CIs and bimodal devices who completed the original cMBEA. Results confirmed that musical perception changes with the type of instrument and is better for music transposed to higher rather than lower frequencies for children with normal hearing but not for children using bilateral CIs. Overall, the modified version of the cMBEA revealed that modifications to music do not overcome the limitations of the CI to improve music perception for children.

Keywords: deafness, cochlear implant, electrical stimulation, Montreal Battery of Evaluation of Amusia (MBEA), bilateral, memory

INTRODUCTION

In the present study, we used a modified version of the *child's Montreal Battery of Evaluation of Amusia* (cMBEA) (Peretz et al., 2003, 2013) to assess music perception in children using bilateral cochlear implants. Our overall aim was to help children with bilateral CIs discriminate fundamental aspects of music. To do this, we modified the complement of instruments used in the cMBEA and added pieces which were shifted in frequency.

Music in Childhood

Music is considered by many to be a universal language and has been present throughout history in every culture. Musical abilities develop in the early months of life (Trehub, 2001). Infants can detect changes in various aspects of musical stimuli, such as *contour* (pitch direction), *interval* (pitch changes that preserve melodic contour), *scale* (tonality), and rhythm. Despite differences in the acoustic features of music and speech (Smith et al., 2002) and hemispheric specializations for spectral and temporal processing (Zatorre et al., 2002), musical development parallels language development and may be critical to language acquisition in humans (Brandt et al., 2012; Norman-Haignere et al., 2019). In fact, musical training increases cortical plasticity, which can strengthen common subcortical circuits and lead to widespread benefits in diverse non-musical skills, such as speech perception in noise, auditory attention, and auditory working memory (Jäncke, 2012; Kraus et al., 2012).

Music perception is a difficult task, which recruits diverse brain regions (Limb et al., 2010). The melodic (pitch-based *what*) and temporal (time-based *when*) dimensions of music are analyzed in parallel by separate neural subsystems (Peretz et al., 2003). The auditory cortex plays a major role in the processing of pitch relations, while temporal relations are also computed by distinct regions, such as the motor cortex, cerebellum, and basal ganglia (Peretz and Zatorre, 2005). Specifically, the right auditory cortex is specialized for pitch processing, whereas the left auditory cortex plays a more important role in rhythm perception (Zatorre et al., 2002).

Music Perception in Cochlear Implant Users

Music perception in listeners with normal hearing is facilitated by the presence of low-order resolved harmonics (Plomp, 1967), which are not well-represented by CI devices with poor frequency and temporal fine structure resolution, due in part to few electrodes, current spread, envelope-based processing, and low stimulation rates (e.g., Zeng, 2002). CIs provide fewer than eight effective channels, but music and pitch perception continue to improve when channels increase (up to ~60) in normal listeners (Kong et al., 2004; Mehta and Oxenham, 2017). Although current spread prevents distortion of binaural processing by small place mismatches, it also reduces the number of independent channels represented by the CI, thereby limiting the capacity for pitch discrimination and music perception (Jiam and Limb, 2019). New speech processing strategies attempt to provide better fine temporal resolution but with little effect on music perception (Magnusson, 2011).

Given effects of CI processing on music, it is not surprising that adults receiving cochlear implants rated their music appreciation and enjoyment as decreasing from a mean of 8.7/10 before hearing loss to 2.6/10 after implantation (Leal et al., 2003; Mirza et al., 2003). The first French patient to receive electrical stimulation from within the cochlea famously described the changes in stimulation from different cochlear places (in order to stimulate changes in pitch perception) as "the turning of a roulette wheel" (Djourno and Eyries, 1957; Djourno et al., 1957). Studies since then have shown that CI users tend to perceive rhythm in music more accurately than pitch or timbre (McDermott and McKay, 1997; Gfeller et al., 2002b; McDermott, 2004; Bruns et al., 2016). The minimum interval that CI users can discriminate is larger than seven semitones on average, compared with well under 1 semitone for NH peers (Gfeller et al., 2002a; Mary Zarate et al., 2012; Bruns et al., 2016). When presented with pairs of sound sequences varying in rhythm, but not pitch, and asked to determine whether they are the same or different, adult CI users achieved a mean score of 88% (Gfeller and Lansing, 1991). Similarly, melodies with more rhythmic patterns were more easily recognized (Schulz and Kerber, 1994). Increased activation in the frontal cortex during melody versus rhythm perception may reflect greater mental effort (Limb et al., 2010).

Children with CIs perform even more poorly on music perception and recognition tests than adult CI users (Jung et al., 2012) but their ratings of musical enjoyment can be high nonetheless (Drennan et al., 2015). Children are better able to hear changes in rhythm than aspects of music which require spectral resolution [e.g., scale, contour, or interval (Hopyan et al., 2012) or harmony (Zimmer et al., 2019)]. Music perception is slightly better in those children who had some residual hearing during the period prior to implantation (Hopyan et al., 2012). Children can successfully combine residual acoustic hearing in one ear with electrical hearing through a CI in the other ear (bimodal hearing) to discriminate differences between music excerpts (Polonenko et al., 2017). Children who have access to hearing in both ears through two CIs or a hearing aid in one ear and CI in the other (bimodal) are able to discriminate some musical changes better than children who use one CI alone

(Polonenko et al., 2017). The ability to use mode (i.e., pitch) cues to judge emotion in music increases with longer periods of acoustic hearing prior to implantation and better residual hearing in the non-implanted ear (Hopyan et al., 2012; Giannantonio et al., 2015). Music perception and singing also appear to improve for children with CIs who receive musical training (Giannantonio et al., 2015; Polonenko et al., 2017; Yang et al., 2019). Moreover, there are reports of individual CI users who have good music perception (Maarefvand et al., 2013), suggesting possibilities for improved music listening through CIs.

The Montreal Battery of Evaluation of Amusia for Testing Music Perception in Cochlear Implant Users

The *Montreal Battery of Evaluation of Amusia* (MBEA) test (Peretz et al., 2003) has proven to be a sensitive, reliable, and valid tool for identifying impaired music perception in individuals with amusia (Vuvan et al., 2018) as well as in adult and child CI users (Cooper et al., 2008; Hopyan et al., 2012; Polonenko et al., 2017; Lima et al., 2018). The child's MBEA (cMBEA) has slight differences from the adult version (MBEA) (Peretz et al., 2013); the melodies are shorter (~7 notes rather than ~10), there are fewer test items (20 rather than 30 in each subtest), the metric test is not included, and 10 different instruments are used to make the test more engaging for children. The cMBEA has five subtests: *Scale, Contour, Interval, Rhythm,* and *Memory*. Half of the trials in the first four subtests contain identical pairs of melodies, while the other trials are melodies that differ by one note. Children indicate whether the pairs are the "same" or "different." Note differences can be out-of key (Scale subtest), a change in pitch directions (Contour subtest), a change in note interval within the same the key and contour of the melody (Interval subtest), or a change in grouping of note durations (Rhythm subtest). In the fifth and final subtest, single melodies are presented; half were previously presented in the first four subtests and the other half are new melodies. Children indicate whether each melody is "old" or "new."

The musical excerpts in the cMBEA have fundamental frequencies ranging from 247 to 988 Hz. The perception of these melodies could be compromised in CI users for a number of reasons. First, as discussed above, there are limited numbers of effective cochlear implant frequency channels (Rubinstein, 2004) to represent the spectral components of the musical stimuli with restricted representation of low frequencies. Second, the range of frequencies contained in the music are represented by electrodes that sit in more basal areas of the cochlea than predicted by frequency-position functions (Greenwood, 1990; Stakhovskaya et al., 2007). This can increase the pitch heard by cochlear implant users. Third, there may be decreasing populations of spiral ganglia available for electrical stimulation in more basal than apical areas of the cochlea in deafness (Leake et al., 1992; Nadol, 1997) which could further compromise central representation of the musical pieces in the MBEA. These factors may explain why adults with CIs judge higher frequency music to be distorted or shrill compared to lower frequency music (Gfeller et al., 2002a). The effects of shifting the spectra of music to lower or higher frequencies on music perception through a CI remains to be determined.

There may also be aspects of the MBEA stimuli which restrict music perception in CI users. Cooper et al. (2008) noted that some musical excerpts in the MBEA have fundamental frequencies which fall below the range of frequency channels in most CIs and recommended transposing these melodies up two octaves to maximize place pitch perception. On the other hand, Gfeller et al. (2002b) found that pure tone frequency discrimination in a group of adult CI users was better at 1600 Hz than 3200 Hz which suggests that an opposite approach, transposing music to lower frequencies might have benefits. Cooper et al. (2008) also noted that melody transposition below the lower limit of fundamental frequencies used in the MBEA would help to define the limits of temporal pitch coding in CI users.

The complement of instruments that are used to play the cMBEA stimuli could also have unique effects on children using CIs. In the adult version of the test, all music was played by piano whereas the child version contains 10 instruments (including piano) to help maintain test engagement (Peretz et al., 2013). It is clear that children using CIs have more difficulties than their normal hearing peers distinguishing between different instruments (Roy et al., 2014) but potential effects of different instruments on cMBEA performance in either group of children has not been studied to our knowledge.

Children with normal hearing do show clear musical preferences. For example, there are gender-based biases that can influence what instrument children choose to play (O'Neill and Boultona, 1996) and infants prefer happy music which has large pitch changes (Corbeil et al., 2013). These preferences could be affected by deafness and CI use. Adults with CIs rate the timbre quality as being different between different types of instruments (Gfeller et al., 2002b) and exhibit poor pitch perception for piano tones in particular (Galvin et al., 2008). It is possible that there are different effects of instrument on music perception in children with CIs given child-based musical preferences and the limited access to acoustic musical input in early sensitive periods of development.

In the present study, we examined whether modifications to musical excerpts in the cMBEA could help children with CIs better discriminate music. Our specific hypothesis was that better scores on the cMBEA can be achieved by children using CIs by removing piano excerpts and including music excerpts with modified spectra.

MATERIALS AND METHODS

This study was conducted under the approval of the Hospital for Sick Children's Research Ethics Board which adheres to the Tri-Council Policy Statement: Ethical Conduct for Research Involving Humans.

Participants

A modified version of the Child's MBEA test (modified cMBEA) was administered to 37 children: 23 with normal hearing and

14 with bilateral CIs. Demographic details for the CI users are detailed in **Table 1**. All child CI users were recruited from the Cochlear Implant Program at the Hospital for Sick Children in Toronto and had bilateral severe-to-profound sensorineural hearing loss that occurred in childhood; hearing loss was progressive in three children. Two children (CI22 and CI29) had a period of usable residual hearing prior to implantation (aided or unaided thresholds of $\leq$ 40 dB HL at any test frequency). Six children (CI2-8) received their first devices at median 1.74 years of age (range = 0.73–4.96) and were provided with second devices after 5.53 years of unilateral CI stimulation (0.9, 11.23) (sequential bilateral implantation), and 8 children (CI15-29) received their implants simultaneously at a median of 3.12 years of age (range 0.79–12.15). Children received different device generations (Nucleus 24CA, 24CS, or 24RE) and speech processors using the advanced combined encoder (ACE) strategy.

High resolution computed tomography scans confirmed normal cochlear anatomy in all but two children: child CI2 had a Mondini malformation (incomplete partition type II) and child CI22 had an enlarged left vestibular aqueduct. Four children had GJB2 gene mutations causing deficiencies in Connexin 26 gap junction protein (Propst et al., 2006), while smaller subsets had Usher Syndrome (n = 2) and received ototoxic medications at a young age (n = 1). The etiology of deafness was unknown in the remaining seven children.

A group of 23 children with normal hearing (NH) also completed the modified cMBEA. They were matched to the bilateral CI group in terms of age [$t(35)$ = 0.17, p = 0.87]. The NH and CI groups also reported taking music lessons or classes over similar periods of time, although the range was wider in the NH group [$t(32.47)$ = 1.35, p = 0.19; NH mean = 3.05 $\pm$ 3.39 years; CI mean = 1.96 $\pm$ 1.47 years]. Results of these children were compared to scores from previously reported groups of children who completed the original (unmodified) version of the cMBEA (Hopyan et al., 2012; Polonenko et al., 2017). As detailed in **Table 2**, the Polonenko data include children who used bilateral CIs and bimodal devices and the Hopyan data focused on children with bilateral deafness who used a unilateral CI. Both studies included their own control groups of children with normal hearing (NH). The age at testing was remarkably similar across all groups. Age at implantation was similar in children receiving bilateral CIs (BCI) and they had similar inter-implant periods. Children using unilateral CIs (UCI) received their implants at slightly older ages than the children receiving bilateral CIs (UCI_Hopyan: 5.0 $\pm$ 2.9 years, BCI_Steel: 3.4 $\pm$ 3.3 and BCI_Polonenko: 1.7 $\pm$ 1.2 years), reflecting CI candidacy at this earlier period of the Toronto SickKids implant program. Children using bimodal devices (BM) were also slightly older at implantation (BM_Polonenko: 7.3 $\pm$ 4.4 years) given their access to sound through hearing aids in the non-implanted ear. Duration of time-in-sound was calculated as the sum of the duration of CI experience and pre-implant residual hearing in children using CIs and as age for children with normal hearing. Children with CIs had slightly less time in sound than their normal hearing peers.

The Modified Child's Montreal Battery of Evaluation of Amusia

A modified version of the cMBEA (Lebrun et al., 2012) was created to evaluate music perception. The cMBEA consists of five subtests: *Scale, Contour, Interval, Rhythm,* and *Memory* (detailed in the Introduction), with fundamental frequencies ranging from 247 to 988 Hz. The 10 test trials, which were composed of piano tones in the original child's MBEA, were removed, because CI users exhibit poor pitch perception for piano tones (Galvin et al., 2008) and 20 additional trials were added to test effects of frequency shifts. High frequency transpositions aimed to give better access to fundamental frequencies of

TABLE 1 | Participant demographic information.

Child	Etiology	CI1			CI2		Inter-implant delay (years)	Age at test (years)	Bilateral CI experience (years)
		Age (years)	Ear	Device	Age (years)	Device			
CI2	Unknown	1.21	R	24CA	8.49	24RE	7.29	13.99	5.39
CI3	Connexin26	2.27	L	24CA	5.58	24RE	3.31	12.14	6.48
CI4	Usher	1.12	L	24CS	4.90	24RE	3.77	11.63	6.67
CI5	Usher	0.73	R	24RE	1.62	24RE	0.90	8.91	7.22
CI6	Unknown	4.96	L	24CS	15.40	24RE	10.44	17.95	2.50
CI8	Unknown	2.92	R	24RE	14.15	24RE	11.23	17.97	3.76
CI15	Connexin26	1.73	Bilateral	24RE	1.73	24RE	0	8.21	6.38
CI18	Unknown	1.28	Bilateral	24RE	1.28	24RE	0	8.20	6.82
CI20	Unknown	4.54	Bilateral	24RE	4.54	24RE	0	9.84	5.19
CI22	Ototoxicity	12.15	Bilateral	24RE	12.15	24RE	0	16.97	4.76
CI23	Connexin26	0.79	Bilateral	24RE	0.79	24RE	0	5.95	5.08
CI24	Unknown	4.51	Bilateral	24RE	4.51	24RE	0	8.62	4.04
CI25	Connexin26	0.95	Bilateral	24CA	0.95	24CA	0	9.45	8.40
CI29	Unknown	8.44	Bilateral	24RE	8.44	24RE	0	13.83	5.27

Demographic data for 14 bilateral cochlear implant (CI) users who completed the modified cMBEA (group: BCI_Steel).

TABLE 2 | Demographics of children who completed the modified and unmodified child versions of the MBEA.

	Group	Study	Child MBEA	Devices	*N*	Age at test (years)	Age at CI-1 (years)	Inter-implant delay (years)	Time in sound (years)
CI Users	BCI_Steel	Steel	Modified	Bilateral	14	11.7 ± 3.9	3.4 ± 3.3	2.6 ± 4.1	8.9 ± 3.0
	BCI_Polonenko	Polonenko	Original	Bilateral	26	10.5 ± 1.7	1.7 ± 1.2	2.5 ± 2.8	8.8 ± 1.9
	BM_Polonenko	Polonenko	Original	Bimodal	8	11.0 ± 2.3	7.3 ± 4.4	n/a	9.2 ± 1.8
	UCI_Hopyan	Hopyan	Original	Unilateral	23	12.5 ± 3.9	5.0 ± 2.9	n/a	9.1 ± 3.9
Normal hearing	NH_Steel	Steel	Modified		23	11.9 ± 3.2	n/a	n/a	11.9 ± 3.2
	NH_Polonenko	Polonenko	Original		16	11.8 ± 3.0	n/a	n/a	11.8 ± 3.0
	NH_Hopyan	Hopyan	Original		23	11.7 ± 2.9	n/a	n/a	11.7 ± 2.9

Unilateral cochlear implant (UCI), bilateral cochlear implant (BCI), bimodal (BM), normal hearing (NH).

MBEA musical excerpts and to better mimic cochlear frequency-position (Greenwood, 1990; Stakhovskaya et al., 2007) whereas transposition to lower frequencies might alleviate adverse responses to high pitches in music (Gfeller et al., 2002a), take advantage of and better pure tone frequency discrimination at lower than higher frequencies (Gfeller et al., 2002b), and help to define the limits of temporal pitch coding in implant users (Cooper et al., 2008). Two high frequency trials and two low frequency trials were added to each of the five subtests, resulting in 22 trials in each subtest (110 trials). Four trials in each subtest (20 total) were randomly selected for frequency modification. Sample Manager v3.4.1 (Audiofile Engineering, 2011) was used to raise the fundamental frequency of 10 of these trials by 2 octaves and lower the fundamental frequency of 10 trials by 1 octave. Musical stimuli, ranging from 60 to 70 dB SPL, were presented in a 2.13 m × 2.13 m sound-attenuating booth and played through Windows Media Player on a Dell Vostro 1520 laptop computer and external Centrios speaker system (model no. 1410106) at zero degrees azimuth. Levels were calibrated in dBA using a sound-level meter (Larson-Davis 800B). Listeners were seated 1 m away from the speakers.

Following modifications, the modified cMBEA was comprised of 110 test trials and 10 practice trials and lasted approximately 35 min in duration. Each subtest contained 22 test trials. Subtests were applied in the following order: Scale, Counter, Interval, Rhythm, and Memory. Practice trials preceded each subtest and contained stimuli from the original cMBEA which were representative of each subtest. For the first four subtests, half of the trials contained identical pairs of melodies, while the other half consisted of melodies that differed by one note. Children indicated whether the pairs of melodies that they heard were the same or different by pressing one of two buttons. Half of the fifth and final subtest the surprise/incidental memory test, contained melodies previously presented in the first four subtests, while the other half consisted of new melodies. For this subtest, children were asked whether they had heard the melody presented in the preceding subtests or if it was novel. The number of correct discriminations were summed, creating a "correct discrimination" score. These scores are presented as a percentage of total trials.

Data Analyses

Mixed model regressions were conducted on the correct discrimination scores using the lme4 (Bates et al., 2015) and lmerTest (Kuznetsova et al., 2017) packages in R and Rstudio (Version 1.0.153) (R Core Team, 2018). ANOVAs and pairwise *post hoc* analyses were implemented using the Satterthwaite method to estimate denominator degrees of freedom for t-statistics of the mixed models. Significance was defined at $p < 0.05$. Figures were created using the ggplot2 package (Wickham, 2016).

RESULTS

Figure 1 plots the individual (dots) and mean ± SE (bar) scores for the groups of children who completed the modified cMBEA (Steel groups) compared to previously published results of children who completed the original version of the cMBEA (Hopyan et al., 2012; Polonenko et al., 2017). Mixed model regression analyses with fixed effects of subtest and group and random intercept for participant revealed significant effects of subtest [$F(4,504) = 8.5$, $p < 0.0001$], group [$F(6,126) = 34.7$, $p < 0.0001$] and an interaction between subtest and group [$F(24,504) = 2.6$, $p < 0.0001$]. Relevant statistical comparisons of the interaction effect are shown in **Table 3**. The scores of children with normal hearing across studies are shown in **Figure 1A**.

There was no significant difference between the scores of children with normal hearing who completed the modified versus original versions of the cMBEA (NH_Steel vs. NH_Polonenko: $t(126) = -0.37$, $p > 0.05$; NH_Steel vs. NH_Hopyan: $t(126) = -0.38$, $p > 0.05$). Findings in all three normal hearing groups were consistent: all had significantly poorer scores on the Scale subtest compared to at least one other subtest ($p < 0.05$ as detailed in **Table 3**) and there were no significant differences between the three different NH groups for any of the five subtests or the total scores ($p > 0.05$). Thus, there was no significant effects of the modified version of the cMBEA for children with normal hearing.

Results from the four groups of children using CIs are shown in **Figure 1B**. As expected, all groups showed significantly poorer scores relative to all three groups of children with normal hearing across subtests and total score ($t > 4.3$, $p < 0.00001$). As previously reported, children with unilateral CIs (Hopyan et al., 2012) and children with bilateral CIs (Polonenko et al., 2017) perceived changes in the Rhythm subtest better than other subtests. This was also true of children with bilateral CIs who completed the

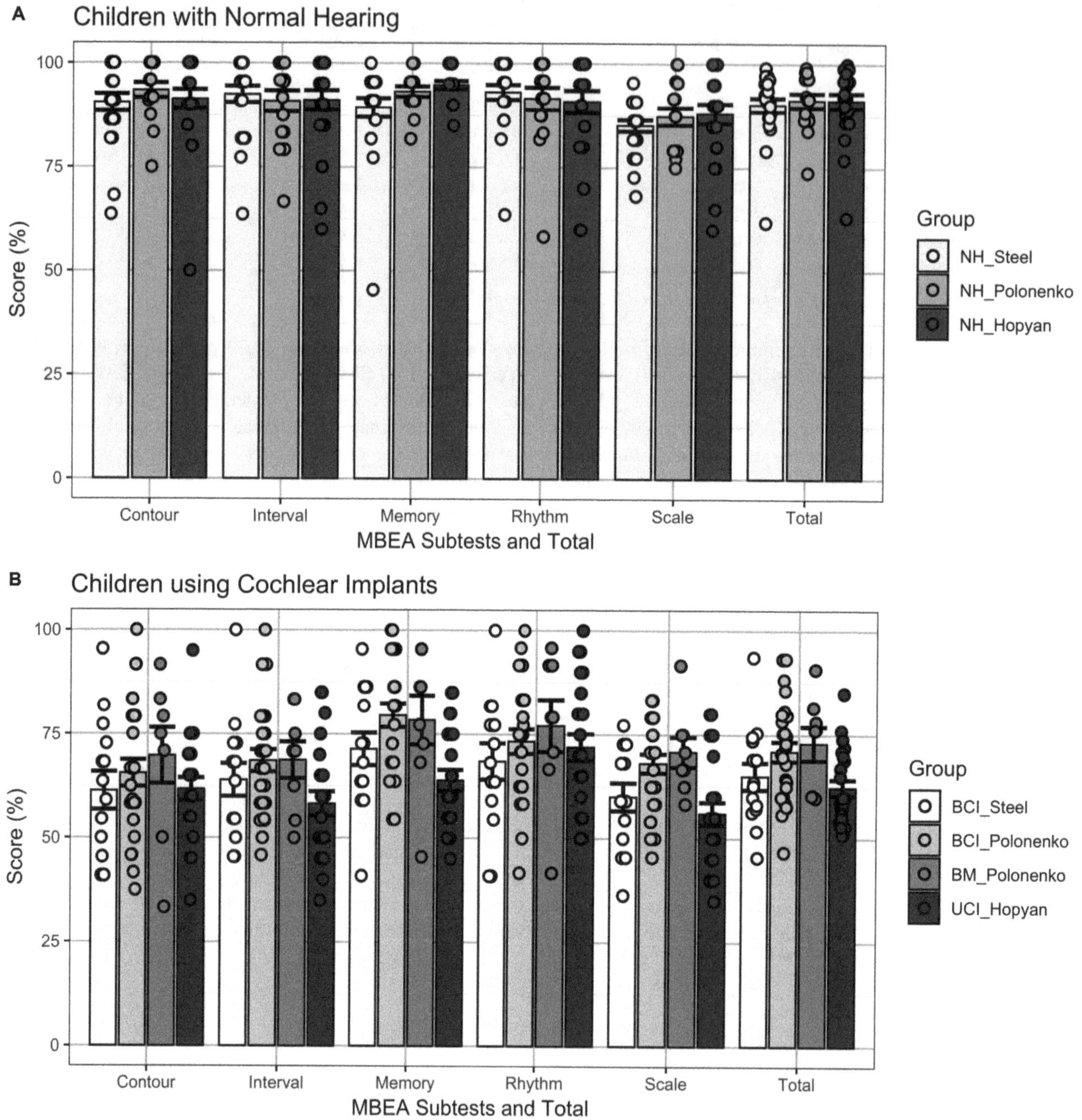

FIGURE 1 | (A) Individual (dots) and mean ± SE (bar) scores on cMBEA subtests and the total Score (Total) are shown for three groups of children with normal hearing: children completing the modified cMBEA (NH_Steel), and children who completed the original version (NH_Polonenko and NH_Hopyan). All three groups scored more poorly on the Scale subtest than the other subtests ($p < 0.05$) but there were no significant differences between groups on any of the five subtests or the total score ($p > 0.05$). **(B)** Individual (dots) and mean ± SE (bar) scores on cMBEA subtests and the total score are shown for four groups of children who use cochlear implants. Children with bilateral CI who completed the modified cMBEA (BCI_Steel) and children with Bilateral CIs (BCI_Polonenko), with Bimodal devices (BM_Polonenko) and Unilateral CIs (UCI_Hopyan) who completed the original version of the test from previous studies. Scores were lower than in the children with normal hearing ($p < 0.0001$) with best scores in the rhythm subtests in all groups ($p < 0.001$). In addition, better memory scores were found in the BCI_Polonenko and BM_Polonenko groups than the UCI_Hopyan group ($p < 0.001$ and $p = 0.004$, respectively) and a trend for better memory for the BCI_Steel group relative to the UCI_Hopyan group was found ($p = 0.07$).

modified version of the cMBEA (Steel group). Scores on the memory subtest were also of note: as previously reported, children with bilateral CIs and bimodal users (Polonenko et al., 2017) were able to recall music on the memory subtest better than children with unilateral CIs (Hopyan et al., 2012). Children with bilateral CIs who completed the modified version of the cMBEA showed a similar strength in the memory subtest but the trend toward improvement relative

TABLE 3 | Significant comparisons of subtest:group interaction.

Group	Subtest comparisons			df	*t*-Value	*p*-Value	Significance
Subtest comparisons by group							
NH_Steel	Scale		Contour	504	−0.42	0.034	*
	Scale		Interval	504	−2.39	0.004	**
	Scale		Rhythm	504	−2.98	0.002	**
NH_Polonenko	Scale		Contour	504	−0.18	0.043	*
NH_Hopyan	Scale		Memory	504	−1.82	0.007	**
BCI_Steel	Scale	-	Rhythm	504	−2.14	0.009	**
	Scale	-	Memory	504	−5.06	<0.001	***
	Contour	-	Rhythm	504	−0.84	0.026	*
	Contour	-	Memory	504	−3.76	0.002	**
BCI_Polonenko	Scale	-	Rhythm	504	−0.60	0.027	*
	Scale	-	Memory	504	−6.82	<0.001	***
	Contour	-	Rhythm	504	−3.12	0.001	**
	Interval	-	Rhythm	504	−0.09	0.046	*
	Rhythm	-	Memory	504	−1.59	0.008	**
BM_Polonenko	Scale	-	Memory	504	0.77	0.075	.
UCI_Hopyan	Scale	-	Rhythm	504	−10.95	<0.001	***
	Scale	-	Memory	504	−2.90	0.002	**
	Contour	-	Rhythm	504	−5.30	<0.001	***
	Interval	-	Rhythm	504	−8.77	<0.001	***
	Interval	-	Memory	504	−0.73	0.024	*
	Rhythm	-	Memory	504	12.96	0.001	**

Group comparisons	Subtest			df	*t*-Value	*p*-Value	Significance
Subtest comparisons across implant groups							
BCI_Steel vs. other CI groups	Memory	-	Memory:BCI_Polonenko	300	−0.076	0.048	*
	Memory		Memory:UCI_Hopyan	300	15.74	0.073	.
BCI_Polonenko vs. other groups	Scale	-	Scale:UCI_Hopyan	300	18.95	<0.001	***
	Interval	-	Interval:UCI_Hopyan	300	17.29	0.004	**
	Memory	-	Memory:UCI_Hopyan	300	22.57	<0.001	***
BM_Polonenko vs. other groups							
	Scale	-	Scale:UCI_Hopyan	300	24.70	0.004	**
	Scale	-	Scale:UCI_Hopyan	300	24.70	0.004	**
	Memory	-	Memory:UCI_Hopyan	300	24.45	0.004	**

*Significance codes: '***' < 0.001, '**' < 0.01, '*' < 0.05.*

to the Hopyan unilateral CI group did not reach statistical significance ($p = 0.07$).

As shown in **Figure 2**, scores across subtests on the modified cMBEA were averaged for music excerpts played by each type of instrument in children with normal hearing and children using bilateral CIs. Significant effects were found for instrument [$F(8,280) = 3.6$, $p < 0.0001$], group [$F(1,35) = 60.8$, $p < 0.0001$] and the interaction between instrument and group [$F(1,8) = 280$, $p < 0.02$]. Comparisons revealed scores in the NH group which were best for the violin and worst for the vibraphone ($p < 0.05$). Scores in children with bilateral CIs were clearly poorer than in their peers with normal hearing ($p < 0.0001$) and were not significantly different between instruments ($p > 0.05$).

Scores on the musical excerpts that were shifted in frequency are shown for both children with normal hearing and children using bilateral CIs in **Figure 3**. Consistent with overall findings discussed above, scores were significantly poorer in children using bilateral CIs relative to normal hearing peers [$F(1,35) = 59.0$, $p < 0.0001$]. There was also a trend toward differences between high and low frequency shifts [$F(1,35) = 4.1$, $p = 0.05$] which reflected significantly better scores for music shifted to high versus low frequencies (mean ± SD = 90.43 ± 11.47 and 85.22 ± 9.47%, respectively) in children with normal hearing [$t(22) = 2.4$, $p < 0.05$]. Although the mean data suggest the same trends in children with bilateral CI and there was no significant interaction between group and frequency shift [$F(1,35) = 0.044$, $p = 0.83$], the differences in scores between high and low frequency shifts (mean ± SD = 60.00 ± 18.81 and 53.57 ± 20.61%, respectively) were not significant in the CI group [$t(13) = 1.0$, $p > 0.05$].

DISCUSSION

Results indicated that our modifications to musical excerpts in the cMBEA did not help children with CIs achieve better scores

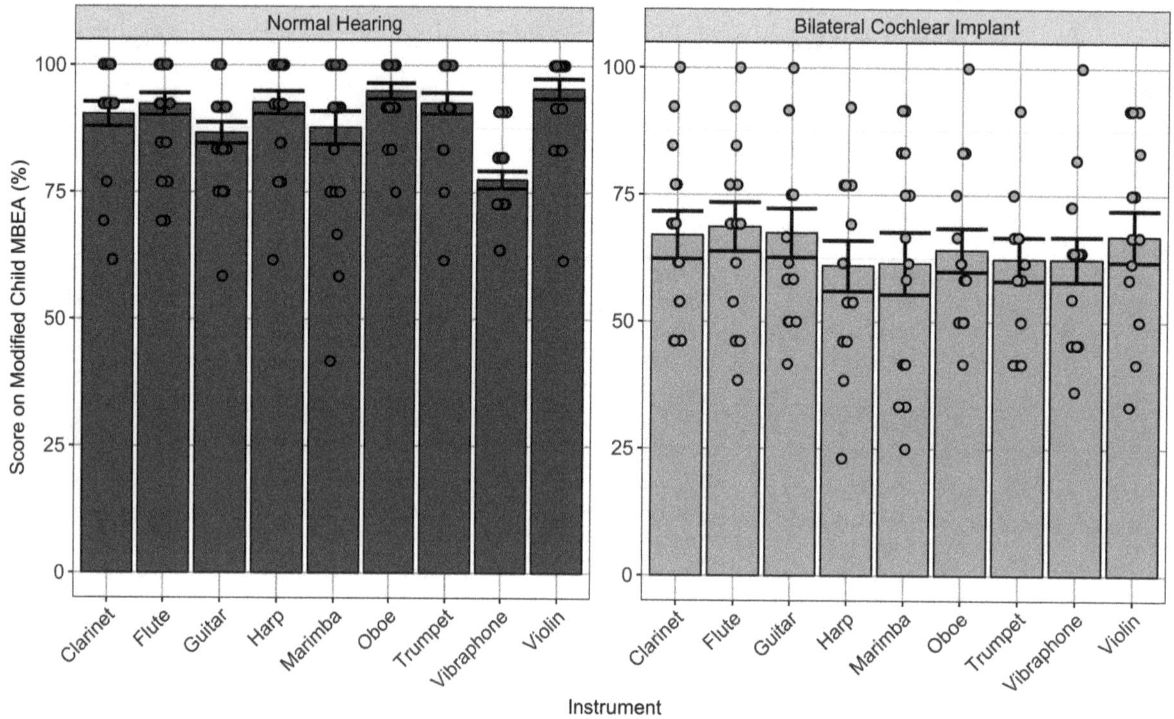

FIGURE 2 | Individual (dots) and mean ± SE (bar) scores on the modified cMBEA stimuli grouped by instrument type. Data from children with normal hearing (NH_Steel), shown on the left, reveal slightly better scores when music was played by the violin ($p < 0.05$). Scores were significantly poorer in children with bilateral CIs (BCI_Steel), shown on the right ($p < 0.0001$), and no significant differences in scores by instrument were found for this group ($p > 0.05$).

on this test of music discrimination. Specifically, performance by children using CIs on the cMBEA when piano excerpts were removed and music excerpts with modified spectra were included was not different from results in other groups who completed the original version of the cMBEA. This finding was counter to the study hypothesis. The group with bilateral CIs who completed the modified cMBEA showed a trend toward improved abilities to remember music compared to a group listening through a unilateral CI but effects were smaller than in previous cohorts of children with bilateral CIs and bimodal devices who completed the original version of the cMBEA. On the other hand, children with normal hearing did show better music perception for some instruments than others and better scores for music shifted to higher frequencies than music shifted to lower frequencies. Overall, the modified version of the cMBEA revealed that modifications to music do not overcome the limitations of the CI for music perception in children. In addition, trends in the present cohort compliment significant findings in previous groups of children using bilateral devices that show that access to hearing in both ears promotes better memory for music compared to children using unilateral CIs.

Modifications to the Child MBEA Do Not Affect Discrimination Scores in Children With Normal Hearing

In the modified cMBEA, piano excerpts were removed and 20 trials of musical excerpts which were either raised or lowered in frequency were added. As shown in **Figure 1A**, these modifications did not affect subtest and total scores in children with normal hearing relative to previous data in similar aged groups who completed the original version of the test. The high scores achieved in all three groups suggest that the distinctions in music tested in the cMBEA are fairly easy for children with normal hearing. Similarly, Vuvan et al. (2018) found that 175 participants aged 16 to 69 years (mean = 29.7 years) with no reported deficits often achieved maximum scores on this test (Vuvan et al., 2018). A slight decrease in score was only found in the Scale subtest and, again, this was a consistent finding across the three groups, confirming that the modified version of the cMBEA had little effect on abilities to detect musical differences in children with normal hearing. The finding that performance was poorer on the Scale subtest may reflect either differences in the discrimination required between the Scale and other subtests or the fact that perception of scale or *tonality* is a more complex and higher-order task than contour and interval perception. The latter point is supported by evidence that musical scale is processed by a specialized system in the prefrontal cortex (Peretz et al., 2003).

The Modified cMBEA Does Not Yield Better Music Perception Scores in Children Using CIs

Data shown in **Figure 1B** reveal that the modified cMBEA yields scores that are consistent with those obtained in children with

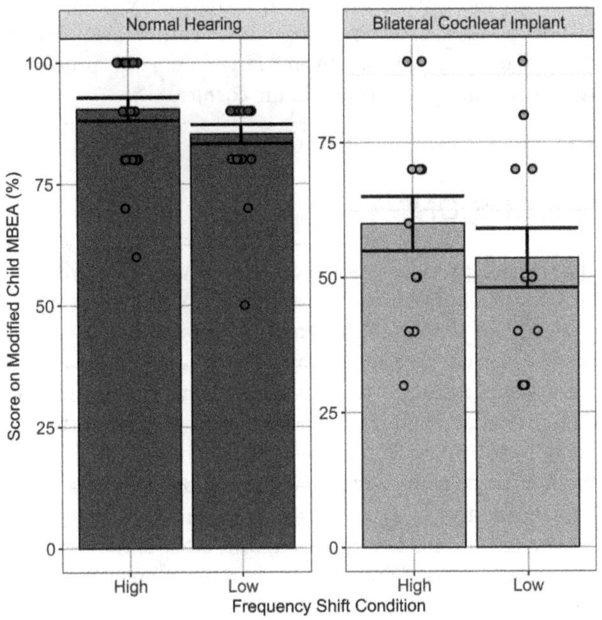

FIGURE 3 | Individual (dots) and mean ± SE (bar) scores on those stimuli in the modified cMBEA which were raised or lowered in frequency. Children with normal hearing (NH_Steel) scored better for music raised to higher frequencies than music lowered in frequency ($p < 0.05$). There was no significant effect for children using bilateral CIs (BCI_Steel) ($p > 0.05$).

bilateral CIs who completed the original cMBEA in previous studies. Clearly, discrimination scores are reduced relative to normal hearing peers in all 4 of the CI groups. As discussed in previous papers, many children using CIs are effectively amusic (Hopyan et al., 2012; Polonenko et al., 2017; Lima et al., 2018) based on score cutoffs of ~75% (Vuvan et al., 2018). Yet, unlike individuals with amusia, individuals with hearing loss who use CIs report frequent engagement with music and that they enjoy listening to music (Mirza et al., 2003; Migirov et al., 2009; Looi et al., 2012). This positive relationship with music could stem from a combination of access to music through their CIs, exposure in social and cultural events, and training (Prevoteau et al., 2018; Riley et al., 2018).

Musical experience in children with early onset hearing loss is likely very different from that of adults who lose their hearing and receive implants later in life. Children with CIs hear music in a unique way. As shown in **Figure 1B**, all of the groups of children with hearing loss were better able to hear changes in the Rhythm subtest as compared with changes on the Scale, Tnterval or Contour subtests. This relative strength was not affected by the modifications to the cMBEA and is consistent with several previous investigations (e.g., Gfeller and Lansing, 1991; Cooper et al., 2008; Hopyan et al., 2012), reflecting adequate temporal resolution through CIs for detecting rhythmic patterns in music (McDermott, 2004). CI users are heavily dependent on rhythm when attempting to identify different melodies (Gfeller et al., 2002a) and struggle to recognize melodies in the absence of rhythm cues (Kong et al., 2004). Rhythm perception may also underlie perception of speech and emotions by CI users (Leal et al., 2003; Hopyan et al., 2011). As Hopyan et al. (2012) noted, music in the Rhythm subtest also contain pitch variations, potentially explaining why children using CIs show poorer scores than normal hearing children on this subtest of the cMBEA. In addition, there may be variability in temporal processing between CI users. Lower gap detection thresholds, one of many possible measure of temporal processing, have been associated with better speech perception in CI users (Muchnik et al., 1994) and perhaps could also predict differences in perception of rhythm in music. Overall, however, the modifications to the cMBEA were either too subtle or targeted the wrong aspects of music to identify relative strengths that children using CIs might have for perceiving music.

Advantage of Bilateral Input Over Unilateral CI for Music Memory

As shown in **Figure 1B**, children using bilateral CIs or bimodal devices did not achieve significantly higher scores than children using unilateral CIs on the Scale, Interval, Contour, or Rhythm subtests of the cMBEA (original and modified versions). While a second CI device enhances many binaural listening abilities, such as spatial unmasking, binaural summation, and sound localization (Litovsky et al., 2012), bilateral implantation does not seem to overcome the CI device limitations that compromise music perception in deaf children. Veekmans et al. (2009) used the Munich Music Questionnaire to assess music enjoyment in post-lingually deafened adults who used both unilateral and bilateral CIs and found that a larger percentage of bilateral CI users reported being able to recognize many elements of music, such as melody and timbre, though the difference was not statistically significant. The authors suggested that bilateral implantation may improve music perception by capturing the better ear and reducing the number of cochlear dead regions across the two ears that are not sufficiently stimulated due to lack of neural integrity. It is possible then that music enjoyment is driven more by sound quality than ability to detect differences between musical excerpts. It is important also to keep in mind that adults with post-lingual deafness, like those in the Veekmans et al. (2009) study, were able to access music normally during early development which provides them advantages for music listening over CI users with pre-lingual deafness (Bruns et al., 2016).

The largest difference between bilateral and unilateral CI users in the present cohorts of children was on the Memory subtest. Scores on the memory subtest were significantly better for the bilateral CI and bimodal users in previous cohorts tested with the original version of the cMBEA compared to unilateral CIs users. The bilateral CI users who completed the modified cMBEA showed a trend toward increased Memory subtest scores related to the scores on the original cMBEA in the unilateral CI group ($p = 0.07$). The relative strength of memory for music by children using bilateral devices may be interpreted as a consequence of reduced listening effort in children who have access to bilateral rather than unilateral hearing (Polonenko et al., 2017). The Memory subtest scores were amongst the highest of all subtests in all groups of children using CIs. Hopyan et al. (2012) have pointed out that superior memory for melodies is a phenomenon unique to CI children given that their adult counterparts do not score better on the Memory subtest compared with other subtests on the MBEA (Cooper et al., 2008). If so, perhaps this skill could be harnessed in therapy to improve music perception in children with CIs.

Music Perception Is Not Better When Particular Instruments or Spectral Changes Are Presented in Children With CIs

Effects of particular instruments and spectral manipulations of music were assessed in children using bilateral CIs and normal hearing peers using a modified version of the cMBEA. Changes in scores, shown in **Figure 2**, showed effects in the children with normal hearing but not in children with bilateral CIs. As shown, scores were highest for music played by violin and poorest when the music was played with the vibraphone in children with normal hearing. This could reflect biases and preferences of each participant, prior musical exposure, or different discrimination skills required by each subtest. By contrast, children with CIs showed no changes in score by instrument, consistent with previous findings that the subtle differences in timbre by instrument are not available to them (McDermott, 2004) or that they are not able to make use of strategies used by adult CI users to discriminate timbre (Kong et al., 2004; Macherey and Delpierre, 2013). With this in mind, it is unlikely that children using CIs have particularly poor perception of piano music. As shown in **Figure 1**, removing the piano pieces did not significantly affect cMBEA scores in children with normal hearing or in children with CIs.

Administering test batteries with more appropriate stimuli for children using CIs, such as wider ranges of stimulus frequencies, may provide a more valid assessment of children's music discrimination ability. The modified cMBEA scores did achieve this objective as scores were poorer for music shifted to lower than higher frequencies. CI users primarily use differences in the place of stimulation within the cochlea, as opposed to the rate of neural firing, to code pitch and changes in pitch (Moore, 2003; Laneau et al., 2004); thus, one solution might be to transpose MBEA melodies up two octaves to maximize place pitch perception or to transpose to lower frequency below the lower limit of fundamental frequencies used in the MBEA in order to define the limits of temporal pitch coding in CI users. This was done in the present study; data shown in **Figure 3** confirm that children with normal hearing were better able to discriminate trials that were raised in frequency compared to those in response to music lowered in frequency. These effects were not found in children using CIs. It is thus likely that the challenges of CI pitch coding are larger than the problem of mismatched place pitch coding in the cochlea.

CONCLUSION

There was no overall advantage to modifying the cMBEA in any of the subtests or the total score in children using CIs, suggesting that the main challenges to CI processing of music cannot be solved by playing music with specific instruments or transposing music to try to minimize mismatches in place-pitch representation in the cochlea. Rather, potential strengths in memory for music in children with CIs might be harnessed in therapy to help improve their perception of music. Future studies might also take advantage of within-subject testing to assess changes in music perception with interventions by using shorter tests of music perception such as the abbreviated version of the cMBEA (Peretz et al., 2013).

ETHICS STATEMENT

The studies involving human participants were reviewed and approved by the Hospital for Sick Children Research Ethics Board. Written informed consent to participate in this study was provided by the participants' legal guardian/next of kin.

AUTHOR CONTRIBUTIONS

MS, MP, SG, and TH collected and analyzed the data, and reviewed the manuscript. BP reviewed and supported the data collection and analyses, and reviewed the manuscript. KG supervised the data collection, analyzed the data, and wrote the manuscript.

ACKNOWLEDGMENTS

We would like to acknowledge the contributions of the participants and their families as well as the Cochlear Implant Program team at the Hospital for Sick Children.

REFERENCES

Audiofile Engineering (2011). *SampleManager v3.4.1.* Available at: https://syntheway.com/Audiofile_Engineering_Sample_Manager.htm

Bates, D., Mächler, M., Bolker, B., and Walker, S. (2015). Fitting Linear Mixed-Effects Models Using lme4. *J. Stat. Softw.* 67, 1406. doi: 10.18637/jss.v067.i01

Brandt, A., Gebrian, M., and Slevc, L. R. (2012). Music and Early Language Acquisition. *Front. Psychol.* 3:327. doi: 10.3389/fpsyg.2012.00327

Bruns, L., Mürbe, D., and Hahne, A. (2016). Understanding music with cochlear implants. *Sci. Rep.* 6, 32026. doi: 10.1038/srep32026

Cooper, W. B., Tobey, E., and Loizou, P. C. (2008). Music Perception by Cochlear Implant and Normal Hearing Listeners as Measured by the Montreal Battery for Evaluation of Amusia. *Ear Hear.* 29, 618–626. doi: 10.1097/AUD.0b013e318174e787

Corbeil, M., Trehub, S. E., and Peretz, I. (2013). Speech vs. singing: infants choose happier sounds. *Front. Psychol.* 4:372. doi: 10.3389/fpsyg.2013.00372

Djourno, A., and Eyries, C. (1957). [Auditory prosthesis by means of a distant electrical stimulation of the sensory nerve with the use of an indwelt coiling.]. *Presse Med* 65, 1417.

Djourno, A., Eyries, C., and Vallancien, B. (1957). [Electric excitation of the cochlear nerve in man by induction at a distance with the aid of micro-coil included in the fixture.]. *C R Seances Soc Biol Fil* 151, 423–425.

Drennan, W. R., Oleson, J. J., Gfeller, K., Crosson, J., Driscoll, V. D., Won, J. H., et al. (2015). Clinical evaluation of music perception, appraisal and experience in cochlear implant users. *Int. J. Audiol.* 54, 114–123. doi: 10.3109/14992027.2014.948219

Galvin, J. J., Fu, Q.-J., and Oba, S. (2008). Effect of instrument timbre on melodic contour identification by cochlear implant users. *J. Acoust. Soc. Am.* 124, EL189–EL195. doi: 10.1121/1.2961171

Gfeller, K., and Lansing, C. R. (1991). Melodic, rhythmic, and timbral perception of adult cochlear implant users. *J Speech Hear Res* 34, 916–920. doi: 10.1044/jshr.3404.916

Gfeller, K., Witt, S., Adamek, M., Mehr, M., Rogers, J., Stordahl, J., et al. (2002a). Effects of training on timbre recognition and appraisal by postlingually deafened cochlear implant recipients. *J Am Acad Audiol* 13, 132–145.

Gfeller, K., Witt, S., Woodworth, G., Mehr, M. A., and Knutson, J. (2002b). Effects of frequency, instrumental family, and cochlear implant type on timbre recognition and appraisal. *Ann Otol Rhinol Laryngol* 111, 349–356. doi: 10.1177/000348940211100412

Giannantonio, S., Polonenko, M. J., Papsin, B. C., Paludetti, G., and Gordon, K. A. (2015). Experience Changes How Emotion in Music Is Judged: Evidence from Children Listening with Bilateral Cochlear Implants, Bimodal Devices, and Normal Hearing. *PLoS One* 10:e0136685. doi: 10.1371/journal.pone.0136685

Greenwood, D. D. (1990). A cochlear frequency-position function for several species—29 years later. *J. Acoust. Soc. Am.* 87, 2592–2605. doi: 10.1121/1.399052

Hopyan, T., Gordon, K., and Papsin, B. (2011). Identifying emotions in music through electrical hearing in deaf children using cochlear implants. *Cochlear Implants Int.* 12, 21–26. doi: 10.1179/146701010X12677899497399

Hopyan, T., Peretz, I., Chan, L. P., Papsin, B. C., and Gordon, K. A. (2012). Children using cochlear implants capitalize on acoustical hearing for music perception. *Front Psychol* 3:425. doi: 10.3389/fpsyg.2012.00425

Jäncke, L. (2012). The Relationship between Music and Language. *Front. Psychol.* 3:123. doi: 10.3389/fpsyg.2012.00123

Jiam, N. T., and Limb, C. J. (2019). Rhythm processing in cochlear implant-mediated music perception. *Ann. N. Y. Acad. Sci.* 1453, 22–28. doi: 10.1111/nyas.14130

Jung, K. H., Won, J. H., Drennan, W. R., Jameyson, E., Miyasaki, G., Norton, S. J., et al. (2012). Psychoacoustic performance and music and speech perception in prelingually deafened children with cochlear implants. *Audiol Neurootol* 17, 189–197. doi: 10.1159/000336407

Kong, Y.-Y., Cruz, R., Jones, J. A., and Zeng, F.-G. (2004). Music perception with temporal cues in acoustic and electric hearing. *Ear Hear.* 25, 173–185. doi: 10.1097/01.aud.0000120365.97792.2f

Kraus, N., Strait, D. L., and Parbery-Clark, A. (2012). Cognitive factors shape brain networks for auditory skills: spotlight on auditory working memory. *Ann. N. Y. Acad. Sci.* 1252, 100–107. doi: 10.1111/j.1749-6632.2012.06463.x

Kuznetsova, A., Brockhoff, P. B., and Christensen, R. H. B. (2017). lmerTest Package: Tests in Linear Mixed Effects Models. *J. Stat. Softw.* 82, 1–26. doi: 10.18637/jss.v082.i13

Laneau, J., Wouters, J., and Moonen, M. (2004). Relative contributions of temporal and place pitch cues to fundamental frequency discrimination in cochlear implantees. *J. Acoust. Soc. Am.* 116, 3606–3619. doi: 10.1121/1.1823311

Leake, P. A., Snyder, R. L., Hradek, G. T., and Rebscher, S. J. (1992). Chronic intracochlear electrical stimulation in neonatally deafened cats: effects of intensity and stimulating electrode location. *Hear Res* 64, 99–117. doi: 10.1016/0378-5955(92)90172-j

Leal, M. C., Shin, Y. J., Laborde, M.-L., Calmels, M.-N., Verges, S., Lugardon, S., et al. (2003). Music perception in adult cochlear implant recipients. *Acta Otolaryngol. (Stockh.)* 123, 826–835.

Lebrun, M. A., Moreau, P., McNally-Gagnon, A., Mignault Goulet, G., and Peretz, I. (2012). Congenital amusia in childhood: a case study. *Cortex* 48, 683–688. doi: 10.1016/j.cortex.2011.02.018

Lima, J. P., de Iervolino, S. M. S., and Schochat, E. (2018). Habilidades auditivas musicais e temporais em usuários de implante coclear após musicoterapia. *CoDAS* 30, e20180006. doi: 10.1590/2317-1782/20182018006

Limb, C. J., Molloy, A. T., Jiradejvong, P., and Braun, A. R. (2010). Auditory cortical activity during cochlear implant-mediated perception of spoken language, melody, and rhythm. *J Assoc Res Otolaryngol* 11, 133–143. doi: 10.1007/s10162-009-0184-9

Litovsky, R. Y., Goupell, M. J., Godar, S., Grieco-Calub, T., Jones, G. L., Garadat, S. N., et al. (2012). Studies on bilateral cochlear implants at the University of Wisconsin's Binaural Hearing and Speech Laboratory. *J Am Acad Audiol* 23, 476–494. doi: 10.3766/jaaa.23.6.9

Looi, V., Gfeller, K., and Driscoll, V. (2012). Music Appreciation and Training for Cochlear Implant Recipients: A Review. *Semin. Hear.* 33, 307–334. doi: 10.1055/s-0032-1329222

Maarefvand, M., Marozeau, J., and Blamey, P. J. (2013). A cochlear implant user with exceptional musical hearing ability. *Int. J. Audiol.* 52, 424–432. doi: 10.3109/14992027.2012.762606

Macherey, O., and Delpierre, A. (2013). Perception of Musical Timbre by Cochlear Implant Listeners: A Multidimensional Scaling Study. *Ear Hear.* 34, 426–436. doi: 10.1097/AUD.0b013e31827535f8

Magnusson, L. (2011). Comparison of the fine structure processing (FSP) strategy and the CIS strategy used in the MED-EL cochlear implant system: Speech intelligibility and music sound quality. *Int. J. Audiol.* 50, 279–287. doi: 10.3109/14992027.2010.537378

Mary Zarate, J., Ritson, C. R., and Poeppel, D. (2012). Pitch-interval discrimination and musical expertise: is the semitone a perceptual boundary? *J. Acoust. Soc. Am.* 132, 984–993. doi: 10.1121/1.4733535

McDermott, H. J. (2004). Music perception with cochlear implants: a review. *Trends Amplif* 8, 49–82. doi: 10.1177/108471380400800203

McDermott, H. J., and McKay, C. M. (1997). Musical pitch perception with electrical stimulation of the cochlea. *J Acoust Soc Am* 101, 1622–1631. doi: 10.1121/1.418177

Mehta, A. H., and Oxenham, A. J. (2017). Vocoder Simulations Explain Complex Pitch Perception Limitations Experienced by Cochlear Implant Users. *J. Assoc. Res. Otolaryngol.* 18, 789–802. doi: 10.1007/s10162-017-0632-x

Migirov, L., Kronenberg, J., and Henkin, Y. (2009). Self-Reported Listening Habits and Enjoyment of Music among Adult Cochlear Implant Recipients. *Ann. Otol. Rhinol. Laryngol.* 118, 350–355. doi: 10.1177/000348940911800506

Mirza, S., Douglas, S. A., Lindsey, P., Hildreth, T., and Hawthorne, M. (2003). Appreciation of music in adult patients with cochlear implants: a patient questionnaire. *Cochlear Implants Int.* 4, 85–95. doi: 10.1179/cim.2003.4.2.85

Moore, B. C. J. (2003). Coding of sounds in the auditory system and its relevance to signal processing and coding in cochlear implants. *Otol. Neurotol. Off. Publ. Am* 24, 243–254. doi: 10.1097/00129492-200303000-00019

Muchnik, C., Taitelbaum, R., Tene, S., and Hildesheimer, M. (1994). Auditory temporal resolution and open speech recognition in cochlear implant recipients. *Scand. Audiol.* 23, 105–109. doi: 10.3109/01050399409047493

Nadol, J. B. Jr. (1997). Patterns of neural degeneration in the human cochlea and auditory nerve: implications for cochlear implantation. *Otolaryngol Head Neck Surg* 117, 220–228. doi: 10.1016/s0194-5998(97)70178-5

Norman-Haignere, S. V., Kanwisher, N., McDermott, J. H., and Conway, B. R. (2019). Divergence in the functional organization of human and macaque auditory cortex revealed by fMRI responses to harmonic tones. *Nat. Neurosci.* 22, 1057–1060. doi: 10.1038/s41593-019-0410-7

O'Neill, S. A., and Boultona, M. J. (1996). Boys' and Girls' Preferences for Musical Instruments: A Function of Gender? *Psychol. Music* 24, 171–183. doi: 10.1177/0305735696242009

Peretz, I., Champod, A. S., and Hyde, K. (2003). Varieties of musical disorders. The Montreal Battery of Evaluation of Amusia. *Ann. N. Y. Acad. Sci.* 999, 58–75. doi: 10.1196/annals.1284.006

Peretz, I., Gosselin, N., Nan, Y., Caron-Caplette, E., Trehub, S. E., and Béland, R. (2013). A novel tool for evaluating children's musical abilities across age and culture. *Front. Syst. Neurosci.* 7:30. doi: 10.3389/fnsys.2013.00030

Peretz, I., and Zatorre, R. J. (2005). Brain Organization for Music Processing. *Annu. Rev. Psychol.* 56, 89–114. doi: 10.1146/annurev.psych.56.091103.070225

Plomp, R. (1967). Pitch of complex tones. *J Acoust Soc Am* 41, 1526–1533.

Polonenko, M. J., Giannantonio, S., Papsin, B. C., Marsella, P., and Gordon, K. A. (2017). Music perception improves in children with bilateral cochlear implants or bimodal devices a. *J. Acoust. Soc. Am.* 141, 4494–4507. doi: 10.1121/1.4985123

Prevoteau, C., Chen, S. Y., and Lalwani, A. K. (2018). Music enjoyment with cochlear implantation. *Auris. Nasus. Larynx* 45, 895–902. doi: 10.1016/j.anl.2017.11.008

Propst, E. J., Papsin, B. C., Stockley, T. L., Harrison, R. V., and Gordon, K. A. (2006). Auditory responses in cochlear implant users with and without GJB2 deafness. *Laryngoscope* 116, 317–327. doi: 10.1097/01.mlg.0000199401.26626.4b

R Core Team. (2018). *R: A language and environment for statistical computing.* Vienna: R Foundation for Statistical Computing.

Riley, P. E., Ruhl, D. S., Camacho, M., and Tolisano, A. M. (2018). Music Appreciation after Cochlear Implantation in Adult Patients: A Systematic Review. *Otolaryngol.-Head Neck Surg.* 158, 1002–1010. doi: 10.1177/0194599818760559

Roy, A. T., Scattergood-Keepper, L., Carver, C., Jiradejvong, P., Butler, C., and Limb, C. J. (2014). Evaluation of a Test Battery to Assess Perception of Music in Children With Cochlear Implants. *JAMA Otolaryngol. Neck Surg.* 140, 540. doi: 10.1001/jamaoto.2014.341

Rubinstein, J. T. (2004). How cochlear implants encode speech. *Curr Opin Otolaryngol Head Neck Surg* 12, 444–448. doi: 10.1097/01.moo.0000134452.24819.c0

Schulz, E., and Kerber, M. (1994). "Music perception with the MED-EL implants," in *Music Perception with the MED-EL Implants. In: Advances in Cochlear Implants*, eds I. J. Hochmair-Desoyer, and E. S. Hochmair (Vienna: Manz), 326–332.

Smith, Z. M., Delgutte, B., and Oxenham, A. J. (2002). Chimaeric sounds reveal dichotomies in auditory perception. *Nature* 416, 87–90. doi: 10.1038/416087a

Stakhovskaya, O., Sridhar, D., Bonham, B. H., and Leake, P. A. (2007). Frequency Map for the Human Cochlear Spiral Ganglion: Implications for Cochlear Implants. *J. Assoc. Res. Otolaryngol.* 8, 220–233. doi: 10.1007/s10162-007-0076-9

Trehub, S. E. (2001). Musical predispositions in infancy. *Ann N Acad Sci* 930, 1–16. doi: 10.1111/j.1749-6632.2001.tb05721.x

Veekmans, K., Ressel, L., Mueller, J., Vischer, M., and Brockmeier, S. J. (2009). Comparison of music perception in bilateral and unilateral cochlear implant users and normal-hearing subjects. *Audiol Neurootol* 14, 315–326. doi: 10.1159/000212111

Vuvan, D. T., Paquette, S., Mignault Goulet, G., Royal, I., Felezeu, M., and Peretz, I. (2018). The Montreal Protocol for Identification of Amusia. *Behav. Res. Methods* 50, 662–672. doi: 10.3758/s13428-017-0892-8

Wickham, H. (2016). *ggplot2: Elegant Graphics for Data Analysis.* New York: Springer-Verlag.

Yang, J., Liang, Q., Chen, H., Liu, Y., and Xu, L. (2019). Singing Proficiency of Members of a Choir Formed by Prelingually Deafened Children With Cochlear Implants. *J. Speech Lang. Hear. Res.* 62, 1561–1573. doi: 10.1044/2019_JSLHR-H-18-0385

Zatorre, R. J., Belin, P., and Penhune, V. B. (2002). Structure and function of auditory cortex: music and speech. *Trends Cogn Sci* 6, 37–46. doi: 10.1016/s1364-6613(00)01816-7

Zeng, F. G. (2002). Temporal pitch in electric hearing. *Hear. Res.* 174, 101–106. doi: 10.1016/s0378-5955(02)00644-5

Zimmer, V., Verhey, J. L., Ziese, M., and Böckmann-Barthel, M. (2019). Harmony Perception in Prelingually Deaf, Juvenile Cochlear Implant Users. *Front. Neurosci.* 13:466. doi: 10.3389/fnins.2019.00466

2

Implicit Processing of Pitch in Postlingually Deafened Cochlear Implant Users

Barbara Tillmann[1,2,3], Bénédicte Poulin-Charronnat[1,2,3,4], Etienne Gaudrain[1,2,3,5], Idrick Akhoun[6], Charles Delbé[1,2,3,4], Eric Truy[2,3,7] and Lionel Collet[2,3]*

[1] CNRS UMR5292, INSERM U1028, Auditory Cognition and Psychoacoustics Team, Lyon Neuroscience Research Center, Lyon, France, [2] University of Lyon, Lyon, France, [3] Université Claude Bernard Lyon 1, Villeurbanne, France, [4] LEAD-CNRS, UMR5022, Université Bourgogne Franche-Comté, Dijon, France, [5] University Medical Center Groningen, University of Groningen, Groningen, Netherlands, [6] School of Psychological Sciences, The University of Manchester, Manchester, United Kingdom, [7] CNRS UMR5292, INSERM U1028, Brain Dynamics and Cognition Team, Lyon Neuroscience Research Center, Lyon, France

***Correspondence:**
Barbara Tillmann
Barbara.Tillmann@cnrs.fr

Cochlear implant (CI) users can only access limited pitch information through their device, which hinders music appreciation. Poor music perception may not only be due to CI technical limitations; lack of training or negative attitudes toward the electric sound might also contribute to it. Our study investigated with an implicit (indirect) investigation method whether poorly transmitted pitch information, presented as musical chords, can activate listeners' knowledge about musical structures acquired prior to deafness. Seven postlingually deafened adult CI users participated in a musical priming paradigm investigating pitch processing without explicit judgments. Sequences made of eight sung-chords that ended on either a musically related (expected) target chord or a less-related (less-expected) target chord were presented. The use of a priming task based on linguistic features allowed CI patients to perform fast judgments on target chords in the sung music. If listeners' musical knowledge is activated and allows for tonal expectations (as in normal-hearing listeners), faster response times were expected for related targets than less-related targets. However, if the pitch percept is too different and does not activate musical knowledge acquired prior to deafness, storing pitch information in a short-term memory buffer predicts the opposite pattern. If transmitted pitch information is too poor, no difference in response times should be observed. Results showed that CI patients were able to perform the linguistic task on the sung chords, but correct response times indicated sensory priming, with faster response times observed for the less-related targets: CI patients processed at least some of the pitch information of the musical sequences, which was stored in an auditory short-term memory and influenced chord processing. This finding suggests that the signal transmitted via electric hearing led to a pitch percept that was too different from that based on acoustic hearing, so that it did not automatically activate listeners' previously acquired musical structure knowledge. However, the transmitted signal seems sufficiently informative to lead to sensory priming. These findings are encouraging for the development of pitch-related training programs for CI patients, despite the current technological limitations of the CI coding.

Keywords: music perception, cochlear implants, implicit investigation method, auditory sensory memory, priming

INTRODUCTION

Satisfactory music perception, emotional, intentional prosody, and tonal language intelligibility remain barriers yet to be overcome by cochlear implant (CI) technology (e.g., Zeng, 2004; McKay, 2005; Gfeller et al., 2007). CIs are surgically implanted devices that directly stimulate the auditory nerve in individuals with profound deafness. However, while the current CI technology can restore speech perception in quiet for most users, the spectral information it is able to transmit is severely limited. One consequence of this limitation is that pitch perception remains very limited compared to normal-hearing (NH) listeners (see, e.g., Moore and Carlyon, 2005, for a review). Melody processing—a major component of music perception—requires some capacity for pitch processing. Various tests for music perception have been proposed to investigate CI users' abilities to use the information provided by electric hearing. These tests include the assessment of listeners' capacities in the discrimination of pitch changes and pitch direction, the identification of melodies and timbres, as well as the processing of rhythms and emotions (e.g., Cooper et al., 2008; Looi et al., 2008; Nimmons et al., 2008; Kang et al., 2009; Brockmeier et al., 2010; Gaudrain and Başkent, 2018; Zaltz et al., 2018). While rhythmic processing is close to normal, CI listeners have been shown to be impaired in tasks requiring pitch discrimination or pitch direction judgments, even though inter-subject variability can be large (for reviews, see McDermott, 2004; Moore and Carlyon, 2005; Drennan and Rubinstein, 2008). For example, pitch discrimination thresholds have been reported to vary from one or two semitones to two octaves, also as a function of frequency (Drennan and Rubinstein, 2008; Jung et al., 2010). Large variability has been also observed in impaired melodic contour processing, with performance ranging from chance level to close-to-normal performance (Galvin et al., 2007; Fuller et al., 2018). Melodic contour processing is also influenced by the timbre of the material (Galvin et al., 2008). When tested for familiar melody recognition and identification, CI listeners are impaired, but helped by rhythm or lyrics. CI listeners' difficulties in recognizing familiar melodies are considerably enhanced when these are presented without lyrics or without the familiar rhythmic pattern.

Interestingly, the poor musical outcome may not only be due to CI technical limitations in transmitting pitch. Lack of training or negative attitudes to the new electric sound might also affect music perception (e.g., Trehub et al., 2009). Indeed, useable pitch information seems to be coded, given that training and exposure have been shown to provide improvements in music perception and appreciation (Leal et al., 2003; Lassaletta et al., 2008; Fuller et al., 2018). First, several reports have indicated correlations between self-reported listening habits, such as the amount of music listening, music enjoyment, and perceptual accuracy (e.g., Gfeller et al., 2008; Migriov et al., 2009). Second, several data sets suggest the possibility of training pitch perception in prelingually deaf children (Chen et al., 2010) and postlingually deaf adults (Fu and Galvin, 2007, 2008; Galvin et al., 2007). Training has also been shown to have beneficial effects on the recognition of musical instruments (Driscoll et al., 2009), on musical performance (Yucel et al., 2009; Chen et al., 2010) and on emotion recognition (Fuller et al., 2018).

In currently available studies on CI, pitch and music perception have been investigated with explicit testing methods requiring discrimination, identification, or recognition. These methods do not test for the implicit processing of pitch and music in CI listeners. However, implicit (indirect) investigation methods in various domains have been shown to be more powerful to reveal spared, preserved processing abilities than can be done by explicit investigation methods. For example, experiments using the priming paradigm have provided evidence for spared implicit processes despite impaired explicit functions in either visual or auditory modalities (Young et al., 1988 for spared face recognition in a patient with prosopagnosia; Tillmann et al., 2007 for spared music processing in a patient with amusia).

The priming paradigm investigates the influence of a prime context on the processing of a target event that is either related or unrelated. Its central feature is that participants are not required to make explicit judgments on the relation between prime and target, but to make fast judgments on a perceptual feature of the target (manipulated independently of the relations of interest). Such indirect, implicit tests may shed new light on our understanding of CI listeners' music perception. Our present study tested music perception in CI listeners with a musical priming paradigm. This behavioral experimental method does not require explicit judgments and should be more sensitive to reveal spared pitch processing in these listeners, as suggested by effects of training and exposure.

In addition, while pitch discrimination thresholds in CIs are generally too large to detect the musically relevant difference of one semitone (e.g., Gaudrain and Başkent, 2018), combining multiple tones into a chord may yield different results. Indeed, the interaction of different pitch components, like in a chord, may result in spectro-temporal patterns in the implant that are more detectable than the variation of each of the components in isolation. In other words, while pitch representation in CIs is unlikely to resemble that in NH listeners, the representation of chords may be better preserved across modes of hearing (as suggested, for instance, by Brockmeier et al., 2011).

Measuring brain responses with the methodology of electroencephalography (EEG) can also provide some indirect, implicit evidence for music perception. Koelsch et al. (2004) reported musical structure processing in postlingually deafened, adult CI users who were not required to explicitly judge the tonal structure of musical sequences[1]. Event-related brain potentials (ERPs) were measured for musical events that were either expected (confirming musical structures and regularities, i.e., in-key chords) or unexpected (violating musical regularities, i.e.,

[1] The sequences also contained timbral deviants and participants were required to detect these deviants (65% of correct responses for the CI users vs. 79% for the control group). CI listeners' event-related brain potentials also reflected the detection of the timbre change, even though with smaller amplitude than NH control participants. As the timbres of the used instruments (piano, organ) also differed by their temporal attack, behavioral and neural responses to the timbre change (indicating acoustic irregularity detection) might be based on these temporal envelope changes, in addition to the spectral changes.

Neapolitan sixth chord[2], also referred to as "irregular" chord). Furthermore, the unexpected, irregular chord was more irregular in the fifth position of five-chord sequences (thus in the final position) than in the third position. For control NH participants, the ERPs (in particular an early right anterior negativity, referred to as ERAN) were larger for the irregular chords than for the in-key chords, and even larger for the irregular chords in the fifth position than in the third position. It is thus not only the chord *per se*, but also its structural position in the sequence that raised the violation. For the CI participants, the irregular chords also evoked an ERAN, suggesting that the CI users processed the musical irregularity, even though the amplitudes of the ERAN were considerably smaller than in the NH control participants (leading to a missing ERAN in the third position). According to the authors, the observed ERP patterns indicated that the neural mechanisms for music-syntactic irregularity-detection were still active in CI patients. This finding suggests that CI listeners' knowledge about the Western tonal musical system, which they had acquired prior to deafness, can be accessed despite the poor spectral signal transmitted by the CI. This finding was particularly encouraging for CI users as it indicated that their brains might accurately process music, even though explicitly CI users report difficulties in discriminating and perceiving musical information.

However, since the publication of this work, the domain of music cognition and neuroscience has advanced and pointed out that musical structure violations might introduce new acoustic information in comparison to the acoustic information of the context. The introduction of this new acoustic information provides an alternative explanation to musical irregularity effects based on sensory processing (instead of cognitive processing of musical structures) (see Bigand et al., 2006; Koelsch et al., 2007). Some of the musical violations used to investigate musical structure processing introduced new notes, which had not occurred yet in the sequence. These musical violations, which confounded acoustic violations and context effects, can be explained on a sensory level only. To confirm the influence of listeners' musical structure knowledge (beyond acoustic influences), controlled experimental material is needed. This has been done in more recent behavioral and ERP studies in NH listeners (e.g., Bigand et al., 2001; Koelsch et al., 2007; Marmel et al., 2010), but for CI listeners, this experimental approach is still missing.

Our study fills in this need by testing postlingually deaf adult CI users with experimental musical material that allows the investigation of musical structure processing without acoustic confounds (i.e., the material used in Bigand et al., 2001). The musical sequences in our experiment were eight-chord sequences, with the last chord (i.e., the target chord) being either the expected, tonally regular tonic chord (i.e., related target) or the less-expected, subdominant chord (i.e., less-related target). A cognitive hypothesis predicted faster processing for the expected tonic than for the less-expected subdominant chord. To avoid acoustic confounds, neither the tonic nor the subdominant target occurred in the sequence. Furthermore, the experimental material was constructed in such a way to contrast this cognitive hypothesis of musical structure processing with a sensory hypothesis: Even though neither the tonic nor the subdominant target chord occurred in the sequence, the pitches of the component tones of the less-related subdominant target chord occurred more frequently in the sequence than those of the related tonic target chord. Consequently, faster response times for the less-related chord than for the related chord (thus the reversed pattern of the cognitive hypothesis) would point to sensory priming (also referred to as repetition priming): Sensory information would be simply stored in a sensory memory buffer, leading to facilitated processing of repeatedly presented information. This hypothesis does not require the activation of tonal knowledge, but is based solely on the acoustic features of the presented auditory signal. Alternatively, if the coding of the pitch information transmitted by the CI was too poor to lead either to cognitive or sensory priming, no difference in response times should be observed between the related and less-related targets.

To back up the cognitive and sensory explanations of our experimental material, we present three types of analyses of the experimental material. These analyses compared the related and less-related conditions for (1) the number of shared tones (pitch classes[3]) between target and prime context; (2) the overlap in harmonic spectrum; and (3) the similarity of acoustic information between the target and the prime context in terms of pitch periodicity (as in Koelsch et al., 2007; Koelsch, 2009; Marmel et al., 2010)[4]. While these analyses are originally designed to represent the normal auditory system, we also implemented versions of (2) and (3) through a simulation of electrical stimulation by a cochlear implant.

In the present musical priming study investigating CI listeners, musical sequences, which ended on either the related tonic target or the less-related subdominant target (as described above), were presented as sung material, with a sequence of sung nonsense syllables (e.g., /ka//sha/etc). The last chord was sung on the syllable /di/ or /du/. Participants had to discriminate syllables by judging as fast as possible whether the last chord was sung on /di/ or /du/. This well-established musical priming implicit method allows measuring response times, supposed to reflect processing times of the last chord. For various populations of NH listeners, previous studies have shown the influence of tonal knowledge on processing speed and thus supported the cognitive hypothesis: Response times were faster for the related tonic chord than for the less-related subdominant chord. This result has been observed not only for English and French

[2]The "Neapolitan sixth chord" is a variation of the subdominant chord (an in-key chord), but contains two out-of-key notes (in the tonality of C major, these are the notes *a♭* and *d♭* in the chord: *a♭ – f – d♭*). When this chord is used as a substitution of a subdomimant chord, it sounds unusual, but not wrong (as in the third position of the sequences by Koelsch et al., 2004). However, when used as a substitution of a tonic chord, it sounds wrong (as in the fifth position of the sequences by Koelsch et al., 2004).

[3]A pitch class is defined as a set of pitches at different pitch heights that are separated by octaves (i.e., an interval defined by multiples of the fundamental frequency of a tone), for example the tones at 220, 440, and 880 Hz all belong to the pitch class of A.

[4]For the experimental material of Koelsch et al. (2004), these three analyses are presented as Supplemental Digital Content.

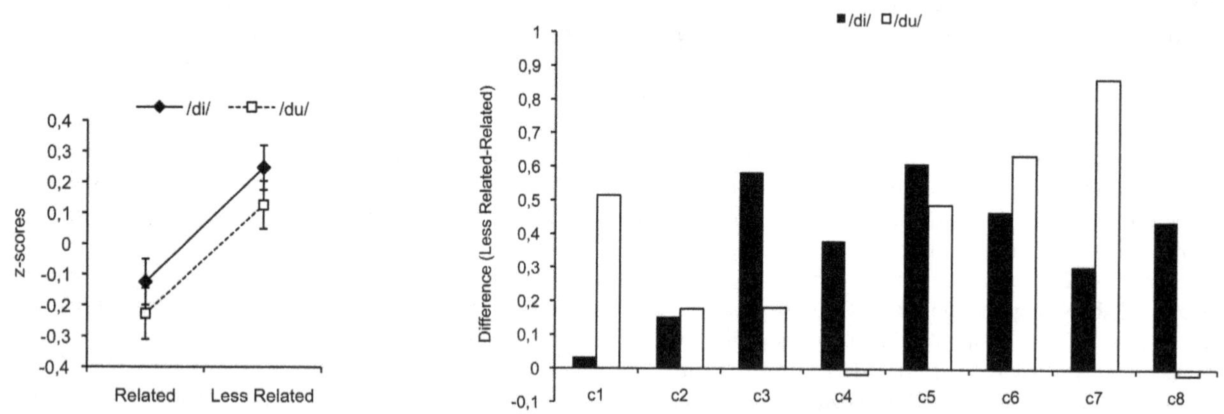

FIGURE 1 | Average data of the 8 control participants in Tillmann et al. (2008) on the left, and their individual data on the right [this group of control participants had a mean age of 65 (±10) years]. For comparable data patterns of group of students, see Bigand et al. (2001) and Tillmann et al. (2008), of groups of children, see Schellenberg et al. (2005), and of another group of control participants as well as their individual data patterns, see Tillmann et al. (2007). Positive and negative values indicate facilitated processing for related and less-related targets, respectively.

college students (musicians and non-musicians, Bigand et al., 2001; Tillmann et al., 2008), but also for 6-year-old children (Schellenberg et al., 2005), cerebellar patients (Tillmann et al., 2008), and amusic patients (Tillmann et al., 2007). **Figure 1** represents this data pattern for the control group tested in Tillmann et al. (2008) (on the left) and for the individual participants (on the right), with positive values indicating faster response times for the related tonic chord than for the less-related subdominant chord. Note that we here plotted the individual data patterns from Tillmann et al. (2008) as this allows us to show the consistency of the priming pattern in control participants (particularly important as our present study did not include NH participants). Based on Koelsch et al. (2004) conclusions, we expected to observe the same data pattern for the CI users than previously observed for the NH users. The faster processing of the related tonic chord would indicate that the transmitted signal of the CI is sufficient to activate listeners' musical knowledge acquired prior to deafness. The construction of our material is such that another pattern of results is also informative of the underlying processes. The reverse data pattern, where the less-related subdominant chord is processed faster, would indicate that the transmitted signal allows accumulation of sensory information in a short-term memory buffer, which then influences processing times (based on repetition priming). Finally, if the limited spectral resolution available through implants is not sufficient to provide relevant information to the CI user's brain, then processing times should not differ between the two priming conditions.

MATERIALS AND METHODS

Participants

Seven CI patients were tested in the present experiment using their own processor without their contralateral hearing aid. They were all postlingually deafened adult CI users who were implanted unilaterally (see **Table 1** for participants' characteristics, including information of the implant type, speech processor, coding strategy, and stimulation rate). Only one of the participants (ci7) reported having some musical training (9 years, starting at the age of 11, with 8 years of piano and 1 year of guitar), and reported currently practicing music about 1 h per week. All participants provided written informed consent to the study, which was conducted in accordance with the guidelines of the Declaration of Helsinki, and approved by the local Ethics Committee (CPP Sud-Est II). They were paid a small honorarium to thank them.

Materials

The 48 chord sequences of Bigand et al. (2001) were used (with permission). These eight-chord sequences ended on either the tonally related tonic chord or the less-related subdominant chord (defining the target). The tonal relatedness of the final chords (the targets) was manipulated by changing the last two chords of the musical sequences (defining either a pair of dominant chord followed by tonic chord or a pair of a tonic chord followed by a subdominant chord). A further control was performed over the entire set of sequences, the material was constructed in such a way that a given chord pair (containing the target) defined the ending of the sequences in both related and less-related conditions. For example, when the first six chords (prime context) instill the key of C Major, the chord pair G-C functions as a dominant chord followed by a tonic chord. If, however, the prime context instills the key of G Major, the same chord pair functions as a tonic chord followed by a subdominant chord. Accordingly, over the experimental set, the 12 possible major chords served as related and less-related targets depending on the prime context.

Each of the first seven chords sounded for 625 ms and the target chord sounded for 1250 ms. The chord sequences were composed in such a way that the target chord never occurred in the sequence (see below for further analyses of the acoustic similarity between prime and target for the two experimental

TABLE 1 | Demographics of the seven participants.

CI Participant	Gender	Age (years)	Hearing Loss			Implanted Ear	Duration CI use (years)	Contralateral hearing Aid	Implant	Speech processor	Strategy	Stimulation Rate
			Onset Time	Age at Deafness	Duration before implantation (years)							
ci_1	F	68	Progressive	20	30	L	1	Y	CI24RE	Freedom SP	ACE 10 max	1200 Hz
ci_2	F	69	Progressive	25	15	R	1	Y	CI24RE	Freedom SP	ACE 12 max	1200 Hz
ci_3	F	47	Congenital and progressive	10	33	R	9	Y	CI24RE	Freedom SP	ACE 12 max	1200 Hz
ci_4	M	32	Early	56	20	R	2	Y	CI24RE	Freedom SP	ACE 10 max	1200 Hz
ci_5	F	32	Early	66	24	L	-	N	CI24RE	Freedom SP	ACE 10 max	900 Hz
ci_6	F	30	Progressive	25	11	L	-	Y	CI24M	Esprit 3G	CIS 12 channels	900 Hz
ci_7	F	33	Progressive	23	21	L	1	Y	CI24RE	Freedom SP	ACE 10 max	1200 Hz

Onset time refers to the onset time of profound deafness (early: deafness begun in childhood, but after the development of spoken language (thus postlingually); congenital and progressive: the subject had a hearing loss at birth, but was hearing-aid fitted when 10-years old as the hearing-loss worsened).

conditions). Example sequences are available as Supplemental Digital Content.

The sequences were sung on CV-syllables by sampled voice sounds (using Vocal-Writer software, Woodinville, WA, United States). Chords were generated by the simultaneous presentation of 3 or 4 synthetized utterances of the same syllable with different fundamental frequencies, which corresponded to the component tones of the chords. The succession of the synthetic syllables did not form a meaningful, linguistic phrase (e.g., /da fei ku ʃo fa to kei/), and the last syllable (i.e., of the target) was either /di/ or /du/ to define the experimental task. The experimental session consisted of 50% of sequences ending on the related tonic target (25% being sung with /di/, 25% with /du/) and 50% ending on the less-related subdominant target (25% with /di/, 25% with /du/). The experiment was run on Psyscope software (Cohen et al., 1993).

Procedure

The sequences were presented over two loudspeakers (placed at about 80 cm in front of the participant, left and right from the screen of the laptop computer, thus at an azimuth of 45 degrees) at about 70 dB SPL, which was perceived as comfortable loudness level. The participants listened through the microphone of the processor using their everyday program and settings. The experiment was run in the main sound-field room of the University of Lyon CI clinic center.

The participants were asked to decide as quickly and as accurately as possible whether a chord was sung on /di/ or /du/ by pressing one of two keys. Incorrect responses were accompanied by an auditory feedback signal and a correct response stopped the sounding of the target. Participants were first trained on 16 isolated chords (50% sung on /di/ or /du/, respectively). The training phase was repeated in case the task was not understood, notably for difficulties to perceive the difference between the syllables or responding too slowly. Participants were encouraged to give their response while the target chord was still sounding, but a later time out was used (2800 ms) to not pressurize the participants too strongly. In the next phase of the experiment, the eight-chord sequences were explained to the participants with an example sequence and participants were asked to perform the same task on the last chord of each sequence. After four practice sequences, the 48 sequences were presented in random order twice in two blocks, separated by a short break. Two participants performed only one block (ci2, ci7). A short random-tone sequence was presented after each response to avoid carry-over effects between trials. The experiment lasted about 15 to 20 min.

AUDITORY PROPERTIES AND PERCEPTUAL PROCESSING

When musical violations used to investigate musical structure processing introduce new tones, which had not occurred yet in the context, they confound the processing of acoustic violations with the cognitive processing of musical structures. The processing of these musical violations could thus be explained on a sensory level only, without the need for the involvement of listeners' knowledge of musical structures (acquired prior to deafness). Experimental material must thus be constructed in such a way to control acoustic influences and disentangle them from cognitive influences (linked to listeners' musical structure knowledge). In this section, we first present analyses of the acoustic and estimated perceptual similarities between the prime context and the related/less-related target in three ways, as previously done in the studies investigating NH listeners. We then present simulations that take in consideration potential changes due to the implication of the implant. None of the simulations predict facilitated processing for the related tonic chord in comparison to the less-related subdominant chord.

Analyses of the Acoustic Similarity Between the Prime Context and the Target in Related and Less-Related Conditions

To check for acoustic influences, we analyzed our material in terms of (1) the number of pitch classes shared between targets and contexts as a function of the condition (related vs. less-related), (2) the spectral overlap of targets and contexts (simulating a place coding of pitch information), and (3) periodicity overlap in auditory short-term memory (simulating a temporal coding of pitch information). These analyses simulated different plausible pitch representations (place vs. time coding) and their integration over time. All analyses showed that acoustic influences would predict facilitated processing for the less-related subdominant chord. This prediction thus contrasts with cognitive, musical structure processing, which predicts facilitated processing for the related tonic chord.

Overlap in Pitch Classes Between Target and Context

To analyze the number of pitch classes shared between the target and the first seven chords (the context), we calculated (a) for each sequence, the number of occurrence of the target's pitch classes in the first seven chords, and (b) the average over the sequence sets in the two conditions: The resulting mean was higher for the less-related condition (14.75 ± 2.05) than for the related condition (12.25 ± 2.93), $t(11) = 2.61$, $p = 0.03$. This finding thus represents a sensory advantage for the less-related subdominant targets and contrasts with the cognitive (tonal) advantage for the related tonic targets.

Spectral Contrast

To estimate the spectral overlap between target and context, we compared the spectra obtained from the first seven chords (of each sequence) with the spectra obtained from the corresponding target chord. The spectra were obtained by averaging the spectrogram computed over either the context or the target with FFT-time windows of 186 ms and 50%-window overlap (93 ms). Two metrics were used to judge the similarity of prime and target spectra: a correlation and an Euclidian distance. Because correlations are very sensitive to edge effects, the spectra were limited to the range 100 to 8000 Hz, and the overall spectral slope was compensated, in each sequence, based on the average of the target and prime spectra. The Euclidian distance was calculated on the spectrum expressed in decibels. Average correlation (Fisher-transformed, Fisher, 1921) and Euclidian distance values obtained for the sequence sets in the related and less-related conditions were then compared (**Figure 2A**). We analyzed those results with a repeated measures ANOVA with the factors syllable and relatedness. Correlation values were higher for the less-related condition than for the related condition [$F(1,11) = 7.74, p < 0.05, \eta_g^2 = 0.20$] thus confirming the acoustic advantage of the less-related subdominant chord. However, while the Euclidian distance did not significantly depend on the relatedness [$F(1,11) = 0.75$, $p = 0.41, \eta_g^2 = 0.02$], it did depend on the nature of the target syllable [$F(1,11) = 87.9$,

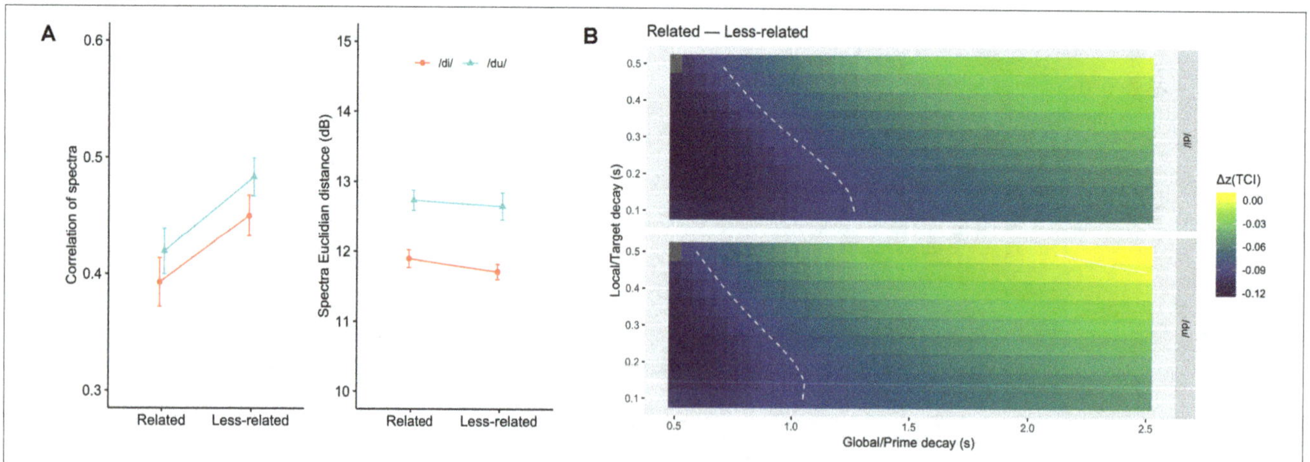

FIGURE 2 | (A) Average spectral correlation (left) and Euclidian distance (right) for the related and less-related condition, and for the two target syllables. Higher correlations, and smaller Euclidian distances, are compatible with more sensory priming. **(B)** Difference in Fisher transformed tonal contextuality index between related and less-related conditions, as a function of syllable, and global and local decays. The solid line represents the value 0.0 where the two types of context have the same TCI. The dashed lines represent the critical limit beyond which differences can be considered significant.

$p < 0.001, \eta_g^2 = 0.46$]. All other effects and interactions were non-significant [$ps > 0.22$].

Pitch Periodicity in a Model of Auditory Short-Term Memory: Tonal Contextuality Index

To further test the acoustic influences in the experimental material, we used Leman (2000) model (as implemented in the IPEMtoolbox v1.02 by Leman et al., 2005) that stores auditory information in a short-term memory buffer. Acoustic input is first processed in a frontend module mimicking the peripheral auditory system (Van Immerseel and Martens, 1992). The output is then processed with a pitch module that extracts periodicities using an autocorrelation approach. Finally, the periodicity output is passed into a memory module. This model relies on the comparison of pitch images of two echoic memories, which differ in duration. With longer memory decays, the pitch images are smeared out, so that the images reflect the context echoic memory, while with a shorter decay the pitch images reflect the target echoic memory. Measuring the differences between the two images by computing their correlation gives an indication of how well the target (local) pitch image acoustically fits with the given (global) context. This measure is referred to as the Tonal Contextuality Index (TCI). In our case, to avoid choosing a specific point sample during the target to compare the periodicity patterns, we averaged them over the duration of the target, both for the short (local) and long (global) memory decays, and correlated these summary images. For the choice of the memory decay durations, as currently no precise information about the dynamics of auditory memory in human listeners are available, our simulations were carried out with local and global decay parameters varying systematically by steps of 0.05, from 0.1 to 0.5 s and from 0.5 to 2.5 s, for the local and global decay parameters, respectively, in order to explore a large parameter space of the model.

For the present analyses, the audio files of the 48 chord sequences were given as input to the model. TCI was calculated for each sequence and transformed into z-values using Fisher's transformation (Fisher, 1921). The spaces of the differences between the TCI of the two targets are reported in **Figure 2B** for each target syllable. In these figures, positive Δz(TCI) values indicate that the related condition yields stronger contextuality than the less-related condition, and negative values reflect the opposite. Here all Δz(TCI) values were negative, indicating stronger TCI for subdominant targets than for tonic targets, thus predicting facilitated processing for the less-related targets. In **Figure 2B**, it can be seen that significantly negative values are found for short global decay values, but no significant positive values were observed. To further assess the role of relatedness on TCI, we analyzed the TCI data with a linear-mixed model with relatedness and syllable as fixed factors and tonality, local decay and global decay as random intercepts (p-values were obtained with Satterthwaite's method). The model yields a significant effect of relatedness [$F(1{,}17605) = 578.6, p < 0.0001$], confirming that the less-related condition produced higher TCIs than the related one. The effect of syllable was also significant [$F(1{,}17605) = 137.4, p < 0.0001$] and so was the interaction [$F(1{,}17605) = 5.78, p = 0.016$]: the TCI was higher for /du/ than for /di/, but the that difference was less important in the less-related condition.

These results, thus confirm that the facilitated processing for tonic targets reported for NH participants by Bigand et al. (2001) and others (Schellenberg et al., 2005; Tillmann et al., 2007, 2008) reflect the influence of listeners' knowledge about musical structures on target chord processing (see also Bigand et al., 2003).

In sum, the results of these three analyses confirmed that sensory and cognitive hypotheses make contrasting predictions for our experimental material: The sensory hypothesis predicts facilitated processing for the less-related targets, while the cognitive hypothesis predicts facilitated processing for the related targets. These predictions are in agreement with the alternative hypotheses made here above for the CI users: If the CI users show faster response times for the less-related subdominant chord, this finding would suggest the influence of the contextual auditory information (stored in a memory buffer) on target chord processing. If, however, CI users show faster response times for the related tonic chord, this finding would suggest the influence of CI users' musical knowledge (acquired prior to deafness).

Analyses of the Electrical Similarity Between the Prime Context and the Target in Related and Less-Related Conditions

In the previous sections, we examined the potential influence of sensory factors, rather than cognitive, on the priming effect induced by the material. Both the spectral contrast model (see section "Spectral Contrast") and the tonal contextuality model (see section "Pitch Periodicity in a Model of Auditory Short-Term Memory: Tonal Contextuality Index") assume a NH frontend. In the case of implant stimulation, the simultaneously presented tones that produce a chord interact and can generate other patterns. In other words, situations that would not induce sensory priming in NH listeners may very well do so in CI listeners.

To evaluate this possibility, we implemented a frontend mimicking a cochlear implant and the pattern of neural activation generated by electrical stimulation (Gaudrain et al., 2014). The model is based on the Nucleus Matlab Toolbox (Cochlear Ltd.), which generates patterns of electrical stimulation along the electrode array of the implant. The generated electrical field is then propagated in the cochlea to mimic current spread (Bingabr et al., 2008). Neural activation probability resulting from this electrical field is then calculated using approaches adapted from Rattay et al. (2001). This time-place image is used first to examine the spectral contrast between prime and target, and then to evaluate the tonal contextuality.

Spectral Contrast

As shown in **Figure 3A**, calculating the same metrics as in the section "Spectral Contrast," i.e., correlation of detrended spectra, and Euclidian distance, again, there was no significant difference between the related and less-related conditions [for the correlation $F(1{,}11) = 1.13, p = 0.31, \eta_g^2 = 0.03$; for the Euclidian distance $F(1{,}11) = 0.18, p = 0.68, \eta_g^2 = 0.003$]. The nature of

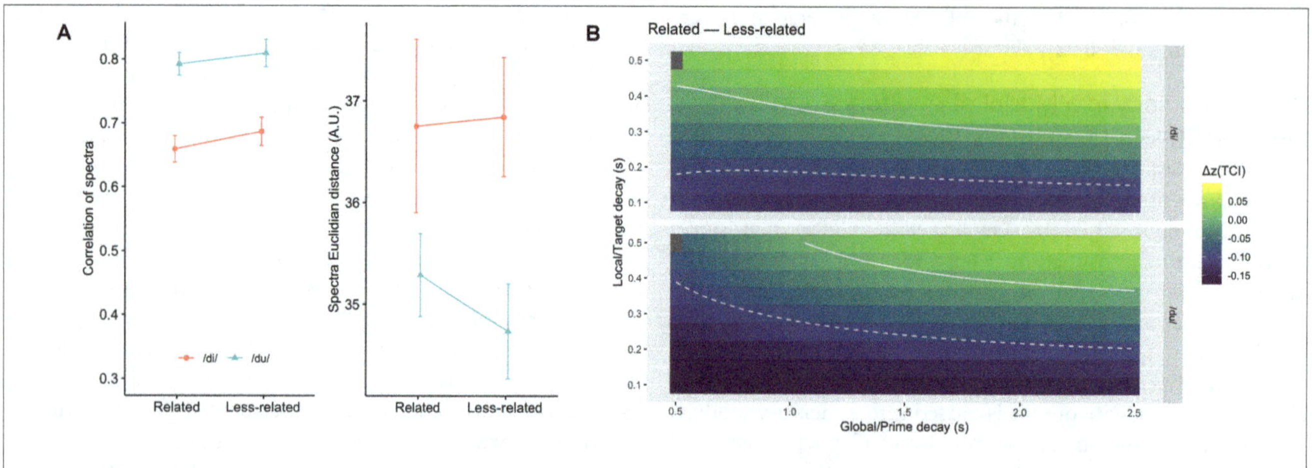

FIGURE 3 | Same as **Figure 2** for the CI model. **(A)** Average spectral correlation (left) and Euclidian distance (right) for the related and less-related conditions, and for the two target syllables. Higher correlations, and smaller Euclidian distances, are compatible with more sensory priming. **(B)** Difference in Fisher transformed tonal contextuality index between related and less-related conditions, as a function of syllable, and global and local decays. The solid line represents the value 0.0 where the two types of context have the same TCI. The dashed lines represent the critical limit beyond which differences can be considered significant.

the syllable had a significant effect on both measures [for the correlation $F(1,11) = 64.2, p < 0.001, \eta^2_g = 0.40$; for the Euclidian distance $F(1,11) = 19.0, p < 0.01, \eta^2_g = 0.17$]. No interaction was significant.

Tonal Contextuality Index

The electrically induced neural activation image was used as auditory image to feed into the pitch module of the IPEMtoolbox in order to extract periodicity structures. The rest of the model (memory decay and TCI computation) was identical to the one used for the acoustic/NH model.

The results, shown in **Figure 3B**, indicate that no combination of local and global memory decay yields positive Δz(TCI) beyond the critical value. When applying the same linear-mixed model as in the section "Pitch Periodicity in a Model of Auditory Short-Term Memory: Tonal Contextuality Index," the effect of relatedness was found to be significant [$F(1,35318) = 165.2, p < 0.0001$], with the less-related condition having a globally higher TCI. The effect of syllable was also significant [$F(1,35318) = 20.4, p < 0.0001$] and so was the interaction [$F(1,35318) = 48.6, p < 0.0001$]: the TCI was higher for /du/ than for /di/, but the that difference was less important in the less-related condition.

From this analysis, it appears that, like for the NH model, the CI model predicts faster response times for the less-related condition than for the related condition.

RESULTS

Percentages of correct responses were high overall, with an average accuracy of 95% (ranging from 92 to 100%). Because of differences in average response latency between participants (ranging from 561 ms to 1567 ms) and with the goal to focus on differences between related and less-related targets, correct response times were individually normalized to *z*-scores with a mean of 0 and a standard deviation of 1 (**Figure 4**, left). *z*-Scores were analyzed with a 2 × 2 ANOVA with Musical Relatedness (related/less related) and Target Syllable (di/du) as within-participant factors. The main effect of Musical Relatedness was significant, $F(1,6) = 23.32$, $p = 0.003$, MSE = 0.02, indicating faster processing for less-related targets than for related targets. Overall, responses were faster for the syllable /di/ than /du/, $F(1,6) = 19.26$, $p = 0.005$, MSE = 0.13, as previously observed for NH listeners (Bigand et al., 2001). The interaction between Musical Relatedness and Target Syllable was not significant ($p = 0.55$).

Figure 4 (right) displays differences between less-related and related targets for the two target syllables for each participant. Positive values indicate faster processing for related targets, and negative values indicate faster processing for less-related targets. Faster processing for less-related targets was observed for all participants (except /du/ for ci5).

DISCUSSION

Our study investigated the perception of musical structures by postlingually deaf adult CI users. These listeners were mostly non-musicians without formal musical training. As shown in numerous studies in music cognition domain (e.g., Bigand and Poulin-Charronnat, 2006), NH non-musician listeners acquire implicit knowledge about the Western tonal musical system by mere exposure to music in everyday life and thanks to the cognitive ability of implicit learning (see also Tillmann et al., 2000). The postlingually deaf adult CI users participating in our present study had thus acquired this kind of implicit musical knowledge prior to deafness. We were investigating whether the signal quality of the CI—despite its poor spectral cues—is sufficient to activate this previously acquired implicit musical knowledge and to influence chord processing. We used a behavioral approach based on an indirect investigation method. The priming paradigm avoids asking for direct explicit

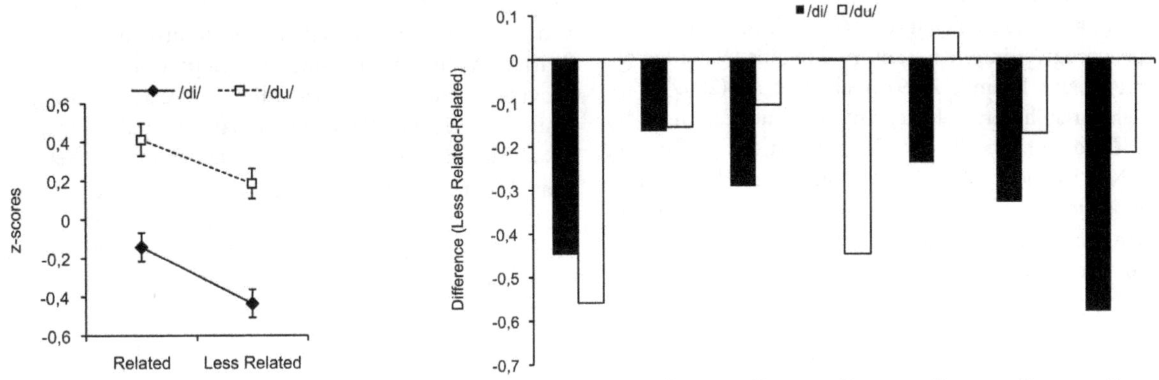

FIGURE 4 | Average data of the CI participants on the left and their individual data on the right. Positive and negative values indicate facilitated processing for related and less-related targets, respectively.

judgments about the musical material, and takes advantage of implicit investigation. For music perception, the power of this implicit method has been previously shown by reporting musical structure knowledge in an amusic patient despite explicit music processing deficits (Tillmann et al., 2007) and in children as young as at the age of 6 years (Schellenberg et al., 2005), while explicit investigation methods had estimated the required age at 10 years (Imberty, 1981).

Based on our previous research, we used sung-chord sequences. The required priming task was a syllable-identification task (with syllables differing by one phoneme). The high accuracy we observed here showed that the CI users could perform this task without difficulty. The experimental material was constructed in such a way that three different data patterns could be expected, each indicating different underlying processes: (1) Faster processing of the related tonic chord would indicate that the transmitted signal of the CI is sufficient to activate listeners' musical knowledge acquired prior to deafness; (2) faster processing of the less-related subdominant chord would indicate that the transmitted signal allows accumulation of sensory information in a short-term memory buffer, which then influences processing times (based on repetition priming); and (3) equal processing times for both chords would rather suggest that the limited spectral resolution available through implants is not sufficient to provide relevant information to the CI user's brain.

The observed data pattern (see **Figure 4**) clearly supports the second hypothesis: Processing was facilitated for the less-related target, which is the target that benefited from sensory priming. This finding suggests that the signal transmitted via electric hearing was too different from the signal based on acoustic hearing, so that it did not automatically activate listeners' previously acquired musical structure knowledge. However, the signal seems sufficiently informative to lead to sensory priming.

This conclusion seems to contradict the conclusion of Koelsch et al. (2004) based on ERPs in CI users, suggesting that tonal knowledge can be reached via electric hearing. We thus performed three acoustic analyses (pitch class, spectrum, pitch periodicity) also for the experimental material of Koelsch et al. (2004; see Supplemental Digital Content), notably to investigate acoustic similarities of the target with its preceding context. These analyses allowed us to resolve this contradiction. They showed that the material used by Koelsch et al. (2004) does not allow disentangling sensory and cognitive contributions in chord processing and the position effect. A more parsimonious explanation would thus be based on acoustic influences only. A similar argument has been made later by Koelsch et al. (2007), thus leading the authors to use new musical material with more subtle musical structure manipulations. However, this new material had not yet been used in an EEG study investigating CI users.

Our present findings support the hypothesis that despite the poor coding of spectral information, the CI transmits some pitch-related information of the musical material. Interestingly, based on our analyses, the observed sensory priming does not seem to be based on the individual pitches used, that is the spectral content *per se* (see section "Spectral contrast"). Instead, the sensory priming may be based on periodicity pattern similarity, as evidenced by the tonal contextuality index analysis (see section "Tonal Contextuality Index"). This is rather encouraging for implant users because, while their perception of pitch in natural sounds is very limited (e.g., in syllables, Gaudrain and Başkent, 2018 found discrimination thresholds for F0 between 4 and 20 semitones), it seems that when multiple tones are combined into chords, it makes periodicity patterns arise, to a degree that they can induce priming. This may suggest that, perhaps counter-intuitively, perception of chord sequences in CIs may be a more manageable goal than melody recognition. This finding thus integrates into other studies, suggesting that listeners can benefit from information provided by electric hearing even for music perception. Notably, studies have shown benefits of increased, self-imposed music exposure and of training programs to exploit the transmitted signal in music and pitch perception (e.g., Galvin et al., 2007). Converging evidence comes from the music appraisal of prelingually deaf CI listeners who are missing the comparison with music perception based on acoustic hearing (e.g., Trehub et al., 2009). Prelingually deaf children seem to find music interesting and enjoyable (Trehub et al., 2009; Looi and She, 2010) and children's engagement with music may also enhance their progress in other auditory domains (Mitani et al., 2007; Rochette and Bigand, 2009). Galvin et al. (2009) have shown a high variability in melodic contour identification across CI users, with some musically experienced CI users performing as well as NH listeners. Most importantly, they showed that training on melodic contour (using visual support) improves performance in melodic contour identification in CI users, even though the transmitted signal was not changed. It is worth further clarifying that with "pitch" we are here referring to the acoustic information that is related to the pitch percept in NH listeners. Indeed, we need to acknowledge that we do not know whether this is a subjective pitch percept for the CI listeners, as it is for NH listeners, but can ascertain it is related to that acoustic information.

Our findings together with other data sets on the beneficial effects of musical training and musical exposure are thus encouraging for the development of pitch-related training programs for CI patients. Indeed, in parallel to the technological efforts aiming to improve the coding strategies implemented in the CI device, efforts need to be made for training programs in order to improve how the brains of CI users are exploiting the transmitted signal.

Training programs might need to work differently for postlingually deaf adult CI users and prelingually deaf child CI users. Because of the differences between acoustic and electric hearing, adults find music often disappointing or unacceptable, leading to changes in listening habits and decreased subjective enjoyment in comparison to prior to deafness (McDermott, 2004; Lassaletta et al., 2008; Looi and She, 2010). In contrast, the child implant users find music interesting and enjoyable (Trehub et al., 2009; Looi and She, 2010). The postlingually deaf adult CI users have acquired cognitive patterns and schemata for speech and music based on their previously normal (or impaired, but aided) hearing. However, the information provided by the CI is different, in particular for the coding of the spectro-temporal fine structure. The prior knowledge, which was developed based on the information available in acoustic hearing, might thus create perceptual filters and cognitive schema of "pitch" in music, which result in costs for picking out the relevant information from the transmitted signal. In contrast to the postlingually deaf adult CI users, early-implanted children CI users have developed their speech and music patterns based on the information in the electric hearing. As they are missing the comparison to the information provided by acoustic hearing, they appreciate and enjoy music, while for the postlingually implanted adults the CI version of music is only a poor representation of their memory. Training programs would thus need to increase exposure leading to the construction of newly shaped perceptual filters and schemata. The findings of our present study provide some further grounds for this training by showing that some pitch information is implicitly processed by the adult CI users. They thus have implications for rehabilitation programs, notably by encouraging training strategies that rely on spared implicit processing resources.

ETHICS STATEMENT

All participants provided written informed consent to this study, which was conducted in accordance with the guidelines of the Declaration of Helsinki, and approved by the local Ethics Committee (CPP Sud-Est II).

AUTHOR CONTRIBUTIONS

BT, BP-C, IA, and LC contributed to the conception and design of the study. BT, BP-C, and IA acquired the data. BT, BP-C, EG, and CD performed the statistical analysis and modeling. ET and LC provided access to the patients and related information. BT wrote the first draft of the manuscript. EG and CD wrote the simulation sections of the manuscript. All authors contributed to the manuscript revision, and read and approved the submitted version.

ACKNOWLEDGMENTS

We thank Fabien Seldran for the help with the experimental setup.

REFERENCES

Bigand, E., Delbé, C., Poulin-Charronnat, B., Leman, M., and Tillmann, B. (2014). Empirical evidence for musical syntax processing? Computer simulations reveal the contribution of auditory short-term memory. *Front. Syst. Neurosci.* 8:94. doi: 10.3389/fnsys.2014.00094

Bigand, E., and Poulin-Charronnat, B. (2006). Are we "experienced listeners"? A review of the musical capacities that do not depend on formal musical training. *Cognition* 100, 100–130. doi: 10.1016/j.cognition.2005.11.007

Bigand, E., Poulin, B., Tillmann, B., and D'Adamo, D. (2003). Cognitive versus sensory components in harmonic priming effects. *J. Exp. Psychol. Hum. Percept. Perform.* 29, 159–171.

Bigand, E., Tillmann, B., Poulin, B., D'Adamo, D. A., and Madurell, F. (2001). The effect of harmonic context on phoneme monitoring in vocal music. *Cognition* 81, 11–20.

Bigand, E., Tillmann, B., and Poulin-Charronnat, B. (2006). A module for syntactic processing in music? *Trends Cogn. Sci.* 10, 195–196. doi: 10.1016/j.tics.2006.03.008

Bingabr, M., Espinoza-Varas, B., and Loizou, P. C. (2008). Simulating the effect of spread of excitation in cochlear implants. *Hear. Res.* 241, 73–79. doi: 10.1016/j.heares.2008.04.012

Brockmeier, S. J., Fitzgerald, D., Searle, O., Fitzgerald, H., Grasmeder, M., Hilbig, S., et al. (2011). The MuSIC perception test: a novel battery for testing music perception of cochlear implant users. *Cochlear Implants Int.* 12, 10–20. doi: 10.1179/146701010X12677899497236

Brockmeier, S. J., Peterreins, M., Lorens, A., Vermeire, K., Helbig, S., Anderson, I., et al. (2010). Music perception in electric acoustic stimulation users as assessed by the Mu.S.I.C. Test. *Adv. Otorhinolaryngol.* 67, 70–80. doi: 10.1159/000262598

Chen, J. K. C., Chuang, A. Y. C., McMahon, C., Hsieh, J. C., Tung, T. H., Li, L. P., et al. (2010). Music training improves pitch perception in prelingually deafened children with cochlear implants. *Pediatrics* 125, E793–E800. doi: 10.1542/peds.2008-3620

Cohen, J., MacWhinney, B., Flatt, M., and Provost, J. (1993). PsyScope: an interactive graphic system for designing and controlling experiments in the psychology laboratory using Macintosh computers. *Behav. Res. Methods Instrum. Comput.* 25, 257–271. doi: 10.3758/bf03204507

Cooper, W. B., Tobey, E., and Loizou, P. C. (2008). Music perception by cochlear implant and normal hearing listeners as measured by the montreal battery for evaluation of Amusia. *Ear Hear.* 29, 618–626. doi: 10.1097/AUD.0b013e318174e787

Drennan, W. R., and Rubinstein, J. T. (2008). Music perception in cochlear implant users and its relationship with psychophysical capabilities. *J. Rehabil. Res. Dev.* 45, 779–790. doi: 10.1682/jrrd.2007.08.0118

Driscoll, V. D., Oleson, J., Jiang, D., and Gfeller, K. (2009). Effects of training on recognition of musical instruments presented through cochlear implant simulations. *J. Am. Acad. Audiol.* 20, 71–82. doi: 10.3766/jaaa.20.1.7

Fisher, R. A. (1921). On the 'probable error' of a coefficient of correlation deduced from a small sample. *Metron* 1, 3–32.

Fu, Q. J., and Galvin, J. J. (2007). Perceptual learning and auditory training in cochlear implant recipients. *Trends Amplif.* 11, 193–205. doi: 10.1177/1084713807301379

Fu, Q. J., and Galvin, J. J. (2008). Maximizing cochlear implant patients' performance with advanced speech training procedures. *Hear Res.* 242, 198–208. doi: 10.1016/j.heares.2007.11.010

Fuller, C. D., Galvin, J. J., Maat, B., Başkent, D., and Free, R. H. (2018). Comparison of two music training approaches on music and speech perception in cochlear implant users. *Trends Hear.* 22:2331216518765379. doi: 10.1177/2331216518765379

Galvin, J. J., Fu, Q.-J., and Nogaki, G. (2007). Melodic contour identification by cochlear implant listeners. *Ear Hear.* 28, 302–319. doi: 10.1097/01.aud.0000261689.35445.20

Galvin, J. J., Fu, Q.-J., and Oba, S. (2008). Effect of instrument timbre on melodic contour identification by cochlear implant users. *J. Acoust. Soc. Am.* 124, EL189–EL195. doi: 10.1121/1.2961171

Galvin, J. J., Fu, Q.-J., and Shannon, R. V. (2009). Melodic contour identification and music perception by cochlear implant users. *Ann. N. Y. Acad. Sci.* 1169, 518–533. doi: 10.1111/j.1749-6632.2009.04551.x

Gaudrain, E., and Başkent, D. (2018). Discrimination of voice pitch and vocal-tract length in cochlear implant users. *Ear Hear.* 39, 226–237. doi: 10.1097/AUD.0000000000000480

Gaudrain, E., Stam, L., and Baskent, D. (2014). "Measure and model of vocal-tract length discrimination in cochlear implants," in *Proceedings of the 2014 International Conference on Audio, Language and Image Processing*, Shanghai, 31–34. doi: 10.1109/ICALIP.2014.7009751

Gfeller, K., Oleson, J., Knutson, J. F., Breheny, P., Driscoll, V., Olszewski, C., et al. (2008). Multivariate predictors of music perception and appraisal by adult cochlear implant users. *J. Am. Acad. Audiol.* 19, 120–134. doi: 10.3766/jaaa.19.2.3

Gfeller, K., Turner, C., Oleson, J., Zhang, X., Gantz, B., Froman, R., et al. (2007). Accuracy of cochlear implant recipients on pitch perception, melody recognition and speech reception in noise. *Ear Hear.* 28, 412–423. doi: 10.1097/aud.0b013e3180479318

Imberty, M. (1981). Acculturation tonale et structuration perceptive du temps musical chez l'enfant. Basic musical functions and musical ability. *R. Swed. Acad. Music* 32, 81–130.

Jung, K. H., Cho, Y. S., Cho, J. K., Park, G. Y., Kim, E. Y., Hong, S. H., et al. (2010). Clinical assessment of music perception in Korean cochlear implant listeners. *Acta Otolaryncol.* 130, 716–723. doi: 10.3109/00016480903380521

Kang, R., Nimmons, G. L., Drennan, W., Longnion, J., Ruffin, C., and Nie, K. (2009). Development and validation of the University of Washington clinical assessment of music perception test. *Ear Hear.* 30, 411–418. doi: 10.1097/AUD.0b013e3181a61bc0

Koelsch, S. (2009). Music-syntactic processing and auditory memory: similarities and differences between ERAN and MMN. *Psychophysiology* 46, 179–190. doi: 10.1111/j.1469-8986.2008.00752.x

Koelsch, S., Jentschke, S., Sammler, D., and Mietchen, D. (2007). Untangling syntactic and sensory processing: an ERP study of music perception. *Psychophysiology* 44, 476–490. doi: 10.1111/j.1469-8986.2007.00517.x

Koelsch, S., Wittfoth, M., Wolf, A., Müller, J., and Hahne, A. (2004). Music perception in cochlear implant users: an event-related potential study. *Clin. Neurophysiol.* 115, 966–972. doi: 10.1016/j.clinph.2003.11.032

Lassaletta, L., Castro, A., Bastarrica, M., Pérez-Mora, R., Herrán, B., Sanz, L., et al. (2008). Changes in listening habits and quality of musical sound after cochlear implantation. *Otolaryngol. Head Neck Surg.* 138, 363–367. doi: 10.1016/j.otohns.2007.11.028

Leal, M. C., Shin, Y. J., Laborde, M. L., Calmels, M. N., Verges, S., Lugardon, S., et al. (2003). Music perception in adult cochlear implant recipients. *Acta Otolaryngol.* 123, 826–835.

Leman, M. (2000). An auditory model of the role of short-term memory in probe-tone ratings. *Music Percept.* 17, 435–463.

Leman, M., Lesaffre, M., and Tanghe, K. (2005). *IPEM Toolbox for Perception-Based Music Analysis Version 1.02.* Available at: https://www.ugent.be/lw/kunstwetenschappen/en/research-groups/musicology/ipem/finishedprojects/ipem-toolbox.htm (accessed April 24, 2019).

Looi, V., McDermott, H., McKay, C., and Hickson, L. (2008). Music perception for cochlear implant users compared with that of hearing aid users. *Ear Hear.* 29, 421–434. doi: 10.1097/AUD.0b013e31816a0d0b

Looi, V., and She, J. (2010). Music perception of cochlear implant users: a questionnaire and its implications for a music training program. *Int. J. Audiol.* 49, 116–128. doi: 10.3109/14992020903405987

Marmel, F., Tillmann, B., and Delbé, C. (2010). Priming in melody perception: tracking down the strength of cognitive expectations. *J. Exp. Psychol. Hum. Percept. Perform.* 36, 1016–1028. doi: 10.1037/a0018735

McDermott, H. J. (2004). Music perception with cochlear implants: a review. *Trends Amplif.* 8, 49–82. doi: 10.1177/108471380400800203

McKay, C. M. (2005). Spectral processing in cochlear implants. *Aud. Spectr. Process.* 70, 473–509. doi: 10.1016/s0074-7742(05)70014-3

Migriov, L., Kronenberg, J., and Henkin, Y. (2009). Self-reported listening habits and enjoyment of music among cochlear implant recipients. *Ann. Otol. Rhinol. Laryngol.* 118, 350–355. doi: 10.1177/000348940911800506

Mitani, C., Nakata, T., and Trehub, S. E. (2007). Music recognition, music listening, and word recognition by deaf children with cochlear implants. *Ear Hear.* 28, S38–S41.

Moore, B. C. J., and Carlyon, R. P. (2005). "Perception of pitch by people with cochlear hearing loss and by cochlear implant users," in *Pitch, Neural Coding and Perception*, eds C. J. Plack, A. J. Oxenham, R. R. Fay, and A. N. Popper (New York, NY: Springer), 234–277. doi: 10.1007/0-387-28958-5_7

Nimmons, G. L., Kang, R. S., Drennan, W. R., Longnion, J., Ruffin, C., Worman, T., et al. (2008). Clinical assessment of music perception in cochlear implant listeners. *Otol. Neurotol.* 29, 149–155. doi: 10.1097/mao.0b013e31812f7244

Rattay, F., Lutter, P., and Felix, H. (2001). A model of the electrically excited human cochlear neuron. I. Contribution of neural substructures to the generation and propagation of spikes. *Hear. Res.* 153, 43–63. doi: 10.1016/s0378-5955(00)00256-2

Rochette, F., and Bigand, E. (2009). Long-term effects of auditory training in severely or profoundly deaf children. *Ann. N. Y. Acad. Sci.* 1169, 195–198. doi: 10.1111/j.1749-6632.2009.04793.x

Schellenberg, E. G., Bigand, E., Poulin-Charronnat, B., Garnier, C., and Stevens, C. (2005). Children's implicit knowledge of harmony in Western music. *Dev. Sci.* 8, 551–566. doi: 10.1111/j.1467-7687.2005.00447.x

Tillmann, B., Bharucha, J. J., and Bigand, E. (2000). Implicit learning of tonality: a self-organizing approach. *Psychol. Rev.* 107, 885–913. doi: 10.1037//0033-295x.107.4.885

Tillmann, B., Justus, T., and Bigand, E. (2008). Cerebellar patients demonstrate preserved implicit knowledge of association strengths in musical sequences. *Brain Cogn.* 66, 161–167. doi: 10.1016/j.bandc.2007.07.005

Tillmann, B., Peretz, I., Bigand, E., and Gosselin, N. (2007). Harmonic priming in an amusic patient: the power of implicit tasks. *Cogn. Neuropsychol.* 24, 603–622. doi: 10.1080/02643290701609527

Trehub, S. E., Vongpaisal, T., and Nakata, T. (2009). Music in the lives of deaf children with cochlear implants. *Ann. N. Y. Acad. Sci.* 1169, 534–542. doi: 10.1111/j.1749-6632.2009.04554.x

Van Immerseel, L. M., and Martens, J. (1992). Pitch and voiced/unvoiced determination with an auditory model. *J. Acoust. Soc. Am.* 91, 3511–3526. doi: 10.1121/1.402840

Young, A. W., Hellawell, D., and DeHaan, E. H. F. (1988). Cross-domain semantic priming in normal subjects and a prosopagnosic patient. *Q. J. Exp. Psychol.* 40A, 561–580. doi: 10.1080/02724988843000087

Yucel, E., Sennaroglu, G., and Belgin, E. (2009). The family-oriented musical training for children with cochlear implants: speech and musical perception results of two year follow-up. *Int. J. Pediatr. Otorhinolaryngol.* 73, 1043–1052. doi: 10.1016/j.ijporl.2009.04.009

Zaltz, Y., Goldsworthy, R. L., Kishon-Rabin, L., and Eisenberg, L. S. (2018). Voice discrimination by adults with cochlear implants: the benefits of early implantation for vocal-tract length perception. *J. Assoc. Res. Otolaryngol.* 19, 193–209. doi: 10.1007/s10162-017-0653-5

Zeng, F.-G. (2004). Trends in cochlear implants. *Trends Amplif.* 8, 1–34. doi: 10.1177/108471380400800102

APPENDIX

Analyses of the Acoustic Similarity Between the Harmonic Context and the Target in Regular and Irregular Conditions of Koelsch et al. (2004)

We ran the three analyses investigating the acoustic similarity between contexts and targets also with the material of Koelsch et al. (2004), which is currently the only paper that tested musical structure processing in CI patients with an indirect investigation method. A total of 260 tonal harmonic sequences made up of five chords were generated as a MIDI file from the authors' description.[5] An audio file was then synthetized using a piano timbre. Duration of the first four chords was 600 ms, while the fifth chord sounded for 1200 ms. Sequences were presented in six blocks to the model. Each block was in a different tonal key (*C, D, E, F#, Ab,* and *Eb* keys). To conform to the experimental procedure reported by the authors, echoic memory state was reset between each block, but not between each sequence within a block.

Overlap in Pitch Class Between Targets and Contexts

We analyzed the number of pitch classes shared between a target chord and its preceding chords, as a function of target type and target position within the sequence. We used the MIDI file generated as described above. The mean number of pitch classes shared between target and preceding context was higher for the tonic regular condition (5.4 $\pm$ 3.29) than for the irregular condition (1.35 $\pm$ 1.34). More interestingly, the difference between regular and irregular targets was stronger for the fifth position (6.41) than for the third position (1.68), revealing a sensory advantage for the regular targets at the fifth position. Consequently, the cognitive (tonal) advantage for regular targets over irregular targets was confounded with acoustic similarity.

Spectrum Analyses

We estimated the spectral overlap between the target chords and their respective harmonic contexts. For each sequence of the material of Koelsch et al. (2004)'s study, the spectrum obtained from the target chord was correlated with the spectrum obtained from preceding chords. The spectra were obtained by averaging the spectrogram computed over the contexts and targets with FFT-time windows of 186 ms and 50%-window overlap (i.e., 93 ms). A Position (3 vs. 5) $\times$ Chord Type (Regular vs. irregular) ANOVA on average correlation values showed not only main effects of both Position, $F(1,256) = 308.51$, MSE = 0.175, $p < 0.0001$, and Chord type, $F(1,256) = 359.82$, MSE = 0.204, $p < 0.0001$, but—most importantly—a significant interaction, $F(1,256) = 24.65$, MSE = 0.014, $p < 0.0001$: The difference between regular and irregular chords was stronger for position 5 than for position 3, $t(64) = 5.55$, $p < 0.0001$ (see **Appendix Figure 1A** here below), thus confirming a sensory advantage at position 5.

Pitch Periodicity in Auditory Short-Term Memory

We here ran the implementation of Leman (2000) model and its IPEM toolbox as used in Bigand et al. (2014) and its graphical presentation of the local and global parameters and Tonal Contextuality index (TC). For the material of Koelsch et al. (2004), the differences between regular chords (i.e., in-key) and irregular chords (i.e., Neapolitan sixth chord) are reported in **Appendix Figures 1B,C** here below, for positions 3 and 5, respectively. Irrespective of position within the sequence, irregular chords elicited a stronger dissimilarity in short-term pitch memory than did regular, in-key target chords (as illustrated by the hot colors, TC of the in-key chords were higher than for the irregular chords, i.e., $TC_{in-key} - TC_{irregular} > 0$). In addition, the size of the dissimilarity mirrored the size of the ERAN, thus accounting for the effect of position: Simulations predicted stronger dissimilarity for the irregular chords occurring at the syntactically incorrect position (i.e., at position 5; **Appendix Figure 1C**), compared to the syntactically correct position (i.e., at position 3; **Appendix Figure 1B**). The stronger dissimilarity of the target at position 5 in terms of TC is illustrated in **Appendix Figure 1D** that reports a (positive) difference between position 5 minus position 3. In sum, the sensory model accounts for the data pattern observed in Koelsch et al. (2004), suggesting that in this study the effect of position in participants' data might have a sensory rather than a cognitive origin.

To summarize these analyses, for the experimental material used in Koelsch et al. (2004), cognitive and sensory hypothesis made the same predictions, that is, a cost of processing is expected for the musically irregular chord, in particular in the fifth position. The three types of analyses thus reveal that we cannot conclude whether CI participants' ERPs reflected the violation of information accumulated in a sensory memory buffer or the activation of musical knowledge (see Koelsch et al., 2007, for a similar argument for this experimental material in NH listeners).

[5]In each harmonic sequence, the first chord was always the tonic. Chords at the second position were tonic, mediant, submediant, subdominant, dominant to the dominant, secondary dominant to mediant, secondary dominant to submediant, or secondary dominant to supertonic. Chords at the third position were subdominant, dominant, dominant 6–4 chord or Neapolitan sixth chord. Chords at the fourth position were always the dominant seventh chord. Finally, chords at the fifth position were either a tonic or a Neapolitan sixth chord. Neapolitan chords at the third position never followed a secondary dominant. Neapolitan chords at the fifth position never followed a Neapolitan chord at the third position. Both Neapolitan chords occurred with a probability of 25% (resulting in the presentation of 65 Neapolitans at the third, and 65 at the fifth position).

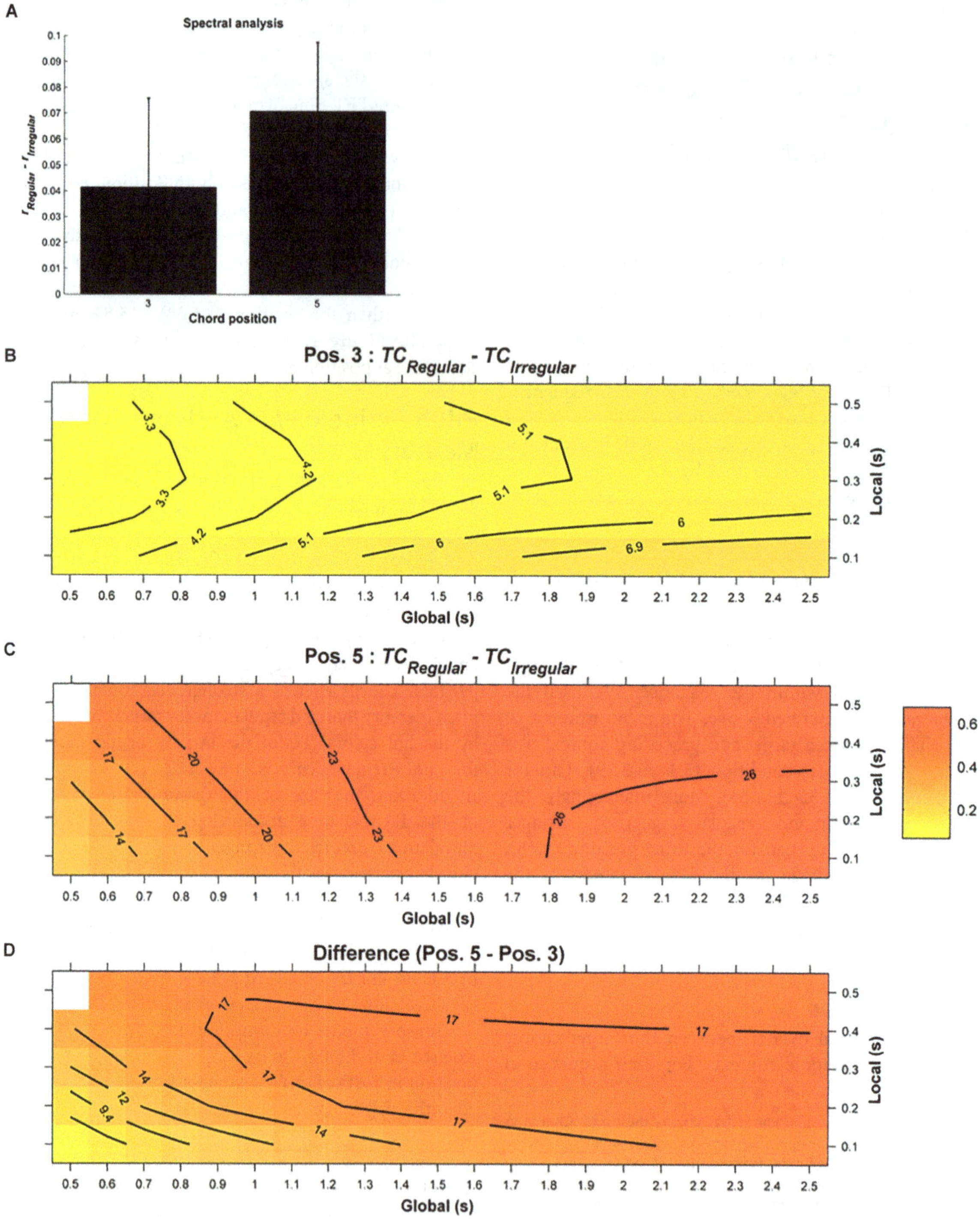

APPENDIX FIGURE 1 | Results of the acoustic analyses for the material Koelsch et al. (2004), presenting differences between the regular and irregular chords for positions 3 and 5, for the harmonic spectrum **(A)** and the model of Leman **(B–D)**. For panels B and C, the mean differences between the tonal contextuality of the target chords ($TC_{regular} - TC_{irregular}$) are presented as a function of the local and global context integration windows. Positive, negative, and non-significant differences are represented by hot (i.e., red), cold (i.e., blue), and white colors, respectively (two-tailed paired *t*-test, $p < 0.05$; *t*-values are reported as contours). A positive difference indicates that the pitch similarity in the sensory memory induced by the related target is stronger than that of the less-related target. Panel D completes this presentation with the difference for positions 5 and 3.

3

Design and Evaluation of a Real-Time Audio Source Separation Algorithm to Remix Music for Cochlear Implant Users

Sina Tahmasebi, Tom Gajęcki and Waldo Nogueira*

Department of Otolaryngology, Medical University Hannover and Cluster of Excellence "Hearing4all", Hanover, Germany

Correspondence:
Sina Tahmasebi
Tahmasebi.Sina@mh-hannover.de

A cochlear implant (CI) is a surgically implanted electronic device that partially restores hearing to people suffering from profound hearing loss. Although CI users, in general, obtain a very good reception of continuous speech in the absence of background noise, they face severe limitations in the context of music perception and appreciation. The main reasons for these limitations are related to channel interactions created by the broad spread of electrical fields in the cochlea and to the low number of electrodes that stimulate it. Moreover, CIs have severe limitations when it comes to transmitting the temporal fine structure of acoustic signals, and hence, these devices elicit poor pitch and timber perception. For these reasons, several signal processing algorithms have been proposed to make music more accessible for CI users, trying to reduce the complexity of music signals or remixing them to enhance certain components, such as the lead singing voice. In this work, a deep neural network that performs real-time audio source separation to remix music for CI users is presented. The implementation is based on multi-layer perception (MLP) and has been evaluated using objective instrumental measurements to ensure clean source estimation. Furthermore, experiments in 10 normal hearing (NH) and 13 CI users to investigate how the vocals to instruments ratio (VIR) set by the tested listeners were affected in realistic environments with and without visual information. The objective instrumental results fulfill the benchmark reported in previous studies by introducing distortions that are shown to not be perceived by CI users. Moreover, the implemented model was optimized to perform real-time source separation. The experimental results show that CI users prefer vocals 8 dB enhanced with the respect to the instruments independent of acoustic sound scenarios and visual information. In contrast, NH listeners did not prefer a VIR different than zero dB.

Keywords: music source separation, deep learning, neural networks, multi-layer perception, real-time, cochlear implant

1. INTRODUCTION

A cochlear implant (CI) is a medical electronic device that is surgically implanted in the inner ear and can provide hearing sensations to people suffering from profound hearing loss. CIs allow the patients to understand speech in quiet and even in a noisy background. However, music appreciation is still challenging for CI users, as it requires a good pitch perception and melody recognition (McDermott, 2004; Limb and Roy, 2013). CI devices typically transmit 12–22 spectral channels, each modulated slowly in time. This representation provides enough information for speech understanding in quiet conditions and rhythmic perception of music. However, this representation is not enough to support speech understanding in noise or melody recognition, as melody recognition requires complex pitch perception, which in turn depends strongly on access to spectral and temporal fine structure cues (McDermott, 2004; Macherey et al., 2011). This work investigates the use of a real-time algorithm to make music more accessible for CI users.

Previous research in the area of music enhancement for CI users has focused on reducing music complexity (Nagathil et al., 2017) or on amplifying vocals relative to the background instruments (Buyens et al., 2014; Pons et al., 2016; Gajęcki and Nogueira, 2018). Spectral complexity reduction of music was investigated based on dimensionality reduction techniques, such as principal component analysis and a partial-least squares analysis. Enhancement of singing voice has been investigated based on the finding that CI users prefer singing music remixed such that the vocals are boosted by 6 dB with respect to the background instruments (Buyens et al., 2014). In this context several source separation algorithms have been proposed to separate the vocals from the instruments and remix these components accordingly. Previous approaches used a harmonic/percussive sound separation (HPSS; Buyens et al., 2014) algorithm, non-negative matrix factorization (NMF), multi-layer perceptrons (MLP), deep recurrent neural networks (DRNN), and convolutional autoencoders (DCAE) in order to separate different sources within an audio mixture (Pons et al., 2016; Gajęcki and Nogueira, 2018). However, all these algorithms were implemented in non-real-time fashion to perform source separation.

A key factor in the design of source separation methods for music enhancement is the distortions that these algorithms introduce in the processed signals. These distortions are typically quantified through objective instrumental measures, such as the signal-to-distortion ratio (SDR), the signal-to-artifacts ratio (SAR), and the signal-to-interference ratio (SIR) (Vincent et al., 2010). Gajęcki and Nogueira (2018) investigated the maximum levels of artifacts and distortions accepted by CI users to remix music with enhanced vocals. They demonstrated that source separation algorithms with an SDR > 0.69 dB and an SAR > 4.42 dB were suitable for remixing singing pop music for CI users.

In order for the source separation algorithm to operate in real-time, algorithmic complexity and latency need to be minimized. Regarding latency, even delays in the order of tens of milliseconds can cause a de-synchronization between the visual and the acoustic information provided by the CI. Stone and Moore (2003) measured maximum non-noticeable latency for hearing aid devices of around 15–20 ms for speech signals. The international telecommunication union (ITU) performed several subjective evaluations (ITU, 2008) and reported the acceptable and the detectable lip synchronization error. This error was assessed by means of the time delay between the visual feedback and acoustic information provided by a person speaking. Their results revealed that the measured time delay detectability was 125 ms and the threshold of acceptability was 185 ms, respectively, with respect to perfect lip synchronization when audio lagging behind the video. Furthermore, Hay-McCutcheon et al. (2009), in a similar study, investigated the audiovisual asynchrony for CI users. In this study, the measured minimum noticeable audiovisual asynchrony was around 200 ms, when the video was leading the audio. These values could be taken as an upper boundary for the design of a real time source separation algorithm.

Previous source separation algorithms to remix music for CIs have been evaluated under laboratory settings using clean digital recordings. It remains a question whether these algorithms are usable in real music events in which reverberation influences the acoustics. Moreover, these source separation algorithms were evaluated only using pre-processed sounds. It is therefore interesting to investigate whether these algorithms are usable in real-time giving the users the possibility to continuously modify the level difference between the singing voice and the instruments to reach a final decision on their preference.

Although music experiments are typically investigated only through sound, it is very important to consider that CI users have access to both hearing and visual cues. It has been shown that when congruent visual and auditory cues are processed together, perceptual accuracy is enhanced in both normal hearing (NH) and in hearing-impaired listeners (Perrott et al., 1990; Ross et al., 2007; Landry et al., 2012). The importance of vision in lip reading the singing voice, which helps in understanding the lyrics, the fact that CI users can see the instruments being played, as well as the information provided by the performance can significantly enhance their perception (Plant, 2015). It therefore remains a question of whether source separation algorithms used to enhance the vocals are necessary if visual information is available.

In this work, we implement and evaluate a deep neural network (DNN) to perform real-time music source separation to improve music appreciation of CI users in realistic acoustic scenarios. The model is based on an MLP and is trained to automatically identify the lead singing voice contained in western pop music to remix it accordingly to the subjects' preference. Prior to assessing individual balance preferences, objective instrumental measures will be used to make sure that the source separation algorithm fulfills the benchmark proposed by Gajęcki and Nogueira (2018). Finally, the balance between music and singing voice will be assessed by means of experimental tests were subjects will indicate their preferred vocals-to-instruments-ratio (VIR), which is defined as the ratio between the power of the vocal signal and the instruments signal in dB, with and without visual cues. As the experiments were meant to be as realistic as possible, 360° video and 3D audio were provided to the listeners. In this context, the subjects should be able to move their heads toward the singer or to the background instruments and therefore they should be provided with consistent acoustic and visual cues.

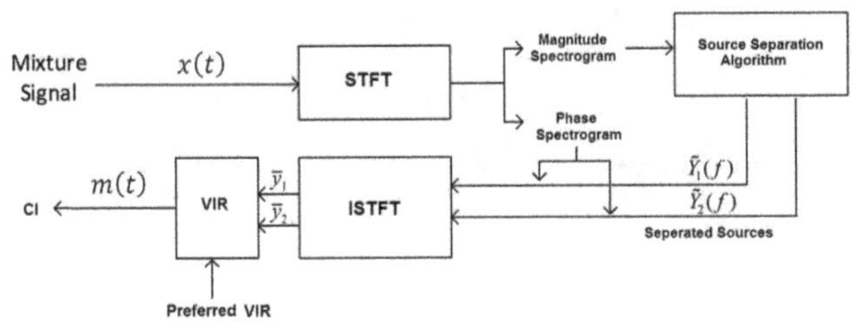

FIGURE 1 | Block diagram of the source separation algorithm.

2. METHODS AND MATERIALS

2.1. Music Source Separation and Remix Algorithm

Figure 1 shows a block diagram representing the data-flow of the used music source separation and remixing framework. The input signal $x(t)$ consists of the original mixture, of vocals and instruments and the output signal $m(t)$ is a remixed version of the input signal that is delivered to the CI speech processor at discrete time t. The desired VIR is applied to the estimated signals to be then remixed and delivered to the CI listener.

The music source separation process starts by feeding the magnitude spectrogram of the input mixture to the source separation algorithm. For a vocal signal $y_1(t)$ and an instruments signal $y_2(t)$ we construct a corresponding mixture signal $x(t) = y_1(t) + y_2(t)$. We compute the short-time Fourier transform of length 1024 samples to obtain the spectrums $Y_1(k)$, $Y_2(k)$, $X(k)$ for frame k. Since the time-domain audio signals are real, we used half of the spectral length, as dropping the negative frequencies does not lead to any information loss, which leads to a spectral size of 513 bins. For inverting the spectrum of $Y_1(k)$ and $Y_2(k)$, back into the time domain, we used the phase of the mixture spectrum and applied the inverse STFT with overlap-add to synthesize the music signal, for both the vocals and instruments components. **Figure 1** illustrates the block diagram of the algorithm. The ability that MLPs have to approximate any input/output map made them one of the most popular network architectures (Panchal et al., 2011). Furthermore, as MLPs require relatively low computation complexity, they became the first choice of this study to perform music source separation. The number of input and output units is directly related to the size of the analysis window. We used an STFT with a window length of 1,024 samples, an overlap of 75%, and a Hamming window to transform, which leads to a spectrum with a dimension of 513 bins. In order to exploit the temporal dependency in the music signals, three consecutive frames with two frames overlap were used as input to the network resulting in an input size of 513*3. During the source separation process, we specify multiple parameters, that have a direct effect on separation quality and are linked to the network's structure. The depth of the MLP was set to one hidden layer with 1,024-units and a rectified linear unit (ReLU) activation function, which resulted in a three layer network with an input size of 513*3 units and output layer of 1,026 (2*513) units which corresponds to the two spectrums of vocal and instruments signal. After selecting the number of hidden layers and units in each layer, a proper training algorithm was used to minimize the algorithm error by fitting the model to the training data. During training, the fixed parameters were: the batch size which was set to 128 and the initial learning rate which was set to 0.005. The adaptive moment estimation algorithm (Adam) (Kingma and Ba, 2014) was used as the optimization algorithm. A hundred epochs were used to train the network, where after each epoch, the learning rate was decreased by 0.9 and the training data were shuffled. To avoid over-fitting, a dropout layer with a probability of 80% was applied. Three consecutive frames were used as input to exploit the temporal context in the audio signals. However, introducing more frames to the network did not improve the objective instrumental measurement values.

2.2. Audio Material Used to Train the Neural Network

In this work, we use three audio data sets to perform the objective and experimental evaluations in NH and CI users of the investigated audio source separation algorithms. The data sets will be described in the following lines.

- **iKala Data Set:** The first data set introduced by Chan et al. (2015) namely iKala contains 252 30-s tracks of vocal and backing track music with a sample rate of 44,100 Hz. Each music track is a stereo recording, with one channel for the singing voice and the other for background music. All music tracks have been performed by professional musicians and six singers, of which three were female and three males. The iKala data set contains non-vocal time passages where the source separation algorithm assumes the presence of vocals and having non-vocal time passages in the data set may challenge the algorithm. The presence of vocals in the instruments signal and long non-vocals regions were the reasons that in experimental settings 30 music tracks of data set have been excluded, making the total number of music tracks in the iKala data set equal to 222.
- **The MUSDB Data Set:** MUSDB data set was the second data set with 150 professionally mixed songs from different genres, each including four stereo sources (bass, drums, vocals and a group of other instruments) used in this work. The data set was divided into the training and the testing data set with 100 and 50 songs, respectively.
- **Buyens Shared Data Set:** As the third data set, six popular music pieces (Buyens et al., 2014) that have been used in previous CI studies to create and report a benchmark (Pons et al., 2016; Gajęcki and Nogueira, 2018) have been also used in this study.
- **Custom Data Set with Virtual Acoustics:** All the previous data sets were studio recordings with no spatial characteristics. In order to have a DNN which can be used in a realistic sound scenario, it was necessary to train the model with a data set that included spatial characteristics. To create a music data set with such characteristics, TASCAR was used to simulate realistic sound scenarios (Grimm et al., 2015). TASCAR is a toolbox to create virtual acoustics in real-time. TASCAR toolbox is based on an image source model that simulated localized

TABLE 1 | Details about created sound scenarios.

Sound scenario	Dimensions in meters (x, y, z)	Damping factor	Reflection coefficient	Virtual receiver position (x, y, z)
1	(30, 30, 8)	0.70	0.25	At the center (0, 0, 0)
2	(20, 20, 7)	0.80	0.20	At the center (0, 0, 0)

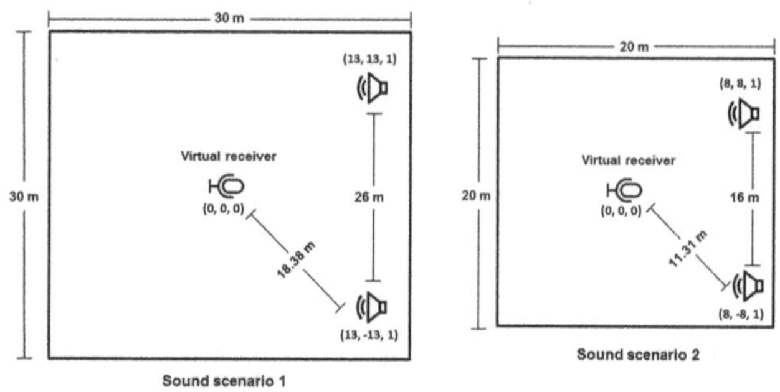

FIGURE 2 | Visualization of the created sounds scenarios. **(Left)** Sound scenario 1 consisting of large reverberant room (T20 = 0.24 s, T60 = 0.65 s); **(Right)** Sound scenario 2 consisting of a smaller and less reverberant room (T20 = 0.18 s, T60 = 0.5 s).

sources, reflections and a diffuse sound model for adding background recordings and reverberation. The image source model rendered an image source for each combination of the primary sound source and a reflecting surface, provided that the primary source was not behind the surface. To playback the content of a virtual scene created by TASCAR on an arbitrary playback device, Ambisonics decoding must be performed to get the signals for the channels of the playback system. The acoustic scene was rendered and played through an array of 16 loudspeakers. In order to assess the effect of different sound scenarios on the performance of the DNN model, two rooms with different dimensions and acoustic characteristics were rendered through the 16 loudspeaker setup and the TASCAR toolbox. A reverberant room with a T20 = 0.24 s and T60 = 0.65 s and a smaller and less reverberant room with a T20 = 0.18 s and T60 = 0.5 s were used in the experiments.

In each sound scenario a virtual receiver with an omnidirectional characteristic is defined which captures the sound in that space. The real receiver (CI user or dummy head) was placed in the center of the loudspeaker layout in the lab and received the sound corresponding with the position of the virtual receiver in each defined sound scenario. The virtual environment consisted of two loudspeakers reproducing stereo mixes aiming at resembling a music concert amplified with a public address system (PA system). The room impulse response was modeled by the toolbox using the reflection coefficient and a damping factor shown in **Table 1**. **Figure 2** shows a visualization of the created sound scenarios.

A Nucleus speech processor (Cochlear, Sydney, Australia), mounted on a dummy head at the height of 1.4 m was placed in the center of loudspeaker layout to record the custom data set. While TASCAR was running on a Linux operating system, another PC, which was connected to the Nucleus speech processor through a sound card, was recording the simulated sound field. The custom data set was exclusively used to train, validate and, test the MLP using objective instrumental measures.

2.2.1. Training, Validation, and Testing Data Set

To have a uniform data set, the signals contained in the MUSDB set, which had different lengths, were chopped in 30 s long samples and were mixed with the iKala data set. Finally, we distributed the iKala and MUSDB data sets into the training, validation and testing sets. During this study, 60% of the iKala and MUSDB data sets were used as the training data set, 20% as the validation data set and 20% as testing data set. Moreover, the music signals shared by Buynes were added to the testing data set.

2.3. Experiments in Normal Hearing Listeners and Cochlear Implant Users

This study consisted of two experiments. In the first one, the effect of having different sound scenarios on VIR preferences was investigated. In the second one, the effect of having visual cues on VIR preferences was investigated.

2.3.1. Subjects

Thirteen bilateral CI users with different musical backgrounds and 10 NH subjects participated in the study. The demographic information of the tested CI subjects is presented in **Table 2**. From the 13 CI users only 10 CI subjects participated in each experiment as indicated in the same table. All subjects gave informed consent to the project as approved by the Medical University Hannover Institutional Review Board. The subjects were asked to turn off any program on the speech processor and use the audio cable as input. None of the subjects had residual hearing except for Subject S07, who had bilateral residual hearing up to 250 Hz. This particular subject was also asked to wear soft foam earplugs to minimize acoustic leakage. In the first perceptual experiment, ten NH subjects participated in the study as a control group.

2.3.2. Test Setup Used in Listening Experiments

The experiments were conducted monaurally using the better performing side of each subject. Sound material was presented in a double-walled sound-treated room using 16 active (self-amplified) loudspeakers (Genelec 8030B, Helsinki, Finland), which were organized in a circle with a radius of 1.25 m and were driven by an A16 MKII digital to analog converter connected to a PC with Ubuntu Xenial 14.04 operating system. Subjects were seated in the center of the loudspeaker array and the audio material was always presented at a level corresponding to 65 dB SPL at the position of the participant's head.

TABLE 2 | Information of the CI subjects, who took part in the experiments.

Subject id	Age	Cause of deafness	Duration of deafness	Implant experience on tested side	Sound processor	Brand
S01[a,b]	65–70	Unknown	9Y	21Y	Opus2	MEDEL
S02[a,b]	80–85	Genetic	4M	7Y	Opus2	MEDEL
S03[a,b]	55–60	Sudden deafness	2M	4Y	Naida	AB
S04[a,b]	60–65	Unknown	6Y	13M	CP910	Cochlear
S05[a,b]	70–75	Sudden deafness	29M	3Y	CP910	Cochlear
S06[a]	65–70	Unknown	3.5Y	5Y	Harmony	AB
S07[a]	65–70	Unknown	4M	12Y	CP910	AB
S08[a,b]	20–25	Otitis media	4Y	20Y	CP910	Cochlear
S09[a]	60–65	Unknown	5Y	4Y	CP910	Cochlear
S10[a,b]	20–25	Unknown	0M	18M	Naida	AB
S11[b]	70–75	Unknown	4Y	4Y	CP910	Cochlear
S12[b]	65–70	CRS	31Y	6Y	CP910	Cochlear
S13[b]	20–25	Meningitis	4 M	18Y	CP910	Cochlear

Time data are expressed in years (Y) or in months (M).
[a]Participated in the first part of experiment 1 [b]Participated in the second part of experiment 1. CRS, congenital rubella syndrome.

TABLE 3 | Music tracks used in experiment 1.

Song id	Data set	Song name	Genre
M1	iKala	21058_chorus	Pop
M2	iKala	31104_verse	Pop
M3	iKala	31118_chorus	Pop
M4	iKala	54236_chorus	Pop
M5	MUSDB	Secretariat—Over The Top	Pop rock
M6	MUSDB	Georgia Wonder—Siren	Folk rock
M7	MUSDB	The Long Wait—Dark Horses	Folk
M8	Popular music	Hey Jude (The Beatles) (excerpt A)	Pop, country music
M9	Popular music	Hey Jude (The Beatles) (excerpt B)	Pop, country music
M10	Popular music	Dock of the Bay (Otis Redding)	Pop, classic soul

TABLE 4 | Music tracks used in experiment 2.

Song id	Song name	Genre
CasA	Cassiopeia (excerpt 1)	Electronic
CasB	Cassiopeia (excerpt 2)	Electronic
CasC	Cassiopeia (excerpt 3)	Electronic
KönigA	Der König in Thule (excerpt 1)	Sung poetry
KönigB	Der König in Thule (excerpt 2)	Sung poetry
KönigC	Der König in Thule (excerpt 3)	Sung poetry

The microphone of a Nucleus speech processor (Cochlear, Sydney, Australia) was used to capture the presented audio signals during all subjective tests. The microphone had an omnidirectional characteristic and no beamforming was used during the tests. The captured signals were then processed through the algorithm and presented to the subject's speech processor. A preamplifier was used to amplify the captured signal which was routed to the subject's own processor, in direct-in mode, through a 3.5 mm audio cable. During the tests, the microphone on the subject's CI was disabled.

The subjects were asked to adjust a slider that controlled the VIR using the left and right arrow keys on a keyboard while listening to the music. The slider had 24 steps each corresponding to 1 dB on a logarithmic scale from −12 to +12 dB VIR. In order to prevent any bias, initial VIR for each song presentation was randomly chosen and the subjects were kept blinded to the initial VIR. Afterward, the subjects adjusted the VIR to their preferred setting.

For NH subjects, instead of a CI, a headphone (DT 770, Beyerdynamic, Heilbronn, Germany) was used to present the music tracks. The music tracks presented to the NH subjects were captured with the same microphone on the Nucleus speech processor. The headphone was calibrated to present each music piece at 65 dB SPL using only one side, at the self-reported preferred ear.

2.3.3. Music Material Used in Listening Experiments

Music tracks shown in **Tables 3, 4** have been used in experiment 1 and 2, respectively. The music excerpts used in experiment 1 had a duration of 5 s, whereas the ones used in experiment 2 were 45 s in duration. The pieces selected for experiment 2 had clear vocals with simple music accompaniment (electronic in "Cassiopeia" and a flute and a tuba in "der König in Thule") and in that sense were similar to the pieces used in experiment 1.

2.3.3.1. Virtual test scenarios in experiment 1

The TASCAR library was used in experiment 1 to add spatial characteristics to the studio-quality music tracks. In this experiment the two sound scenarios presented in **Figure 2** were used to assess the VIR preferences of NH listeners and CI users.

2.3.3.2. Virtual test scenarios in experiment 2

Six music excerpts from live recordings in a concert was used in the experiment 2 (Nogueira, 2019). In comparison to the before-mentioned data sets, which were recorded with studio quality and had no spatial characteristics, these music excerpts were spatially recorded using the Eigenmic 32 microphone (Summit, New Jersey, USA). These music tracks already contained the spatial characteristics of a concert hall.

2.3.4. Experiment 1: Online Vocals to Instruments Ratio Adjustment

In the first experiment, 5-s excerpts of ten signals from three data sets were used (**Table 3**). Each excerpt was calibrated at 65 dB SPL and was played in a loop until the subject adjusted the VIR slider in their favored position. Subjects had no time limits to adjust the VIR for each music track and were allowed to have a break whenever they desired. After the test, subjects were asked to fill in a questionnaire providing their musical background experiences or knowledge and music genre preference. This procedure including the stimulus length was chosen based on previous studies (Pons et al., 2016; Gajęcki and Nogueira, 2018). This experiment was divided into two parts. In the first part of the experiment, NH listeners and CI users were asked to adjust the VIR for a test data set. In this part, the VIR was modified keeping the level of the instruments fixed while modifying the level of the vocals. In the second part of the experiment, the VIR was altered by modifying the level of the vocals and the instruments in opposite directions to keep the overall presentation level constant at 65 dB SPL. The second part of this experiment was included to exclude potential effects due to variations in loudness.

2.3.5. Experiment 2: Effect of Visual Information on VIR Preferences

The goal of this experiment was to examine whether visual feedback affects the VIR preferences of the CI recipients. This experiment was divided into two parts. The music pieces 4 of a concert were presented to the subjects, once without visual information, and once with visual information through a set of Oculus Rift (Facebook, Irvine, California, USA) virtual reality (VR) headset. Each music excerpt was repeated until the subjects adjusted the VIR at their favored value. As mentioned in section 2.3.3, the music pieces were recorded with an Eigenmic 32 microphone array that has 32 microphones, capable of providing 4-th order Ambisonics. Reaper (Cockos, New York, USA) on an Ubuntu PC was used as a digital workstation to process the audio material. The audio signals were captured by an Eigenmic 32 microphone array and during the tests they were first encoded to 4-th order Ambisonics and then decoded to the layout used in the testing lab. GoPro player (GoPro, San Mateo, California, USA) on a Windows (Microsoft, Redmond, Washington, USA) PC was deployed to present the visual materials of the concert. As the digital workstation and the GoPro player use different synchronization protocols, a third party application, which was able to send and receive OSC and UDP messages, was used to synchronize both audio and video. For this experiment, the VIR was applied in the same way as in the second part of the previous experiment; i. e. by modifying the level of the vocals and the instruments in opposite directions to keep the overall presentation level constant at 65 dB SPL. During the second part of the test, the Nucleus speech processor was fixed on the Oculus Rift VR headset. It is worth mentioning that five subjects wore eyeglasses, which they took off during this experiment.

3. RESULTS

3.1. Objective Instrumental Measures

Figure 3 shows the objective results for music tracks used in the first perceptual experiments. Mean SDR and SAR of the music tracks in sound scenario 1, which was a larger room with more diffusive and reverberant characteristics, with 5.5 dB is around 0.3 dB worse than the mean SDR obtained in the second room. However, the SAR values obtained in the first sound scenario (8.8 dB) were slightly better than in the second sound scenario (8.7 dB). Both sound scenarios fulfill the benchmark reported by Gajęcki and Nogueira (2018), where the lower bounds for SDR and SAR were reported with 0.69 and 4.42 dB, respectively. It is worth mentioning that the room characteristics cause changes in the music tracks, which leads to different objective results after source separation, which can be seen in **Figure 3**.

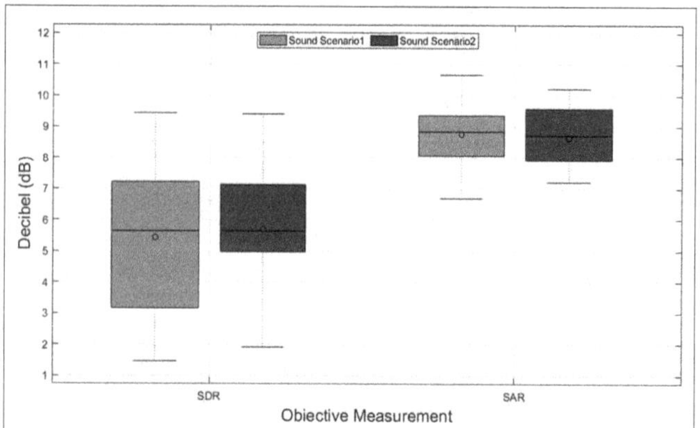

FIGURE 3 | Results of the objective instrumental measurements based on the signal-to-distortion-ratio (SDR) and the signal-to-artifacts-ratio (SAR) in decibels (dB) for two sound scenarios across music tracks.

3.2. Experiment 1: Online Vocals to Instruments Ratio Adjustment

Figure 4 presents the individual and group VIR preferences of the first part of experiment 1 for CI users (top panels) and NH listeners (bottom panel) for two virtual sound scenarios. The line and the circle in the boxes represent the median and the mean, respectively. On average, the VIR mean across CI users was 8.2 and 8.5 dB and across NH listeners was −2 and −1.7 dB for sound scenarios 1 and 2, respectively. Note that for CI users S1, S6, and S7 no box can be seen in specific sound scenarios as the plots for these subjects collapsed to a single line due to small variance in their results. These subjects adjusted the VIR in more than 75 % of the cases to the same value. R Studio (Boston, Massachusetts, USA) software was used to conduct the statistical analysis. First, the VIR preferences of CI users and NHs were tested against the null hypothesis that the preferred VIR was equal to zero dB. This was done for the two parts of the experiment for each tested sound scenario by means of two-tailed t-tests.

For the first part of the experiment, where the VIR was set by modifying the vocals with respect to the instruments, the CI group showed a preference for positive VIRs for the first ($Mean =$ 8.5 dB, $SD = 2.4$ dB, $p < 0.001$) and second sound scenarios ($Mean = 8.2$ dB, $SD = 2.5$ dB, $p < 0.001$). The NH group, on the other hand, did not show any evidence of preferring a balance different from the original mix (VIR=0 dB) for the first sound scenario ($Mean = -2$ dB, $SD = 3.2$ dB, $p < 0.086$) nor for the second sound scenario ($Mean = -1.75$ dB, $SD = 2.8$ dB, $p < 0.082$). Finally, none of the tested groups' preferred VIR depended on the sound scenario ($p = 0.297$ for the CI users and $p = 0.7$ for the NH group).

Figure 5 presents the individual and group VIR preferences of the second part of experiment 1 for CI users (top panels) and NH

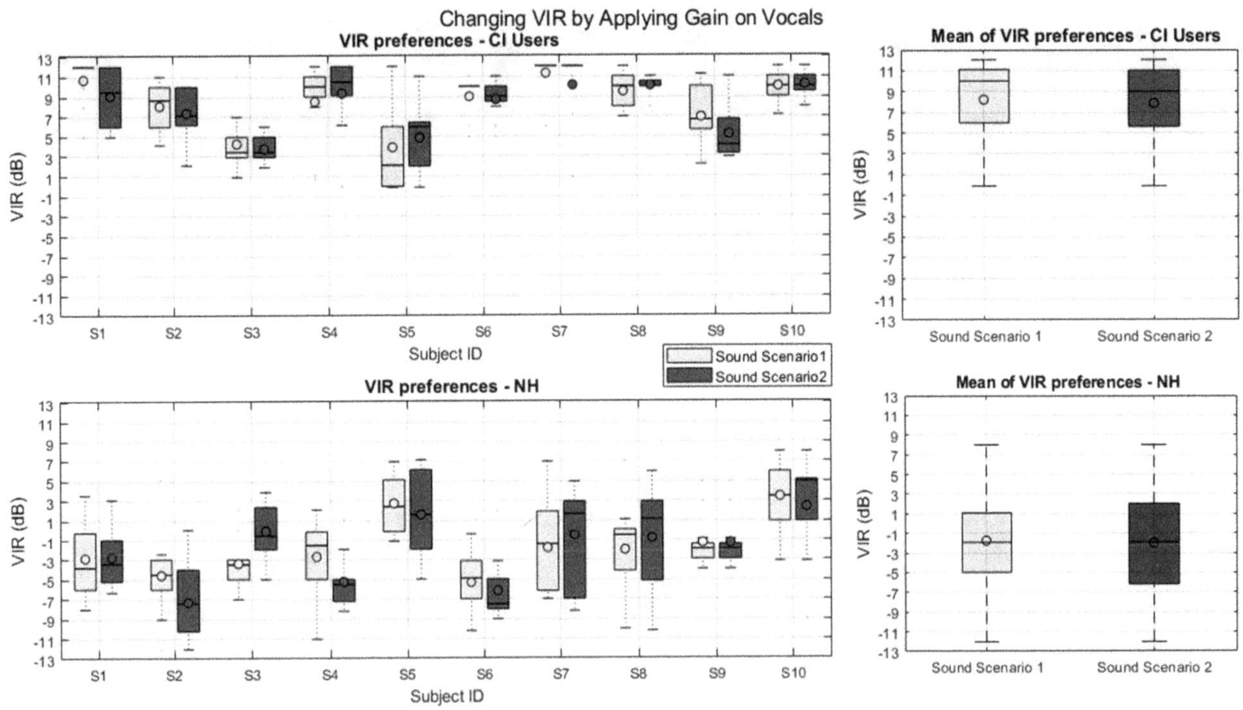

FIGURE 4 | VIR values from part one of experiment 1: Changing VIR by applying gain on vocals. **(Top left)** VIR preferences of CI users, **(Top right)** mean VIR of CI users, **(Bottom left)** VIR preferences of NH subjects, **(Bottom right)** mean VIR of NH subjects.

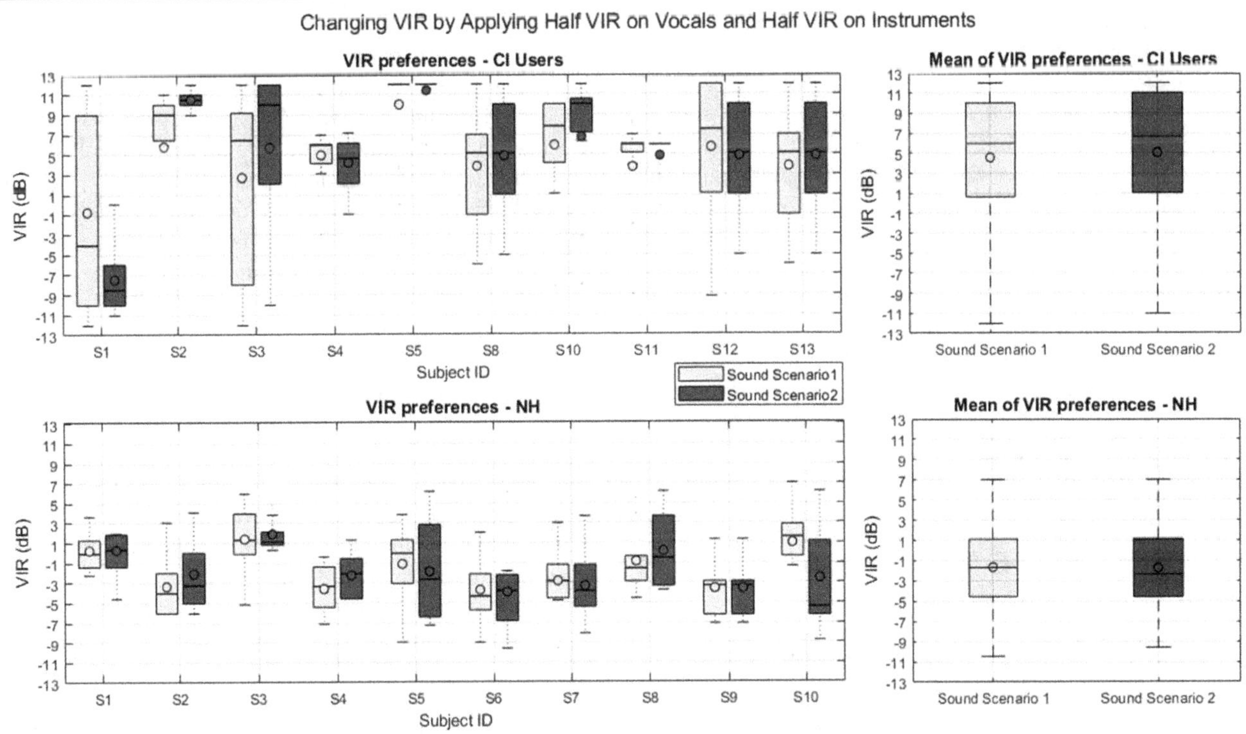

FIGURE 5 | VIR values from part two of experiment 1: Changing VIR by Applying Half VIR on Vocals and Half VIR on Instruments. **(Top left)** VIR preferences of CI users, **(Top right)** mean VIR of CI users, **(Bottom left)** VIR preferences of NH subjects, **(Bottom right)** mean VIR of NH subjects.

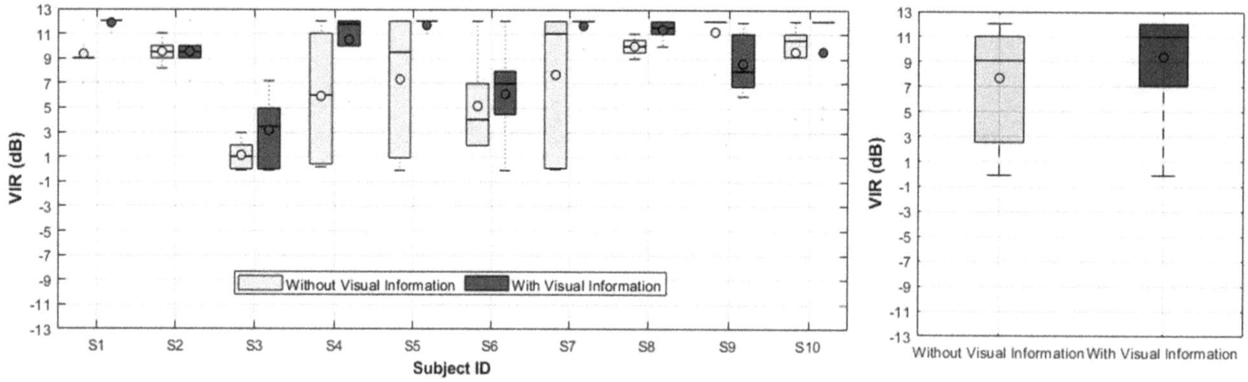

FIGURE 6 | (Left) VIR values from 10 CI users in Experiment 2. **(Right)** Mean VIR across subjects and music tracks for Experiment 2.

listeners (bottom panel) for two virtual sound scenarios. Note that for CI users S1, S6, and S7 no box-plot could be created as they adjusted the VIR in more than 75 % of the cases to the same value. In the second part of experiment 1 subject S5 with around 11 dB and subject S1 with −4 dB had the highest and lowest mean VIR preferences. Subject S1 was the only CI user with a negative mean VIR preferences in all experiments.

For this part of the experiment, where the VIR was set by altering the singing voice and the background instruments level simultaneously in opposite directions. The CI group showed also a preference for positive VIRs for the first ($Mean = 4.6$ dB, $SD = 2.7$ dB, $p < 0.001$) and second sound scenarios ($Mean = 5.3$ dB, $SD = 5.1$ dB, $p = 0.0093$). The NH group, again, did not show any evidence of preferring a balance different from the original mix (VIR = 0 dB) for the first sound scenario ($Mean = -1.6$ dB, $SD = 2$ dB, $p = 0.0194$) nor for the second sound scenario ($Mean = -1.7$ dB, $SD = 1.9$ dB, $p = 0.0194$). For this part of the experiment, again, non of the tested groups' preferred VIR depended on the sound scenario ($p = 0.024$ for the CI users and $p = 0.027$ for the NH group).

To conclude the statistical analysis for this first experiment, a final t-test analysis was performed to assess if the measured VIRs depended on the VIR adjustment method (i.e., balancing the vocals alone or adjusting both signals in opposite directions), two-tailed t-tests were performed comparing the VIRs measured between the VIR adjustment methods for each group. The t-tests revealed that the measured VIRs did not depend on the VIR adjustment method for none of the tested groups $p < 0.001$.

3.3. Experiment 2: Effect of Visual Information on VIR Preferences

The individual VIR preferences set by the CI group in the second experiment are presented in **Figure 6** (left). **Figure 6** (right) shows the mean VIR across subjects and music excerpts for both conditions. The line and the circle in the boxes represent the median and the mean, respectively. As shown in **Figure 6**, the individual results for the condition without visual information show a larger variance in comparison to the condition with visual information. Similarly to experiment 1 the results from subjects S1, S5, S7, S9, and S10 in some specific sound scenarios are collapsed into a line due to very small variance in their responses.

The results of both conditions (i.e., with and without visual information) were statistically significant with respect to the original mix (VIR = 0 dB), as revealed by a two-tailed t-test ($p < 0.005$). When comparing the mean VIR between both conditions, however, no significant differences were found ($p = 0.024$).

4. DISCUSSION

In this work, a real-time source separation algorithm based on a DNN has been designed to enhance the singing voice in pop western music for CI users. The real-time implementation allowed the investigation of remixing music for CI users under realistic acoustic environments and with the presence of additional visual information. Moreover, for the first time, the subjects were able to modify the amount of vocal enhancement online in contrast to previous studies that only used pre-processed sounds. The results of the current study confirm that CI users prefer the vocals enhanced with respect to the instruments even if the music contains reverberation and visual information is available.

The proposed algorithm to remix music for CI users is based on an MLP with an input layer with 513 × 3 units, one hidden layer and an output layer with dimension 1,026. Based on the proposed benchmark by Gajęcki and Nogueira (2018), CI users should not be able to notice the degradation in sound quality caused by the source separation algorithm when the SDR and SAR are larger 0.69 and 4.42 dB, respectively. The proposed algorithm obtained an SDR of 8 dB using the iKala test data set and an SDR of 5.5 and 3 dB for the MUSDB and the Buyens data sets, respectively. Moreover, the source separation algorithm could be implemented in the front end of a sound coding strategy as its algorithmic latency is determined by the hop size of the used STFT. In our implementation, we used a hop size equal to 25% of the STFT's window length resulting in 6 ms algorithmic latency. The algorithm was implemented in MATLAB and run at 44,100 Hz sample rate in a 64 bit Windows 10 PC with an Intel (Santa Clara, California, USA) Core i7 4.3 GHz CPU and 16 GB RAM resulting in a computation time of 2 ms for each audio frame, well below the algorithmic latency to ensure real time processing. Hay-McCutcheon et al. (2009) measured and reported the minimum noticeable audiovisual asynchrony for CI users. The outcomes of that research revealed that CI users were insensitive to an asynchrony of up to 200 ms when the video was leading the audio. Considering that result and the latency caused by our system (around 100 ms), we assume that the audiovisual asynchrony of our system was not noticeable for the tested CI subjects. Moreover, it is worth mentioning that during listening experiments, none of the subjects expressed any reaction regarding the audiovisual asynchrony caused by the latency.

Ten bilateral CI users participated in two perceptual experiments. The first experiment showed that even if reverberation is added to the music scene, CI users prefer the vocals enhanced with respect to the background instruments. Two methods were used to alter the VIR, in the first method the instruments were kept constant while the singing voice was modified. Under this condition, CI users set the VIR to 8.2 and 8.5 dB for a low and a high reverberant room, respectively. Note that, as one of the subjects (S7) had bilateral residual hearing in the low frequencies, earplugs were used to attenuate the sounds transmitted through his/her acoustic hearing. Still, the attenuation was probably not enough to completely attenuate the low-frequency acoustic sounds causing the subject to set the VIR to high values to be able to perceive the voice enhancement more clearly.

In this same condition, NH listeners set the VIR to −2 and −1.7 dB for the low and the high reverberant room, respectively. The main limitation of this method to alter the VIR is that the presentation level increased with increasing VIR and therefore, presentation level was a confounding factor. For this reason, the experiment was repeated modifying the VIR by altering the singing voice and the background instruments level simultaneously but in opposite directions to keep the music presentation level constant. In this second condition, CI users preferred a VIR of 5.3 and 4.6 dB in the low and the high reverberant sound scenario, respectively. In contrast, NH listeners did not prefer the vocals to be enhanced. Previous studies (Buyens et al., 2014; Pons et al., 2016) showed that CI users find music more enjoyable when the vocals are enhanced by 6 dB on average. The larger vocal enhancement observed in the current study may be explained by the introduced reverberation which causes more difficulties in perceiving the singing voice and in turn results in CI users requiring an even further enhancement of the singing voice.

In the second experiment, the impact of visual information was examined by comparing the VIR preferences of CI users with and without using VR headset. The results of the experiment show no significant difference between the measured VIR with and without visual information. These results indicate that the use of source separation to remix music in CI listeners to enhance the singing voice may be applicable also for music listening in live concerts, performances, theaters, religious ceremonies or any other social event related to music that contains visual information.

It is important to mention that each subject had distinct VIR preferences and that the preferred VIR even varied from music track to music track. These results indicate that each CI recipient needs a subject-specific remixed music track for a better music appreciation. For this reason, it is important to expose the VIR parameter of the source separation algorithm such that the CI listener can adjust it to its own needs. Here one can foresee that the wireless communication to smartphones or the use of remote controls with such a parameter exposed could be very beneficial to make music more accessible for CI users (Nogueira et al., 2019).

5. CONCLUSION

This work introduced a real-time music source separation algorithm using a multilayer perceptron (MLP) to separate the singing voice from the background elements in music for CI users in realistic sound scenarios. Objective results show that the implemented neural network fulfills the benchmark reported by Gajęcki and Nogueira (2018) and therefore, we assume that the degradation caused by this algorithm is not noticeable by CI recipients. Results from the experimental measures in CI users show that neither the presence of visual information nor different sound scenarios have an impact on VIR adjustment by CI recipients. Our experiments confirm that CI recipients find music more enjoyable when the vocals are enhanced with respect to the instruments and that this can be achieved by real-time audio source separation based on a neural network.

ETHICS STATEMENT

The studies involving human participants were reviewed and approved by the Medical University Hannover Institutional Review Board. The patients/participants provided their written informed consent to participate in this study.

AUTHOR CONTRIBUTIONS

ST contributed with the study design, measurements, algorithm design, implementation, and writing the manuscript. TG contributed in the algorithm development, study design, and writing the manuscript. WN contributed with the project and study design, algorithm development, and writing the manuscript.

ACKNOWLEDGMENTS

Special thanks to all CI users from the German Hearing Center (DHZ) of the Medical University of Hannover (MHH) and also to the NH subjects that volunteered to participate in the extensive experiments. The authors would also to thank Wim Buyens for sharing the audio excerpts and Giso Grimm for developing TASCAR library used for this work.

REFERENCES

Buyens, W., van Dijk, B., Moonen, M., and Wouters, J. (2014). Music mixing preferences of cochlear implant recipients: a pilot study. *Int. J. Audiol.* 53, 294–301. doi: 10.3109/14992027.2013.873955

Chan, T.-S., Yeh, T.-C., Fan, Z.-C., Chen, H.-W., Su, L., Yang, Y.-H., et al. (2015). "Vocal activity informed singing voice separation with the ikala dataset," in *Proceedings of the 1998 IEEE International Conference on Acoustics, Speech and Signal Process* (Brisbane, QLD), 718–722. doi: 10.1109/ICASSP.2015.7178063

Gajęcki, T., and Nogueira, W. (2018). Deep learning models to remix music for cochlear implant users. *J. Acoust. Soc. Am.* 143, 3602–3615. doi: 10.1121/1.5042056

Grimm, G., Luberadzka, J., Herzke, T., and Hohmann, V. (2015). Toolbox for acoustic scene creation and rendering (TASCAR): render methods and research applications. *Acta. Acust. United Ac.* 1–10.

Hay-McCutcheon, M., Pisoni, D., and Hunt, K. (2009). Audiovisual asynchrony detection and speech perception in hearing-impaired listeners with cochlear implants: a preliminary analysis. *Int. J. Audiol.* 48, 321–333. doi: 10.1080/14992020802644871

ITU (2008). *Recommendation ITU-T J.248: Requirements for Operational Monitoring of Video-to-Audio Delay in the Distribution of Television Programs.* Geneva: International Telecommunication Union.

Kingma, D., and Ba, J. (2014). "Adam: a method for stochastic optimization," in *International Conference on Learning Representations, 2015* (San Diego, CA).

Landry, S., Bacon, B. A., Leybaert, J., Gagné, J.-P., and Champoux, F. (2012). Audiovisual segregation in cochlear implant users. *PLoS ONE* 7:e33113. doi: 10.1371/journal.pone.0033113

Limb, C., and Roy, A. (2013). Technological, biological, and acoustical constraints to music perception in cochlear implant users. *Hear. Res.* 308, 13–26. doi: 10.1016/j.heares.2013.04.009

Macherey, O., Deeks, J. M., and Carlyon, R. P. (2011). Extending the limits of place and temporal pitch perception in cochlear implant users. *J. Assoc. Res. Otolaryngol.* 12, 233–251. doi: 10.1007/s10162-010-0248-x

McDermott, H. J. (2004). Music perception with cochlear implants: a review. *Trends Amplif.* 8, 49–82. doi: 10.1177/108471380400800203

Nagathil, A., C., Weihs, K. N., and Martin, R. (2017). Spectral complexity reduction of music signals based on frequency-domain reduced-rank approximations: an evaluation with cochlear implant listeners. *J. Acoust. Soc. Am.* 142, 1219–1228. doi: 10.1121/1.5000484

Nogueira, W. (2019). "Evaluation of new music compositions in live concerts by cochlear implant users and normal hearing listeners," in *International Symposium on Computer Music Multidisciplinary Research* (Marseille), 294–305.

Nogueira, W., Nagathil, A., and Martin, R. (2019). Making music more accessible for cochlear implant listeners: recent developments. *IEEE Signal Process. Mag.* 36, 115–127. doi: 10.1109/MSP.2018.2874059

Panchal, G., Ganatra, A., Kosta, Y., and Panchal, D. (2011). Behaviour analysis of multilayer perceptrons with multiple hidden neurons and hidden layers. *Int. J. Comp. Theory Eng.* 3, 332–337. doi: 10.7763/IJCTE.2011.V3.328

Perrott, D. R., Saberi, K., Brown, K., and Strybel, T. Z. (1990). Auditory psychomotor coordination and visual search performance. *Percept. Psychophys.* 48, 214–226. doi: 10.3758/BF03211521

Plant, G. (2015). Musical favors: reintroducing music to adult cochlear implant users. *Cochlear Implants Int.* 16, S5–S12. doi: 10.1179/1467010015Z.000000000271

Pons, J., Janer, J., Rode, T., and Nogueira, W. (2016). Remixing music using source separation algorithms to improve the musical experience of cochlear implant users. *J. Acoust. Soc. Am.* 140, 4338–4349. doi: 10.1121/1.4971424

Ross, L. A., Saint-Amour, D., Leavitt, V. M., Molholm, S., Javitt, D. C., and Foxe, J. J. (2007). Impaired multisensory processing in schizophrenia: Deficits in the visual enhancement of speech comprehension under noisy environmental conditions. *Schizophr. Res.* 97, 173–183. doi: 10.1016/j.schres.2007.08.008

Stone, M. A., and Moore, B. C. J. (2003). Tolerable hearing aid delays. III. Effects on speech production and perception of across-frequency variation in delay. *Ear Hear.* 24, 175–183. doi: 10.1097/01.AUD.0000058106.68049.9C

Vincent, P., Larochelle, H., Lajoie, I., Bengio, Y., and Manzagol, P.-A. (2010). Stacked denoising autoencoders: learning useful representations in a deep network with a local denoising criterion. *J. Mach. Learn. Res.* 11, 3371–3408. doi: 10.5555/1756006.1953039

4

Adult Cochlear Implant Recipients' Perspectives on Experiences with Music in Everyday Life: A Multifaceted and Dynamic Phenomenon

Kate Gfeller[1,2,3], Virginia Driscoll[1,3] and Adam Schwalje[3]*

[1] School of Music, College of Liberal Arts and Sciences, The University of Iowa, Iowa City, IA, United States, [2] Department of Communication Sciences and Disorders, College of Liberal Arts and Sciences, The University of Iowa, Iowa City, IA, United States, [3] Iowa Cochlear Implant Clinical Research Center, Department of Otolaryngology, The University of Iowa Hospitals and Clinics, Iowa City, IA, United States

***Correspondence:**
Kate Gfeller
kay-gfeller@uiowa.edu

Background: Cochlear implants (CIs), which have been designed primarily to support spoken communication of persons with severe to profound hearing loss, are highly effective in supporting speech perception in quiet listening conditions. CI users as a group achieve significantly poorer perception and appraisal of music, and speech perception is compromised when background music is present, though outcomes vary considerably across recipients. A number of factors have been identified that contribute to variable music listening experiences, but many questions remain, particularly regarding experiences in everyday life from the perspective of CI users.

Purpose: The purpose of this study was twofold: The first aim was to explore the perspectives of adult CI recipients regarding two experiences with music in everyday life: purposeful music listening and background music that competes with spoken conversation. The second aim was to develop a framework of everyday music experiences based upon CI perspectives that could inform future rehabilitative practices and research initiatives.

Methods: Qualitative and patient-engaged research methodologies were used to emphasize the perspectives of the CI users. Participants included 40 experienced adult CI users ranging in age from 19 to 81 enrolled in 13 CI centers. Participants completed on-line semi-structured open-ended questionnaires regarding purposeful music listening and background music in conjunction with spoken communication. Responses were analyzed using an iterative inductive coding process consistent with grounded theory methodology. The interrelated themes that emerged from the data were then organized into a model synthesizing components from models on music response and self-management for persons with chronic health conditions.

Outcomes: Data analyses informed the development of a Dynamic Problem Solving Model for Management of Music Listening Environments adapted from Hill-Briggs (2003) Problem Solving Model of Chronic Illness Self-Management. Key findings were: (1) Music listening is a dynamic, multifaceted experience; satisfactory listening depended upon optimal combinations of factors; (2) Music listening is effortful, but the extent of satisfaction is influenced by expectations and self-management of the situation; (3) CI users have limited access to resources for optimizing music experiences. Many CI users would consider rehabilitation, but level of commitment and priorities differ across CI users.

Keywords: cochlear implant, adults, music, problem solving, patient-centered research

INTRODUCTION

Cochlear implants (CIs) are designed primarily to support spoken communication and awareness of environmental sounds. Several decades of research and development to upgrade implant technology have resulted in enhanced speech perception, especially in quiet listening conditions, but many CI users still achieve poor outcomes for speech recognition in noise and for perception of music (Eskridge et al., 2012; Gfeller et al., 2012; Looi et al., 2012; Philips et al., 2012; Limb and Roy, 2014; Drennan et al., 2015; Dritsakis et al., 2017).

Most information regarding music perception and enjoyment by CI recipients has been generated through laboratory studies testing basic perceptual attributes (pitch, melody, timbre, rhythm) (e.g., Drennan et al., 2015 (for reviews, see Looi et al., 2012; Philips et al., 2012; Limb and Roy, 2014) or surveys using closed-ended (fixed response) questions deemed important by researchers (Gfeller et al., 2000; Mirza et al., 2003; Lassaletta et al., 2008; Migirov et al., 2009; Looi and She, 2010; Philips et al., 2012; Drennan et al., 2015). Nearly 30 decades of research indicates while some musical sounds are more accessible than others, CI users as a group have poor perception of pitch and timbre, and time spent listening to music typically declines following implantation (Gfeller and Lansing, 1991, 1992; Pijl, 1995; Fujita and Ito, 1999; Looi et al., 2012; Limb and Roy, 2014; Drennan et al., 2015). Interestingly, perceptual accuracy is not a strong predictor of music appreciation and CI users are variable in music perception and enjoyment (Gfeller et al., 2008; Philips et al., 2012; Wright and Uchanski, 2012; Drennan et al., 2015).

Factors contributing to variability include age, cognitive processing, residual hearing, hearing aid use, and music training (Gfeller et al., 2008, 2010, 2012). The impact of these factors varies as a function of the musical stimuli and response task (e.g., Gfeller et al., 2008, 2010; Fuller et al., 2018).

While accuracy does not typically improve from mere exposure over time (Gfeller et al., 2010), some aspects of perception and appraisal improve in response to focused listening practice or formal training, though outcomes are variable (for review, see Looi et al., 2012; Fuller et al., 2018). Despite potential benefits, music training is not commonly offered in typical clinical practice (Looi and She, 2010; Philips et al., 2012; Dritsakis et al., 2017).

Most studies of music and CIs have focused on purposeful listening. In everyday life, music also functions as background music for ambience or to enhance mood. Several studies indicate that background music has a negative impact on speech perception, but the impact varies depending upon the specific music (Eskridge et al., 2012; Gfeller et al., 2012; Başkent et al., 2014). Music and speech also interact through song lyrics (Collister and Huron, 2008). Hearing device users have particular difficulty understanding song lyrics if the SNR between sung lyrics and background accompaniment is too low (Gfeller et al., 2009; Wilhelm, 2016).

These studies have provided important information regarding basic aspects of music perception of CI users, with particular emphasis on device efficacy and assessment of "endpoint" outcomes in with controlled samples, stimuli, and environments (Pisoni et al., 2017). However, many questions remain concerning CI user variability in music experiences. Furthermore, laboratory testing cannot fully elucidate the challenges that CI recipients face when listening to music in everyday life (Philips et al., 2012; Pisoni et al., 2017).

Understanding the experiences that cochlear implant users face in everyday listening experiences with music is challenging in part because of the inherently complex and dynamic nature of music listening. Consider the following:

(1) Music in real life comprises rapidly changing and seemingly infinite combinations of collative properties of frequency, duration, timbre, and amplitude, resulting in ongoing changes in complexity and organized within different stylistic grammars. The listener's perceptual organization, enjoyment, and symbolic meaning are affected by the extent of their familiarity with particular songs or genre, which is influenced by enculturation and training (Hargreaves and North, 2010). Furthermore, in everyday life, the functions of music vary (e.g., entertainment, part of cultural rituals, for relaxation etc.), as well as response tasks (casual listening, focused attention, etc.) (Sloboda, 2010; Hargreaves and North, 2010). In public settings, listeners often have limited control over which music is played and under what conditions (Sloboda, 2010; Hargreaves and North, 2010). Consequently, CI users are likely to be exposed to music with complex collative properties, including selections or styles that are unfamiliar.

(2) In real life, listening environments for music vary enormously (e.g., outdoor performances, concert halls, bars, personal listening devices, etc.), and the conditions change over time. For example, the number and configuration of other people in the environment, the sound waves within an acoustical space, and competing noise such as traffic or air handling systems will fluctuate over time.

(3) Music is commonly paired with speech through song lyrics or as background to spoken conversations in social settings

(Gfeller et al., 2009, 2012); on-going changes occur in the focus and function of the music (Sloboda, 2010). In some instances, the listener attempts to understand sung lyrics against a background accompaniment (Gfeller et al., 2009; Wilhelm, 2016). Sometimes music is ambient background sound; the listener's primary task is to extract the conversation (Gfeller et al., 2012). Music and conversation may co-occur in a task requiring split attention. For example, at a bar with live music, the listener's attention shifts back and forth between listening to a jazz combo and the voices of their conversation partners.

(4) Listeners differ from one another and over time, not only as a function of auditory profile, but in psychosocial characteristics that impact listening (Hughes et al., 2018). People with hearing loss differ in self-efficacy and cognitive resources available for managing a complex listening environment or auditory signal (Smith and West, 2006; Gregory, 2011; Smith, 2014; Pisoni et al., 2017). Personal capacity for processing sounds will also change as a function of fatigue, age, or familiarity with the stimuli (Gfeller et al., 2008; Hargreaves and North, 2010; Başkent et al., 2014; Pisoni et al., 2017).

In summary, music experiences in everyday life are multifaceted and dynamic and thus challenging to represent in highly controlled experiments. To date, few studies with CI users have examined real-life situations involving music or addressed CI users' perspectives and priorities for managing or improving music experiences (Looi and She, 2010; Plant et al., 2015).

While no singular research approach can fully address the complexities associated with real-life music experiences of CI recipients, some research methods are associated with *greater* emphasis on experiences as perceived by the target population. Two such approaches are patient-centered and qualitative research methodologies. Patient-centered research methodology seeks meaningful input from patients and other stakeholders (e.g., family members, advocates) throughout the research process (Clancy and Collins, 2010; Hickam et al., 2013; Brodt et al., 2015; Forsythe et al., 2017). Stakeholder input has been attributed with greater likelihood that the research questions and interpretation will reflect the perspectives and priorities of the target population, and that the methods will facilitate strong rates of enrollment, retention, and protocol compliance (Domecq et al., 2014; Frank et al., 2014; Sheridan et al., 2017).

The use of qualitative research in health care has risen markedly over the past 25 years (Bradley et al., 2007; Mather et al., 2018). Qualitative research can help reveal patients' own experiences of illness and health care, as opposed to categories pre-determined by researchers, and can highlight previously unidentified issues worthy of future hypothesis testing. Qualitative research is particularly suitable for questions related to natural settings, such as coping with health problems in everyday life, thus complementing research questions better suited toward controlled experiments (Bradley et al., 2007; Creswell, 2014; Mather et al., 2018).

While there is no singularly appropriate way to conduct qualitative research, it has several hallmark characteristics. Questions are examined primarily through words rather than numbers. The data are reported in narratives, with liberal reporting of the participants' own words; the researcher attempts to remain open to the participants' perspectives (Savenye and Robinson, 1996; Bradley et al., 2007; Creswell, 2014). Qualitative research questions tend to be broad and exploratory in nature in order to encourage participants to share their experiences within the context of their daily lives and communities (Creswell, 2014). Rather than starting with a theory and an *a priori* hypothesis, qualitative researchers generate or inductively develop theory or pattern of meaning from the views of the participants.

The general process for analysis involves coding the data into categories and themes, and interpreting themes for relationships and core concepts. These are examined in relation to existing theories and literature. The researcher's own experiences and background will shape their interpretation of finding, consequently, the authors reveal in the document prior experiences that may influence their interpretations; the use of first-person voice in describing the research process is common (Strauss and Corbin, 1994; Savenye and Robinson, 1996; Bradley et al., 2007; Creswell, 2014).

In-person or phone interviews, focus groups, and semi-structured questionnaires are often utilized in qualitative research to obtain rich narratives from participants (Savenye and Robinson, 1996; Creswell, 2014; Mather et al., 2018). However, in-person interviews or focus groups can raise challenges in gathering information from a geographically diverse sample. In addition, interviews can be challenging when conducting research with people with significant hearing loss. The propensity for misunderstandings due to competing noise, accents, or speech impediments, among other issues, can undermine clear communication and interact with the accuracy of their responses (Tates et al., 2009). Online questionnaires comprising open-ended items are reasonable alternatives for gathering interview data, particularly when seeking input from a geographically diverse population (Creswell, 2014).

Several recent studies have used qualitative methods to better understand the real-life experiences of cochlear implant users. Hughes et al. (2018) utilized a grounded theory analysis to explore listening effort in everyday spoken communication before and after implantation (Hearing aid use vs. CI use). Participants included 15 adult HA/CI users and two caregivers (ages 42–84). The participants responded to open-ended questions regarding listening effort. The conversations were transcribed, and units of meaning were coded and analyzed for themes. The analyses described the mental energy required to attend to and process spoken communication, and adaptation and compensatory strategies required to maintain control over their listening environment.

The analyses revealed that the CI improved the auditory signal enough to enable more successful communication. Using a CI moderated, but *did not remove* the requirements for listening effort. Listening effort, fatigue, and stress were problems with both HA and CI use, particularly in multi-speaker conversations. The degree of effort varied depending upon the level of background noise, information complexity, and speaker characteristics. CI users were more likely to "accept" the fatigue and effort required if the listening task helped them to maintain social connectedness. The authors reported that qualitative methods provided a more holistic and nuanced conceptualization of effortful listening in everyday life, and highlighted the importance of social connectedness as a motivation for sustained effort.

In some instances, qualitative research is used to better understand outcomes from prior experimental studies or standardized tests. Harris et al. (2016) used qualitative methods to better understand the highly variable patterns of rehabilitation strategies initiated by adult CI users in real life. A diverse group of 23 adult CI users completed open-ended questionnaire items and interviews; the data were analyzed using thematic content analysis. The analyses revealed that personal motivation and social support were critical to self-initiated rehabilitation, and emphasized the importance of the CI users' attitudes and behaviors in optimizing CI benefit beyond basic device maintenance and mapping. Very few audiologists had offered information about or resources for rehabilitation.

Though not related specifically to music enjoyment, these studies (Harris et al., 2016; Hughes et al., 2018) present examples of qualitative research that focus on everyday listening experiences of CI recipients, emphasizing psychosocial factors and enhanced outcomes in real life. They also illustrate various methodological approaches suitable for examining everyday experiences and perspectives of CI recipients.

Focusing more specifically on the music experiences of CI users, Bartel et al. (2011) conducted qualitative case studies of 5 cochlear implant recipients from in their clinic who self-reported music as a major issue following cochlear implantation. Data were gathered through individual semi-structured interviews comprising questions about musical background, experiences with music prior to hearing loss (e.g., social life, profession etc.), and post-implant music appreciation. Grounded theory was used for data analyses. All participants considered music an important part of their lives prior to deafness; all experienced sub-optimal music appreciation after implantation—especially decreased sound quality and enjoyment. The five participants reported a wide range of satisfaction with music post-implantation and emphasized the need for careful listening. Participants expressed hope that rehabilitation might improve music experiences, but the study did not include questions about improving music listening.

Dritsakis et al.'s (2017) qualitative study also focused on music listening and CI users, but concentrated on the relationship between music and quality of life. The researchers enrolled 30 adult CI users between ages 18 and 81 representing a wide range of patient characteristics and musical background. As part of six focus group discussions, participants were asked broad, open-ended questions about music and quality of life. The transcribed conversations were analyzed using a deductive approach called template analysis. Pre-determined coding categories of physical, psychological, and social well-being based upon the Quality of Life Model of the World Healthcare Organization were used in the analyses.

Participants reported that music contributed to quality of life by influencing positive emotions, relaxation, reminiscence, and reduced isolation similar to experiences reported in research about persons with normal hearing. However, the participants also described unpleasant feelings and limited participation in music-related and routine activities because of difficulties with music perception and enjoyment. Background music with conversation required additional concentration and effort, and hindered social opportunities. The authors concluded that quality of life could be enhanced by improved music experiences, and recommended greater access to music rehabilitation. While this study emphasized positive and negative aspects of music listening and quality of life, strategies for, or barriers to optimizing music experiences were beyond the scope of the paper.

In summary, nearly 30 years of research indicates that adult CI users as a group have impaired perception and appraisal of music, though CI users are highly variable on many measures. Most research outcomes to date reflect endpoint outcomes in relation to device or user characteristics as examined in highly controlled studies.

These studies are essential to our understanding of CI benefit and the development of future technology. However, many questions remain regarding the real life music experiences of CI recipients, and those factors that contribute to positive vs. negative experiences with music. Few studies have focused on the psychosocial factors that influence music listening. Are there individual listener attitudes or behaviors that improve or undermine music listening, or that buffer disappointing outcomes? Do CI users have concerns that have been inadvertently overlooked in prior research? This study was initiated with hopes that the experiences and perspectives of CI users would offer fresh perspectives on those factors that support or undermine music experiences in everyday life.

The purpose of this study was twofold: The first aim was to explore the perspectives of adult CI recipients on two experiences with music in everyday life: purposeful music listening and background music that competes with spoken conversation in social settings. The second aim was to develop a conceptual framework based upon the perspectives of CI users that could inform rehabilitation practices and future research initiatives.

MATERIALS AND METHODS

Approach

Because the purpose of this study was to better understand the perspective of adult cochlear implant users in everyday life, we chose two methodological approaches that would emphasize the viewpoints of the CI users themselves in naturalistic settings: patient-centered and qualitative research methods. Patient-centered research methodology seeks meaningful input from patients and other stakeholders in all phases of research (Hickam et al., 2013), which can result in findings that more fully reflect the perspectives and priorities of the target population (Domecq et al., 2014; Sheridan et al., 2017).

Stakeholder input was gathered in the initial development of our study, including one of the co-authors (A. Schwalje) who has a hearing loss, several CI users and family members affiliated with our center, and representatives of advocacy groups (State of

Iowa Department of Disabilities, Association of Adult Musicians with Hearing Loss, University of Iowa Office for Student with Disabilities). Their input informed the development of research questions, questionnaire items, protocol, and data analyses.

Consistent with qualitative methodology, the research questions were broad, oriented toward the participants' perspectives, and focused on naturalistic phenomena. Data were gathered through open-ended questionnaires, and data analysis comprised an iterative inductive process through which the data from the questionnaires revealed themes and core concepts.

In keeping with qualitative research methodology, we provide the context regarding the experiences of the authors that could influence their perspectives. The authors all had postgraduate training and professional experience as musicians. All three authors had professional experience testing or treating CI patients, and had engaged in on-going conversations with CI users regarding music and their CIs. The third author, who was a professional musician prior to becoming a physician, has a moderate progressive hearing loss and uses hearing aids.

Additional qualitative approaches associated with various portions of the inquiry will be described throughout the paper.

Participants

Qualitative research utilizes purposive sampling in which participants are selected who represents particular phenomena relevant to the research questions (Savenye and Robinson, 1996; Creswell, 2014). Cochlear implant users comprise a diverse group with regard to auditory profile, life experiences, and musical experiences. Therefore, enrollment criteria were broad: CI users 19 years or older who have had at least 12 months CI use and who spoke English as a first language. While brand or model of device was initially taken into consideration, aside from the preservation of residual hearing, group data have not revealed particular devices or strategies as clearly superior for music perception (Gfeller et al., 2008; Looi et al., 2012). Thus, device type was not specified in enrollment criteria.

The University of Iowa Human Subjects Review Board approved enrollment procedures. Participants were identified through the Iowa Cochlear Implant Clinical Research Center's CI Registry and through announcements posted on websites for CI recipients. Invitations including informed consent procedures were sent out to those who met criteria.

To ensure a diverse sample with regard to music perception and involvement, we examined the Iowa CI Registry database to ascertain distributions of pitch ranking tests (Pitch Discrimination Test, Gfeller et al., 2002) and a questionnaire of music background and involvement (Iowa Music Questionnaire, Gfeller et al., 2000). This perusal revealed a wide distribution of results on both measures, thus increasing the likelihood of enrolling a diverse sample with regard to music perception and enjoyment.

Invitations to CI users outside the center were posted on listservs and web postings including the following: Hearing Loss Association of the Americas (HLAA), the Association of Adult Musicians with Hearing Loss (AAMHL), or through word of mouth (e.g., informed by their audiologist). Those individuals interested contacted the center to participate. Each participant provided their consent in response to a letter of consent, and was then sent a link to the questionnaire.

Forty adults consented to participate, including 28 patients from the Iowa Cochlear Implant Research Center and 12 from other CI centers. This sample size was greater than enrollments recommended in textbooks about grounded theory analysis (20–30 being considered adequate, Creswell, 2014). The age range was 19–81 years at time of testing. Participants used the following devices: traditional long electrode devices (LE) (n = 22), hybrid (A + E) (n = 12), and single sided deafness (SSD, deaf ear stimulated by CI, normal hearing on the contralateral side) (n = 6). This provided a continuum of participants with regard to residual hearing, an important factor in music perception. The sample also included individuals with different onset of hearing loss and age at implantation. Twenty-eight had lost hearing well into adulthood; 12 had pre- or perilingual deafness and had reached adulthood by the time of this study. The average length of CI use was 12.25 years, ranging from 2.44 to 28.07 years.

While qualitative research does not conduct hypothesis testing of independent variables, themes that emerge from the data can reveal trends of subgroups within the population. Therefore, we examined different coding patterns from the subgroups (pre- vs. postlingual deafness, LE, hybrid, SSD) in later iterations the analyses.

The Semi-Structured Questionnaire

Cochlear implant recipients' perspectives were gathered through an on-line questionnaire. Open-ended questions were used to encourage participants to share rich and detailed thoughts, attitudes, and experiences, as opposed to responding to closed-ended (limited set) researcher-derived categories of response. A semi-structured approach, common in qualitative studies in health care, was used to encourage thorough responses closely related to the main research question (Creswell, 2014; Mather et al., 2018).

Initial questions for the online questionnaire were created by the authors. CI recipients, audiologists, and persons from advocacy groups examined drafts of the interview questions; their feedback was used to identify omissions and for input on recruitment, enrollment, and protocol implementation.

The questionnaire items reflected the primary research aims of the study, and included the following subtopics: (1) music enjoyment/experiences before hearing loss and after implantation; (2) speech and background music; (3) technology and music or music and speech; (4) music through CIs; (5) listening environments; (6) accommodations and strategies; (7) rehabilitation tools; (8) informational resources and counseling; and (9) aspirations for improved CI benefit with music. Closed-ended items were included to gather demographic information on the hearing profile, musical background, age, length of use, and type of implants used. The instructions and open-ended questions presented appear in **Supplementary Appendix A**.

Protocol

An online questionnaire was chosen for several reasons: (1) It facilitated enrollment of individuals from multiple centers, thus representing a variety of clinical experiences; (2) Individual responded without influence of the opinions of others (which arguably can be advantageous, such as focus groups); (3) An on-line response mode reduced the possible impact of auditory deficits that might interfere with in-person group conversations; (4) Online response were downloaded directly into a database, thus avoiding possible errors in transcription or note taking. Prior research also indicates that outcomes from on-line inquiries are similar to or even superior to outcomes from in-person focus groups (Tates et al., 2009).

After informed consent was obtained, participants were contacted by e-mail with a password-protected link to a website using a Qualtrics^{XM} questionnaire platform. Participants were given 4 weeks to complete the on-line questionnaire. Each participant was paid $20 per hour for up to 2 h of time spent in completing their responses.

Each individual's responses were automatically downloaded from the Qualtrics^{XM} platform into a protected database and stored using an alphanumeric ID. Each respondent's information formed a unit of analysis. Questionnaire responses were copied to word documents and assigned a respondent code to prevent any bias toward familiarity with respondents or their device configuration.

Analysis of Interview Data

The method for analysis was grounded theory (GT). The underlying premise of GT is that any potential theory is grounded in the coded data as opposed being based on *a priori* hypotheses. Consistent with GT, the analysis consisted of an iterative and reflexive process described below (see **Figure 1**).

The interview data were first read carefully multiple times by the authors to get a general sense of the data. In qualitative research, the text is dense and rich, and not all information can be included. Thus, researchers aggregate data into a small number of themes (Savenye and Robinson, 1996; Creswell, 2014). Proceeding line-by-line, the first two authors used open coding to break the data into meaningful units at the word, phrase, or sentence level. Each participant's responses were analyzed independent of the individual questions because responses may apply to multiple questions.

Each unit of meaning was assigned a conceptual label or code to define meaning, actions, and to facilitate exploration of relationships between codes. Codes may include expected concepts from past literature as well as codes not anticipated (Savenye and Robinson, 1996; Bradley et al., 2007; Creswell, 2014). Responses that fit under multiple codes were included under each relevant code.

The first two authors completed a second round of coding (focused coding) to group similar concepts; those codes were once again grouped into more abstract, high level categories which are referred to as themes (Bradley et al., 2007). For example, codes of pitch, complexity, and timbre were grouped under a higher-level category of "structural components of music." Codes such as "structural components of music" and "environment" could be grouped under themes such as "pleasant" or "unpleasant." In some instances, a code fit under more than one theme. For example, the code, "loudness" was not only a structural feature of music but also related to codes of unpleasant experiences. During the first two rounds of coding, the readers were blinded to participant identity or device subgroup.

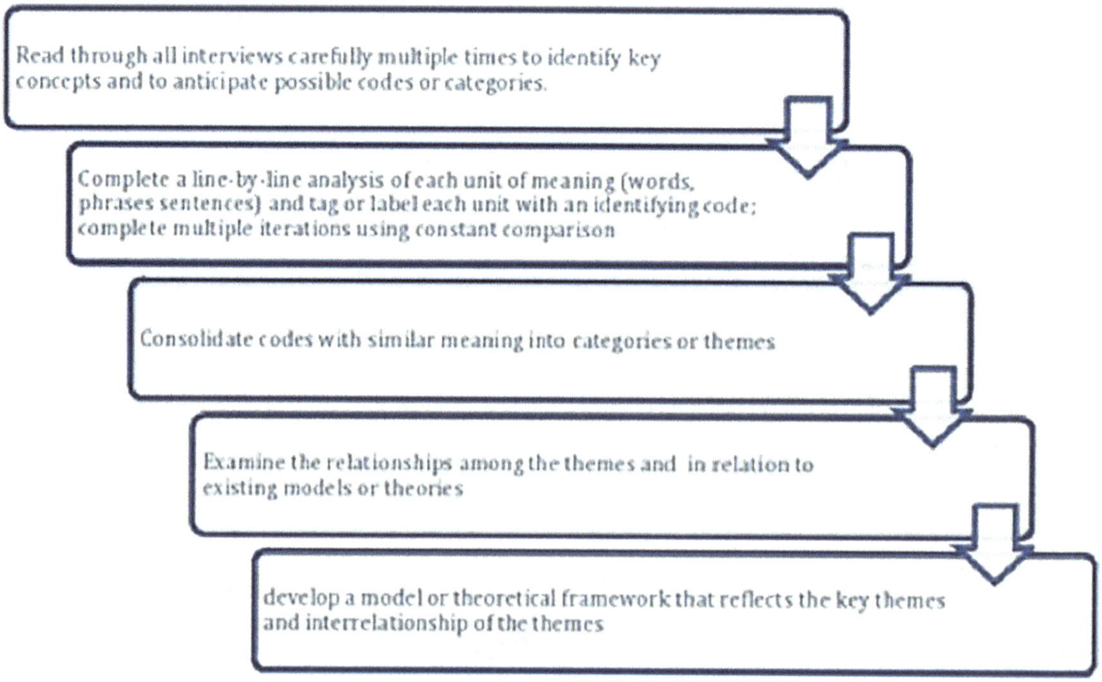

FIGURE 1 | Flowchart of steps in the qualitative analysis.

Although qualitative methods focus primarily on the words, magnitude coding can help determine the most prominent and important themes (Saldaña, 2013). Frequency (i.e., number of occurrences) and extensiveness (number of respondents) of responses were calculated (Attride-Stirling, 2001; Miles et al., 2014) (see **Supplementary Appendix B**). Following the first two rounds of coding, the first two authors examined the data in relation to device subgroups (LE, Hybrid, SSD) for possible trends related to hearing configuration. The most prominent themes and the relationships among themes were conceptualized through core categories or central concepts, which represented the main themes (Creswell, 2014; Hughes et al., 2018).

Consistent with GT methodology, further literature review followed data analysis to support and further develop the theoretical categories originating from the data (Savenye and Robinson, 1996; Creswell, 2014; Hughes et al., 2018). This included models or theories from music psychology, audiology, and health psychology (e.g., self-management of chronic illness).

Verification of coding was established through ongoing discussion between the first two authors regarding the quality and consistency of coding. In addition, an outside reviewer (a research assistant from the lab not involved in this project) analyzed a 20% subset of responses to verify the coding used. Responses from the outside evaluator were highly consistent with the initial analysis; no categories or codes were recommended for addition or deletion and any differences in coding choices were resolved through discussion.

Validation of content was achieved through member checking (Creswell, 2014). This involved sharing a summary of themes from the analysis with the participants, to determine whether the themes reflected their comments. Thirty of the 40 participants responded to the invitation to participate in member checking, and confirmed the themes to be representative of their questionnaire responses.

Consistent with grounded theory methods, the results were reported in narrative description of the primary themes or concepts and dissenting opinions, with liberal use of direct quotes from the participants as exemplars (Creswell, 2014).

RESULTS

Codes and Themes

Across the 40 participants, the 27 open-ended questionnaire items yielded a total of 601 individual responses comprising 1655 lines of typed text, numbering 21,520 words. **Supplementary Appendix B** presents the coding definitions as well as the themes, codes, and sub-codes that resulted from three rounds of inductive coding. This appendix presents the number of and percent of participants represented in each code. While qualitative data relies primarily on narratives to report the results, magnitude coding can assist in identifying the most prominent themes or codes. By examining the prevalence of and relationships among codes and themes, we identified three core categories. Core categories are central concepts that appear frequently, represent main themes, and are related to one another (Creswell, 2014; Hughes et al., 2018). These core categories appear below.

Core Categories

Core Category 1: Music Listening Is a Dynamic, Multifaceted Experience, With Satisfactory Listening Conditional to Optimal Combinations of Factors

Music experiences in everyday life involved dynamic interaction of the CI recipient's auditory profile, the auditory signal (music, music and speech), social context, and the environment. These components changed over time, and were often beyond the control of the listener.

Particular factors (e.g., music, environment, and social context) were not inherently positive or negative, but rather conditional to prevailing circumstances over time as they interacted with the listener's auditory profile. Qualifiers such as "it depends upon," "it varies," "sometimes," "it differs when/if" were commonly found in relation to both positive and negative experiences. For example, under the code of "environment," one participant described a sub-code of "outdoor concerts" as pleasant and conducive to enjoyment. Contextual details revealed that this outdoor concert was held in an open, quiet park and the CI user was seated in optimal proximity to the performers. In contrast, another participant described an outdoor concert as a poor listening environment, noting that the concert venue was in close proximity to noisy traffic, and the social context of the concert was a noisy audience. Codes and themes from the data related to this core category appear in **Figure 2**.

Core Category 2: Music Listening Was Effortful, but the Extent of Satisfaction Was Influenced by Expectations and Self-Management of the Situation

Most participants described music listening as effortful or requiring attention; fatigue, cognitive overload, and emotional frustrations were associated with negative experiences or avoidance behaviors. While many listening conditions were beyond the control of the CI user, participants varied in their response to and success in handling challenging conditions. Experiences in managing music listening comprised several themes, including strategies used to engineer the listening situation (e.g., music, environment, technology), barriers that impeded enjoyment (e.g., environment, lack of resources), and personal characteristics (e.g., attitudes, perseverance, avoidance) that influenced the listeners' responses to evolving circumstances, and attitudes toward those experiences.

Core Category 3: CI Users Have Limited Access to Resources for Optimizing Music Experiences

Most participants had limited awareness of, or access to training programs, assistive listening devices, or other resources for enhancing music experiences. The overwhelming majority (90%) expressed a desire for more resources to improve music experiences. However, participants described excessive cost, lack of access, and time required for training as barriers to rehabilitation. Level of commitment (e.g., willingness to dedicate time and money) and priorities for training content varied across participants.

Together, these core categories indicated that satisfactory outcomes in everyday music experiences were not only a function of the musical sounds, the auditory profile of the listener, and the

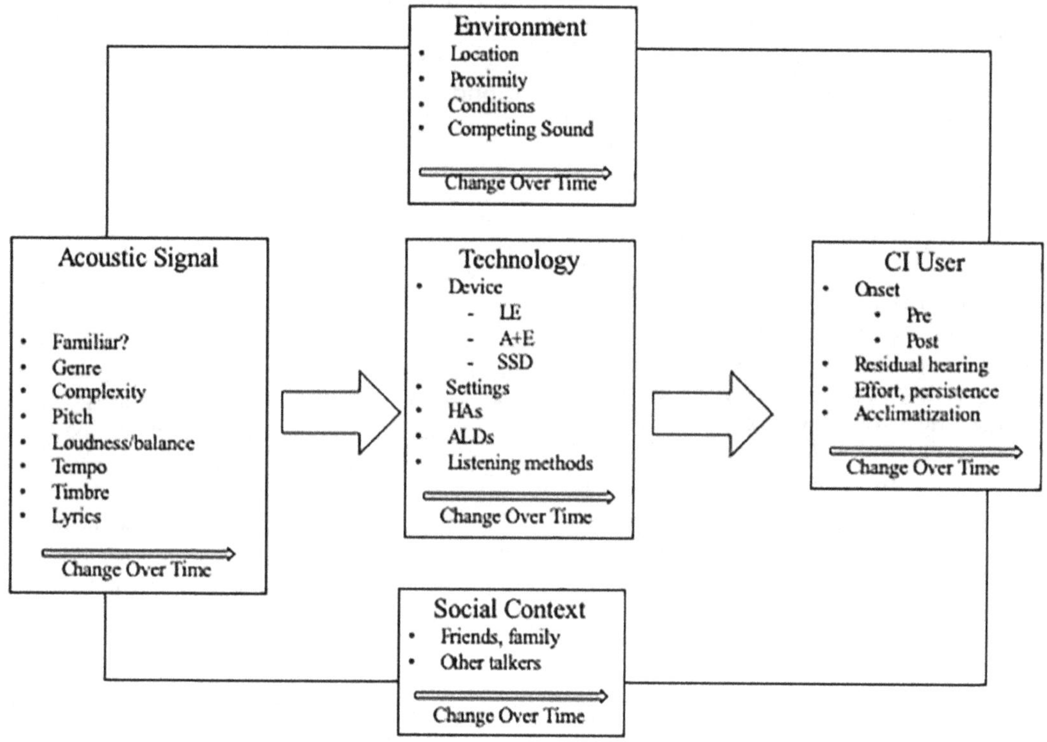

FIGURE 2 | Codes and themes associated with core category 1.

listening environment, but also attitudes and behaviors required for managing or coping with the degraded signal, especially in inhospitable listening environments. Unfortunately, resources to help CI users improve listening enjoyment were not readily available to many of these participants.

In order to address the second aim of this study, we developed a conceptual framework, based upon the CI users' perspectives that could inform future research and rehabilitation.

Generating a Conceptual Framework for Rehabilitative and Research Options

Consistent with grounded theory, we conducted an additional literature review after the initial coding process to examine themes, categories and their interrelationships as they related to existing models and theories. A model from psychology of music, the Reciprocal Feedback Model of Musical Response (RFM-MR) (Hargreaves and North, 2010), conceptualized the reciprocal nature of music, the listening situation, and the listener, resulting in physical, cognitive, and emotional responses to music. The RFM-MR reflected many codes and themes associated with our first core category, but did not address the perceptual limitations imposed by hearing loss or the CI, which severely undermines perception and enjoyment of the collative characteristics of music. The RFM-MR also did not address strategies or resources required to manage difficult listening conditions.

Until medical and technological solutions can more nearly restore "normal" musical sounds, CI recipients seeking more satisfying music listening are left to manage their circumstances by establishing realistic expectations and rehabilitative and compensatory efforts. These can be facilitated by the internal (cognitive and emotional) state of the listener (Krueger and Casey, 2009). The Hill-Briggs Problem Solving Model of Chronic Illness Self-Management reflected many codes and themes associated with core categories 2 and 3 (see **Figure 3**).

Hill-Briggs developed her model to guide disease self-management training and interventions for diabetics, drawing extensively from cognitive psychology, educational research/learning theory, and social problem solving. While diabetes is clearly different from hearing loss in etiology and treatment, both diabetes and hearing loss are chronic conditions that require symptom management in the absence of a cure. Psychological and behavioral factors play a critical role for both populations (Hill-Briggs, 2003; Harris et al., 2016; Young-Hyman et al., 2016; Hughes et al., 2018).

Diabetes can be managed to differing extents by diet, exercise and medication, but compliance with protocols and complete control can be challenging; even individuals who are highly compliant experience medical complications (e.g., loss of vision, nerve pain) and frustration (Hill-Briggs, 2003; Young-Hyman et al., 2016). Furthermore, dietary options associated with social environments and the desire to "fit in" can undermine compliance with nutritional guidelines and exercise. Personal factors such as fatigue or motivation also impact successful management.

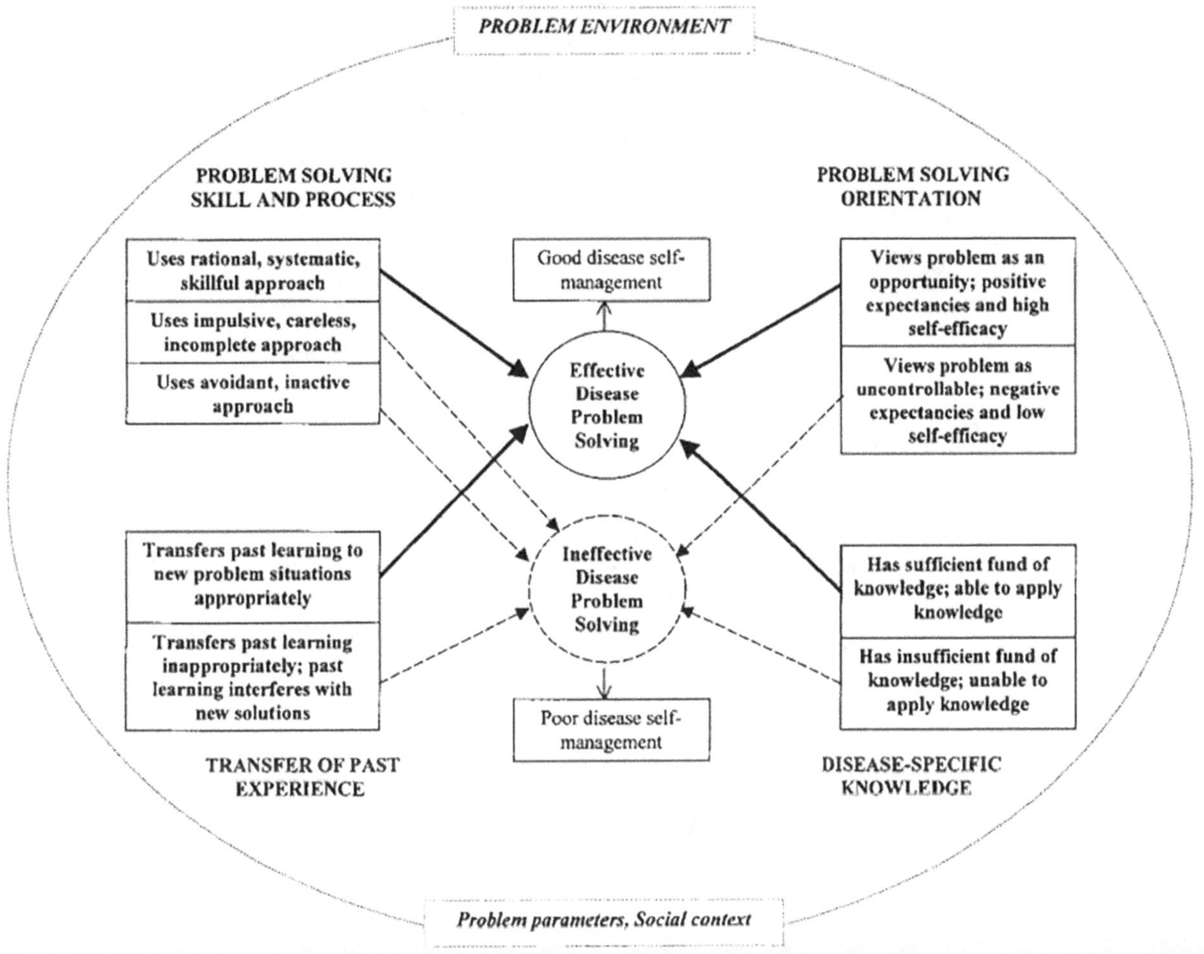

FIGURE 3 | Hill-Briggs (2003) problem solving model of chronic illness self-management.

Cochlear implants provide access to sound, but they do not cure hearing loss or replicate normal hearing. The CI user is responsible for device maintenance and use, compensating for poor auditory input, and negotiating the many noisy environments found in everyday life. CI users may face choices of "smiling and nodding" in noisy and tiring listening conditions, or avoiding those circumstances altogether; avoidance contributes to social isolation, which has implications for quality of life and emotional well-being (Philips et al., 2012; Hughes et al., 2018). Environments with music are particularly problematic because CI technology is not well suited to conveying key structural components of music (for review, see Limb and Roy, 2014). These challenges described for diabetics and CI users respectively, influence the extent to which the individuals, even with cutting edge medical interventions, will thrive and enjoy satisfactory social integration.

Model Development

While the RFM-MR (Hargreaves and North, 2010) focused on music, the listening situation, and the listener, the Hill-Briggs (2003) model focused on cognitive, affective, and behavioral responses to a chronic health condition within a social environment. Examining the emerging themes and core concepts from our data analysis in relation to these two models, we synthesized the relevant components of the two models to conceptualizes the CI users' perception of music in everyday life in a model that we call A Dynamic Problem Solving Model for Management of Music Listening Environments (DPSM-MMLE) (see **Figure 4**).

The outer elliptical components of the model (auditory profile, environment, music and music and speech, and social context) reflect the reciprocal process as conceptualized in the RFM-MR (Hargreaves and North, 2010). The broad category of "Problem Parameters" from the Hill-Briggs model was changed to "Music and Music and Speech," the focus of the research question. Given the diversity among CI users (e.g., age of onset, residual hearing) in relation to music listening, we included a component of "Auditory Profile."

The listener's responses to or handling of the music experiences appear within the ellipses: cognitive, affective and behavioral processes associated with self-efficacy, problem solving and self-management associated with the Hill-Briggs

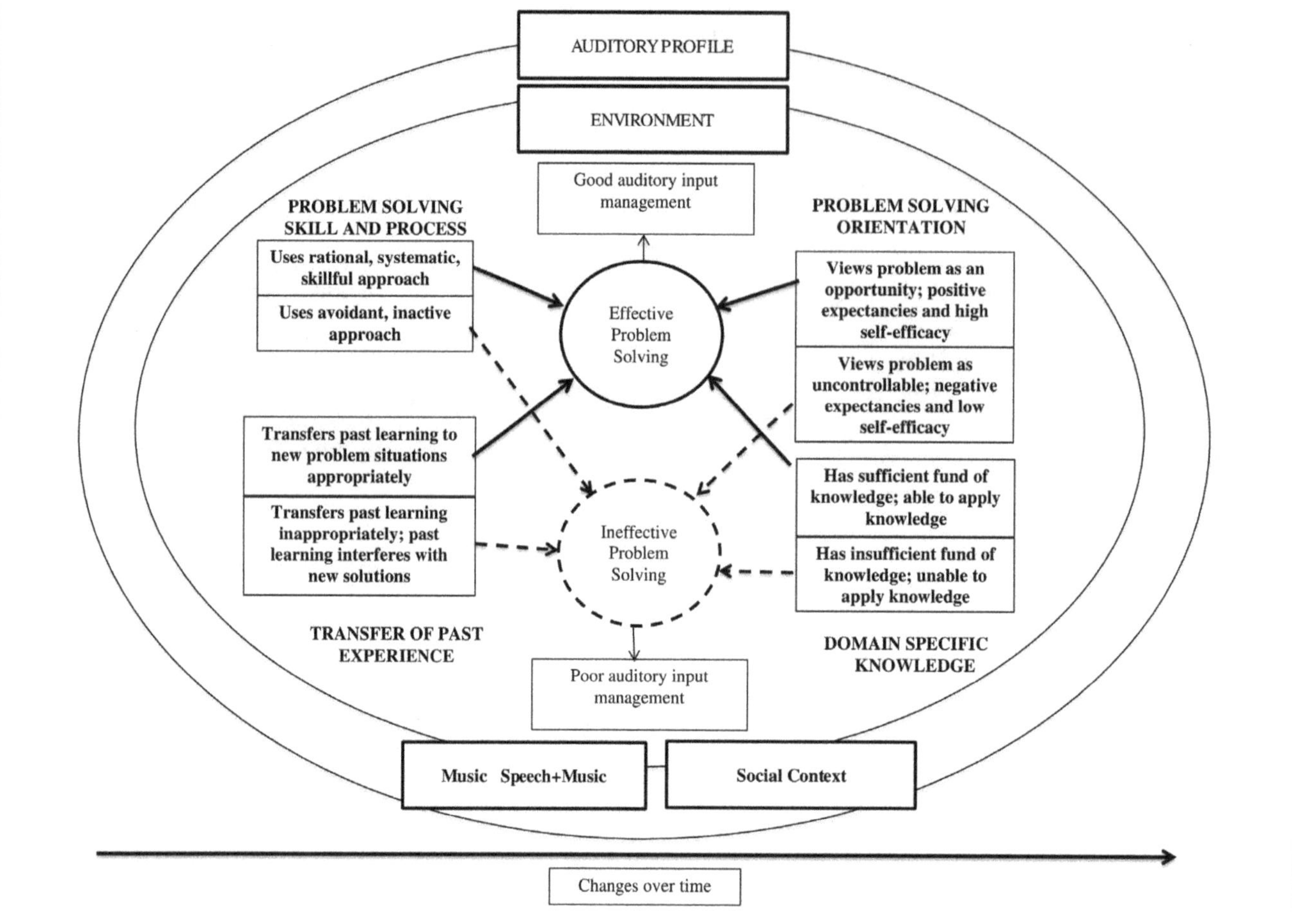

FIGURE 4 | Dynamic problem solving model for management of music listening environments adapted from Hill-Briggs (2003).

model (Hill-Briggs, 2003). In the adapted model, the category of "Disease Specific Knowledge" from Hill-Briggs's model was modified to reflect knowledge of hearing loss and CI technology in relation to music ("Domain Specific Knowledge"). Finally, to emphasize the dynamic and reciprocal nature of music, listening environments, and listener attributes and actions (e.g., neuroplasticity, changing attitudes and behaviors) we added the component of "Changes Over Time."

Consistent with qualitative methods, the following section presents narratives and exemplar quotes describing the core categories, themes and codes as conceptualized within the Dynamic Problem Solving Model (DPSM-MMLE) for Management of Music Listening Environments.

Core Categories and Themes Conceptualized Within the Dynamic Problem Solving Model for Management of Music Listening Environments

Core Category 1: Music listening is a dynamic, multifaceted experience, with satisfactory listening conditional to optimal combinations of factors

Four components of the DPSM-MMLE (outer ellipses) reflecting Core Category 1 were: (1) music and music in speech, (2) environment, (3) auditory profile, and (4) social context. As noted in the introduction, each of these components is dynamic—that is, characterized by change. Furthermore, music listening is multifaceted in that all of these components interact. Music heard in everyday life (as opposed to controlled stimuli in experiments) is inherently dynamic and multifaceted in that it can include from one to as many as hundreds of individual musicians (such as in a large symphony or choral performance) performing together on rapidly changing combinations of pitch, rhythm, timbre and dynamics; these structural elements will continue to change second by second in overall complexity and familiarity to the listener. These musical combinations interact more or less successfully with the processing characteristics of the hearing device(s), and are impacted by the changing room acoustics, concurrent social interactions, and the presenting cognitive processing capabilities of the listener.

As documented in prior studies, CI users typically have impaired perception of some musical features, particularly pitch, melody, and timbre, even when presented as highly controlled individual components. By in large, loud environments are uncomfortable or distorted. These participants responses, while consistent with those findings, offered a more nuanced picture specific to everyday experiences, namely that there is a continuum of positive to negative experience for each of these factors (environment, musical features, auditory profile, social context) contingent upon the specific combination of elements at any given point in time. These factors were to a considerable extent beyond the control of the CI user.

The conditional and multifaceted nature of music listening was illustrated in the following quotes:

> "Experience with music and with the CI varies greatly with factors such as the quality of the speakers and whether I'm familiar with the music. If I'm listening to a song I'm familiar with on Bose speakers in a quiet small room, it is a great experience. If I'm listening to an unfamiliar song on a cell phone, it is an awful experience that requires a lot of effort" (Postlingual LE).

This participant described not only the impact of elements of the music impact but also the importance of manner of listening and the location. Another traditional implant recipient and a hybrid user elaborated on the impact the sound environment can play.

> "I feel like the difficulty of speech and music increases a lot with increasing environmental factors, such as the size of the room/area, or the number of people speaking, or the number of instruments involved. It requires a great deal of effort to enjoy music or understand speech toward the high end of the spectrum of unfavorable environmental factors" (Postlingual LE).

> "It depends on the situation. At the symphony, it is easy to enjoy. In a restaurant or department store, it is difficult to understand the spoken word when music is playing. At a social gathering, music makes it difficult to understand conversation. Music is easy to listen to by itself but mix in conversation and it is difficult to hear either conversation or music" (Hybrid, Postlingual).

This quote illustrates the dynamic interaction of specific musical elements, the CI, and the listener's present energy status. "There are some tones that are clear as a bell and some tones with static-like noise to them. Some days seem better than others. Maybe I get tired?" (Hybrid, Postlingual).

Specific to music characteristics, participants emphasized particular features of music that influenced music listening. The most prominent codes were: (1) prior familiarity with the music "I do not understand any of the words during songs unless I already know the song;" (2) complexity of the music; and (3) loudness: "Fast paced and loud is difficult, where soft and slower are more easily understood. Men's voices are easier to understand than a women's high voice." (LE, Prelingual). Many found familiar music easier to understand, and "new" music difficult or impossible to understand. Participants used mental recall of familiar music along with most accessible structural components to piece together the degraded signal.

> "I was in a toy store and over the speakers they were playing The Mickey Mouse Song. I used to watch the Mickey Mouse Club when I was 5–7 years old and just loved the show. At first I ignored the music but then I recognized the beat and suddenly I realized what the song was. I could hear the lyrics and the memory of that song came flooding back to me. I stood there with my mouth open. That was an awesome moment."

Regarding complexity, 67.5% of participants indicated that music with fewer instruments or voices, or made up of simpler melodies, harmonies or rhythms were easier to perceive and organize. Participants reported, "If there are a lot of instruments playing together, it just sounds like noise" and "The more complex the musical harmonies and music types, the worse it sounded".

Some musical genres were associated with more accessible components. For example, one participant stated, "Country music is best to understand because the background music isn't so loud. You can hear the words better. If I try rap or rock it is hard. I would say it depends more on the song (the level of background music playing)" (LE, Prelingual).

Eighty-five percent of participants described one or more structural features of music as barriers to enjoyment. Nearly half (47.5%) described loud music as a barrier to satisfactory listening, whether as part of purposeful music listening or in combination with speech. Poor balance among components within one piece of music, such as an accompaniment too loud for the vocalist, or melody line was problematic. Only 17.5% specifically mentioned pitch (frequency range, matching a pitch, or recognizing melodies) as a barrier to music enjoyment.

With regard to speech and background music, background music was described in negative terms, particularly when loud in relation to the target conversation partner(s).

> "Depending upon the situation [background] music doesn't have an impact on my conversations with people because it's soft and calming. However, at a bar. . .it's harder to hear in a social conversational setting because . . . they generally have it turned up louder than they need to have it" (LE, Prelingual).

The impact of loud music was repeated across all participants: "Depending on how loud the music is, I do have challenges understanding people in group settings." "It is very difficult to understand and carry on a conversation when music is playing at a restaurant or social gathering."

Environment. Ninety percent of the participants described the environment as a barrier to satisfactory listening. For example, sitting too close to sound speakers could make the sound intolerably loud, or drown out the voice of one's conversation partner. In contrast, being seated too far from a performer could make perception problematic. Problem environments were considered a barrier across all subcategories of CI users (onset, device type).

> "Location of the music makes a big difference in music enjoyment. I have purposefully avoided going to live concerts. If I try to listen to music and there are other conflicting sounds such as machines running or people speaking in the background, then it becomes a waste of time. For me, the best environment would be listening to music on a car radio with the car parked in a parking lot and the windows rolled up with the motor turned off. That's zero interference and I can control the volume and sound on the car radio" (Postlingual LE).

Social context. Music experiences often occur in social circumstances as entertainment, cultural enrichment, or as background ambience (Sloboda, 2010). Thus, social context is an important aspect of music experiences, and can be either negative or positive in nature. The participants commonly described social events as negative experiences due to multiple talkers. Although ambient music in social settings is typically intended to create a pleasant social environment, ambient music can function as a masker to the speech of conversation partners. "It is very difficult to understand and carry on a conversation when music is playing at a restaurant or social environment" (Postlingual LE).

Many participants expressed frustration regarding situations requiring focused attention to both speech *and* music (such as live music at a club), which resulted in unsatisfactory outcomes for both. Participants described undesirable options of either putting up with loud sounds and having to "nod and guess," or avoiding many social situations altogether. Social settings combining music and speech tended to be problematic for all subgroups of the participants, regardless of the differences in residual hearing (LE, SSD, Hybrids).

"Awful! The problem is that virtually all good restaurants are noisy." This was the response from one postlingually deaf LE participant. Another stated, "Bars can be awful. Either too loud to hear people talking or all the people talking makes it so I can't clearly understand the music" (post LE). When trying to participate in situations where background music was present, fatigue was a factor: "I often get exhausted from trying to hear and will just zone out." (Post LE) "Oh boy, carrying on a conversation in a noisy setting is difficult work." (Hybrid LE)

Participants also described the problems associated with background music in the context of film scores for movies or TV: "I can do one or the other... I have never been able to listen to two things at the same time... For TV, I still rely heavily on the CC [closed captioning]."

While the noise that accompanies many social gatherings was problematic, other comments revealed positive aspects of social context. Approximately a quarter of the participants (27.5%) indicated that social support from others in one's group helped CI users to cope with difficult listening situations. As one participant with single sided deafness stated, "I've trained my friends to sit on my good ear side so I can hear them talk and also hear music." Another participant shared, "If I'm in a social situation at someone's home, I may ask them to turn off the music as it interferes with my ability to understand speech" (Postlingual LE).

More than a third (37.5%) of the participants discussed the benefits of information shared among CI users, such as information on assistive listening devices (ALDs), strategies, and resources. A hybrid user reported, "I have 3 uncles who got the cochlear implant prior to myself, and I spent several hours discussing the ins and outs of the device with them, therefore they have been my primary resource." Another participant with pre-lingual deafness stated, "It was always interesting in HLAA groups to hear about other deaf/hard of hearing individuals' experiences in complex listening environments and what they did or did not do to fix the problem."

Auditory profile. Trends across the subgroups (LE-Pre or postlingual, Hybrid, SSD) indicated that the listener's auditory profile and hearing devices had an important impact on music listening, depending upon the particular musical features presented. However, participants within all device configuration groups described music listening as effortful, particularly if the music components were complex or the listening environment was noisy. Postlingually deaf individuals often mentioned the use of top-down processing to make sense of degraded input, while prelingually deaf individuals tended to describe music as more enjoyable than the other subgroups; they seemed more satisfied with what they could access through their CIs.

Residual hearing. Persons with SSD and hybrid devices had greater residual hearing, which had a synergistic impact on electric hearing. While very few comments included specific reference to pitch, melody, harmony, or timbre, persons with more residual hearing (e.g., SSD or Hybrid users) tended to find greater enjoyment in pitch-based components of music.

Device configuration. Most differences in perceptual accuracy or enjoyment were associated with residual hearing or onset of hearing loss, rather than technical choices. Very few participants offered comments regarding the CI brand or signal processing scheme, though a few did report device-related enhancements, such as this prelingually deaf LE user: "I could not imagine life without music. Since getting the Nucleus 6, I notice an improvement in hearing the word/lyrics in the songs such as country music. Very enjoyable."

More common were general comments regarding the limitations of CI, signal processing, or ALDs. "I have found that programming for music is lacking (Postlingual LE). "The quality I have now [with my CI] does not make music sound rich and full." (Postlingual LE) "I have tried to have a music program placed onto my processors. To be honest, the software used to program these must be very bad" (Postlingual LE). "I have never liked any of the automatic programs... I have tried these devices with CD players and get either a buzz, too soft as well as distortion" (Postlingual LE).

Participants described Roger Pens (small wireless microphones that looks like a pen) and other mini mics most frequently as helpful ALDs. A small proportion used hearing aids in conjunction with their CIs; those using hearing aids generally described them as helpful. However, described enhancements of technology were often conditional to specific kinds of music or listening situations.

Changes over time. As prior research indicates, music perception and enjoyment does not normalize as a result of mere exposure and on-going CI use, however, extended and focused listening time can enhance music listening (Gfeller et al., 2010). As noted earlier, music listening experiences are inherently dynamic, with musical combinations, environmental factors, and the listener's internal state changing over time. Related to this concept, one participant noted that she could function well at the ceremonial part of a wedding, but as soon as the reception begin, the loud music made coping impossible and she was "forced to leave." In addition, changes over time related to the listener's internal capacities. The participants described changes in energy, cognitive or emotional resources, or acclimatization to the device or signal processing that influenced music enjoyment.

One participant described changes in acclimatization to the signal over the course of time:

> "The first 3 months after activation was extremely difficult. As time went on, it became easier. About 9 months it started sounding "normal" again. I was still missing things but my brain adjusted to the new sound and it was becoming enjoyable again rather than effortful. Now at 1.5 year, it is easy and enjoyable probably 90% of the time" (Hybrid, Postlingual).

Another listener, with a traditional device also shared their sentiment.

> "For 3 years I struggled just to get decent sound in this ear [second implant]. But after more and more programming, it slowly improved (not as good as the first [CI] through)...At first, I couldn't tell if I got the correct notes [while playing the piano]...but interestingly I found that once my fingers remembered the fingering, the scales sounded right" (Postlingual, LE).

Looking across themes and codes associated with Core Category 1, a major theme that emerged is that music listening was effortful. As one participant stated, "After implantation, I needed to totally relearn music." This theme emphasizes that technology alone did not facilitate meaningful listening experiences with music; attitudinal and behavioral characteristics of and strategies used by the CI recipient were as important. That is the focus of the following section.

Core Category 2: Music listening was effortful, but extent of satisfaction was influenced by expectations and self-management of the situation

Most participants described music listening as effortful. However, the extent of satisfaction in listening could be mediated by the internal capacity of the CI user to cope successfully or manage the music, environment, social context, or use of ALDs. Considering relationships of strategies (uses of technology, musical choices, social support, and attitude) and the barriers that undermined satisfactory listening, these themes were examined in relation to self-management approaches identified in health psychology (Hill-Briggs, 2003). The following section summarizes themes and codes that reflect the following quadrants within the ellipses of the DPSM-MMLE: domain specific knowledge; transfer of past experience to new situations; problem solving skills, and problem solving orientation. The themes and codes that emerged from the data appear in **Figure 5**.

Domain-specific knowledge. Self-management of challenging circumstances required adequate knowledge of hearing loss and hearing devices as they interacted with music components, as well as resources for optimizing music (e.g., training programs, accommodations). These participants possessed the greatest amount of domain specific knowledge about CIs, hearing aids, lip reading, closed captioning, and ALDs. While 89.47% indicated that they would like to have access to music training, most were unfamiliar with options or unsuccessful in acquiring resources. Problems with access are discussed in greater depth later in this paper (Core Category 3).

Transfer of past learning. The ability to recall and apply past knowledge appropriately to new situations is an important aspect of problem solving (Hill-Briggs, 2003), though transfer is predicated on sufficient knowledge of relevant information. Participants described examples of transfer of knowledge related to hearing loss (e.g., lip reading, closed captioning) as well as music. In some cases, past information was not fully relevant (Hill-Briggs, 2003). For example, some applications of ALDS were unsuccessful, particularly in relation to music listening.

Many relied on closed captioning for TV or movies. A number (32.5%) of participants used lip-reading not only to understand conversation partners in noisy environments, but also to understand song lyrics. For one participant, lip reading paired with technology was useful in live concerts.

> "I enjoy going to concerts, but in order for me to follow along with the lyrics, I have to look at the big screen to see their lips. Overall I enjoy my concert experiences and I will continue to go to more because I enjoy country music because that's the type of music I enjoy best" (LE post).

Knowledge of specific music also helped: "Having as much information as possible about the music being played is a trick of mine. I'll look at the set list ahead of time to know what is coming next" (LE Prelingual).

Problem solving skills and process. The data revealed important differences among the participants with regard to problem solving skills and processes (e.g., avoidance vs. systematic, skillful approaches). Active strategies used for management or coping included: (1) using technological options such as Roger Pens, closed captioning, adjusting the volume/sensitivity, (2) personal effort, including lip reading, assertiveness, effortful/active listening, repeated listening, (3) careful music selection (familiar music, or more accessible genres), and (4) controlling the listening environment (proximity, listening conditions). However, these strategies required initiative, trial and error, effort and a personal orientation toward problem solving, which is discussed later in this paper.

The effectiveness of particular problem solving strategies varied as a function of the hearing history, device characteristics, musical background, and willingness to seek social support. For example, comments regarding using one's memory of music to "piece together" previously familiar music were associated with postlingually deaf participants. "Where there is background music, I ask the people I am with what song is playing and then pull from auditory memory" (LE pre).

Many of the participants used avoidance of problem situations (52.5%) or the sound source (37.5%) as a passive strategy for coping. It was highlighted by these participants, "I don't go out very much because it's very difficult to hear in social settings" (Prelingual LE). "I have purposely avoided going to live concerts because I know I would not enjoy it." Another hybrid recipient reported, "Social situations with music (wedding receptions)—I leave." In regards to movie theaters, one prelingual participant shared, "I purposely do not go to the movie theater because I know I would not enjoy it" (LE, Prelingual).

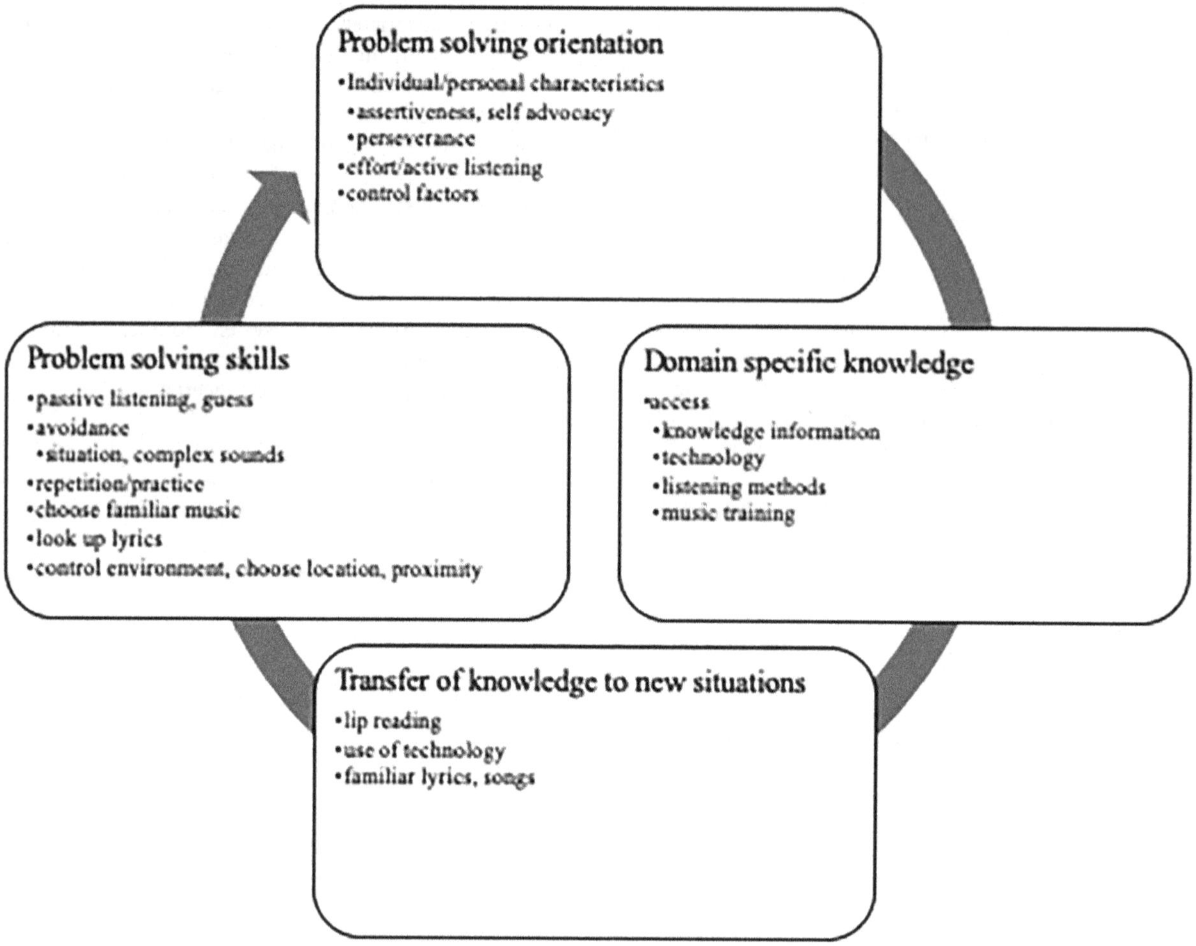

FIGURE 5 | Codes and themes associated with core category 2.

Possessing relevant knowledge does not automatically result in effective transfer or knowledge or effective problem solving (Hill-Briggs, 2003). More positive attitudes toward challenges have been described as problem solving orientation.

Problem solving orientation. Coding revealed that CI users differed considerably with regard to their problem solving orientation. Problem solving orientation in this context referred to a strong sense of self-efficacy, viewing problems as opportunities, and positive expectancies. Comments from 42.5% of the group reflected some level of self-efficacy, that is, confidence in the ability to handle a situation; those with strong self-efficacy took initiative to improve listening circumstances. For example, one CI recipient stated,

> "I feel it is up to the CI user to step up and ask what the conversation is about. and make them [conversation partners] aware of my presence. Training should include straightforward discussion with CI users that they need to take control in their conversational groups" (LE post).

Another added, "I believe, in order for the cochlear implant to work, you have to be an active participant in working/training yourself to listen with it." A third, highlighting the need for self-advocacy shared, "I've been known to ask the hosts to turn [loud music] down/off, and it usually ends up that other people thought it was too loud as well but didn't want to say anything." (Postlingual LE) This sentiment was echoed by another, "If I'm going to be in a restaurant, I will often ask for a corner or a quiet table. Sometimes I will ask to have the music lowered (Postlingual LE).

Another CI recipient implanted as a child stated, "I usually ask if we can go to a more quiet place, or I try my best to read lips."

In some instances, problem solving orientation involved positive expectancies more than strategies or accommodations. "I go to a lot of rock concerts and while I may not have complete quality sound that I can enjoy without lots of effort, I have not made it a factor when determining whether to go to a show or not" (perilingual LE).

In contrast, the following quotes, just a few of many, illustrate a lack of control or low self-efficacy: "Sometimes I'm just lost and can't wait to go home" (Postlingual hybrid recipient). "I do avoid noisy environments and sometimes avoid a situation altogether" (Postlingual LE).

Core Category 3: CI users have limited access to resources for optimizing music experiences

This core category related to the component of Domain Specific Knowledge, one of the four central quadrants of the DPSM-MMLE. A key concern of these participants (82.5%) was a lack of accessible and/or affordable resources for dealing with everyday listening experiences involving music. Sixty-five percent of the participants indicated that they were unaware of resources or information to enhance CI benefit, and that rehabilitation was not addressed in regular audiology appointments. As one participant noted, "There is often a gap between the medical community, including doctors, audiologists and manufacturers of hearing devices and the real world of living with a hearing loss." Another stated, "What would help? Audiologists who believe that listening to music with CIs is possible."

Ninety percent of participants indicated that they would like to improve music listening. Of that group, 72.2%, especially LE and hybrid users, indicated that they would be interested in trying music training, especially computer-based training. These themes are illustrated by the following comments:

> "I would suggest that there be more emphasis placed on the emotional adjustment to living with a CI. I received my implant in December of 2016 and is just now feeling settled. It was a tumultuous first year. I worked very hard to remain positive" (Post hybrid).

> "I think that everyone who is implanted and then with every change of the implants (hybrid to full electronic) should be able to go to rehab much like those who have problems with their physical body. If you were able to go weekly and someone was able to explain the features of the implant over and over and could help you track your progress that would be helpful!" (Post hybrid).

This desire was echoed: "I would like to see a speech/hearing rehabilitation/therapy program that CI users could access in person with trained professionals to become proficient at using every possible technology available for the CI's to improve their overall listening experience" (Post hybrid).

Many participants expressed uncertainty on where to find resources, noting limited counseling time with audiologists, and lack of non-commercial websites that include information about music, especially for adults. Over half the participants (57.5%) indicated that cost would be a barrier to training or purchasing ALDs that might enhance music listening. The participants described an "acceptable" range of cost for training programs as "free" to less than $100. Nearly three quarters (73.68%) indicated that they would prefer computer-based training that they could complete from home at their own convenience, though some desired social support (e.g., on-line feedback) as part of that training.

> "I would be more comfortable doing it online if it is self-paced and measures my progress. It would be helpful if I could communicate with a person to ask questions and maybe share my progress and experience with other CI users."

Nearly half (47.3%) remarked that time required for training, even if affordable, would be difficult to accomplish along with normal life responsibilities. Those expressing interest in training indicated that they would be interested in training for a few half hour or hour sessions, several time a week for a few weeks duration.

With regard to content, some expressed concern that available training programs lack relevance to their real-life needs. The top priorities (>25%) for improvement were: understanding lyrics (63.16%), enjoying personally favorite genre (55.25%), improved listening of more complex music (31.58%), and more normal sound quality (28.9%).

DISCUSSION

The first aim of this study was to explore the perspectives of adult CI recipients regarding music in everyday life, in essence, asking them to "think outside the booth." Core categories that emerged from the data included: (1) the dynamic, multi-faceted, and "conditional" nature of music listening; (2) problem solving attitudes and behaviors that support enhancement or coping; and (3) the limited resources currently available for helping CI users to optimize music experiences in real life. The components associated with these core categories were organized into a framework, the Dynamic Problem Solving Model for Management of Music Listening Environments.

The results of this study confirmed that many prior music-CI studies address priorities of CI users, as well as revealing concern that some CI recipient priorities have heretofore have received limited research attention. Consistent with prior research studies, these participants reported difficulties perceiving and enjoying many aspects of music and understanding speech in background music. The range of responses was also consistent with variability documented among CI recipients for music outcomes (Gfeller et al., 2008, 2010, 2012; Looi et al., 2012; Başkent et al., 2014; Limb and Roy, 2014; Drennan et al., 2015).

Not all their priorities were in line with research trends to date, however. For example, present-day research tends to emphasis "endpoint" results specific to device or processing categories (Philips et al., 2012; Pisoni et al., 2017); these participants offered very few comments regarding specific brands or models of CIs or signal processing. They focused more on environmental, social and psychological challenges associated with music experiences, which have received limited attention in extant research.

Regarding music, although pitch perception has been a strong emphasis for many studies, these participants most frequently named music complexity and familiarity as issues influencing their music experiences; background music was described as a major impediment to satisfactory conversations. Relatively speaking, only a modest body of research has focused on these concerns to date (e.g., Gfeller et al., 2003, 2005, 2012; Eskridge et al., 2012; Başkent et al., 2014). Familiarity and complexity (including the complexity of speech and music) are interesting variables in relation to signal processing, as well as the auditory profile and cognitive processes of listeners, and present factors ripe for deeper exploration.

Highly controlled studies that focus on the underlying mechanisms of electric hearing and music are essential, and must remain a high priority for device development and basic science. However, until a more "normal" musical signal can be conveyed through electric hearing, the experiences of these CI users suggests the need for a complimentary agenda of research and clinical counseling. That agenda should more fully tap into the dynamic and multifaceted nature of music listening in real world conditions, as well as rehabilitation or accommodations for managing noisy public places or complex sounds.

This recommendation should not be viewed as an "either or" situation. The phenomenon of hearing loss and CI use is complex and multifaceted. Thus many research foci and approaches are necessary to move hearing science forward, while also optimizing real-world listening experiences for the many CI users who continue to live with past and current-generation technology.

The participants in this study highlighted psychosocial aspects of music experiences, particularly effort and coping, foci that have received scant attention in prior studies of CIs and music. The effort that these participants described in music experiences was similar to outcomes reported in recent studies of speech communication (e.g., Harris et al., 2016; Pichora-Fuller et al., 2016; Hughes et al., 2018). Listening goals often depend on the amount of cognitive energy expended, with greater energy required when the quality of the signal is poor (Pichora-Fuller et al., 2016); a degraded signal is common for many musical sounds. Situations requiring effort beyond the listener's current capacity may be unsustainable and result in withdrawal from social experiences including music. As noted by Dritsakis et al. (2017), avoidance of music has negative implications for quality of life.

Conversely, some individuals with similar listening abilities may consider the same situations as motivational challenge and, thus, choose to persevere (Pichora-Fuller et al., 2016). Thus, clinical guidance for rehabilitation or counseling should take into account the problem-solving orientation of the individual and motivational factors that promote active listening and problem solving, such as social connection and preferred or culturally relevant music.

The prevalence of remarks from these CI users regarding effortful listening in noisy environments is a concern, not only from a communication standpoint but also in relation to physical and emotional health of CI users. According to Sarafino and Smith (2016), individuals experience greater stress when (1) circumstances are perceived as outside of one's control; (2) when effort is accompanied by distress; (3) when social connections are undermined; (4) when the individual lacks resources; and (5) when functioning in noisy environments. These stressors were all associated with music experiences described by these participants. Chronic stressors are associated with higher prevalence of medical problems and reduced quality of life (Sarafino and Smith, 2016). Thus, the concerns expressed by these CI users have implications for general well-being and should be addressed in rehabilitation, along with hearing device optimization. This also suggests the need for public advocacy and education regarding "listener friendly" environments.

The dynamic nature of music listening as expressed by these CI users brings to mind the term, "coping," which has been defined by some as a dynamic process in which people try and manage the perceived discrepancy between life demands and the resources they need to manage stressful situations. When coping with a difficult situation, the individual has ongoing transactions with the environment in which they are required to appraise and re-appraise the influential factors and response options. Thus coping is an on-going and ever changing process (Sarafino and Smith, 2016). This suggests that counseling CI users regarding music listening should include not only helpful "listening tips," but should also include guidance to enhance self-efficacy, realistic expectations, flexible problem solving, and provision of access to useful information, including training programs, that can be accessed on an on-going basis.

An unexpected result of this study was the top priorities of these CI users for music training. Ninety percent indicated the desire to have training programs, but emphasized that the content should be practical, and should include personally meaningful listening tasks. Thus, analytic exercises of isolated structural components intended to enhance basic auditory processing might be complemented with tasks that recipients see as relevant to daily life.

Most training studies, to date, have focused on enhancing pitch perception, or melody and timbre recognition (see review, Looi et al., 2012). Surprisingly the musical component most frequently identified by this sample was ability to hear sung lyrics. Perception of sung lyrics against background accompaniment constitutes a speech in noise task, thus training for song lyrics could offer a challenging but relevant rehabilitative task beneficial to speech as well as music perception.

These participants varied in what content and format they desired for training, suggesting the need for a clinically useful menu of options with regard to purpose, content, and prerequisite skills. For example, particular forms of information may be more or less accessible depending upon the specific CI user based upon past music training or onset of hearing loss (e.g., reading music notation, mental representation of "normal" pitch).

Participants also emphasized that their busy lives precluded intensive time commitments for training. Most of the participants interested in training were willing to train for approximately 30 min, several times a week, over one or two weeks. Neuroplasticity requires ample repetition over time. Thus, the concern regarding time commitment brings up important questions of how much training is required for measurable improvements, and protocol components that support compliance and persistence. Individual priorities should be considered when counseling CI users on music-based training options.

The participants in our sample revealed a range of responses to music experiences from active problem solving to avoidance and withdrawal. Attitudes and behaviors toward rehabilitation are in part a function of the individual's problem solving orientation.

What factors are associated with a strong problem solving orientation? Can a problem solving orientation be encouraged or taught?

Future studies and clinical guidance may be informed by research and clinical approaches in psychology. According to cognitive psychologist Albert Bandura (2010), self-efficacy is the belief in one's capabilities to organize and execute the course of action required to manage situations. It is determined by motivation, amount of effort extended in, how long you will persist in the face of adversity, and belief that you can ultimately succeed. These beliefs are related to one's sense of mastery in past tasks relevant to the target goal, modeling by others, social persuasion, social support, and positive emotional state. An examination of methods for developing self-efficacy may be clinically useful avenues for future counseling of CI recipients.

The results of this study indicate a need for accessible information that audiologists can quickly and easily share with their patients and families. These participants' comments regarding lack of input from audiologists on rehabilitation was consistent with findings by Harris et al. (2016). It is also possible that busy audiologists, who must typically focus on speech outcomes, may lack time to delve into factors influencing music perception and enjoyment. This gap between research knowledge and clinical application may reflect in part fiscal and system pressures associated with healthcare delivery. According to one study, more than 50% of audiologists have 90 min or less to take care of audiograms, speech testing, mapping and troubleshooting during audiology visits. Little if any time remains for counseling on unique challenges such as music listening (Dunn, 2018). Thus, it is of little surprise that audiologists do not provide information and guidance about music and complex listening environments.

These participants and prior studies have noted limited reimbursement for rehabilitative strategies for adult hearing device users following implantation or device acquisition. This lack of rehabilitation is notable, in that CIs can have direct costs of more than three times the cost of a knee replacement, yet the typical adult hearing device recipient in the United States often does not have access to a structured rehabilitation program (Harris et al., 2016). Professional organizations and audiologists might advocate for rehabilitation programs for adult CI recipients to optimize CI use in challenging listening conditions. In addition, these findings may suggest the need for assessment protocols that more fully document outcomes in real-world environments as well as speech perception in controlled test environments. The themes from this study may provide a foundation for the development of an assessment tool for evaluating successful outcomes in real-life conditions.

This study has limitations that should be discussed. While concerted efforts were made to recruit a diverse sample with regard to music experiences and background, it is possible that this study tended to attract CI users for whom music is personally important. The participants were primarily residents of the United States, thus their experiences are more likely consistent with health care and social practices within the United States. These enrollment patterns may limit the relevance of these results to the larger population of CI users. While inter-rater reliability and member checking were used to verify and validate the analyses, the questions and analyses were subject to the viewpoints of the authors and consultants, whose perspectives on CIs and music may not represent the range of important perspectives on this topic. Consistent with principles of qualitative methodology, this study was not intended to provide objective "truths" confirmed though testable hypotheses. Further research is needed to test the impact and applicability of the themes that emerged from this sample to other subgroups and the larger CI population.

In closing, through the voices of these CI users, we see a glimpse into the everyday music experiences and the challenges associated with using a helpful but imperfect listening device for music. Music continues to be a challenge for the many thousands of CI and HA users who will continue to rely on current technology (Gfeller et al., 2012). The Dynamic Problem Solving Model for Management of Music Listening Environments offers a useful organizational tool for considering relevant variables for research on real-life music experiences, and clinical initiatives that are consistent with the priorities of the CI users in everyday life. Possible initiatives might include experiments that more nearly reflect the dynamic and multifaceted nature of real-life listening environments, rehabilitative programs that include psychosocial factors, the development of user-friendly resources, and public advocacy for listener-friendly public spaces.

The comments from these CI users reveal that satisfactory music experiences in real life are complex in nature, and a simple "how to" list for improvement is unlikely to "fix" the problems. However, audiologists may provide helpful guidance by discussing or having at hand available links to websites or reader-friendly articles (unrelated to device marketing) that clarify why music listening is challenging, and strategies from other CI users. These resources might emphasize and explain the dynamic nature of music listening and the need for on-going problem solving. Strategies might include enrollment of one's social network, use of ALDs for specific situations, self-directed training programs, and options for managing the listening environment. Different approaches, including rehabilitation, accommodations, judicious choice of music and listening environment, and avoidance of particularly difficult situations all have potential benefits, depending upon the dynamic combination of music, environment, and listener characteristics.

DATA AVAILABILITY STATEMENT

The datasets for this study will not be made publicly available because the study protocol was approved by the University IRB on the condition that data were not to be shared with members not a part of the research team as participants could be identified based upon their responses. They did not provide consent for such identification.

ETHICS STATEMENT

This study was carried out in accordance with the requirements of the University of Iowa Human Subjects Institutional Review Board. All participants were provided with an invitation to participate and a letter of consent. Those who wished to participate responded to VD and informed consent was implied. This protocol was approved by the University of Iowa Human Subjects Institutional Review Board.

AUTHOR CONTRIBUTIONS

All authors contributed to the conceptualization of the patient-centered methodology and the development of the measurement tool. KG was primary author for the grant application that supported this project. AS had primary oversight for the development of the online focus group protocol and recruitment of participants. VD had primary oversight for first and second cycle coding and inductive analyses of the dataset. KG had primary oversight for the deductive coding and the development of the model proposed in this manuscript. KG and VD were primary authors of the manuscript, and AS contributed feedback.

ACKNOWLEDGMENTS

We thank Carolyn Wanat, Ph.D., Pamela Wesely, Ph.D., and Jane Engeldinger, MD, for consultation on research methods and model development and to Laura Beth Reznicek, Miranda Aldrich, and Hae Sun Kim for assistance with coding verification and manuscript preparation. We also thank Dr. Hill-Briggs for granting permission for adaptation of her model of self-management of chronic illness.

REFERENCES

Attride-Stirling, J. (2001). Thematic networks: an analytic tool for qualitative research. *Qual. Res.* 1, 385–405. doi: 10.1177/146879410100100307

Bandura, A. (2010). "Self-efficacy," in *The Corsini Encyclopedia of Psychology*, eds I. B. Weiner, and W. E. Craighead (Hoboken, NJ: John Wiley & Sons, Inc), 1–3.

Bartel, L. R., Greenberg, S., Friesen, L. M., Ostroff, J., Bodmer, D., Shipp, D., et al. (2011). Qualitative case studies of five cochlear implant recipients' experience with music. *Cochlear Implants Int.* 12, 27–33. doi: 10.1179/146701010x486435

Başkent, D., van Engelshoven, S., and Galvin, J. J. III (2014). Susceptibility to interference by music and speech maskers in middle-aged adults. *J. Acoust. Soc. Am.* 135, EL147–EL153. doi: 10.1121/1.4865261

Bradley, E. H., Curry, L. A., and Devers, K. J. (2007). Qualitative data analysis for health services research: developing taxonomy, themes, and theory. *Health Serv. Res.* 42, 1758–1772. doi: 10.1111/j.1475-6773.2006.00684.x

Brodt, M., Norton, M., Christine, K., and Kratchman, A. (2015). So much more than a "pair of brown shoes": triumphs of patient and other stakeholder engagement in patient-centered outcomes research. *Pat. Exp. J.* 2, 43–49. doi: 10.35680/2372-0247.1057

Clancy, C., and Collins, F. S. (2010). Patient-Centered outcomes research institute: the intersection of science and health care. *Sci. Transl. Med.* 2:37cm18. doi: 10.1126/scitranslmed.3001235

Collister, L. B., and Huron, D. (2008). Comparison of word intelligibility in spoken and sung phrases. *Empir. Musicol. Rev.* 3, 109–125. doi: 10.18061/1811/34102

Creswell, J. W. (2014). *A Concise Introduction to Mixed Methods Research*. Thousand Oaks, CA: SAGE publications.

Domecq, J. P., Prutsky, G., Elraiyah, T., Wang, Z., Nabhan, M., Shippee, N., et al. (2014). Patient engagement in research: a systematic review. *BMC Health Serv. Res.* 14:89. doi: 10.1186/1472-6963-14-89

Drennan, W. R., Oleson, J. J., Gfeller, K., Crosson, J., Driscoll, V. D., Won, J. H., et al. (2015). Clinical evaluation of music perception, appraisal and experience in cochlear implant users. *Int. J. Audiol.* 54, 114–123. doi: 10.3109/14992027.2014.948219

Dritsakis, G., van Besouw, R. M., and O'Meara, A. (2017). Impact of music on the quality of life of cochlear implant users: a focus group study. *Cochlear Implants Int.* 18, 207–215. doi: 10.1080/14670100.2017.1303892

Dunn, C. (2018). "Post-implant immediate and long-term care," in *CI2018 Emerging Issues in Cochlear Implantation* (Washington, DC: American Cochlear Implant Alliance).

Eskridge, E. N., Galvin, J. J. III, Aronoff, J. M., Li, T., and Fu, Q. J. (2012). Speech perception with music maskers by cochlear implant users and normal-hearing listeners. *J. Speech Lang. Hear Res.* 55, 800–810. doi: 10.1044/1092-4388(2011/11-0124)

Forsythe, L. P., Frank, L. B., Workman, T. A., Hilliard, T., Harwell, D., and Fayish, L. (2017). Patient, caregiver and clinician views on engagement in comparative effectiveness research. *J. Comp. Effect. Res.* 6, 231–244. doi: 10.2217/cer-2016-0062

Frank, L., Basch, E., and Selby, J. V. (2014). The PCORI perspective on patient-centered outcomes research. *JAMA* 312, 1513–1514.

Fujita, S., and Ito, J. (1999). Ability of nucleus cochlear implantees to recognize music. *Ann. Otol. Rhinol. Laryngol.* 108(7 Pt 1), 634–640. doi: 10.1177/000348949910800702

Fuller, C. D., Galvin, J. J. III, Maat, B., Başkent, D., and Free, R. H. (2018). Comparison of two music training approaches on music and speech perception in cochlear implant users. *Trends Hear.* 22, 1–22. doi: 10.1177/2331216518765379

Gfeller, K., Buzzell, A., Driscoll, V., Kinnaird, B., and Oleson, J. (2009). "The impact of voice range and instrumental background accompaniment on recognition of song lyrics," in *Proceedings of the 7th Asia Pacific Symposium on Cochlear Implants and Related Sciences*, Singapore, 35–40.

Gfeller, K., Christ, A., Knutson, J., Witt, S., and Mehr, M. (2003). The effects of familiarity and complexity on appraisal of complex songs by cochlear implant recipients and normal hearing adults. *J. Music Ther.* 40, 78–112. doi: 10.1093/jmt/40.2.78

Gfeller, K., Christ, A., Knutson, J. F., Witt, S., Murray, K. T., and Tyler, R. S. (2000). Musical backgrounds, listening habits, and aesthetic enjoyment of adult cochlear implant recipients. *J. Am. Acad. Audiol.* 11, 390–406.

Gfeller, K., Jiang, D., Oleson, J. J., Driscoll, V., and Knutson, J. F. (2010). Temporal stability of music perception and appraisal scores of adult cochlear implant recipients. *J. Am. Acad. Audiol.* 21, 28–34. doi: 10.3766/jaaa.21.1.4

Gfeller, K., and Lansing, C. (1992). Musical perception of cochlear implant users as measured by the primary measures of music audiation: an item analysis. *J. Music Ther.* 29, 18–39. doi: 10.1093/jmt/29.1.18

Gfeller, K., and Lansing, C. R. (1991). Melodic, rhythmic, and timbral perception of adult cochlear implant users. *J. Speech Hear. Res.* 34, 916–920. doi: 10.1044/jshr.3404.916

Gfeller, K., Oleson, J., Knutson, J. F., Breheny, P., Driscoll, V., and Olszewski, C. (2008). Multivariate predictors of music perception and appraisal by adult cochlear implant users. *J. Am. Acad. Audiol.* 19, 120–134. doi: 10.3766/jaaa.19.2.3

Gfeller, K., Olszewski, C., Rychener, M., Sena, K., Knutson, J. F., Witt, S., et al. (2005). Recognition of "real-world" musical excerpts by cochlear implant recipients and normal-hearing adults. *Ear Hear.* 26, 237–250. doi: 10.1097/00003446-200506000-00001

Gfeller, K., Turner, C., Mehr, M., Woodworth, G., Fearn, R., Knutson, J. F., et al. (2002). Recognition of familiar melodies by adult cochlear implant recipients and normal-hearing adults. *Cochlear Implants Int.* 3, 29–53. doi: 10.1179/cim.2002.3.1.29

Gfeller, K., Turner, C., Oleson, J., Kliethermes, S., and Driscoll, V. (2012). Accuracy of cochlear implant recipients in speech reception in the presence of background music. *Ann. Otol. Rhinol. Laryngol.* 121, 782–791. doi: 10.1177/000348941212101203

Gregory, M. (2011). Tools for enabling communication partners. *Hear. J.* 64, 44–46.

Hargreaves, D. J., and North, A. C. (2010). "Experimental aesthetics and liking for music," in *Handbook of Music and Emotion: Theory, Research, Applications*, eds P. N. Juslin, and J. A. Sloboda (Oxford: Oxford University Press), 515–546. doi: 10.1093/acprof:oso/9780199230143.003.0019

Harris, M. S., Capretta, N. R., Henning, S. C., Feeney, L., Pitt, M. A., and Moberly, A. C. (2016). Postoperative rehabilitation strategies used by adults with cochlear implants: a pilot study. *Laryngoscope Investig. Otolaryngol.* 1, 42–48. doi: 10.1002/lio2.20

Hickam, D., Totten, A., Berg, A., Rader, K., Goodman, S., and Newhouse, R. (2013). *The PCORI Methodology Report.* Washington: PCORI.

Hill-Briggs, F. (2003). Problem solving in diabetes self-management: a model of chronic illness self-management behavior. *Ann. Behav. Med.* 25, 182–193. doi: 10.1207/s15324796abm2503_04

Hughes, S. E., Hutchings, H. A., Rapport, F. L., McMahon, C. M., and Boisvert, I. (2018). Social connectedness and perceived listening effort in adult cochlear implant users: a grounded theory to establish content validity for a new patient reported outcome measure. *Ear Hear.* 39, 922–934. doi: 10.1097/AUD.0000000000000553

Krueger, R., and Casey, M. (2009). *Focus Groups: A Practical Guide to Applied Science.* Thousand Oaks, CA: Sage.

Lassaletta, L., Castro, A., Bastarrica, M., Perez-Mora, R., Herran, B., Sanz, L., et al. (2008). Changes in listening habits and quality of musical sound after cochlear implantation. *Otolaryngol. Head Neck Surg.* 138, 363–367. doi: 10.1016/j.otohns.2007.11.028

Limb, C. J., and Roy, A. T. (2014). Technological, biological, and acoustical constraints to music perception in cochlear implant users. *Hear. Res.* 308, 13–26. doi: 10.1016/j.heares.2013.04.009

Looi, V., Gfeller, K., and Driscoll, V. (2012). Music appreciation and training for cochlear implant recipients: a review. *Semin. Hear.* 33, 307–334. doi: 10.1055/s-0032-1329222

Looi, V., and She, J. (2010). Music perception of cochlear implant users: a questionnaire, and its implications for a music training program. *Int. J. Audiol.* 49, 116–128. doi: 10.3109/14992020903405987

Mather, M., Hamilton, D., Robalino, S., and Rousseau, N. (2018). Going where other methods cannot: a systematic mapping review of 25 years of qualitative research in Otolaryngology. *Clin. Otolaryngol.* 43, 1443–1453. doi: 10.1111/coa.13200

Migirov, L., Kronenberg, J., and Henkin, Y. (2009). Self-reported listening habits and enjoyment of music among adult cochlear implant recipients. *Ann. Otol. Rhinol. Laryngol.* 118, 350–355. doi: 10.1177/000348940911800506

Miles, M. B., Huberman, A. M., and Saldaña, J. (2014). *Qualitative Data Analysis: A Methods Sourcebook.* Thousand Oaks, CA: SAGE Publications.

Mirza, S., Douglas, S. A., Lindsey, P., Hildreth, T., and Hawthorne, M. (2003). Appreciation of music in adult patients with cochlear implants: a patient questionnaire. *Cochlear Implants Int.* 4, 85–95. doi: 10.1179/cim.2003.4.2.85

Philips, B., Vinck, B., De Vel, E., Maes, L., D'Haenens, W., Keppler, H., et al. (2012). Characteristics and determinants of music appreciation in adult CI users. *Eur. Arch. Otorhinolaryngol.* 269, 813–821. doi: 10.1007/s00405-011-1718-1714

Pichora-Fuller, M. K., Kramer, S. E., Eckert, M. A., Edwards, B., Hornsby, B. W., Humes, L. E., et al. (2016). Hearing impairment and cognitive energy: the framework for understanding effortful listening (FUEL). *Ear Hear.* 37, 5S–27S. doi: 10.1097/aud.0000000000000312

Pijl, S. (1995). Musical pitch perception with pulsatile stimulation of single electrodes in patients implanted with the Nucleus cochlear implant. *Ann. Otol. Rhinol. Laryngol. Suppl.* 166, 224–227.

Pisoni, D. B., Kronenberger, W. G., Harris, M. S., and Moberly, A. C. (2017). Three challenges for future research on cochlear implants. *World J. Otorhinolaryngol.Head Neck Surg.* 3, 240–254. doi: 10.1016/j.wjorl.2017.12.010

Plant, G., Bernstein, C. M., and Levitt, H. (2015). Optimizing performance in adult cochlear implant users through clinician directed auditory training. *Semin. Hear.* 36, 296–310. doi: 10.1055/s-0035-1564460

Saldaña, J. (2013). *The Coding Manual for Qualitative Researchers.* London: Sage.

Sarafino, E. P., and Smith, T. W. (2016). *Health Psychology: Biopsychosocial Interactions*, 9th Edn. Hoboken, NJ: John Wiley & Sons.

Savenye, W. C., and Robinson, R. S. (1996). "Qualitative research issues and methods: an introduction for educational technologists," in *Handbook of Research for Educational Communications and Technology*, eds D. H. Jonassen, and P. Harris (Mahwah, NJ: Lawrence Erlbaum Associates), 1171–1195.

Sheridan, S., Schrandt, S., Forsythe, L., Hilliard, T. S., and Paez, K. A. (2017). The PCORI engagement rubric: promising practices for partnering in research. *Ann. Fam. Med.* 15, 165–170. doi: 10.1370/afm.2042

Sloboda, J. A. (2010). "Music in everyday life: the role of emotions," in *Handbook of Music and Emotion: Theory, Research, Applications*, eds P. N. Juslin, and J. A. Sloboda (New York, NY: Oxford University Press), 493–514.

Smith, S. L. (2014). Promoting self-efficacy in patient-centered audiologic rehabilitation for adults with hearing loss. *Perspect. Aural Rehabil. Instrum.* 21, 24–32.

Smith, S. L., and West, R. L. (2006). The application of self-efficacy principles to audiologic rehabilitation: a tutorial. *Am. J. Audiol.* 15, 46–56. doi: 10.1044/1059-0889(2006/006)

Strauss, A., and Corbin, J. (1994). Grounded theory methodology. *Handb. Qual. Res.* 17, 273–285.

Tates, K., Zwaanswijk, M., Otten, R., van Dulmen, S., Hoogerbrugge, P. M., Kamps, W. A., et al. (2009). Online focus groups as a tool to collect data in hard-to-include populations: examples from paediatric oncology. *BMC Med. Res. Methodol.* 9:15. doi: 10.1186/1471-2288-9-15

Wilhelm, L. A. (2016). *Accessibility of Music Experiences for Individuals With Age-Related Hearing Loss.* Ph.D.thesis, The University of Iowa, Iowa.

Wright, R., and Uchanski, R. M. (2012). Music perception and appraisal: cochlear implant users and simulated cochlear implant listening. *J. Am. Acad. Audiol.* 23, 350–365; quiz379. doi: 10.3766/jaaa.23.5.6

Young-Hyman, D., De Groot, M., Hill-Briggs, F., Gonzalez, J. S., Hood, K., and Peyrot, M. (2016). Psychosocial care for people with diabetes: a position statement of the American Diabetes Association. *Diabetes Care* 39, 2126–2140.

5

Early Deafened, Late Implanted Cochlear Implant Users Appreciate Music More than and Identify Music as Well as Postlingual Users

Christina Fuller[1,2,3*], *Deniz Başkent*[1,2] *and Rolien Free*[1,2]

[1] *Department of Otorhinolaryngology, Head and Neck Surgery, University Medical Center Groningen, University of Groningen, Groningen, Netherlands,* [2] *Research School of Behavioral and Cognitive Neurosciences, Graduate School of Medical Sciences, University of Groningen, Groningen, Netherlands,* [3] *Department of Otorhinolaryngology, Treant Zorggroep, Emmen, Netherlands*

Correspondence:
Christina Fuller
c.d.fuller@umcg.nl

Introduction: Typical cochlear implant (CI) users, namely postlingually deafened and implanted, report to not enjoy listening to music, and find it difficult to perceive music. Another group of CI users, the early-deafened (during language acquisition) and late-implanted (after a long period of auditory deprivation; EDLI), report a higher music appreciation, but is this related to a better music perception?

Materials and Methods: Sixteen EDLI and fifteen postlingually deafened (control group) CI users participated in the study. The inclusion criteria for EDLI were: severe or profound hearing loss onset before the age of 6 years, implantation after the age of 16 years, and CI experience more than 1 year. Subjectively, music perception and appreciation was evaluated using the Dutch Musical Background Questionnaire. Behaviorally, music perception was measured with melodic contour identification (MCI), using two instruments (piano and organ), each tested with and without a masking contour. Semitone distance between successive tones of the target varied from 1 to 3 semitones.

Results: Subjectively, the EDLI group reported to appreciate music more than postlingually deafened CI users. Behaviorally, while clinical phoneme recognition test score on average was lower in the EDLI group, melodic contour identification did not significantly differ between the two groups. There was, however, an effect of instrument and masker for both groups; the piano was the best-recognized instrument, and for both instruments, the masker with non-overlapping pitch was best recognized.

Discussion: EDLI group reported higher appreciation of music than postlingual control group, even though behaviorally measured music perception did not differ significantly between the two groups. Both surprising findings since EDLI CI users would be expected to have lower outcomes based on the early deafness onset, long duration of auditory deprivation, and on average lower clinical speech scores. Perhaps, the music perception difficulty comes from similar electric hearing limitations in both groups. The higher subjective appreciation in EDLI might be due to the lack of a musical memory, with no ability to compare music heard via the CI to acoustic music perception. Overall, our findings support a benefit from implantation for a positive music experience in EDLI CI users.

Keywords: early-deafened, late-implanted, cochlear implant, melody, postlingually deafened, implant outcome

INTRODUCTION

Music is an important daily-life auditory signal that can directly impact emotions, and also often plays an essential role in social entertainment and interactions (Boucher and Bryden, 1997; Drennan and Rubinstein, 2008; Salimpoor et al., 2009; Patel, 2014). The perception of the music signal, rich in acoustic cues, is unfortunately still challenging for users of cochlear implants (CIs) (e.g., McDermott, 2004; McDermott and Oxenham, 2008; Limb and Roy, 2014). In transmission of acoustic signals to the auditory nerve via electric hearing of the implant, due to the limitations of electric stimulation, the signal transmitted via CI is reduced to slow-varying envelopes delivered at a limited spectral resolution, whereby most fine cues needed for optimal music perception are lost (McDermott, 2004; Limb and Roy, 2014; Başkent et al., 2016). Another limiting factor for music perception is perhaps the functioning of the central and peripheral auditory pathway. Within the population of CI users, individuals have different neuronal survival (number of spiral ganglion cells) and/or morphological changes of nerve fibers (e.g., demyelination of the neuron soma of the spiral ganglion cells) (Nadol et al., 2001; Gassner et al., 2005; Seyyedi et al., 2014), due to different etiologies, age, and different periods of auditory deprivation (Teoh et al., 2004; Fallon et al., 2008; Peterson et al., 2010). These factors result in CI users having difficulties perceiving the richness of music, and especially of pitch and timbre (McDermott, 2004; McDermott and Oxenham, 2008; Limb and Roy, 2014), due to the limitations of the electric stimulation, combined with overall state of health of their auditory pathways.

Many music perception studies with CIs have been conducted with the typical implant user: a postlingually deafened (meaning, deafened after language acquisition) person that is implanted later in life. The overall outcomes show that, with the exception of rhythm identification, all other aspects of music perception (pitch, timbre and melody) are poorer in CI users than in normal hearing listeners, and that listening to music with the implant is also subjectively reported to be unsatisfying (Gfeller et al., 2000, 2002; Leal et al., 2003; McDermott, 2004; Galvin et al., 2007; Lassaletta et al., 2007, 2008b; Looi et al., 2012; Limb and Roy, 2014). Compared to hearing aid listeners CI users perform worse for music perception, apart from rhythm recognition (Looi et al., 2008). In case of a combined electrical and acoustical stimulation, frequency discrimination was better in hybrid listeners, instrument identification, and detection as bad between hybrid and CI only listeners (Brockmeier et al., 2010), whereas for real world music excerpts the hybrid and NH listeners outperform the CI user (Gfeller et al., 2006).

In this study, we focus on a relatively new and less typical group of CI users; the early-deafened, late-implanted (EDLI) CI user. EDLI CI users are deafened during language acquisition (defined as deafness onset between 0 and 6 years in this study, based on literature), and only implanted after a longer period of auditory deprivation (implantation at or older than 16 years of age in this study, translating to at least 10 years of auditory deprivation) (Goorhuis-Brouwer and Schaerlaekens, 2000; van Dijkhuizen et al., 2011; Fuller et al., 2013; Heywood et al., 2016). The perception and appreciation of music in this EDLI CI group is mostly unknown. Yet, surprisingly, Fuller et al. (2013) showed that EDLI implant users reported higher appreciation of music compared to postlingually deafened CI users. More specifically, EDLI participants indicated that music sounds pleasant with a CI and rated the perceived quality of music higher than the postlingually deafened CI users did.

One reason for the discrepancy in subjectively reported music appreciation between the EDLI group and typical CI users might be that EDLI implantees rate music better due to a lack of an acoustical musical memory to compare the degraded signal of electric stimulation to, in contrast to postlingual CI users who often report music to sound worse than what they were used to before implantation (Mirza et al., 2003; Limb and Roy, 2014). Another difference between EDLI CI users and postlingually deafened CI users is the different development of auditory pathways and additionally the longer period of auditory deprivation at a young age in the early-deafened individuals. EDLI CI users have developed hearing loss during childhood, defined approximately between 1 and 6 years of age (Waltzman and Cohen, 1999; Sharma et al., 2002; Waltzman et al., 2002; Fallon et al., 2008; Peterson et al., 2010; Gordon et al., 2013), a timeframe during which the brain is best capable of speech and language development. If an individual develops hearing loss during this period a different shaping of the pathways for speech and language processing, as well as for music perception, might occur. Visual language development might interact with the auditory cortex (Champoux et al., 2009; Sandmann et al., 2012). Further the auditory cortex might not effectively process acoustical speech input (Teoh et al., 2004; Lazard et al., 2010). Due to this different development of the auditory pathways, some studies suggest that implantation might not be beneficial in this group, at least not for speech perception (Connell and Balkany, 2006; Medina et al., 2017). In fact, in clinical practice, up until recently, early-deafened individuals were not frequently implanted because of the expected low benefit of implantation for speech outcomes (Heywood et al., 2016). Next to the different neuronal network development in EDLI CI users, the long period of auditory deprivation (in our study at least 10 years) might also be influencing the outcome of implantation (Lazard et al., 2012; Blamey et al., 2013). In postlingually deafened and implanted individuals, the effect of auditory deprivation shows a negative influence on post-implantation speech perception (Lazard et al., 2012; Blamey et al., 2013). Literature suggests that speech perception is even poorer in the EDLI group than in the postlingually deafened group (Teoh et al., 2004; van Dijkhuizen et al., 2011). Some studies suggest to not implant individuals if they have had a 10 years or longer period of auditory deprivation (Connell and Balkany, 2006). Surprisingly, other studies show good implantation results with very low numbers of spiral ganglion cells (Blamey, 1997; Khan et al., 2005, Nadol et al., 2001), while others showed that a higher number of spiral ganglion cells are related to better speech recognition scores post-mortem (Seyyedi et al., 2014). Recently EDLI candidates have been implanted more, for example in the United Kingdom (Heywood et al., 2016). While results for speech perception remain—in general- lower than in postlingually deafened CI users, overall outcomes are still promising as this group often report improvements in quality of life as a result of implantation (Teoh et al., 2004; Santarelli et al., 2008; van Dijkhuizen et al., 2011; Fuller et al., 2013; Heywood et al., 2016).

To comprehensively investigate music perception and appreciation in EDLI CI users, in this study, we used both subjective and psychophysical measures. We investigated the subjective appreciation and perception of music and the psychophysical perception of music using melodic contour identification in EDLI implant users, in comparison to the control group of typical postlingual CI users. The research questions were: (1) Can we replicate our finding that EDLI CI users show a higher subjective music appreciation?; (2) If so, is the subjective music appreciation linked to a better psychophysical music perception?; (3) Are these subjective and psychophysical outcomes correlated, to investigate the potential relevance of the two measures to each other.

MATERIALS AND METHODS

Participants

Sixteen EDLI CI users, as the test group (age range 23–75 years; seven female; demographic details presented in **Table 1**), and fifteen postlingually deafened CI users, as the control group (age range 48–75 years; five female; demographic details in **Table 2**), participated in the study. Four EDLI users overlapped with the earlier study by Fuller et al. (2013), but otherwise the test population differed between the two studies. All participants were native Dutch speakers and had 1 year or more CI experience. We aimed the two groups to be age- and gender-matched as much as possible, but despite this effort age still remained a significant factor [$F_{(1,31)} = 27.99$, $p < 0.001$], with EDLI participants being significantly younger than the control group. The inclusion criteria for EDLI were based on previous literature (Goorhuis-Brouwer and Schaerlaekens, 2000; Sharma et al., 2002; Connell and Balkany, 2006; van Dijkhuizen et al., 2011, 2016; Fuller et al., 2013; Heywood et al., 2016):

1. Severe or profound hearing loss onset before the age of six,
2. Implanted after the age of 16 years.

TABLE 1 | Participant details of the EDLI CI users.

Participant number	Age (years)	Onset of hearing loss (years)	Hearing aid use since (years)	Language	SIR	CI use (years)	Etiology	Clinical speech score (%)
1	72	3	5	Dutch	5	10	Genetic	67
2	38	0	3	Frisian/Dutch	5	12	LVAS	85
3	41	0	0	Dutch/Frisian	3	2	Pendred Syndrome	95
4	64	0	6	Dutch	5	7	Unknown	82
5	62	5	5	Dutch	5	2	Meningitis	63
6	46	4	6	Dutch	5	16	Unknown	81
7	65	0	6	Dutch	5	13	Maternal rubella	90
8	67	0	4	Dutch	4	4	Meningitis	64
9	67	1	1	Dutch	4	5	Meningitis	40
10	62	0	<6	Sign language	3	6	Unknown	30
11	75	1	59	Dutch	5	5	Meningitis	45
12	55	0	4	Dutch with sign	3	1.5	Maternal rubella	60
13	23	0	3	Dutch with sign	4	7.5	Unknown	72
14	58	4	9	Dutch	4	7	Maternal rubella	69
15	62	0	3	Dutch	5	5	Asfyxia	85
16	63	4	21	Dutch	5	15	Unknown	78

TABLE 2 | Participant details of the postlingually deafened CI users.

Participant number	Age (years)	Onset of hearing loss (years)	Hearing aid use since (years)	Language	SIR	CI use (years)	Etiology	Clinical speech score (%)
1	68	18	40	Dutch	5	5	Genetic	67
2	49	39	39	Dutch/Frisian	5	4	Trauma	90
3	69	61	61	Dutch/Frisian	5	7	Sudden deafness	75
4	69	46	46	Dutch	5	7	Ménière disease	90
5	69	32	32	Dutch	5	6	Trauma	93
6	68	50	50	Dutch	5	3	Genetic	88
7	49	34	34	Dutch	5	3	Genetic	90
8	74	31	31	Dutch	5	3	Unknown	69
9	66	18	18	Dutch	5	3	Genetic	79
10	65	55	57	Dutch/Frisian	5	2	Genetic	72
11	66	40	40	Dutch	5	2	Unknown	69
12	48	>18	27	Dutch	5	6	Labyrinth dysp.	93
13	66	45	42	Dutch	5	4	Unknown	78
14	75	33	39	Dutch	5	13	Unknown	78
15	74	50	50	Dutch	5	9	Otosclerosis	100

The inclusion criteria for postlingually deafened control CI users were:

1. Severe hearing loss onset after the age of 18, in order to ensure no overlapping period of early deafness with the EDLI participants.

The age of hearing loss onset was defined based on two sources, namely, the information the participants provided and their medical records. An important factor to note here is that all EDLI users implanted at our clinic were selected for implantation according to a special clinical protocol that is based on a speech intelligibility rating (SIR) (Samar and Metz, 1988) of the implant candidate's speech production, which has been shown to be an influencing factor on speech perception outcome (van Dijkhuizen et al., 2011). A score of three or higher (1–5 scale) indicates implantation candidacy; a score of 3 meaning: "Speech is difficult to understand; however the gist of the content can be understood."; and 5 meaning: "Speech is completely intelligible." The speech intelligibility is judged by an experienced speech therapist in our clinical team, and coupled to an expected outcome of implantation for speech. The clinicians use three outcome measures: (1) sound perception, no or minimal improvement of speech perception; (2) support of speech perception, some improvement in speech perception; (3) improved speech perception. Due to an expected lower implantation outcome, the patients scoring a SIR score 2 or lower receive a negative advise for implantation, which means that the person does not receive the CI. Apart from the language development aspect, EDLI users are additionally advised based on the audiological CI criteria, as well as the amount of auditory stimulation, intrinsic motivation, and medical history. Therefore, the selection of EDLI participants in this study might be biased towards relatively high implantation outcomes due to this specific selection procedure.

As a further characterization of our test and control groups of CI users we have also extracted clinical speech perception scores from the medical records. The test used in our clinic is based on recognition of phonemes in meaningful Dutch consonant-vowel-consonant words from the Nederlandse Vereniging van Audiologie (NVA) corpus, developed by Bosman and Smoorenburg (1995). During regular clinical visits, a list of 12 words spoken by a female speaker is presented at 75 dBA in free field in a sound-treated audiology booth. The 75 dBA level of loudness, a level representative of "loud" speech, was chosen here because a score for all users from both groups was available from our clinical database. The phoneme correct score of the last 11 words is calculated per visit per CI user. From these scores measured post-implantation, we selected the last known score from the clinic, as this would most realistically reflect speech perception performance of the participant around the time of this study. Note that the speech perception scores were not part of inclusion criteria in the present study, and were only used as a characterization of participants. And also worth noting that while these are clinical speech perception scores they are tested by different audiologists in different clinical booths during regular clinical outpatient visits, hence, some variation in these scores is expected also due to such external and circumstantial factors. The timing of these tests was at least 1 year after implantation.

Figure 1 shows the outcomes for the latest clinical speech scores per group. The mean score for EDLI participants was 69%, for postlingually deafened CI users 82%. In the EDLI group a wider range in scores is observed (30–95%), whereas in the postlingual participant group a more consistent higher score range is observed (67–100%). A t-test showed a significant

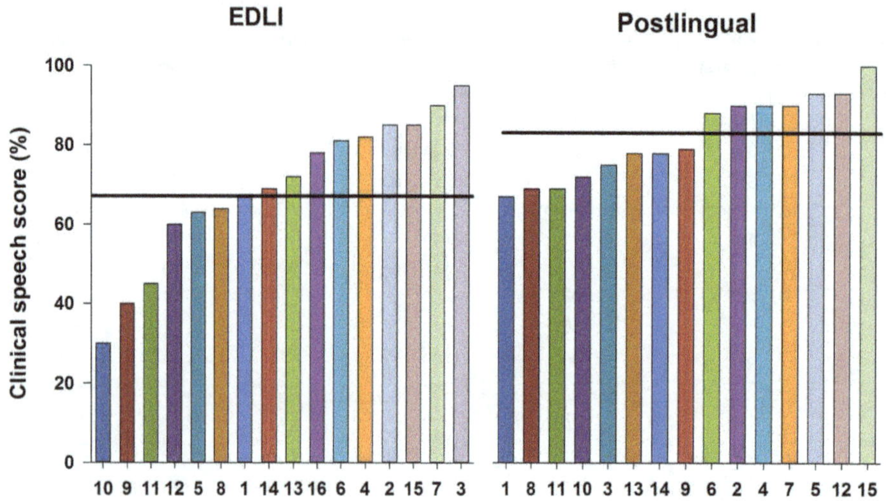

FIGURE 1 | The clinical speech scores shown per individual for the EDLI participant group on the left and for the postlingually deafened control group on the right. The scores are arranged from lowest to highest score in each panel, from left to right. The numbers on the x-axis represent the individuals as numbered in **Tables 1**, **2**. The horizontal line represents the mean score per group.

difference between the clinical speech scores of the two groups [$F_{(1,29)} = -2.38$; $p = 0.02$].

The Medical Ethical Committee of the University Medical Center Groningen (UMCG) reviewed and approved the research protocol. Before data collection started, all participants were given detailed information about study protocols. All participants provided written informed consent in accordance with the Declaration of Helsinki. Financial reimbursement based on the protocol of the Otorhinolaryngology Department of UMCG was provided for participation.

General Procedures

There were two parts of the study. Subjective music appreciation was assessed via a questionnaire, which also included questions on satisfaction and listening habits. Music perception was assessed via a psychophysical test, namely melodic contour identification.

Dutch Musical Background Questionnaire

The Dutch Musical Background Questionnaire (DMBQ) is a translated (to Dutch) and edited version of the Iowa Musical Background Questionnaire (Gfeller et al., 2000). The questionnaire has three parts that measure: satisfaction with listening to music, self-perceived quality of music, and self-reported perception of the elements of music.

In this study, we chose three outcome measures from within these parts of the questionnaire:

1. Self-perceived quality of music,
2. Satisfaction with listening to music,
3. Music listening habits.

We chose these outcome measures: first to be able to compare the outcomes with those of Fuller et al. (2013); second since these outcomes represent the subjective music appreciation and enjoyment, the second most important outcome factor after speech as reported by CI users (Gfeller et al., 2000; Drennan and Rubinstein, 2008; Philips et al., 2012).

Participants, following informed consent, filled the questionnaires via a website digitally either at home or on a laptop at the outpatient clinic. The total time to fill the questions was about 10 min. Thirteen EDLI participants and 11 post-lingual CI participants filled the questions.

Self-perceived quality of music

The self-perceived quality of music is an indication of how music sounds under the best conditions with a CI. Visual analog scales (VASs) are used for 14 opposite adjective descriptors (unpleasant-pleasant, mechanical-natural, fuzzy-clear, does not sound like music-sounds like music, complex-simple, difficult to follow-easy to follow, dislike very much-like very much). The 10 centimeter scales range from 0 (negative quality) to 10 (positive quality). In this study, an average across the seven scales was taken to quantify the self-perceived quality of music.

Satisfaction with listening to music

The satisfaction of listening to music after implantation was measured using one item. The question was: Indicate which statement best describes how your enjoyment of listening to music has or has not changed after implantation. CI users could score three different outcomes:

1) Little or no satisfaction with listening to music,
2) The sound of music is okay or improving over time,
3) Music sounds pleasant.

The items were then scored on a scale of 0 (no satisfaction) to 2 (most satisfaction).

Music listening habits
Habits for listening to music were compared between before (retrospectively) and after implantation in both groups. Two questions were used:

1) I would describe myself as a person who often chooses to listen to music.
   Respondents indicated their agreement with the statement on a rating scale of one ("strongly disagree") to four ("strongly agree").
2) How many hours per week do you listen to music?
   This was scored on a rating scale of one to four: one = 0–2 h, two = 3–5 h, three = 6–8 h, and four = more than 9 h.

By adding these two items, one score before and one score after implantation were calculated for music listening habits. The total score, thus, could range from 2 (min. music listening) to 8 (max. music listening).

Melodic Contour Identification

The Melodic Contour Identification (MCI) test was originally developed by Galvin et al. (2007) and used multiple times in CI studies (Galvin et al., 2007, 2008, 2009, 2012; Fuller et al., 2014, 2018), measuring the identification of nine different melodic contours. By using different instruments the effect of timbre, and by using a masker contour the effect of melody masker can be investigated. The MCI test in this study was configured as in Fuller et al. (2014) to be able to compare the outcomes of our present study with our former study that measured MCI in postlingually deafened CI users. The test consisted of five-tone melodic contours with a total of nine different pitch directions: "Rising," "Flat," "Falling," "Flat-Rising," "Falling-Rising," "Rising-Flat," "Falling-Flat," "Rising-Falling," "Flat-Falling"). 220 Hz was the lowest note per contour. A 1, 2, or 3 semitone distance between the successive notes in the contours was used. Each note was 250 ms long, and the silent interval between notes was 50 ms. Two instruments were used: piano and organ, as in Galvin et al. (2008). MCI was measured with and without a competing contour, the "masker." The masker was always the "flat" contour played by the piano (Galvin et al., 2009). The maskers differed in pitch: a pitch [A3 (220 Hz)] overlapping with target, and another pitch [A5 (880 Hz)] non-overlapping with target. A total of six conditions were tested: (1) piano target alone (no masker), (2) piano target with the A3 piano masker, (3) piano target with the A5 piano masker, (4) organ target alone (no masker), (5) organ target with the A3 piano masker, and 6) organ target with the A5 piano masker. Both masker and target started at the same time, meaning the notes of both were played at the same time.

Melodic contour identification setup
The psychophysical test MCI was conducted in an anechoic chamber at UMCG. Participants were asked to set their CI to their normal daily modus and volume. This setting was not changed during testing. In case of a bimodal participant, they were asked to remove the hearing aid from the contralateral ear during testing. CI users were seated facing a single speaker (Tannoy Precision 8D; Tannoy Ltd., UK) at one-meter distance. The stimuli were presented using MATLAB 2016a (The Mathworks, inc., USA) implemented on a Mac computer (MacOS, El Capitain; Apple, California, USA) and via an Audiofire 4 Audio Recording Interface with preamplification (Echo Audio Corporation, California, USA) and a DA10 digital-to-analog converter (Lavry Engineering Inc.). The stimuli were presented at 65 dB SPL, indicating an audible and comfortable, daily level of loudness. Furthermore, this level is in line with former studies, making a fair comparison possible. After an update of testing room, the stimuli were presented using an Apple Mac mini (MacOS, High Sierra; Apple, California, USA), MATLAB 2018a (The Mathworks, inc., USA), and a MOTU UltraLite-mk4 soundcard.

Melodic contour identification procedure
The contours were visually depicted on a touchscreen monitor [GPEG AOD (Advantech, USA)], which was placed 1 m in front of the participant. After listening to the audio contours, the participants directly indicated via the touchscreen the matching visual contour on the screen, and the results were stored immediately via MATLAB. During training, the participants identified one round of nine contours using three repetitions, a total of 27 contours per instrument without the masker, during which visual feedback was provided. The order of testing during data collection was: piano without a masker, then with the piano with A3, followed by the piano with the A5 masker. After the three piano conditions the same procedure was followed for the organ. During data collection, the nine contours were presented in random order, and were repeated three times per round, thus 27 contours per round. A total of $6 \times 27 = 162$ contours were played in the testing phase, during which no feedback was provided. A percentage correctly identified contours was calculated per condition by the MATLAB software automatically. The total testing time was 30 min.

Statistics
IBM SPSS Statistics 23 was used for the statistical analysis. *T*-tests defined the differences between the groups for the outcomes of the questionnaires. Split-plot repeated measures analysis of variance (ANOVA) was used to analyse the differences between the EDLI group and the postlingually deafened CI users for MCI with a Greenhouser-Geisser correction. Within subject factors were presence of masker (masker, no masker) and instrument (piano, organ). For the satisfaction with listening to music comparison between both groups a Chi-square test with a Monte Carlo simulation was run. For listening habits a Kruskal-Wallis test was computed. Two-tailed Pearson correlations were conducted between the subjective and psychophysical outcomes. A $p < 0.05$ was considered significant.

RESULTS

Subjective—Dutch Musical Background Questionnaire

Self-Perceived Quality of Music

Figure 2 shows the results for the self-perceived quality of music for the EDLI group (in red) and postlingually deafened CI users (in white). Results show a higher perceived quality of the sound

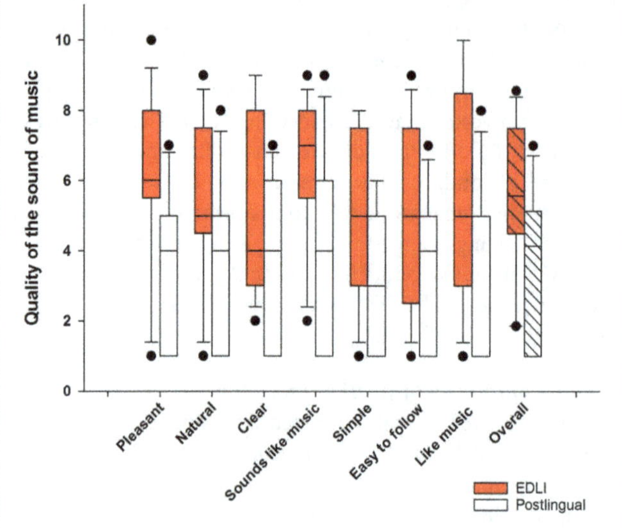

FIGURE 2 | The self-perceived quality of music for EDLI (in red) and postlingually deafened CI users (in white). The boxes represent the 25–75 percentile, the lines the median values, and the error bars the 10–90 percentile. The dots indicate the outliers.

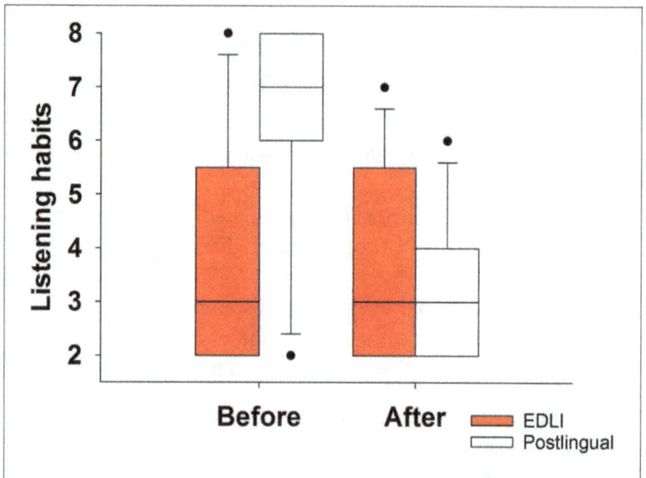

FIGURE 3 | The music listening habits before and after implantation for EDLI and postlingually deafened CI users. The box descriptions are similar to those of **Figure 2**.

TABLE 3 | The percentages of both groups for the satisfaction with listening to music after implantation.

	EDLI (n = 13)	Postlingual (n = 11)
Little or no satisfaction with listening to music	31% (n = 4)	8% (n = 1)
The sound of music is okay or improving over time	46% (n = 6)	92% (n = 10)
Music sounds pleasant	23% (n = 3)	0% (n = 0)

of music for EDLI CI users compared to postlingually deafened CI users. To calculate whether there is a difference in overall quality of music, we averaged over all seven scales to create an overall quality of music outcome score (boxes most on the right side in **Figure 2**). An analysis of variance (ANOVA) with group as a between-subjects factor and the quality of music as within-subjects factor was performed. A significant main effect for group was shown [$F_{(1,22)}$ =6.41, p = 0.02]. No significant effect was shown for the quality of music or the interaction between group and quality of music. It should be noted that not all participants filled the questionnaires. For the EDLI group 13 participants filled the questionnaire, in the control group 11.

Satisfaction With Listening to Music

Table 3 shows the percentages of both groups for the satisfaction with listening to music after implantation. Notable is the difference in distribution between the two groups, as almost all postlingually deafened CI users are in the second category and none in the last, while the EDLI CI users are diffuse across all three categories. Further, 23% of EDLI CI participants reported music to sound pleasant while no postlingual CI participant reported music to sound pleasant. A Chi-square test with a Monte Carlo simulation was run that showed a significant difference in the distribution between the groups X^2 $(2, N = 24 = 5.67, p = 0.049)$.

Music Listening Habits

Figure 3 shows the self-reported music listening habits before and after implantation for EDLI CI users and postlingual CI users. Postlingually deafened CI users reported to listen to music more before implantation compared to the EDLI participants, but they reported their listening habits drop after implantation. A Kruskal Wallis test was performed to compare the listening habits before and after implantation between the groups. A significant difference was shown before implantation $(1, N = 24 = 8.22, p = 0.04)$ and no difference after implantation $(1, N = 24 = 0.035, p = 0.85)$.

Psychophysical—Melodic Contour Identification

Figure 4 shows the results for the MCI test for piano and organ (left and right panels, respectively). The three different conditions from left to right are: no masker, A3 overlapping pitch masker, A5 non-overlapping pitch masker. Performance was worst for the overlapping pitch condition for both instruments in both groups. A split-plot repeated measure analysis of variance (RM ANOVA) with group (two levels; EDLI, postlingually deafened) as between-subjects factor, and instrument (two levels; piano, organ) and masker (three levels; no masker, A3 masker, and A5 masker) as within-subjects factors was performed. The complete analysis is shown in **Table 4**. There were main significant effects for instrument [$F_{(1,29)} = 6.03; p < 0.02$], with the organ being the best recognized instrument, and masker [$F_{(1.61,46.57)} = 14.25; p < 0.001$], with the A3 masker being the most difficult condition. No significant main effect was found for group [$F_{(1,29)} = 0.10; p = 0.76$]. No significant interactions were observed. The observed power was low for the group effect, indicating that larger participant groups would be needed for a potential difference between the two groups' performance.

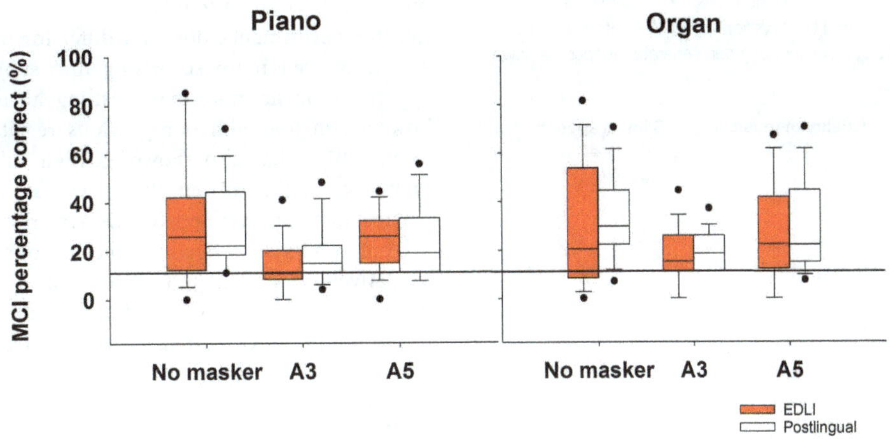

FIGURE 4 | The average percentage correct scores for the melodic contour identification for the piano (left) and organ (right) shown for both groups. From left to right in each panel the masker is shown: no masker, A3 overlapping pitch masker, A5 non-overlapping pitch masker. The box descriptions are similar to those of **Figure 2**. The thick horizontal line represents chance level.

TABLE 4 | The results of the split-plot repeated measures ANOVA for MCI.

Between-subjects factor		Observed power
Group	$F_{(1,29)} = 0.10; p = 0.76$	0.06
Within-subjects factors		
Instrument	$F_{(1,29)} = 6.03; p < 0.02^*$	0.66
Masker	$F_{(1.61,46.67)} = 14.25; p < 0.001^*$	0.99
Instrument x Masker	$F_{(1.89,54.68)} = 0.26; p = 0.72$	0.01
Instrument x Group	$F_{(1,48)} = 0.45; p = 0.51$	0.10
Masker x Group	$F_{(1.61,46.57)} = 0.26; p = 0.72$	0.09
Instrument x Masker x Group	$F_{(1.89,54.68)} = 1.01; p = 0.37$	0.21

**significant ($p < 0.05$).*

Correlations Between Subjective and Psychophysical Measures

A correlational analysis using Spearmans correlation test (two-tailed) was performed between the overall reported music quality and the outcomes of the MCI and the clinical speech scores for both groups (see **Table 5**). No systematic correlations were found. For EDLI participants, a significant positive correlation between the quality of music and the piano A3 masker was shown, but none with the clinical speech scores. For the postlingually deafened participants, no correlations were shown between the subjective and psychophysical measures.

DISCUSSION

The purpose of the study was to investigate the subjective music appreciation and psychophysical music perception in EDLI CI users and to compare these results to the more typical group of postlingually deafened CI users. Most of previous research with EDLI CI users had been done on speech perception. Even though implantation outcome or speech perception were not part of inclusion criteria in the present study, our observations based on clinical speech scores using phoneme-in-word identification were in line with this previous literature on EDLI implant users; our test group of EDLI users perform lower on the clinical speech perception test than our postlingually deafened control CI users and the test group shows a wider variation in outcomes. These differences likely indicate the effects from long-term auditory deprivation in EDLI participants. Based on the lower speech outcomes found in our study group and reported in literature (Teoh et al., 2004; Santarelli et al., 2008; van Dijkhuizen et al., 2011), we expected the EDLI participants to have lower performance in melody identification as well, especially since music is considered an even more complex acoustical signal than speech (McDermott, 2004; McDermott and Oxenham, 2008; Limb and Roy, 2014). Despite this expectation based on previous literature, Fuller et al. (2013) did, surprisingly, show that EDLI CI users subjectively report to enjoy listening to music more than postlingually deafened participants report. Consistently with our former study, EDLI participants of the present study also subjectively reported a higher quality of music than postlingually deafened CI users. There was no difference between the two groups in listening habits after implantation, whereas postlingually deafened CI users reported to listen to music before implantation significantly more than EDLI CI users. Interestingly, EDLI CI users reported to be more satisfied with listening to music after implantation compared to postlingual CI users. For the psychophysical test of music perception, namely, the melodic contour identification, against our expectation, EDLI implant users performed as well as postlingually deafened CI users. EDLI participants thus scored the perceived quality of music higher, and reported to be more satisfied with listening to music than postlingual CI participants, even though the psychophysical music outcomes for MCI were comparable between the groups.

Subjective Results—Dutch Musical Background Questionnaire

Psychophysically both groups performed the same for music perception, but subjectively, surprisingly, EDLI users judged the overall, subjective quality of music significantly higher

TABLE 5 | Correlational analyses between the subjective outcomes of the quality of music clinical speech scores, and the psychophysical MCI outcomes for both piano and organ, shown for EDLI and control group separately (upper and lower parts, respectively).

EDLI	Quality of music	Clinical speech scores
Piano	$r = 0.574$	$r = 0.240$
	$p = 0.07$	$p = 0.48$
	$N = 11$	$N = 11$
Piano A3 masker	$r = 0.683$	$r = -0.04$
	$p = 0.02$*	$p = 0.90$
	$N = 11$	$N = 11$
Piano A5 masker	$r = 0.447$	$r = 0.349$
	$p = 0.17$	$p = 0.29$
	$N = 11$	$N = 11$
Organ	$r = 0.480$	$r = 0.321$
	$p = 0.14$	$p = 0.34$
	$N = 11$	$N = 11$
Organ A3 masker	$r = 0.453$	$r = 0.244$
	$p = 0.16$	$p = 0.47$
	$N = 11$	$N = 11$
Organ A5 masker	$r = 0.455$	$r = 0.304$
	$p = 0.16$	$p = 0.36$
	$N = 11$	$N = 11$
Clinical speech scores	$r = -0.033$	X
	$p = 0.92$	X
	$N = 13$	X
Postlingual		
Piano	$r = -0.333$	$r = 0.191$
	$p = 0.32$	$p = 0.57$
	$N = 11$	$N = 11$
Piano A3 masker	$r = 0.148$	$r = 0.317$
	$p = 0.66$	$p = 0.34$
	$N = 11$	$N = 11$
Piano A5 masker	$r = 0.181$	$r = 0.234$
	$p = 0.59$	$p = 0.49$
	$N = 11$	$N = 11$
Organ	$r = -0.131$	$r = 0.027$
	$p = 0.70$	$p = 0.94$
	$N = 11$	$N = 11$
Organ A3 masker	$r = 0.037$	$r = 0.092$
	$p = 0.91$	$p = 0.79$
	$N = 11$	$N = 11$
Organ A5 masker	$r = 0.143$	$r = 0.119$
	$p = 0.68$	$p = 0.73$
	$N = 11$	$N = 11$
Clinical speech scores	$r = -0.084$	X
	$p = 0.81$	X
	$N = 11$	X

*significant.

than postlingually deafened CI users. Thus, our clinical speech outcomes, which were significantly lower for EDLI group than that of the postlingual control group, confirmed our group to be an EDLI group that fits with the lower expected outcomes from literature. In contrary to this expectation, it is a surprising finding that the performance does not differ for melody identification, and it is even more surprising that subjectively EDLI users appreciate music more than postlingual users. This finding is, however, in line with our previous results reported in Fuller et al. (2013) that also showed a high subjective appreciation of music. In the current study, we included only four EDLI participants that overlapped with our previous study, hence the present results successfully replicated our former results with a relatively new EDLI test population. The positive subjective music appreciation shown by Fuller et al. (2013) and replicated in our study, hence, provide strong evidence that EDLI have a more positive experience of music with the implant.

Not only the quality of music is more positively judged by the ELDI group, but there was also a higher satisfaction with listening to music with the implant. Compared to our former study the EDLI participants of this study are less satisfied; while in this study 23% ticked the "music sounds pleasant" box 60% did so in the previous study. This is however still more positive than the postlingually deafened participants, since none of them indicated that music sounds pleasant. Supporting the latter, other studies have also shown multiple times that the typical CI user is unsatisfied with listening to music (Gfeller et al., 2000; Lassaletta et al., 2008b; Looi and She, 2010).

One might argue that these differences are due to a lack of musical memory from acoustic hearing in EDLI CI users, and that therefore they judge the quality of music to a different scale than postlingually deafened CI users that likely use acoustical music memory as an anchor for their judgments of music quality with an implant (Galvin et al., 2009; Limb and Roy, 2014). Two observations from this study give support to this idea. Firstly, while postlingual CI users reported a large drop in their music listening habits from pre- to post-implantation, EDLI participants reported no change in music listening from pre- to post-implantation. Hence, it is possible that this relative negative change in music listening in postlingual group is an indication of less appreciation of music post-implantation in comparison to pre-implantation acoustic hearing, while EDLI show no such effect. Secondly, that there were no systematic correlations between subjective music appreciation measures and psychophysically measured MCI scores perhaps also indicate that what is subjectively reported relies more on psychological factors, instead of actual perceptual performance with music. On the other hand, alternatively, another influencing factor might be specific to our test population at UMCG, due to our clinical implantation protocol at our implant center in Groningen. The clinical protocol calls for a strict selection of implant candidates and only the EDLI candidates with best SIR scores are implanted. As a result, potentially some of our EDLI participants might have had some acoustic input with a (likely power) hearing aid, as vibrations of low frequencies, or some hearing with very loud music. Of course, given the level of hearing loss reported by participants or in the medical charts for this group, likely the quality of music via these means was different than that with a CI. Most postlingually deafened CI users definitely had a longer period of usable acoustical hearing and thus richer musical experience than the EDLI participants. For clinical speech scores, however, we did find a difference between the two groups, showing the EDLI perform worse for speech perception, perhaps due to a different language acquisition experience during childhood, and in line with what literature suggests. For music perception, however, there might be another explanation. Perhaps the auditory pathways that are involved in the processing of music in the brain: (1) for the actual perception for music; and (2) for the rewarding system related to music appreciation (Blood et al., 1999; Blood and Zatorre, 2001; Peretz et al., 2001), might have been developed differently in EDLI individuals. The limbic and reward regions can cause an emotional response to listening to music, which can be related to familiarity of the musical excerpt (Pereira et al., 2011). If familiarity combined with a musical memory plays a role in the emotional, subjective reaction to music, this might be one of the factors contributing to the difference in music appreciation between the EDLI group and the postlingually deafened participants. Since EDLI CI users have a non-existing or minimal acoustical musical memory, the emotional reaction is supposedly not largely driven by the familiarity from the acoustical memory, but only by the musical memory developed with the CI. Furthermore, this rewarding system might have only been built with the CI, causing only familiarity with listening to music with the CI. Together these experiences might create a more positive response in EDLI participants than postlingually deafened participants for listening to music with a CI.

Listening Habits

The self-reported post-implantation listening habits did show a difference between the two groups of CI users. For postlingually deafened CI users, a decline in listening habits after implantation was shown, as was previously found in various studies (Gfeller et al., 2000; Mirza et al., 2003; Lassaletta et al., 2008a; Migirov et al., 2009; Looi and She, 2010; Philips et al., 2012). This decrease is probably caused by the different experience of listening to music via electrical hearing post-implantation compared to acoustical hearing pre-implantation in this group. There was no significant difference in reported listening habits between the two groups after implantation. Since there was no difference between the two groups in post-implantation listening habits one might argue that there might be other reasons, apart from quality of the sound, or the satisfaction, that cause the (relatively) small amount of time spent on listening to music with a CI. Perhaps listening to music is just very effortful with a CI for all CI users. Since we know the complexity of music makes CI users to perform lower on music identification compared to NH listeners (McDermott and Oxenham, 2008; Limb and Roy, 2014), subjectively CI users also report to prefer less complex music categories compared to NH listeners (Veekmans et al., 2009). Perhaps music is, as is speech in noise perception (Cullington and Zeng, 2011), such an effortful task for CI users, something CI users cannot simply afford to do for many hours a day. A last argument might be that EDLI CI users, since they were suffering from (severe) hearing loss for most of their lives, still do not listen often to music with the implant, as it has not been a large part of their daily life anyway and therefore they simply listen as much as they do before implantation. Last, the EDLI participants were younger then the postlingually deafened CI users and might for this reason appreciate music more, as was shown by Mirza et al. (2003) who showed that younger CI users enjoy music more. Concluding, EDLI CI users show a more positive appreciation of music than postlingually deafened CI users, yet, no differences for listening habits with the implant have been found.

Psychophysical—Melodic Contour Identification

Based on the poorer average implantation outcomes in EDLI CI users for clinical speech perception scores, we expected our EDLI group to also perceive music less well than postlingually deafened CI users. Surprisingly, however, the EDLI and postlingually deafened CI users performed evenly on the melody identification test. The piano was the most difficult instrument to recognize, and the A3 masker with overlapping ground note the most difficult condition for both instruments. The results for the postlingually deafened CI users are in line with former studies (Galvin et al., 2007, 2008, 2009; Fuller et al., 2018). The performance in CI users is lower than in NH listeners that score for all conditions with a mean ranging from 71 (for piano A3) to 80% (for organ without a masker) (Fuller et al., 2014). One interpretation for the lack of difference in performance between the groups might be that the task does not depend on former acoustical, musical input over many years. Some basic pitch perception ability seems to be already developed early in human life. For example, it has been shown in 5 to 11 months old infants that they are capable of distinguishing differing pitch contours, most likely based on sensitivity to temporal cues (Jusczyk and Krumhansl, 1993; Trehub and Hannon, 2006). A well-known example is children preferably listen to child-directed speech, which has exaggerated pitch contours, over adult-directed speech (Fernald and Kuhl, 1987). Given the MCI task stimuli were basic MIDI melodies with no temporal, spectral, vocal, instrumental etc. complexity, perhaps EDLI CI users can sufficiently rely on such an early-developed ability when performing the MCI task with the CI, as do postlingually deafened CI users.

Another reason might be that perhaps the MCI task is independent of the period of auditory deprivation and a different auditory pathway. Perhaps the MCI task measures the ability of the naïve CI user for detection of a semitone sequence; or the MCI captures the real limitations of electric hearing, and does not depend on the differences in auditory pathways, auditory deprivation, or age of deafness. This, however, is contradicted by the finding that MCI performance can be trained in CI users (Galvin et al., 2007, 2012; Patel, 2014; Fuller et al., 2018). One might therefore expect a postlingually deafened participant to have a better auditory pathway for semitone detection than an EDLI CI user. Perhaps in future studies different materials that use more complex melodies, real life music excerpts, or using a range of musical instruments, would show a difference between the groups.

Correlations

To investigate whether the subjective and psychophysical outcomes in our study were associated, and if potential musical appreciation judgment was based on how well a CI user does with music perception, we correlated the subjective measures with the psychophysical measures for melody identification and clinical phoneme identification for both groups. We ran multiple tests, which only showed one significant correlation, something that might be caused by multiple testing, or might be caused by the size of our groups, causing our study to be possibly underpowered. Therefore, we conclude that no systematic correlations were shown. Even though differences were shown between the subjective judgment of both groups, and no differences between the psychophysical behavior, hence, no correlation was shown between the subjective measures and the psychophysical measures.

For speech perception, based on clinical speech scores, also, no correlations with MCI performance or music appreciation were shown for both groups. For the EDLI group this is in line with our former study, where also no correlation was shown between speech perception and music appreciation, but what is newly shown here is the finding that this also does not correlate with MCI performance. Since MCI only measures one aspect of music perception, melody recognition, and it does not measure any other aspects of music, perhaps it is difficult to relate to more real-life outcomes as speech perception and subjective music appreciation, which cover larger aspects of these auditory domains. For postlingually deafened CI users, however, some studies had indicated music perception to be correlated to speech perception. Galvin et al. (2007) specifically showed a correlation between vowel recognition and MCI performance. In their study, the range of semitones used, however, was wider (1–5) and therefore overall performance for MCI was higher, compared to our study where we only used a 1–3 semitone distance, the most difficult test settings. Additionally, our clinical speech perception test is not a vowel test, but a phoneme recognition task. It is possible that identification of an isolated vowel relies more on better decoding of phonetic sounds of speech while identifying phonemes embedded in meaningful words engage other and higher-level mechanisms of speech processing, where other linguistic cognitive factors, such as use of lexical knowledge and context, also play a role.

Another factor of influence is the lack of statistical power due to the limited number of participants in the study and the multiple tests that were run. This might give a biased result for the correlations. In future a higher number of participants is needed to draw a certain conclusion about the correlations between the behavioral and subjective data.

Still, the surprising lack of correlations might indicate that subjective judgment of music appreciation is not entirely determined by perception accuracy, as measured by psychophysical outcomes in both groups, indicating that appreciation is perhaps based on more psychological factors.

Early-Deafened, Late-Implanted Cochlear Implant Users

A potential selection bias is present in our study, even though inclusion criteria for EDLI target group were well-defined based on literature, and average clinical speech score of EDLI group was significantly lower than the average score of the control group, again as would be expected from literature. The source of this potential bias is that EDLI candidates are selected and counseled by our implant team based on certain pre-implantation criteria. For example, based on van Dijkhuizen et al. (2011) who found that the SIR score is related to a better post-implantation speech perception outcome, only participants with a SIR-score 3 or higher are selected for implantation as part of the clinical procedure. A SIR-score 3 or higher indicates that the implant candidate's spontaneous speech is understandable, if necessary, that the listener (speech therapist) is concentrating and perhaps reading lips. Below the score 3, implantation candidate's speech is not understandable, apart from a few words or parts of words. This might have introduced some bias in our study, as our test group perhaps included individuals with the best intelligible speech production. We are aware from the clinical records that there are also EDLI implantees that do not use their CI due to a (either subjective or objective, or both) lack of implantation gain, and EDLI implantees that do not perform well for speech outcomes, but still use the device for sound perception/awareness only. None of these implantees volunteered for this study, leading to EDLI participants who had meaningful clinical speech scores (>30%). Therefore, the EDLI cases of no implant use or no measurable or minimal speech outcome are not represented within our EDLI test group of the present study.

Whether the selection of implantees based on speech scores might have an influence on the music perception and appreciation scores is unknown. An interesting follow-up question might be whether implantees with a SIR-score lower than two, would show the same perceptional and subjective outcomes (related to music) as implantees with a higher SIR-score.

Last, it should be noted that, despite our efforts of matching ages of the two groups, our EDLI users were younger in general than the postlingually deafened control group. Age might therefore be an influencing factor on the outcomes of our study, as a younger age was shown to potentially contribute to higher and better speech and music perception outcomes with a CI in postlingually deafened participants (Sladen and Zappler, 2015).

All in all, the outcomes of this study support implantation in selected early deafened individuals, even after a (relatively long) duration of auditory deprivation. Potential benefits for implantation in EDLI group were supported by our study for music perception, both when subjectively and psychophysically measured. Many of our EDLI CI users, while as a group on average lower in clinical test scores than postlingual CI users, still showed relatively good speech perception benefit, and all EDLI participants had measurable clinical test scores. Hence, in addition to potential gain in speech understanding benefits from implantation, the comparable MCI performance, and the higher subjective judgment of music in EDLI participants indicate additional positive potential outcomes of implantation in this group.

ETHICS STATEMENT

The studies involving human participants were reviewed and approved by Medical Ethical Committee of the University Medical Center Groningen. The patients/participants provided their written informed consent to participate in this study. Written informed consent was obtained from the individual(s) for the publication of any potentially identifiable images or data included in this article.

AUTHOR CONTRIBUTIONS

CF performed the data analysis and wrote the first draft of the manuscript. All authors contributed to manuscript revision, read, approved the submitted version, contributed to conception, and design of the study.

ACKNOWLEDGMENTS

We would like to thank Alejandro Reina, Dana Kort, and Manon Koot for their help with the testing of the participants; John Galvin and Qian-Jie Fu for providing the MCI test.

REFERENCES

Başkent, D., Gaudrain, E., Tamati, T. N., and Wagner, A. (2016). "Perception and psychoacoustics of speech in cochlear implant users," in *Scientific Foundations of Audiology: Perspectives From Physics, Biology, Modeling, and Medicine*, eds A. T. Cacace, E. de Kleine, A. G. Holt, and P. van Dijk (San Diego, CA: Plural Publishing, Inc.), 285–319.

Blamey, P. (1997). Are spiral ganglion cell numbers important for speech perception with a cochlear implant? *Am. J. Otol.* 18 (6 Suppl.), S11–2.

Blamey, P., Artieres, F., Baskent, D., Bergeron, F., Beynon, A., Burke, E., et al. (2013). Factors affecting auditory performance of postlinguistically deaf adults using cochlear implants: an update with 2251 patients. *Audiol. Neurootol.* 18, 36–47. doi: 10.1159/000343189

Blood, A. J., and Zatorre, R. J. (2001). Intensely pleasurable responses to music correlate with activity in brain regions implicated in reward and emotion. *Proc. Natl. Acad. Sci.* 98, 11818–11823. doi: 10.1073/pnas.191355898

Blood, A. J., Zatorre, R. J., Bermudez, P., and Evans, A. C. (1999). Emotional responses to pleasant and unpleasant music correlate with activity in paralimbic brain regions. *Nat. Neurosci.* 2, 382–387. doi: 10.1038/7299

Bosman, A. J., and Smoorenburg, G. F. (1995). Intelligibility of Dutch CVC syllables and sentences for listeners with normal hearing and with three types of hearing impairment. *Audiology* 34, 260–284. doi: 10.3109/00206099509071918

Boucher, R., and Bryden, M. P. (1997). Laterality effects in the processing of melody and timbre. *Neuropsychologia* 35, 1467–1473. doi: 10.1016/S0028-3932(97)00066-3

Brockmeier, S. J., Peterreins, M., Lorens, A., Vermeire, K., Helbig, S., Anderson, I., et al. (2010). Music perception in electric acoustic stimulation users as assessed by the Mu.S.I.C. *Test. Cochlear Implants Hear. Preserve.* 67, 70–80. doi: 10.1159/000262598

Champoux, F., Lepore, F., Gagné, J., and Théoret, H. (2009). Visual stimuli can impair auditory processing in cochlear implant users. *Neuropsychologia* 47, 17–22. doi: 10.1016/j.neuropsychologia.2008.08.028

Connell, S. S., and Balkany, T. J. (2006). Cochlear implants. *Clin. Geriatr. Med.* 22, 677–686. doi: 10.1016/j.cger.2006.04.003

Cullington, H. E., and Zeng, F. G. (2011). Comparison of bimodal and bilateral cochlear implant users on speech recognition with competing talker, music perception, affective prosody discrimination, and talker identification. *Ear Hear.* 32, 16–30. doi: 10.1097/AUD.0b013e3181edfbd2

Drennan, W. R., and Rubinstein, J., T. (2008). Music perception in cochlear implant users and its relationship with psychophysical capabilities. *J. Rehabil. Res. Dev.* 45, 779–789. doi: 10.1682/JRRD.2007.08.0118

Fallon, J. B., Irvine, D. R. F., and Shepherd, R. K. (2008). Cochlear implants and brain plasticity. *Hear. Res.* 238, 110–17. doi: 10.1016/j.heares.2007.08.004

Fernald, A., and Kuhl, P. (1987). Acoustic determinants of infant preference for motherese speech. *Infant Behav. Dev.* 10, 279–293. doi: 10.1016/0163-6383(87)90017-8

Fuller, C. D., Galvin, J. J., Maat, A., Baskent, D., and Free, R. H. (2018). Comparison of two music training approaches on music and speech perception in cochlear implant users. *Trends Hear.* 22:2331216518765379. doi: 10.1177/2331216518765379

Fuller, C. D., Galvin, J. J., Maat, B., Free, R. H., and Başkent, D. (2014). The musician effect: does it persist under degraded pitch conditions of cochlear implant simulations? *Front. Neurosci.* 8:179. doi: 10.3389/fnins.2014.00179

Fuller, C. D., Mallinckrodt, L., Maat, B., Başkent, D., and Free, R. (2013). Music and quality of life in early-deafened late-implanted adult cochlear implant users. *Otol. Neurotol.* 34, 1041–1047. doi: 10.1097/MAO.0b013e31828f47dd

Galvin, J. J., Eskridge, E., Oba, S., and Fu, Q. J. (2012). Melodic contour identification training in cochlear implant users with and without a competing instrument. *Sem. Hear.* 33:399. doi: 10.1055/s-0032-1329227

Galvin, J. J., Fu, Q. J., and Nogaki, G. (2007). Melodic contour identification by cochlear implant listeners. *Ear Hear.* 28, 302–319. doi: 10.1097/01.aud.0000261689.35445.20

Galvin, J. J., Fu, Q. J., and Oba, S. (2008). Effect of instrument timbre on melodic contour identification by cochlear implant users. *J. Acoust. Soc. Am.* 124:EL189-95. doi: 10.1121/1.2961171

Galvin, J. J., Fu, Q. J., and Oba, S. I. (2009). Effect of a competing instrument on melodic contour identification by cochlear implant users. *J. Acoust. Soc. Am.* 125, EL98–103. doi: 10.1121/1.3062148

Gassner, H. G. K., Shallop, J., and Driscoll, C. L. W. (2005). Long-term clinical course and temporal bone histology after cochlear implantation. *Cochlear Implants Int.* 6, 67–76. doi: 10.1179/cim.2005.6.2.67

Gfeller, K., Christ, A., Knutson, J. F., Witt, S., Murray, K. T., and Tyler, R. S. (2000). Musical backgrounds, listening habits, and aesthetic enjoyment of adult cochlear implant recipients. *J. Am. Acad. Audiol.* 11, 390–406.

Gfeller, K., Witt, S., Woodworth, G., Mehr, M. A., and Knutson, J. (2002). Effects of frequency, instrumental family, and cochlear implant type on timbre recognition and appraisal. *Ann. Otol. Rhinol. Laryngol.* 111, 349–356. doi: 10.1177/000348940211100412

Gfeller, K. E., Olszewski, C., Turner, C., Gantz, B., and Oleson, J. (2006). Music perception with cochlear implants and residual hearing. *Audiol. Neurotol.* 11 (Suppl. 1), 12–15. doi: 10.1159/000095608

Goorhuis-Brouwer, S. M., and Schaerlaekens, A. M. (2000). *Taalpathologie En Taaltherapie Bij Nederlandssprekende Kinderen (Handbook Language Development, Language Pathology and Language Therapy in Dutch Speaking Children).* Utrecht, De Tijdstroom.

Gordon, K. A., Jiwani, S., and Papsin, B. C. (2013). Benefits and detriments of unilateral cochlear implant use on bilateral auditory development in children who are deaf. *Front. Psychol.* 4:719. doi: 10.3389/fpsyg.2013.00719

Heywood, R. L., Vickers, D. A., Pinto, F., Fereos, G., and Shaida, A. (2016). Assessment and outcome in non-traditional cochlear implant candidates. *Audiol. Neurotol.* 21, 383–390. doi: 10.1159/000454914

Jusczyk, P. W., and Krumhansl, C. L. (1993). Pitch and rhythmic patterns affecting infants sensitivity to musical phrase structure. *J. Exp. Psychol. Hum. Percept. Perform.* 19, 627–640. doi: 10.1037//0096-1523.19.3.627

Khan, A. M., Handzel, O., Burgess, B. J., Damian, D., Eddington, D. K., and Nadol, J. B. Jr., et al. (2005). Is word recognition correlated with the number of surviving spiral ganglion cells and electrode insertion depth in human subjects with cochlear implants? *Laryngoscope* 115, 672–677. doi: 10.1097/01.mlg.0000161335.62139.80

Lassaletta, L., Castro, A., Bastarrica, M., Perez-Mora, R., Herran, B., Sanz, L., et al. (2008a). Changes in listening habits and quality of musical sound after cochlear implantation. *Otolaryngol. Head Neck Surg.* 138, 363–367. doi: 10.1016/j.otohns.2007.11.028

Lassaletta, L., Castro, A., Bastarrica, M., Pérez-Mora, R., Herrán, B., Sanz, L., et al. (2008b). Musical perception and enjoyment in post-lingual patients with cochlear implants. *Acta Otorrinolaringol.* 59, 228–234. doi: 10.1016/S2173-5735(08)70228-X

Lassaletta, L., Castro, A., Bastarrica, M., Perez-Mora, R., Madero, R., De Sarria, J., et al. (2007). Does music perception have an impact on quality of life following cochlear implantation? *Acta Otolaryngol.* 127, 682–686. doi: 10.1080/00016480601002112

Lazard, D. S., Lee, H. J., Gaebler, M., Kell, C. A., Truy, E., and Giraud, A. L. (2010). Phonological processing in post-lingual deafness and cochlear implant outcome. *Neuroimage* 49, 3443–3451. doi: 10.1016/j.neuroimage.2009.11.013

Lazard, D. S., Vincent, C., Venail, F. P., Van de Heyning, Truy, E., Sterkers, O., et al. (2012). Pre-, per- and postoperative factors affecting performance of postlinguistically deaf adults using cochlear implants: a new conceptual model over time. *PLoS ONE* 7:e48739. doi: 10.1371/journal.pone.0048739

Leal, M. C., Shin, Y. J., Laborde, M., Calmels, M., Verges, S., Lugardon, S., et al. (2003). Music perception in adult cochlear implant recipients. *Acta Otolaryngol.* 123, 826–835. doi: 10.1080/00016480310000386

Limb, C. J., and Roy, A. T. (2014). Technological, biological, and acoustical constraints to music perception in cochlear implant users. *Hear. Res.* 308, 13–26. doi: 10.1016/j.heares.2013.04.009

Looi, V., Gfeller, K., and Driscoll, V. (2012). Music appreciation and training for cochlear implant recipients: a review. *Semin. Hear.* 33, 307–334. doi: 10.1055/s-0032-1329222

Looi, V., McDermott, H., McKay, C., and Hickson, L. (2008). Music perception of cochlear implant users compared with that of hearing aid users. *Ear Hear.* 29, 421–34. doi: 10.1097/AUD.0b013e31816a0d0b

Looi, V., and She, J. (2010). Music perception of cochlear implant users: a questionnaire, and its implications for a music training program. *Int. J. Audiol.* 49, 116–128. doi: 10.3109/14992020903405987

McDermott, H. J. (2004). Music perception with cochlear implants: a review. *Trends Amplif.* 8, 49–82. doi: 10.1177/108471380400800203

McDermott, J. H., and Oxenham, A. J. (2008). Music perception, pitch, and the auditory system. *Curr. Opin. Neurobiol.* 18, 452–463. doi: 10.1016/j.conb.2008.09.005

Medina, M., Polo, R., Gutierrez, A., Muriel, A., Vaca, M., Perez, C., et al. (2017). Cochlear implantation in postlingual adult patients with long-term auditory deprivation. 38:e248–e252. doi: 10.1097/MAO.0000000000001257

Migirov, L., Kronenberg, J., and Henkin, Y. (2009). Self-reported listening habits and enjoyment of music among adult cochlear implant recipients. *Ann. Otol. Rhinol. Laryngol.* 118, 350–355. doi: 10.1177/000348940911800506

Mirza, S., Douglas, S. A., Lindsey, P., Hildreth, T., and Hawthorne, M. (2003). Appreciation of music in adult patients with cochlear implants: a patient questionnaire. *Cochlear Implants Int.* 4, 85–95. doi: 10.1179/cim.2003.4.2.85

Nadol, J. B., Burgess, J. B., Gantz, J. B., Coker, J. N, Ketten, R. D, Kos, I., et al. (2001). Histopathology of cochlear implants in humans. *Ann. Otol. Rhinol. Laryngol.* 110, 883–891. doi: 10.1177/000348940111000914

Patel, A. D. (2014). Can non-linguistic musical training change the way the brain processes speech? The Expanded OPERA Hypothesis. *Hear. Res.* 308, 98–108. doi: 10.1016/j.heares.2013.08.011

Pereira, C. S., Teixeira, J., Figueiredo, P., Xavier, J., Castro, S. L., and Brattico, E. (2011). Music and emotions in the brain: familiarity matters. *PLoS ONE* 6:e27241. doi: 10.1371/journal.pone.0027241

Peretz, I., Blood, A. J., Penhune, V., and Zatorre, R. (2001). Cortical deafness to dissonance. *Brain* 124 (Pt 5), 928–940. doi: 10.1093/brain/124.5.928

Peterson, N. R., Pisoni, D. B., and Miyamoto, R. T. (2010). Cochlear implants and spoken language processing abilities: review and assessment of the literature. *Restor. Neurol. Neurosci.* 28, 237–250. doi: 10.3233/RNN-2010-0535

Philips, B., Vinck, B., De Vel, E., Maes, L., D'Haenens, W., Keppler, H., et al. (2012). Characteristics and determinants of music appreciation in adult CI users. *Eur. Arch. Oto-Rhino-Laryngol.* 269, 813–821. doi: 10.1007/s00405-011-1718-4

Salimpoor, V. N., Benovoy, M., Longo, G., Cooperstock, J. R., and Zatorre, R. J. (2009). The rewarding aspects of music listening are related to degree of emotional arousal. *PLoS ONE* 4:e7487. doi: 10.1371/journal.pone.0007487

Samar, V. J., and Metz, D. E. (1988). Criterion validity of speech intelligibility rating-scale procedures for the hearing-impaired population. *J. Speech Lang. Hear. Res.* 31, 307–316. doi: 10.1044/jshr.3103.307

Sandmann, P., Dillier, N., Eichele, T., Meyer, M., Kegel, A., Pascual-Marqui, R., et al. (2012). Visual activation of auditory cortex reflects maladaptive plasticity in cochlear implant users. *Brain* 135, 555–568. doi: 10.1093/brain/awr329

Santarelli, R. R., De Filippi, E., Genovese, and Arslan, E. (2008). Cochlear implantation outcome in prelingually deafened young adults. *Audiol. Neurotol.* 13, 257–265. doi: 10.1159/000115435

Seyyedi, M., Viana, L. M., and Nadol, J. B. Jr. (2014). Within-subject comparison of word recognition and spiral ganglion cell count in bilateral cochlear implant recipients. *Otol. Neurotol.* 35, 1446–1450. doi: 10.1097/MAO.0000000000000443

Sharma, A., Dorman, M. F., and Spahr, A. J. (2002). A sensitive period for the development of the central auditory system in children with cochlear implants: implications for age of implantation. *Ear Hear.* 23, 532–539. doi: 10.1097/00003446-200212000-00004

Sladen, D. P., and Zappler, A. (2015). Older and younger adult cochlear implant users: speech recognition in quiet and noise, quality of life, and music perception. *Am. J. Audiol.* 24, 31–39. doi: 10.1044/2014_AJA-13-0066

Teoh, S. W., Pisoni, D. B., and Miyamoto, R. T. (2004). Cochlear implantation in adults with prelingual deafness. part II. underlying constraints that affect audiological outcomes: cochlear implantation in adults with prelingual deafness. *Laryngoscope* 114, 1714–1719. doi: 10.1097/00005537-200410000-00007

Trehub, S. E., and Hannon, E. E. (2006). Infant music perception: domain-general or domain-specific mechanisms? *Cognition* 100, 73–99. doi: 10.1016/j.cognition.2005.11.006

van Dijkhuizen, J. N., Beers, M., Boermans, P. P., Briaire, J. J., and Frijns, J. H. (2011). Speech intelligibility as a predictor of cochlear implant outcome in prelingually deafened adults. *Ear Hear.* 32, 445–458. doi: 10.1097/AUD.0b013e31820510b7

van Dijkhuizen, J. N., Boermans, P. B., Briaire, J. J., and Frijns, J. H. M. (2016). Intelligibility of the patients speech predicts the likelihood of cochlear implant success in prelingually deaf adults. *Ear Hear.* 37:e302–10. doi: 10.1097/AUD.0000000000000286

Veekmans, K., Ressel, L., Mueller, J., Vischer, M., and Brockmeier, S. J. (2009). Comparison of music perception in bilateral and unilateral cochlear implant users and normal-hearing subjects. *Audiol. Neurootol.* 14, 315–326. doi: 10.1159/000212111

Waltzman, S. B., and Cohen, N. L. (1999). Implantation of patients with prelingual long-term deafness. *Ann. Otol. Rhinol. Laryngol.* 108(Suppl. 177), 84–87. doi: 10.1177/00034894991080S417

Waltzman, S. B., Roland, J. T. Jr., and Cohen, N. L. (2002). Delayed implantation in congenitally deaf children and adults. *Otol. Neurotol.* 23, 333–340. doi: 10.1097/00129492-200205000-00018

6

Multidimensional Timbre Spaces of Cochlear Implant Vocoded and Non-Vocoded Synthetic Female Singing Voices

Molly L. Erickson**, Katie Faulkner, Patti M. Johnstone, Mark S. Hedrick and Taylor Stone

Department of Audiology and Speech Pathology, University of Tennessee Health Science Center, Knoxville, TN, United States

***Correspondence:**
Molly L. Erickson
merickso@uthsc.edu

Many post-lingually deafened cochlear implant (CI) users report that they no longer enjoy listening to music, which could possibly contribute to a perceived reduction in quality of life. One aspect of music perception, vocal timbre perception, may be difficult for CI users because they may not be able to use the same timbral cues available to normal hearing listeners. Vocal tract resonance frequencies have been shown to provide perceptual cues to voice categories such as baritone, tenor, mezzo-soprano, and soprano, while changes in glottal source spectral slope are believed to be related to perception of vocal quality dimensions such as *fluty* vs. *brassy*. As a first step toward understanding vocal timbre perception in CI users, we employed an 8-channel noise-band vocoder to test how vocoding can alter the timbral perception of female synthetic sung vowels across pitches. Non-vocoded and vocoded stimuli were synthesized with vibrato using 3 excitation source spectral slopes and 3 vocal tract transfer functions (mezzo-soprano, intermediate, soprano) at the pitches C4, B4, and F5. Six multi-dimensional scaling experiments were conducted: C4 not vocoded, C4 vocoded, B4 not vocoded, B4 vocoded, F5 not vocoded, and F5 vocoded. At the pitch C4, for both non-vocoded and vocoded conditions, dimension 1 grouped stimuli according to voice category and was most strongly predicted by spectral centroid from 0 to 2 kHz. While dimension 2 grouped stimuli according to excitation source spectral slope, it was organized slightly differently and predicted by different acoustic parameters in the non-vocoded and vocoded conditions. For pitches B4 and F5 spectral centroid from 0 to 2 kHz most strongly predicted dimension 1. However, while dimension 1 separated all 3 voice categories in the vocoded condition, dimension 1 only separated the soprano stimuli from the intermediate and mezzo-soprano stimuli in the non-vocoded condition. While it is unclear how these results predict timbre perception in CI listeners, in general, these results suggest that perhaps some aspects of vocal timbre may remain.

Keywords: timbre, multidimensional scaling, cochlear implants, vocoding, singing voices

INTRODUCTION

Many post-lingually deafened adults who use cochlear implants (CIs) report that they no longer enjoy listening to music, and poor music perception is often reported as a significant negative factor in self-reported quality of life (Migirov et al., 2009). Cochlear implant signal processing favors the encoding of speech cues and allows users to perceive speech remarkably well using limited spectral and temporal acoustic information (Limb and Roy, 2014). While CI listeners may perceive speech well, some acoustic factors related to the perception of vocal timbre may not be adequately represented in the CI signal.

CI users have difficulty with many aspects of music perception. While rhythm cues are mostly preserved, CI users show deficits in the perception of pitch, melody, and timbre (Limb and Roy, 2014; Drennan et al., 2015; Jiam et al., 2017). Timbre is defined as that auditory attribute that distinguishes two sounds of equal pitch and loudness (ANSI, 1973). This definition must be modified a bit when discussing vocal timbre, which is that auditory attribute that distinguishes two vocal sounds of equal pitch and loudness that are also of approximately the same vowel. Vocal timbre is a perceptual attribute that is related to the acoustic characteristics of the output vocal signal and, therefore, is a function of the interaction of the glottal excitation source with the vocal tract transfer function (Cleveland, 1977; Sundberg, 1994, 2013; Roers et al., 2009).

Perceptually, differences in glottal excitation source spectral slope are believed to be related to the vocal quality dimension of *fluty* vs. *brassy* (Sundberg et al., 2004), while differences in overall resonance frequencies of the vocal tract have been shown to predict perception of Western classical voice categories such as mezzo-soprano and soprano (Cleveland, 1977; Dmitriev and Kiselev, 1979; Erickson, 2004). A clustering of the 3rd, 4th, and 5th resonances, known as the singer's formant cluster (Sundberg, 1974), is associated with perception of *ring* in the voice (Ekholm et al., 1998) and may be related to behavioral modification of vocal tract configuration in either the hypopharyngeal or epilaryngeal area (Sundberg, 1974; Mainka et al., 2015; Story, 2016).

Physiologically, singing voice production often differs greatly from speaking voice production, resulting in differences in timbre between the two modes of voice use. In singing, physiological changes in glottal excitation source, vocal tract length (VTL), and non-vowel related shape of the vocal tract can occur within any given singer based on numerous factors. A detailed description of these factors is beyond the scope of this paper; however, as a starting point, the reader is directed to Johan Sundberg's chapter in *The Psychology of Music* (Sundberg, 2013). Generally, these factors may be described as (a) variations across pitch and loudness (Echternach et al., 2016), (b) variations based on singing style (Sundberg et al., 1993, 1999; Thalén and Sundberg, 2001; Stone et al., 2003; Björkner, 2008; Borch and Sundberg, 2011; Bourne and Garnier, 2012; Guzman et al., 2015; Sundberg and Thalén, 2015; Yang et al., 2015; Bourne et al., 2016; Hallqvist et al., 2017), (c) variations based on vocal register (Titze, 1994; Sundberg and Kullberg, 1999; Sundberg and Högset, 2001; Roubeau et al., 2009), and (d) variations based on the need for a singer's formant cluster (Sundberg, 1974, 1994, 2001, 2013; Dmitriev and Kiselev, 1979; Bloothooft and Plomp, 1986; Barnes et al., 2004; Johnson and Kempster, 2011; Mainka et al., 2015; Story, 2016). Thus, while speakers may keep a relatively constant glottal excitation source spectral slope and exhibit relatively small variations in VTL during speech, successful professional singers must learn to purposefully modify both the glottal excitation source and the vocal tract filter, resulting in vocal productions that are physiologically, acoustically, and perceptually much different from those of speech in many cases. Singers learn to modify both the excitation source of their instrument and the shape of their instrument in order to (a) produce a timbre that is consistent with the desired singing style, and, for many styles, (b) enable the production of pleasing timbre across pitch.

Research examining how well CI users perceive vocal timbre has not been focused on singing voice perception, but instead has focused on speaking voice perception with special attention to talker or gender discrimination or identification. CI users have been shown to have difficulty discriminating speakers (Cleary and Pisoni, 2002; Vongphoe and Feng, 2005; Sjoberg et al., 2017) and, when there is overlap in fundamental frequency, gender (Fu et al., 2005). One aspect of vocal timbre concerns the perception of cues in the acoustic signal that are related to VTL. Recent research has shown that CI users exhibit deficits in their ability to extract VTL cues, which could be a factor contributing to poor speaker and gender identification (Kovačić and Balaban, 2009; Massida et al., 2013; Fuller et al., 2014; Gaudrain and Başkent, 2015; Gaudrain and Baskent, 2018; Zaltz et al., 2018) and could contribute to difficulties in singing voice timbre perception as well.

The primary source of information concerning VTL in singers comes from x-ray data of Western classical singers collected in Dresden during the 1950s (Roers et al., 2009) and by Dmitriev and Kiselev in the 1970s (Dmitriev and Kiselev, 1979). The Dresden x-ray data were collected with the larynx at rest; while the Dmitriev and Kiselev x-ray data were collected during singing. The Dresden data have been analyzed by researchers in Dresden and Stockholm (Roers et al., 2009) using the methods employed by Dmitriev and Kiselev. These researchers found that resting VTLs obtained from sopranos demonstrated a great deal of variability, ranging from just under 130 mm to just over 160 mm. On the other hand, the resting VTLs obtained from mezzo-sopranos demonstrated less variability, ranging from 145 mm to just over 160 mm. There was no statistically significant difference in resting VTL between the two groups. Resting VTL also did not correlate with body height. The data obtained by Dmitriev and Kiselev show a high degree of overlap in the singing VTL of mezzo-sopranos and central sopranos (167–183 mm vs. 168–185 mm, respectively), with only the high sopranos exhibiting much shorter VTLs (153–163 mm). If the central and high soprano data are merged, the variability in the singing VTLs obtained by Dmitriev and Kiselev becomes very similar to the variability in resting VTL observed in the Dresden data. Dmitriev and Kiselev also measured the frequency of "the high singing formants" that occur above 2 kHz and, similarly to the VTL data, observed overlap between mezzo-sopranos and sopranos; with only the high sopranos having distinctly higher upper formant frequencies.

When designing a timbre perception study, researchers can choose to implement an identification task and/or a discrimination task, depending on the goals of the study. Studies utilizing identification tasks in order to examine instrument timbre perception in CI users have found that, generally, when presented with a musical note or song performed on an instrument, CI users demonstrate reduced ability to correctly identify the instrument from either closed or open sets (Schulz and Kerber, 1994; Gfeller et al., 1998, 2002; McDermott, 2004; Looi et al., 2008; Kang et al., 2009). However, identification of a specific instrument requires semantic knowledge of the instrument and an understanding of how the semantic label relates to the acoustics of the instrument. Identification studies do not provide information concerning how well CI users may be able to utilize timbral cues to discriminate between instruments. Multidimensional scaling (MDS) studies, on the other hand, often employ discrimination tasks and allow for the mapping of perceptual spaces without requiring participants to have direct knowledge of semantic labels.

MDS has been used to map the perceptual timbre spaces of instruments (Grey, 1977; Iverson and Krumhansl, 1993; Krimphoff et al., 1994; McAdams et al., 1995; Marozeau et al., 2003; Handel and Erickson, 2004; Caclin et al., 2005) and singing voices (Bloothooft and Plomp, 1988; Erickson, 2003, 2008, 2016, 2020) in normal hearing (NH) populations. In general, MDS studies using real and synthetically constructed instrument tones have revealed that temporal envelope/attack-time (Grey, 1977; Krimphoff et al., 1994; McAdams et al., 1995) and spectral centroid (Grey and Gordon, 1978; Iverson and Krumhansl, 1993; Krimphoff et al., 1994; McAdams et al., 1995; Handel and Erickson, 2004) are the dominant cues for the perception of the dissimilarity of instruments by NH listeners. Additional dimensional correlates found in instrumental MDS studies include spectral fluctuation (Krumhansl, 1989) and frequency vibrato extent (Handel and Erickson, 2004). In singing voices, 1/3 octave spectra (Bloothooft and Plomp, 1988), spectral centroid from 0 to 5 kHz (Erickson, 2008, 2020), spectral centroid from 2 to 5 kHz (Erickson, 2003), and, at higher fundamental frequencies, spectral centroid from 0 to 2 kHz (Erickson, 2020) appear to provide cues useful in judging timbre dissimilarity in voices as does frequency vibrato rate (Erickson, 2003, 2008).

MDS has been used to assess the perception of instrument timbre in NH listeners using vocoded stimuli (Macherey and Delpeirre, 2013) and to assess the perception of instrument timbre in CI users (Kong et al., 2011; Macherey and Delpeirre, 2013). Kong et al. (2011) found that the MDS instrument space produced by pre-lingually and peri-lingually deafened CI users appeared to be most influenced by attack-time cues with spectral centroid cues being less reliable and potentially less salient. However, in a study that examined instrumental MDS dimensions generated by 4 groups (Migirov et al., 2009), NH listeners (Limb and Roy, 2014), NH listeners rating 4-channel vocoded stimuli, Jiam et al. (2017) NH listeners rating 8-channel vocoded stimuli, and (Drennan et al., 2015) post-lingually deafened CI listeners, Macherey and Delpierre (Macherey and Delpeirre, 2013) found similar MDS solutions for all four groups. Dimension 1 organized stimuli according to attack-time. Dimension 2 was correlated with spectral centroid. It should be noted, however, that the CI MDS solution accounted for a smaller amount of variance than did any of the NH solutions and that, contrary to expectations, CI listeners weighted the spectral centroid dimension more strongly and the attack-time dimension less strongly than normal hearing listeners. The results of these two studies suggest that CI listeners may be able to use cues such as attack-time and spectral centroid to discriminate some elements of instrumental timbre. How well these results would generalize to singing voices, which do not differ much in attack-time and which have spectral characteristics that may not differ as much as those found between major classes of instruments, is unknown.

For the current study, an 8-channel noise-band vocoder was used to simulate how CI sound processing alters the perceived timbre of synthetic female singing voices with vibrato for both lower and higher pitched stimuli. NH listeners were presented with both non-vocoded and vocoded synthetic stimuli to examine how their perceptual timbre space was affected by this simulation. It was hypothesized that at lower pitches, 8-channel vocoding would result in the loss of important spectral characteristics, resulting in alterations of the multidimensional perceptual space. However, it was also hypothesized that at higher pitches, the wide spacing of harmonics would cause an under-sampling of the vocal tract transfer function. This under-sampling could cause a lack of spectral peaks in both the non-vocoded and vocoded conditions, theoretically resulting in similar MDS representations in those two conditions.

MATERIALS AND METHODS

Listeners

All listeners provided written informed consent using a procedure approved by the Institutional Review Board of the University of Tennessee, Knoxville. Listeners were recruited from students enrolled in introductory psychology courses at the University of Tennessee, Knoxville and from faculty and students in the University of Tennessee Department of Audiology and Speech Pathology. Listeners were recruited who met the following criteria: (a) bilateral hearing within normal limits ($\geq$20 dB from 500 to 4000 Hz) (ASHA, 1990) and (b) 18 years of age or older. Listeners recruited from Psychology courses were awarded class credit for participating in the study. Psychology students can receive such credit by participating in a variety of studies as well as by writing papers on the topic of research design in lieu of participating in research studies. Thirty listeners were recruited for the experiment; however, one participant did not pass the hearing screening and was removed from the study, resulting in a final N of 29. There were 21 female and 8 male participants with a mean age of 20.17 years and an age range of 18–30 years.

Stimuli

Non-vocoded Synthetic Vocal Stimuli

Non-vocoded synthetic vocal stimuli were generated using a digital source-filter synthesizer. The synthesis model was built using Aladdin Interactive DSP workbench (Hi-Tech

Development, Stockholm, Sweden). Aladdin synthesizes at 16 kHz, so the resulting upper spectral limit was at the Nyquist frequency of 8 kHz.

For the pitches C4 (261.6 Hz), B4 (493.9 Hz), and F5 (698.5 Hz), signals to be used as input to the source-filter synthesizer (henceforth referred to as the excitation source) consisted of a number of harmonics equal to 8000 Hz divided by the fundamental frequency. These harmonics decreased in amplitude by 6 dB/octave, 9 dB/octave, and 12 dB/octave (**Figure 1**). The spectral slopes of these signals (excitation source spectral slopes) were calculated by adding lip radiation (+6 dB/octave) to glottal source spectral slopes that might be produced by female singers based on type or style of singing (12 dB/octave, 15 dB/octave, and 18 dB/octave). All stimuli were constructed with vibrato for the following reasons: (Migirov et al., 2009) due to the length of the study it would not have been possible to include vibrato and non-vibrato stimuli in the MDS analyses; (Limb and Roy, 2014) previous research utilizing non-vocoded and vocoded stimuli revealed nearly identical vibrato and non-vibrato MDS solutions (Jiam et al., 2017; Erickson and Faulkner, 2018); synthetic vibrato stimuli are much more naturalistic and less fatiguing than synthetic non-vibrato stimuli. Excitation source signals were synthesized using a frequency vibrato rate of 5.6 Hz and a frequency vibrato extent of ±50 cents (0.5 semitone). The vibrato rate and extent are values typical of Western classical singing (Hakes et al., 1987).

Excitation source signals were filtered using 3 vocal tract transfer functions, M (mezzo-soprano), S (soprano), and I (intermediate) for the vowel/ɑ/ (**Figure 2**). Each transfer function was constructed using a cascade synthesizer and 8 resonance frequencies. Although 5–6 resonance frequencies would typically fall below the Nyquist frequency of 8 kHz, 8 resonances were used during the synthesis process because vocal tract transfer functions are the sum of overlapping vocal tract resonance filters and, therefore, the transfer function below 8 kHz can be affected by higher resonances. Resonance bandwidths were set to those used in a previous study (Erickson, 2004). Resonance frequencies for the transfer functions M and S were derived from an operatic mezzo-soprano and an operatic light coloratura soprano, respectively, using the following procedure: (Migirov et al., 2009) an 18-pole linear predictive coding (LPC) analysis at the pitch A3 was used to compute preliminary resonance frequencies for the first 8 vocal tract resonances then (Limb and Roy, 2014) resonance frequencies were modified, when necessary, through use of an analysis by synthesis procedure such that the resulting synthetic output spectral peaks corresponded with those of the original target stimulus at pitch A3. Comparisons of the original and synthesized spectra revealed that changes to synthesis bandwidths were not necessary. An intermediate (I) vocal tract transfer function was constructed by calculating intermediate resonance frequencies as follows:

$$ST_I = .5\left(12log_2\frac{R_S}{R_M}\right) \quad (1)$$

$$R_I = R_M\left(2^{ST_I/12}\right) \quad (2)$$

where R_S = the soprano resonance frequency, R_M = the mezzo-soprano resonance frequency, ST_I = the number of semitones midway between R_S and R_M as measured in reference to R_M, and R_I = the resulting intermediate resonance frequency. Resonance frequencies for vocal tract transfer functions M, I, and S are displayed in **Table 1**.

The synthesis procedure resulted in 9 stimuli for each of the following three conditions: C4 not vocoded, B4 not vocoded, and F5 not vocoded. Using Adobe Audition (Salt Lake City, Utah), each stimulus was edited to 1 s in duration and smoothed using spline curves applied to the onsets and offsets, and then normalized in average RMS amplitude. As with real voices, the spectral characteristics of the resulting non-vocoded stimuli were a result of the interaction of the systematically varied

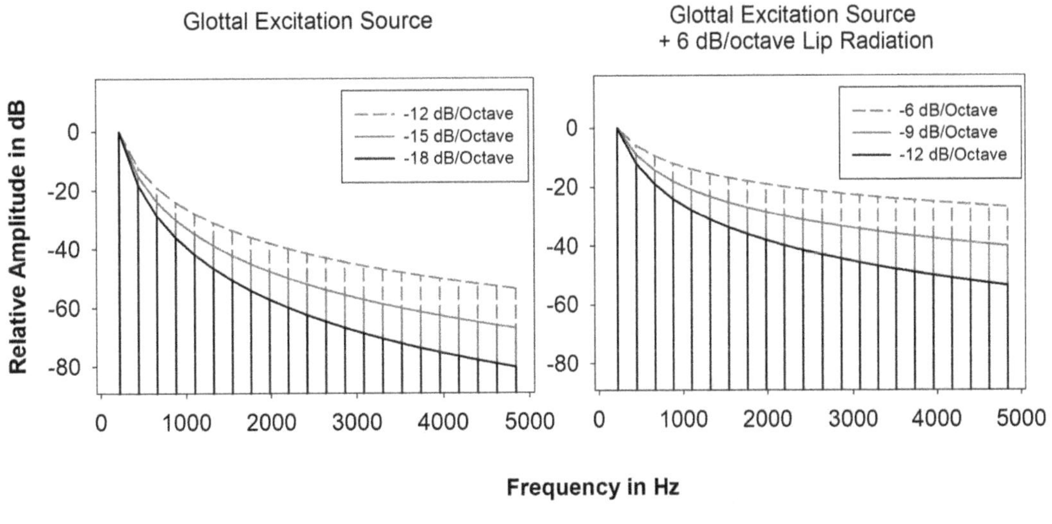

FIGURE 1 | Glottal excitation source spectral slopes without and with +6 dB/octave.

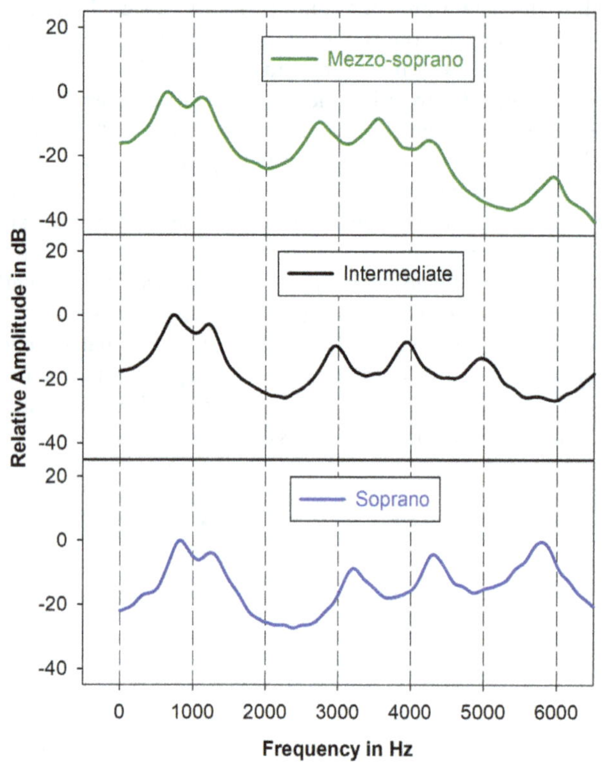

FIGURE 2 | Mezzo-soprano, intermediate, and soprano transfer functions below 6500 Hz. Transfer functions were obtained by stimulating the source-filter synthesizer with white noise and smoothing the output.

TABLE 1 | Resonance frequencies for mezzo-soprano (M), intermediate (I), and soprano (S) stimuli.

Resonance	Frequency in Hz		
	M	I	S
1	625	712	811
2	1158	1227	1300
3	2725	2960	3217
4	3550	3915	4317
5	4300	4991	5793
6	5927	6789	7774
7	7732	8982	10,432
8	10,087	11,882	13,999

excitation source signal and the systematically varied vocal tract transfer function.

Vocoded Stimuli

To create the vocoded stimuli, the 9 stimuli from each of the 3 non-vocoded conditions were processed through an 8-channel noise-band vocoder using the AngelSim^{TM} Cochlear Implant and Hearing Loss Simulator (TigerSpeech Technology, Los Angeles, CA, United States). Input stimuli were filtered into 8 frequency analysis bands using fourth-order band-pass Butterworth filters, the cutoff frequencies of which were determined by a Greenwood function. The temporal envelope in each band was extracted using half-wave rectification and a low-pass fourth-order Butterworth filter with a cutoff frequency of 160 Hz. As with the analysis filters, there were 8 fourth-order band-pass Butterworth carrier filters, the cutoff frequencies of which were identical to the analysis filters. The filtered carrier noise in each band was modulated by the extracted amplitude envelope in the same band. It should be noted that this results in a broadening of each frequency band. The final modulated noise bands were summed to create the vocoded stimuli. Analysis and carrier filter parameter settings are listed in **Table 2**. The vocoding procedure resulted in 9 stimuli for each of the following three conditions: C4 vocoded, B4 vocoded, and F5 vocoded. Vocoded stimuli were normalized in average RMS to the non-vocoded stimuli. Due to the length of the study, it was not possible to include multiple vocoder configurations. The results of this study should be interpreted with that limitation in mind. Also, it cannot be said that a noise-band vocoder would accurately reflect the signal received and processed by CI users.

Experimental Design

Multi-dimensional scaling techniques were employed to determine the perceptual dimensionality of the non-vocoded and vocoded synthetic vocal stimuli. For each of the six conditions, the 9 stimuli were combined into all possible pairs, resulting in a total of 36 pairs for each condition for a total of 216 experimental pairs. Additionally, a practice experiment was created from 20 pairs that spanned a variety of combinations of the experimental stimuli, resulting in 236 stimulus pairs total. A within-subjects designed was used where each participant completed all conditions.

Procedure

The listening experiment took place in a single-walled sound booth (Acoustic Systems RE-144-S, Austin, TX, United States). Stimuli were presented binaurally using Sennheiser HD 545 (Old Lyme, CT, United States) headphones. Prior to the practice session and experiment, listeners were told that they would hear two sounds and that it was their task to indicate how similar or different the two sounds were by using a scroll bar. They were told: (Migirov et al., 2009) if the two sounds were very different, they should drag the scroll bar toward the far right end (Limb and Roy, 2014); if the sounds were the same, they should drag

TABLE 2 | Vocoder analysis and carrier filter parameters of lower cutoff frequency (F_L), higher cutoff frequency (F_U), and bandwidth (ΔF) in Hertz and semitones.

Band	F_L in Hz	F_U in Hz	ΔF in Hz	ΔF in semitones
1	200.0	359.1	159.1	10.13
2	359.1	591.3	232.2	8.63
3	591.3	930.5	339.2	7.85
4	930.5	1425.8	495.3	7.39
5	1425.8	2149.1	723.3	7.10
6	2149.1	3205.3	1056.2	6.92
7	3205.3	4747.7	1542.4	6.80
8	4747.7	7000	2252.3	6.72

the scroll bar all the way to the far left; and (Jiam et al., 2017) if the difference was somewhere between those two extremes they should drag the scroll bar to a corresponding location somewhere between the two ends. Listeners were warned that each stimulus pair would play only once with no opportunity to repeat the pair, so they should be prepared to listen closely for upcoming pairs.

Stimulus pairs in both the practice session and the subsequent experimental session were presented using MEDS (Music Experiment Development System) (UCLA, Los Angeles), an object-oriented development system designed by Roger A. Kendall (Windsor, 2004) that has been widely used in the construction and analysis of perceptual and psychoacoustic experiments. Due to the length of the experiment, stimulus pairs were presented once only. Using a 100-point scroll bar with endpoints labeled "Same" and "Very Different," the listener's task was to indicate the dissimilarity of the paired stimuli. Prior to the MDS experiment, each participant completed the practice session which was composed of 20 randomly ordered stimulus pairs systematically selected to include very similar and very different stimuli of non-vocoded and vocoded pairs across all three pitches. Participant performance on the practice task was monitored and if the researcher felt that the participant did not understand the instructions, the participant was reminded of the experimental task as well as of how to use the scroll bar. After the practice session, listeners completed the MDS experiment. Listeners were presented with counter-balanced blocks, one for each of the six conditions (C4 not vocoded, C4 vocoded, B4 not vocoded, B4 vocoded, F5 not vocoded, and F5 vocoded). This within-subjects designed allowed each participant to act as their own control. Within each block, the 36 pairs were presented in random order.

Acoustic Measures

The current experiment employed several acoustic measures in order to identify those spectral cues that may correlate to specific MDS dimensions. The synthetic stimuli employed in this study have a fixed attack-time, so stimulus onset was not included as an acoustic variable. Because any spectral fluctuation would be a result of frequency modulation of the excitation source which was constant across all stimuli, this also was not included as an acoustic variable. In total, 4 acoustic measures were computed: spectral centroid from 0 to 8 kHz, spectral centroid from 0 to 2 kHz, spectral centroid from 2 to 8 kHz, and energy ratio. The method of calculation for each of these acoustic measures are described in the following sections. Each measure was calculated from the middle of the 1 s sample. All measures were made using the Fast Fourier Transform (FFT) algorithm provided by Praat (Paul Boersma and David Weenink, Institute of phonetic Sciences, University of Amsterdam, The Netherlands) using an analysis window of 0.75 s.

Spectral Centroid Measures

Spectral centroid, a measure of the weighted mean frequencies within a specified frequency range, is frequently used in studies of instrument acoustics (Iverson and Krumhansl, 1993; McAdams et al., 1995; Sandell, 1995; Lakatos, 2000; Schubert et al., 2004). However, this measure is not often used in the study of speaking voice acoustics, where due to the special nature of speech, resonance frequency measures obtained from LPC analysis or spectral peaks measured directly from the output spectral tend to be used. However, in female singing voices, it is difficult to obtain acoustic measures that directly correlate to actual resonance frequencies. As pitch increases, the increasingly wide spacing of harmonics makes it unlikely that these resonance peaks will be represented precisely in the acoustic output spectrum, particularly at fundamental frequency above 350 Hz (Monsen and Engebretson, 1983). For this reason, when vowel is constant, spectral centroid may provide a better measure of the center of spectral mass than those typically used for speech and is a measure that can be employed across the wide range of frequencies that span the female singing voice range. The current study employed three spectral centroid measures, spectral centroid from 0 to 8 kHz, spectral centroid from 0 to 2 kHz, and spectral centroid from 2 to 8 kHz. Spectral centroid from 0 to 8 kHz provides a measure that mathematically corresponds to the center of mass below 8000 Hz and is influenced both by the location of resonance frequencies and spectral slope. Spectral centroid from 0 to 2 kHz provides a measure of the center of mass in the range of the vowel formants. Spectral centroid from 2 to 8 kHz provides a measure of the center of mass in the upper frequencies, a range that has been shown to provide cues to classical singing voice categories when F1 and F2 frequencies are held constant (Berndtsson and Sundberg, 1995) and has been shown to correlate more strongly than other measures to voice category (Frič and Pavlechová, 2018). All spectral centroid measures were calculated after Sandell (1995) using the formula:

$$\frac{\sum_{k=1}^{N} e_k f_k}{\sum_{k=1}^{N} e_k} \qquad (3)$$

where e is the vector of spectral amplitude data points and f is the vector of spectral frequency data points.

Energy Ratio

The singing power ratio (SPR) has been shown to correlate with some aspects of the perception of singing vocal timbre (Omori et al., 1996; Watts et al., 2003). SPR, which is also the Hammarberg Index (Hammarberg et al., 1980) multiplied by -1, is calculated by measuring the ratio of power of the strongest harmonic in the 2–4 kHz frequency range to the power of the strongest harmonic in the 0–2 kHz frequency range and converting to decibels (dB). SPR provides a measure of the degree to which maximum power changes from one frequency range to another and, therefore, provides a measure of output spectral slope independent of the frequency location of spectral peaks. SPR is a difficult measure to employ for noise vocoded stimuli, so the current paper utilized a related output spectral slope measure that does not rely on the measurement of the amplitude of a specific harmonic, the energy ratio (ER). ER was calculated as the ratio of the total energy in the 0–2 kHz range to the total energy in the 2–8 kHz range in dB. Comparison of SPR and ER for the non-vocoded stimuli revealed high positive correlations between these two variables ($R = 0.990–0.999$, $p < 0.001$), suggesting that ER is an appropriate substitute for SPR in this study.

RESULTS

Reliability Analysis

Due to the length of the current study, listeners heard each stimulus once only, so it was not possible to conduct analyses of intra-rater consistency. Inter-rater consistency was measured through computation of intraclass correlation coefficients (ICCs) for each condition using a two-way, random-effects model. Because this study used responses averaged across all listeners (see section Multidimensional Scaling Analysis), the type of ICC employed was "the mean of *k* raters." This type of inter-rater ICC evaluated the consistency of mean responses and ranged from 0.930 to 0.958 (**Table 3**). High inter-rater ICCs based on the consistency of mean responses should not be misinterpreted as suggesting that each individual rater was consistent with all other raters, only that the average was consistent. Single-rater ICCs evaluate how reliable each listener is compared to the other listeners. Single-rater ICCs were poor, ranging from 0.315 to 0.437. Poor single-rater ICCs were not unexpected since each stimulus pair was played only once (see section Multidimensional Scaling Analysis).

Multidimensional Scaling Analysis

Six multidimensional scaling (MDS) analyses were conducted to determine the perceptual dimensionality of the vocal stimuli based on the average responses of listeners to the experimental task. Average responses were used due to the fact that participants heard each stimulus pair once only. By using data representing how an average listener might respond, the effect of response variability including mistakes due to fatigue or lapses of attention were minimized. Separate PROXSCAL analyses were performed for each condition, not vocoded and vocoded, at each pitch, C4, B4, and F5, using IBM SPSS Statistics version 24.0 (IBM, Armonk, NY, United States). All PROXSCAL analyses used ordinal distance measurements with ties allowed and Euclidian metrics. As suggested by Borg and colleagues (Borg et al., 2013), the following model options were used: (Migirov et al., 2009) stress convergence = 0.000001, (Limb and Roy, 2014) minimum stress = 0.0001, (Jiam et al., 2017) maximum iterations = 1000, and an initial model configuration set to multiple random starts = 5000. Because there were only 9 stimuli in each condition, all MDS models were restricted to 2 dimensions. Higher dimensional models would likely have resulted in nearly perfect, but meaningless, fit. A Kruskal's stress type 1 of 0.2 is considered to be a poor fit (Kruskal and Wish, 1978). Model fit was evaluated through analysis of Kruskal's Stress Type 1 (Kruskal, 1964), a measure of how well the MDS solution fits the actual data, and analysis of the amount of dispersion accounted for (DAF), a measure of the variance accounted for by the MDS solution (Borg et al., 2013). Analysis of Stress Type 1 scree plots (**Figure 3**) revealed that for most conditions the best and most parsimonious fit was achieved with 2 dimensions. A Kruskal's stress type 1 of 0.2 is considered to be a poor fit [27]. Analysis of DAF revealed that the 2-dimensional solutions accounted for over 98% of the variance in all conditions. Solutions for all 6 conditions are presented graphically in **Figure 3**. In this figure, as well as throughout the paper, the stimuli are labeled in a manner that indicates the synthesis parameters used to create the stimuli with a letter indicating the vocal tract transfer function (M = mezzo, I = intermediate, and S = light coloratura soprano) and a number indicating the excitation source spectral slope (glottal source spectral slope + lip radiation) in dB/octave (6, 9, and 12). PROXSCAL uses proximity matrices to find a default least squares solution that is arbitrary in orientation and rotationally invariant. All MDS solutions in **Figure 3** are presented in their default orientation except for condition B4 not vocoded, which was rotated counterclockwise 45%, and condition F5 vocoded, which was rotated 25% clockwise. Conditions B4 not vocoded and F5 vocoded displayed dimensionality that was nearly identical to other conditions; however, the dimensional organization was off-axis. Because the dimensionality of MDS solutions is arbitrary and rotationally invariant, rotation of aggregate MDS data points is allowed and is a common practice (Peay, 1988; Giguère, 2006; Borg et al., 2013). Without such rotation, it would not have been possible to compare solutions across conditions (Peay, 1988) or to conduct statistical analyses such as correlations or regressions (Borg et al., 2013). The rotation necessary to align these two off-axis conditions was determined by the following process: (Migirov et al., 2009) matrix rotation was applied using an initial ballpark direction and degree of rotation derived from visual inspection of the MDS plots and (Limb and Roy, 2014) a "brute force" procedure was applied using increments or decrements of 5 degrees until the alignment of data points for these two MDS solutions agreed with those obtain from other conditions.

TABLE 3 | ICC estimates of inter-rater consistency and their 95% confidence intervals based on a mean-rating (k = 29) 2-way random-effects model for all six conditions.

Condition	ICC	95% Confidence Interval	$F(14, 392)$	p
C4 Not vocoded	0.947	0.919–0.969	18.906	<0.001
C4Vocoded	0.930	0.893–0.959	14.327	<0.001
B4Not vocoded	0.954	0.929–0.973	21.715	<0.001
B4Vocoded	0.952	0.926–0.972	20.818	<0.001
F5Not vocoded	0.958	0.935–0.975	23.550	<0.001
F5Vocoded	0.943	0.913–0.967	17.650	<0.001

MDS Results

For both non-vocoded and vocoded conditions at the pitch C4, dimension 1 separated stimuli according to vocal tract transfer functions M, I, and S, while dimension 2 organized the stimuli according to excitation source spectral slope (glottal source spectral slope + lip radiation). The MDS solutions for vocoded stimuli at the higher pitches, B4 and F5 looked very similar to those obtained at the lower pitch, C4. Dimension 1 organized the stimuli according to vocal tract transfer function, M, I, and S, while dimension 2 organize the stimuli according to excitation source spectral slope. On the other hand, the MDS solutions for the non-vocoded stimuli at B4 and F5 looked quite different from those obtained at C4. Dimension 1 did not separate the 3 vocal tract transfer functions, but instead separated the soprano vocal tract transfer function from both the intermediate and

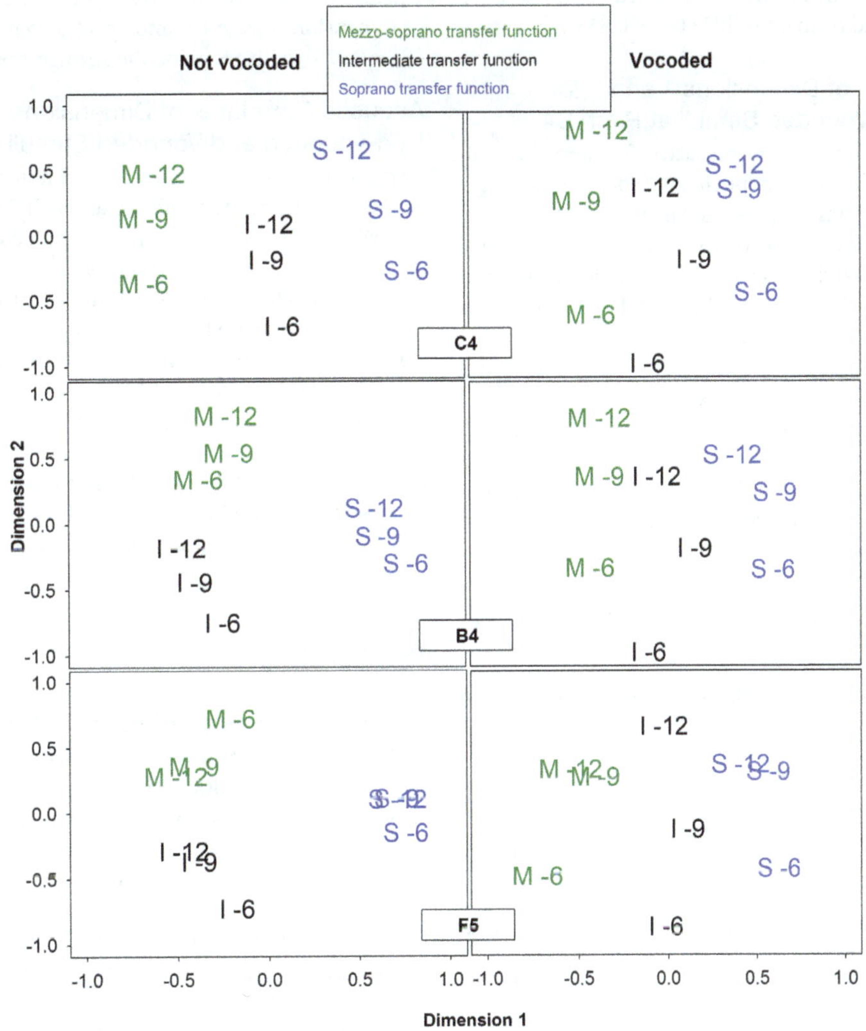

FIGURE 3 | Two-dimensional representations of the MDS perceptual spaces for non-vocoded and vocoded stimuli at pitches C4, B4, and F5. Graph symbols indicate the vocal tract transfer function category of Mezzo-soprano (M), Intermediate (I), or Soprano (S) followed by the glottal excitation source slope.

mezzo-soprano transfer functions. Dimension 2 for the non-vocoded stimuli organized the stimuli according to excitation source spectral slope; however, there was a reversal in order for the mezzo-soprano stimuli at pitch F5.

Relationship of MDS Dimensions to Acoustic Variables

Stepwise regression analyses were performed to see which acoustic measure or combination of measures best predicted each MDS dimension for all conditions. These stepwise regression analyses resulted in models with either 1 or 2 significant predictors. To test collinearity, variance inflation factors (VIFs) (Hocking and Pendelton, 1983; Craney and Surles, 2002) were computed for all 2-predictor models. All 2-predictor models generated VIFs of less than 1.5, with all but one generating VIFs of less than 1.2, indicating that regression coefficients were not likely inflated due to collinearity.

Acoustic Correlates of Dimensions 1 and 2 for Non-vocoded and Vocoded Stimuli at Pitch C4

Stepwise regression analyses were conducted for both the non-vocoded and vocoded stimuli at pitch C4. The results of the stepwise regression analyses are presented in **Table 4**.

The results of stepwise regression analyses for non-vocoded stimuli at pitch C4 suggest that the 2 significant predictors of dimension 1 were spectral centroid from 0-2 kHz and ER (R^2 = 0.944), with spectral centroid from 0 to 2 kHz being the strongest predictor. The 2 significant predictors of dimension 2 were ER and spectral centroid from 2 to 8 kHz (R^2 = 0.976), with ER being the strongest predictor.

The results of stepwise regression analyses for vocoded stimuli at pitch C4 suggest that, as with the non-vocoded stimuli, the 2 significant predictors of dimension 1 were spectral centroid from 0 to 2 kHz and ER (R^2 = 0.863), with spectral centroid from 0 to 2 kHz being the strongest predictor. However, unlike the stepwise regression results for non-vocoded stimuli, the significant predictor of dimension 2 for vocoded stimuli at pitch C4 was spectral centroid from 0 to 8 kHz (R^2 = 0.853).

Acoustic Correlates of Dimensions 1 and 2 for Non-vocoded and Vocoded Stimuli at Pitch B4

Stepwise regression analyses were conducted for both the non-vocoded and vocoded stimuli at pitch B4. The results of the stepwise regression analyses are presented in **Table 5**.

The results of stepwise regression analyses for non-vocoded stimuli at pitch B4 suggest that, as with pitch C4, the 2 significant predictors of dimension 1 were spectral centroid from 0 to 2 kHz and ER (R^2 = 0.943), with spectral centroid from 0 to 2 kHz being the strongest predictor. The significant predictor of dimension 2 was spectral centroid from 0 to 8 kHz (R^2 = 0.621).

The results of stepwise regression analyses for vocoded stimuli at pitch B4 suggest that, as with the non-vocoded stimuli, the 2 significant predictors of dimension 1 were spectral centroid from 0 to 2 kHz and ER (R^2 = 0.985), with spectral centroid from 0 to 2 kHz being the strongest predictor. The 2 significant predictors of dimension 2 were ER and spectral centroid from 2 to 8 kHz (R^2 = 0.979), with ER being the strongest predictor.

Acoustic Correlates of Dimensions 1 and 2 for Non-vocoded and Vocoded Stimuli at Pitch F5

Stepwise regression analyses were conducted for both the non-vocoded and vocoded stimuli at pitch F5. The results of the stepwise regression analyses are presented in **Table 6**.

The results of stepwise regression analyses for non-vocoded stimuli at pitch F5 suggest spectral centroid from 0 to 2 kHz was a significant predictor of dimension 1 (R^2 = 0.848). The 2 significant predictors of dimension 2 were spectral centroid from 2 to 8 kHz and ER (R^2 = 0.854), with spectral centroid from 2 to 8 kHz being the strongest predictor.

The results of stepwise regression analyses for vocoded stimuli at pitch F5 suggest that, as with the non-vocoded stimuli, spectral centroid from 0 to 2 kHz was a significant predictor of dimension 1 (R^2 = 0.729). The significant predictor of dimension 2 was ER (R^2 = 0.819).

TABLE 4 | Prediction of MDS dimensions by acoustic variables using forward regression for non-vocoded and vocoded stimuli at pitch C4.

Non-vocoded stimuli parameter	Dimension 1 R^2 = 0.944		Dimension 2 R^2 = 0.976	
	β	P	β	P
Centroid 0–8 kHz				
Centroid 0–2 kHz	1.027	<0.001		
Centroid 2–8 kHz			−0.303	0.008
ER	−0.655	0.001	−0.784	<0.001
Vocoded stimuli parameter	**Dimension 1 R^2 = 0.863**		**Dimension 2 R^2 = 0.853**	
	β	P	β	P
Centroid 0–8 kHz			−0.923	<0.001
Centroid 0–2 kHz	0.874	0.001		
Centroid 2–8 kHz				
ER	−0.607	0.008		

TABLE 5 | Prediction of MDS dimensions by acoustic variables using forward regression for non-vocoded and vocoded stimuli at pitch B4.

Non-vocoded stimuli parameter	Dimension 1 R^2 = 0.943		Dimension 2 R^2 = 0.621	
	β	P	β	P
Centroid 0–8 kHz			−0.788	0.012
Centroid 0–2 kHz	0.853	<0.001		
Centroid 2–8 kHz				
ER	−0.502	0.002		
Vocoded stimuli parameter	**Dimension 1 R^2 = 0.985**		**Dimension 2 R^2 = 0.979**	
	β	P	β	P
Centroid 0–8 kHz				
Centroid 0–2 kHz	1.001	<0.001	−0.262	0.006
Centroid 2–8 kHz				
ER	−0.553	<0.001	−0.880	<0.001

DISCUSSION

Interpreting the MDS Solutions

MDS provides a means of visualizing relationships between objects in a multi-dimensional space and can serve to test structural hypotheses concerning latent constructs that affect the perception of those objects (Borg et al., 2013). While MDS dimensions sometimes correlate with measured variables, the real interest is often in visualizing how the stimuli group in space, and in the case of the current study, how this grouping might change with vocoding. In the sections that follow, the correlations between some measured acoustic variables and MDS dimensions are discussed. These correlations should not be interpreted as establishing a causal relationship, but instead should be interpreted as measurable acoustic variables that may load on the unmeasurable construct of timbre perception.

TABLE 6 | Prediction of MDS dimensions by acoustic variables using forward regression for non-vocoded and vocoded stimuli at pitch F5.

Non-vocoded stimuli parameter	Dimension 1 R^2 = 0.848		Dimension 2 R^2 = 0.854	
	β	P	β	P
Centroid 0–8 kHz				
Centroid 0–2 kHz	0.921	<0.001		
Centroid 2–8 kHz			−0.986	0.001
ER			0.410	0.049
Vocoded stimuli parameter	**Dimension 1 R^2 = 0.729**		**Dimension 2 R^2 = 0.819**	
	β	P	β	P
Centroid 0–8 kHz				
Centroid 0–2 kHz	0.854	0.003		
Centroid 2–8 kHz				
ER			−0.905	0.001

Pitch C4

It was hypothesized that at lower pitches, 8-channel vocoding would result in the loss of important spectral characteristics, resulting in alterations of the multidimensional perceptual space. While the MDS solutions for the non-vocoded and vocoded stimuli at the pitch C4 looked very similar, some important differences were also observed (see **Figure 3**). The non-vocoded stimuli clustered well based on voice category, occupying distinct spaces along dimension 1. The vocoded stimuli also tended to organize along dimension 1 based on voice category; however, they did not cluster as cleanly, with the I-12 stimulus appearing much closer in distance to the S-12 and S-9 stimuli. All stimuli were organized according to excitation source spectral slope along dimension 2.

Pitches B4 and F5

It was also hypothesized that at the higher pitches, B4 and F5, the wider spacing of harmonics would cause a loss of output spectral peaks in both the non-vocoded and vocoded conditions, theoretically resulting in similar MDS representations. Instead, notable differences between the MDS representations for non-vocoded and vocoded stimuli were seen (see **Figure 3**).

As with the C4 stimuli, non-vocoded stimuli at the pitches B4 and F5 appeared distinctly clustered in the MDS space according to voice category. However, these stimuli were not distributed in the order of voice category along dimension 1. Instead, at these higher pitches (Migirov et al., 2009), the distances between mezzo-soprano and soprano stimuli were less than those observed for pitch C4 and (Limb and Roy, 2014) for some stimulus pairs, the non-vocoded mezzo-soprano and intermediate stimuli were equidistant from the non-vocoded soprano stimuli. To understand these differences, a look at the original aggregate dissimilarities may prove informative. **Table 7** displays a subset of the original aggregate listener dissimilarities where stimulus pairs differed only in voice category. At the pitches B4 and F5, listeners heard mezzo-soprano and soprano stimuli as less dissimilar than they did at the pitch C4. Also, for some stimulus pairs at both B4 and F5, listeners heard mezzo-soprano and intermediate stimuli as equally dissimilar to soprano stimuli. Spectral centroid from 0 to 2 kHz was the strongest predictor of dimension 1 at pitch B4 and was the sole predictor of dimension 1 at the pitch F5. Examination of the spectral energy in the 0–2 kHz range at these higher pitches may (Migirov et al., 2009) provide clues as to why the mezzo-soprano and soprano stimuli were heard as less dissimilar and (Limb and Roy, 2014) why, in some cases, the mezzo-soprano and intermediate stimuli were heard as equally dissimilar to the soprano stimuli. **Figures 4–6** display the spectra for all stimuli with a glottal excitation source of −9 dB/octave for the pitches C4, B4, and F5, respectively. These figures illustrate how under-sampling of the vocal tract transfer function due to widely spaced harmonics can lead to alterations in the perception of dissimilarity. Examination of **Figures 4–6** reveals that generally, but also particularly in the area of 0–2 kHz, spectral details that were present at the pitch C4 were lost at pitches B4 and F5. This loss of spectral information could result in a smaller perceived dissimilarity between mezzo-soprano and soprano stimuli. Also, at these higher pitches, the spectra for the mezzo-soprano and intermediate stimuli from 0 to 2 kHz appear to be very similar, with the first harmonic being higher in amplitude than the second. However, for the soprano stimuli, the first harmonic is equal in amplitude to the second harmonic, possibly contributing to perception that the mezzo-soprano and intermediate stimuli were equally dissimilar to the soprano stimuli. These spectral differences may have contributed to the perceived dissimilarities presented in **Table 7**, which in turn generated the MDS spaces seen in **Figure 3**.

At the pitch F5, other changes in the non-vocoded MDS space begin to emerge. Stimuli having excitation source spectral slopes of −9 dB/octave and −12 dB/octave appeared closely spaced to each other at this pitch.

At the pitches B4 and F5, the MDS spaces for the vocoded and non-vocoded stimuli revealed notable differences in organization, contrary to our hypothesis. Unlike the MDS spaces for the non-vocoded stimuli at the pitches B4 and F5, the MDS spaces for the vocoded stimuli at the pitches B4 and F5 looked similar to those seen at the pitch C4. At the pitch F5, however, the mezzo-soprano and soprano stimuli with excitation source spectral slopes of −9 dB/octave and −12 dB/octave appeared closely spaced to one another, just as in the non-vocoded MDS representation. The finding that the MDS spaces for the vocoded stimuli at pitches B4 and F5 looked similar to the MDS space at pitch C4 is somewhat unexpected and is discussed further in the section that follows.

TABLE 7 | Listener dissimilarity measures for glottal source excitation slopes of −6, −9, and −12 dB/octave at the pitches C4, B4, and F5.

Glottal excitation source slope (dB//Octave)	Voice category pair	Pitch		
		C4	B4	F5
−6	M vs. S	66.45	60.90	61.28
	I vs. S	39.00	50.62	50.21
	M vs. I	40.24	56.45	60.00
−9	M vs. S	63.90	56.21	54.72
	I vs. S	46.03	54.66	53.14
	M vs. I	52.45	53.93	39.86
−12	M vs. S	54.17	52.55	49.72
	I vs. S	41.10	59.24	49.90
	M vs. I	48.59	50.24	35.45

M, Mezzo-soprano; I, Intermediate; S, Soprano.

Effects of Pitch and Location of Vocoder Bands

The effect of vocoding on normal hearing listeners' perception of vocal dissimilarity is likely related to several interacting factors: (a) the pitch of the non-vocoded stimuli, (b) the location of vocal tract resonances, and (c) the center frequency and bandwidth of vocoder filter bands.

Figures 4–6 display the non-vocoded and vocoded spectra for mezzo-soprano, intermediate, and soprano stimuli with an

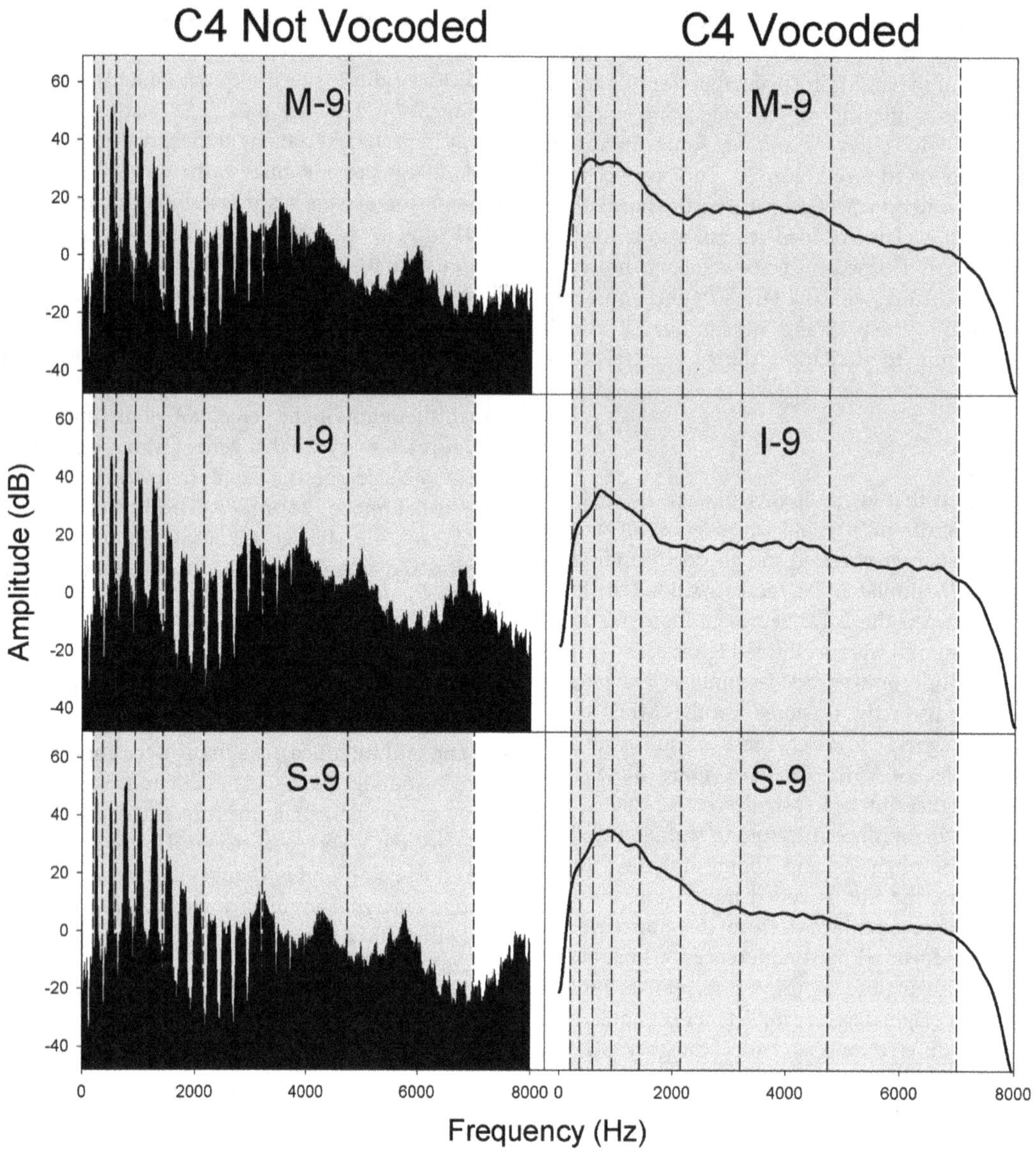

FIGURE 4 | Spectra for non-vocoded and vocoded stimuli for excitation spectral slopes of −9 dB/octave at the pitch C4. The frequency range of vocoding is indicated in gray, while vocoder bands are indicated by vertical dashed black lines. Panel labels indicate the vocal tract transfer function category of Mezzo-soprano (M), Intermediate (I), or Soprano (S) followed by the glottal excitation source slope, −9 dB/octave.

excitation source spectral slope of −9 dB/octave for the pitches C4, B4, and F5, respectively. The frequency range of vocoding is indicated in gray, while vocoder bands are indicated by vertical dashed black lines. Because spectral centroid from 0 to 2 kHz and ER were the strongest predictors of dimension 1 at pitches C4 and B4, and spectral centroid from 0 to 2 kHz was the sole predictor of dimension 1 at the pitch F5, examination of the spectral energy in the 0–2 kHz region for both non-vocoded and vocoded stimuli may prove informative.

At the pitch C4, the closer spacing of harmonics allowed for better representation of resonant peaks in the non-vocoded output spectra. Clear differences in spectral peak location of the non-vocoded stimuli, S-9, I-9, and M-9, in the 0–2 kHz range can be seen. At pitch C4, the first 3 harmonics are each located in a separate vocoder band, resulting in spectral peaks in the vocoded stimuli that seem to correspond reasonably well with those seen in the non-vocoded stimuli. Above 2 kHz, spectral peaks and valleys in the non-vocoded stimuli are located such that when vocoded, these peaks and valleys average out, creating a spectrum from 2 to 7 kHz in the vocoded stimuli that is fairly flat.

At the pitch B4, for the non-vocoded stimuli, the wider spacing of harmonics resulted in a large 1st harmonic amplitude for I-9 and M-9, while for S-9, the 1st and 2nd harmonics are of almost equal amplitude. The fundamental is located in vocoder band 2, while the 2nd harmonic oscillates about the border between bands 3 and 4 and the 3rd harmonic oscillates about the border

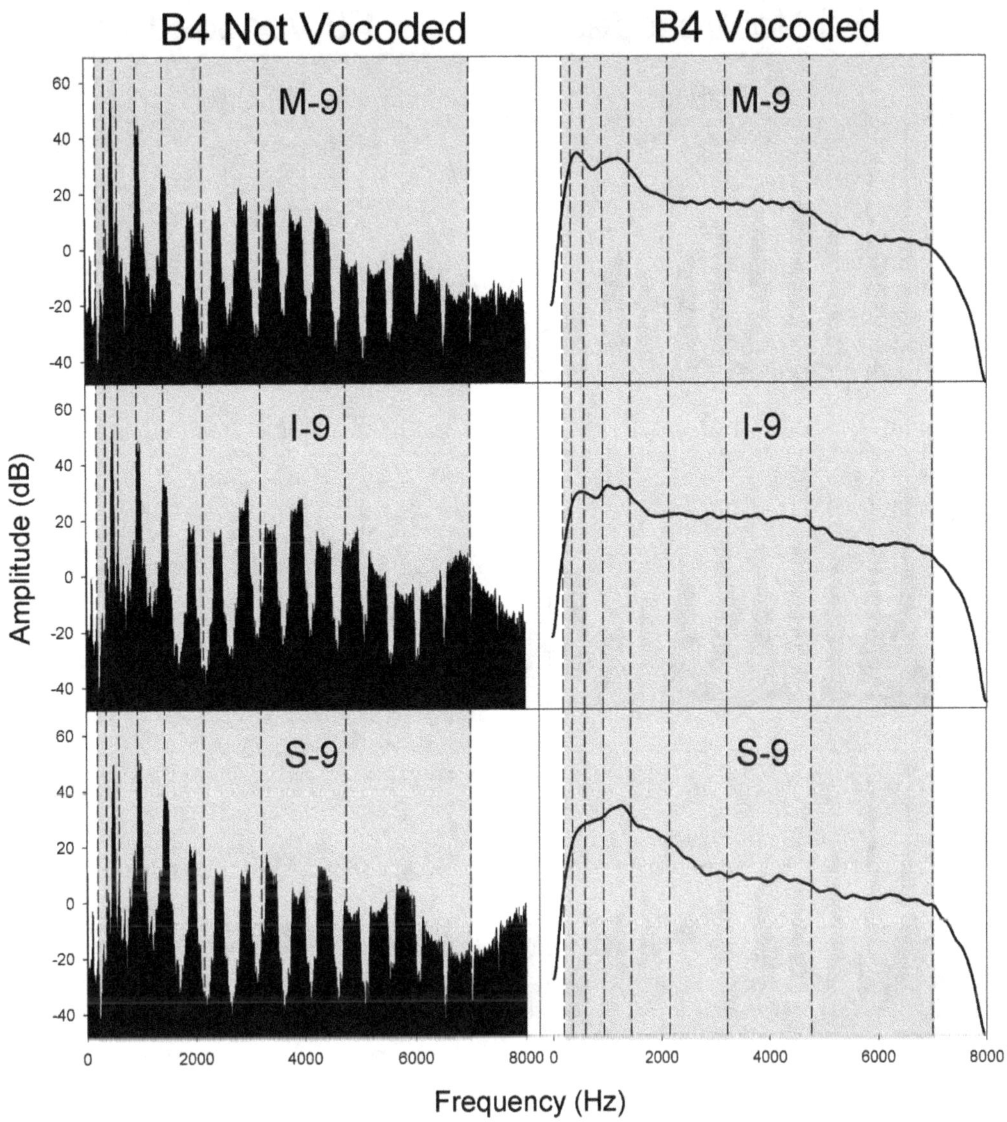

FIGURE 5 | Spectra for non-vocoded and vocoded stimuli for excitation spectral slopes of −9 dB/octave at the pitch B4. The frequency range of vocoding is indicated in gray, while vocoder bands are indicated by vertical dashed black lines. Panel labels indicate the vocal tract transfer function category of Mezzo-soprano (M), Intermediate (I), or Soprano (S) followed by the glottal excitation source slope, −9 dB/octave.

between band 4 and 5. The result is a strong peak in the vocoded spectrum for S-9 that is slightly higher in frequency than that of the non-vocoded S-9 stimulus. The most important effect at B4, however, occurs with I-9 and M-9. The vocoded spectra for these 2 conditions exhibit a second artifactual spectral peak that is not present in the original spectra. This is likely due to the oscillating 2nd and 3rd harmonics crossing into and out of neighboring vocoder filter bands. As with the pitch C4, in the area of 2–7 kHz, the vocoded spectra are relatively flat.

At the pitch F5, for the non-vocoded stimuli, the 1st harmonic is located in vocoder band 3. The 2nd harmonic appears to be located within vocoder band 4 but is also oscillating on the boundary with vocoder band 5. After vocoding, the resulting spectra appear to correspond reasonably well with the non-vocoded spectra in the region of 0–2 kHz. The vocoded spectra above 2 kHz are relatively flat.

The introduction of artifactual spectral peaks in the vocoded condition at pitch B4 for the I-9 and M-9 stimuli may have contributed to the unexpected MDS solutions at this pitch. However, artifactual peaks were not introduced in the vocoded condition at the pitch F5, which exhibited the same phenomenon. Because MDS spaces are only gross approximations of the perceptual space and because dimension 1 was best predicted by a weighted linear combination of both spectral centroid from 0 to 2 kHz and ER at pitch B4, but only by spectral centroid from 0 to 2 kHz at pitch F5, it is difficult to say with certainty that the extra spectral peak in the vocoded condition at pitch B4 was

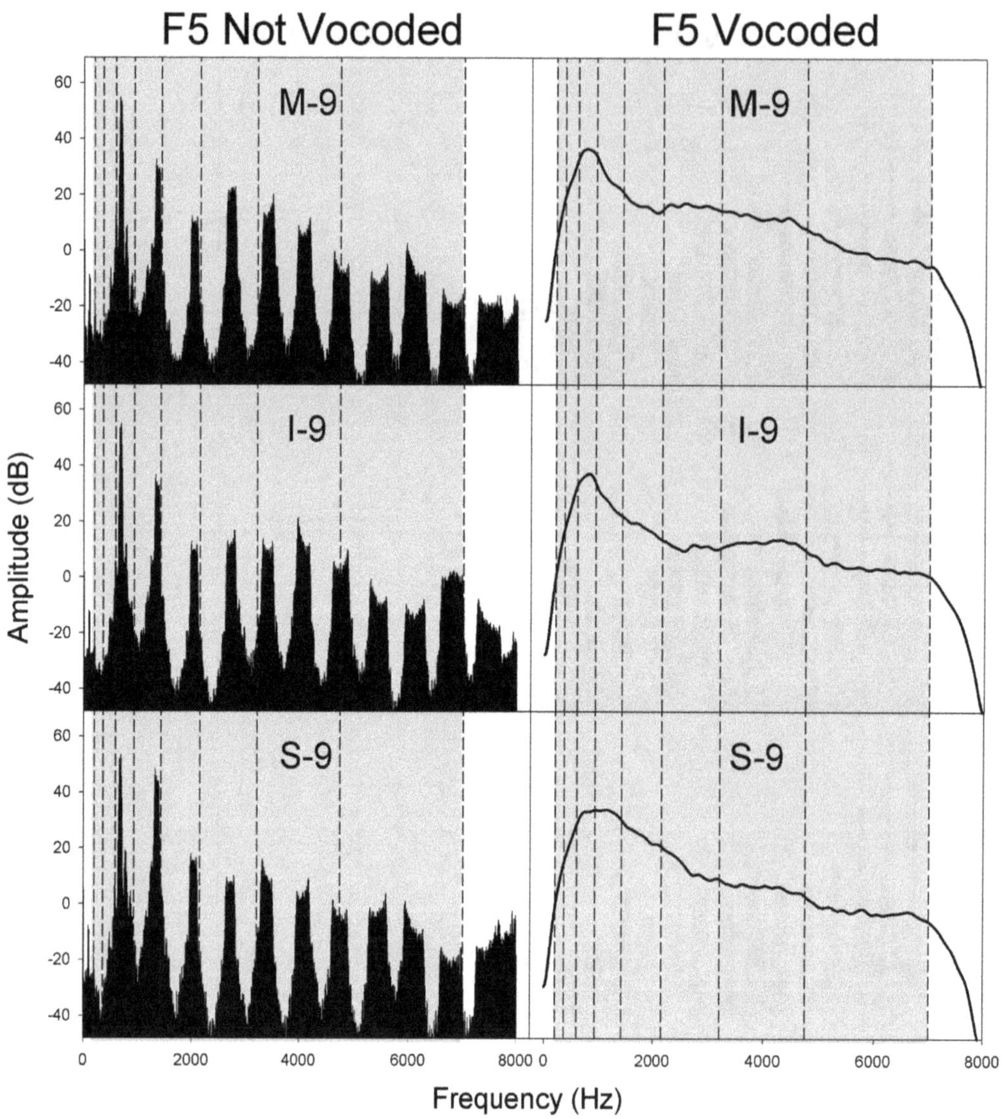

FIGURE 6 | Spectra for non-vocoded and vocoded stimuli for excitation spectral slopes of −9 dB/octave at the pitch F5. The frequency range of vocoding is indicated in gray, while vocoder bands are indicated by vertical dashed black lines. Panel labels indicate the vocal tract transfer function category of Mezzo-soprano (M), Intermediate (I), or Soprano (S) followed by the glottal excitation source slope, −9 dB/octave.

responsible for the differences in organization along dimension 1 between non-vocoded and vocoded stimuli, however, the possible introduction of artifactual spectral peaks, in addition to the possible loss of spectral peaks, during the vocoding process must be considered.

Implications for Cochlear Implant Users

In the current study, there were some instances where normal hearing listeners perceived timbral differences in the non-vocoded conditions that they did not in the vocoded conditions. Conversely, there were situations where introduction of artifactual peaks in the vocoded stimuli may have resulted in normal hearing listeners perceiving timbral differences in the vocoded conditions that they could not perceive in the non-vocoded conditions. Yet, in general, the MDS solutions for non-vocoded and vocoded conditions were similar, suggesting that, for the most part, normal hearing listeners were able to extract some timbral information from the degraded vocoder signal. The degree to which this might happen for CI users will likely depend on the design of the cochlear implant as well as the pitch and resonance characteristics of the singer.

Overall, CI users have poor music perception for many reasons. Device-related factors may affect music perception, including: (a) mismatched frequency-place alignment; (b) spectral smearing as a result of channel interaction and spread of neural excitation; and (c) factors related to the signal processing strategy employed by the device (Limb and Roy, 2014), such as using monopolar vs. all-polar stimulation modes (Marozeau and McKay, 2016). Further, listener factors may limit perception. These listener factors include: (a) variable patterns of nerve survival; (b) electrode array position; and (c) residual acoustic hearing (Bierer and Faulkner, 2010; Limb and Roy, 2014; Pfingst et al., 2015). At the central processing level, there may be extensive changes in the brain as a result of auditory deprivation (Stropahl et al., 2017) as well as altered general cognitive abilities (Holden et al., 2013; Kramer et al., 2018). Therefore, even though timbral cues might be preserved by the initial cochlear implant signal processing, the extent to which each CI user can make use of these cues (i.e., perceptual weighting) may be highly variable (Winn et al., 2016).

One possible device issue that may impact the perception of vocal timbre in CI users concerns spectral slope. Some singing voice styles (Sundberg et al., 1993, 1999; Thalén and Sundberg, 2001; Stone et al., 2003; Björkner, 2008; Bourne and Garnier, 2012; Bourne et al., 2016) and singing voice registers (Sundberg and Kullberg, 1999; Sundberg and Högset, 2001; Roubeau et al., 2009) are differentiated primarily or partially by changes in glottal configuration that manifest in changes in spectral slope. Because CIs typically implement various degrees of amplitude compression, it may not be possible to detect some of the distinctions between voice styles and/or voice production types.

Given the device- and patient-related factors associated with CI use, another approach to improving music perception may be through auditory training. Several studies have shown that following training, CI users have improved their ability to discriminate musical pitch, identify melodic contours, recognize and identify familiar melodies, and identify the timbre of musical instruments (Driscoll, 2012; Galvin et al., 2012; Petersen et al., 2012; Gfeller et al., 2015; Fuller et al., 2018).

Strengths of the Study

One strength of the study is that every participant completed all 6 MDS conditions. Thus, individual differences in the use of the scroll bar or other systematic idiosyncratic behaviors would be expected to be similar across all conditions, allowing each participant to serve as their own control. This allows for the visual comparison of MDS results across conditions.

A second strength of the study is that, while the number of stimuli were necessarily small in each condition, excitation source spectral slopes and vocal tract transfer functions spanned the range typically seen in female singers.

Limitations of the Study

Generally, the current study suffers from the same limitations that befall all studies employing a non-experimental modeling procedure such as MDS. While MDS studies can provide useful insight into how listeners' perceptions are organized, correlating any acoustic parameter to a dimension can be problematic. Thus, while this study found that a linear combination of acoustic variables could predict the MDS dimensions in all conditions very well, this prediction cannot be directly related to human perception, which is a complex phenomenon that likely cannot be reduced to a set of numbers derived from acoustic measurements.

Because each participant completed all conditions, time constraints resulted in several limitations. Each participant by necessity heard all stimulus pairs once only. This required the use of aggregate MDS so that the effect of any errant responses could be minimized. Thus, INDSCAL analyses could not be employed. Additionally, the number of stimuli in each condition had to be restricted to no more than 9, which limits the number of dimensions that can safely be employed in the MDS to two. Finally, additional conditions using a variety of vocoder configurations could not be employed.

The current study utilized 8-channel vocoded stimuli to assess the perceptual dimensionality of singing voice timbre. While vocoders provide a clue as to how the degraded cochlear implant signal might affect the perception of timbral dissimilarity, it cannot be assumed that these results will directly translate to the perception of timbre in cochlear implant populations for reasons highlighted in the previous section.

Future Research

The Role of Context in CI Listener Timbre Perception

While the current study manipulated glottal excitation source slope and vocal tract transfer function, the purpose of the study was to test overall vocal timbre perception. In such studies of vocal timbre, variations in vowel must be kept to a minimum. Even when perceptual studies have been specifically designed to experimentally test a parameter such as voice category perception, researchers have (a) limited the stimuli to just one vowel (Cleveland, 1977; Berndtsson and Sundberg, 1995; Erickson, 2004) or (b) performed a long-time-average spectra (LTAS) over a part or the entirety of a song (Johnson and Kempster, 2011). Future research should examine vocal timbre perception and voice category perception using a variety of vowels and in a variety of contexts.

The Role of Vibrato in the Timbre Perception of CI Listeners

In addition to perceptual information provided by glottal excitation spectral slope and vocal tract transfer function, vibrato may play a role in the ability to hear timbral differences between voices. Vibrato emerges in a Western classical singing voice first as a coherent frequency modulated (FM) voice source which when filtered by the vocal tract produces spectral fluctuations and a secondary amplitude modulation (AM) as harmonics move into and out of vocal tract resonances. Thus, classical vibrato singing is characterized by both FM (also termed frequency vibrato) and AM (also termed amplitude vibrato).

The possible role of vibrato as a timbre cue available to CI listeners has not been well researched. While CI listeners may not be able to hear the fine structure needed to perceive frequency vibrato, the spectral fluctuations associated with vibrato across frequency bands may provide a better representation of timbre than may be available from a non-modulated vocal stimulus (McAdams and Rodet, 1988). These spectral fluctuations may also give rise to the perception of vibrato rate and/or extent, an element of timbre that may assist in the discrimination of voices. Additionally, both the frequency and extent of secondary amplitude modulations could provide salient timbral cues. Future research should examine the role that vibrato may play in timbre discrimination in both NH listeners presented with vocoded stimuli and CI listeners by Migirov et al. (2009) utilizing synthetic stimuli that vary in vibrato rate or (Limb and Roy, 2014) utilizing real singing voices. Given that training has been shown to improve music perception in CI users, the knowledge gained from such studies could be used to develop and test training strategies.

SUMMARY AND CONCLUSION

Vocal tract resonance frequencies have been shown to be a cue to the perception of voice categories such as baritone, tenor, mezzo-soprano, and soprano, while changes in glottal source spectral slope are believed to be related to perception of vocal quality dimensions such as *fluty* vs. *brassy* and are associated with the production of various singing styles and singing registers. For the simulated mezzo-soprano, intermediate, and coloratura soprano voices used in this study, MDS solutions grouped stimuli according to voice category and excitation source spectral slope in all conditions. However, while stimuli tended to be grouped by voice category, such grouping did not always correlate with an MDS dimension. Excitation source spectral slope was generally represented as increasing along dimension 2; however, at the pitch F5 where widely spaced harmonics would not likely line up with vocal tract resonances well, thus obscuring some elements of excitation source spectral slope, this organization did not always hold. While it is unclear how well these timbre percepts would emerge as MDS dimensions for CI listeners, in general, these results suggest that perhaps some aspects of vocal timbre may remain and combined with other information such as vibrato rate, may provide some cues to singer identity.

ETHICS STATEMENT

This study was carried out in accordance with the recommendations of the Institutional Review Board of the University of Tennessee, Knoxville, with written informed consent from all subjects. All subjects gave written informed consent in accordance with the Declaration of Helsinki. The protocol was approved by the Institutional Review Board of the University of Tennessee, Knoxville.

AUTHOR CONTRIBUTIONS

ME, PJ, MH, and KF contributed to the conception and design of the study. ME performed the MDS analyses and wrote the first draft of the manuscript. TS contributed to data analysis and interpretation. PJ, MH, and KF provided expertise concerning cochlear implants and contributed ideas for the introduction and discussion sections. KF wrote a section in the discussion section. All authors contributed to manuscript revision, read and approved the submitted version.

REFERENCES

ANSI (1973). *Psychoacoustical Terminology. S3.20.* New York, NY: American National Standards Institute.

ASHA (1990). Guidelines for screening for hearing impairments and middle ear disorders. *ASHA* 32, 17–24.

Barnes, J., Davis, P., Oates, J., and Chapman, J. (2004). The relationship between professional operatic soprano voice and high range spectral energy. *J. Acoust. Soc. Am.* 116, 530–538. doi: 10.1121/1.1710505

Berndtsson, G., and Sundberg, J. (1995). Perceptual significance of the center frequency of the singer's formant. *Scand. J. Logop. Phoniatr.* 20, 35–41. doi: 10.3109/14015439509098728

Bierer, J. A., and Faulkner, K. F. (2010). Identifying cochlear implant channels with poor electrode-neuron interface: partial tripolar, single-channel thresholds and psychophysical tuning curves. *Ear Hear.* 31, 247–258. doi: 10.1097/AUD.0b013e3181c7daf4

Björkner, E. (2008). Musical theater and opera singing–why do different? A study of subglottal pressure, voice source, and formant frequency characteristics. *J. Voice* 22, 533–540. doi: 10.1016/j.jvoice.2006.12.007

Bloothooft, G., and Plomp, R. (1986). The sound level of the singer's formant in professional singing. *J. Acoust. Soc. Am.* 79, 2028–2033. doi: 10.1121/1.393211

Bloothooft, G., and Plomp, R. (1988). The timbre of sung vowels. *J. Acoust. Soc. Am.* 84, 847–860. doi: 10.1121/1.396654

Borch, D. Z., and Sundberg, J. (2011). Some phonatory and resonatory characteristics of the Rock, Pop, Soul, and Swedish Dance Band styles of singing. *J. Voice* 25, 532–537. doi: 10.1016/j.jvoice.2010.07.014

Borg, I., Groenen, P. J. F., and Mair, P. (2013). *Applied Multidimensional Scaling.* New York, NY: Springer.

Bourne, T., and Garnier, M. (2012). Physiological and acoustic characteristics of the female music theater voice. *J. Acoust. Soc. Am.* 131, 1586–1594. doi: 10.1121/1.3675010

Bourne, T., Garnier, M., and Samson, A. (2016). Physiological and acoustic characteristics of the male music theatre voice. *J. Acoust. Soc. Am.* 140, 610–621. doi: 10.1121/1.4954751

Caclin, A., McAdams, S., Smith, B. K., and Winsberg, S. (2005). Acoustic correlates of timbre space dimension: A confirmatory study using synthetic tones. *J. Acoust. Soc. Am.* 118, 471–482. doi: 10.1121/1.1929229

Cleary, M., and Pisoni, D. B. (2002). Talker discrimination by prelingually deaf children with cochlear implants: Preliminary results. *Ann. Otol. Rhinol. Laryngol. Suppl.* 189, 113–118. doi: 10.1177/00034894021110s523

Cleveland, T. F. (1977). Acoustic properties of voice timbre types and their influence on voice classification. *J. Acoust. Soc. Am.* 61, 1622–1629. doi: 10.1121/1.381438

Craney, T. A., and Surles, J. G. (2002). Model-dependent variance inflation factor cutoff values. *Qual. Eng.* 14, 391–403. doi: 10.1081/qen-120001878

Dmitriev, L., and Kiselev, A. (1979). Relationship between the formant structure of different types of singing voices and the dimensions of the supraglottal cavities. *Folia Phoniatr.* 31, 238–241. doi: 10.1159/000264170

Drennan, W. R., Oleson, J. J., Gfeller, K., Crosson, J., Driscoll, V. D., Won, J. H., et al. (2015). Clinical evaluation of music perception, appraisal and experience in cochlear implant users. *Int. J. Audiol.* 54, 114–123. doi: 10.3109/14992027.2014.948219

Driscoll, V. D. (2012). The effects of training on recognition of musical instruments by adults with cochlear implants. *Semin. Hear.* 33, 410–418. doi: 10.1055/s-0032-1329230

Echternach, M., Burk, F., Burdumy, M., Traser, L., and Richter, B. (2016). Morphometric differences of vocal tract articulations in different loudness conditions in singing. *PLoS One* 11:e0153792. doi: 10.1371/journal.pone.0153792

Ekholm, E., Papagiannis, G. C., and Chagnon, F. P. (1998). Relating objective measurements to expert evaluation of voice quality in Western classical singing: Critical perceptual parameters. *J. Voice* 12, 182–196. doi: 10.1016/s0892-1997(98)80038-6

Erickson, M. L. (2003). Dissimilarity and the classification of female singing voices: A preliminary study. *J. Voice* 17, 195–206. doi: 10.1016/s0892-1997(03)00022-5

Erickson, M. L. (2004). The interaction of formant frequency and pitch in the perception of voice category and jaw opening in female singers. *J. Voice* 18, 24–37. doi: 10.1016/j.jvoice.2003.08.001

Erickson, M. L. (2008). Dissimilarity and the classification of male singing voices. *J. Voice* 22, 290–299. doi: 10.1016/j.jvoice.2006.10.002

Erickson, M. L. (2016). Acoustic properties of the voice source and the vocal tract: Are they perceptually independent? *J. Voice* 30, .e9–.e22.

Erickson, M. L. (2020). Inexperienced listeners' perception of timbre dissimilarity within and between voice categories. *J. Voice* 34, P302.e1–302.E13. doi: 10.1016/j.jvoice.2018.09.012

Erickson, M. L., and Faulkner, K. F. (2018). "Multidimensional timbre spaces of cochler implant vocoded and non-vocoded synthetic female voices," in *Proceedings of The 2nd Music and Cochlear Implants Symposium*, Montreal.

Frič, M., and Pavlechová, A. (2018). Listening evaluation and classification of female singing voice categories. *Log. Phon. Vocol.* [Epub ahead of print].

Fu, Q. J., Chinchilla, S., Nogaki, G., and Galvin, J. (2005). Voice gender identification by cochlear implant users: The role of spectral and temporal resolution. *J. Acoust. Soc. Am.* 118, 1711–1718. doi: 10.1121/1.1985024

Fuller, C. D., Galvin, J. Jr., Maat, B., Baskent, D., and Free, R. H. (2018). Comparison of two music training approaches on music and speech perception in cochlear implant users. *Trends Hear.* 22:2331216518765379.

Fuller, C. D., Gaudrain, E., Clarke, J. N., Galvin, J. J., Fu, Q. J., Free, R. H., et al. (2014). Gender categorization is abnormal in cochlear implant users. *J. Assoc. Res. Otolaryngol.* 15, 1037–1048. doi: 10.1007/s10162-014-0483-7

Galvin, J. Jr., Eskridge, E., Oba, S., and Fu, Q. J. (2012). Melodic contour identification training in cochlear implant users with and without a competing instrument. *Semin. Hear.* 33, 399–409. doi: 10.1111/j.1749-6632.2009.04551.x

Gaudrain, E., and Başkent, D. (2015). Factors limiting vocal-tract length discrimination in cochlea. *J. Acoust. Soc. Am.* 137, 1298–1308. doi: 10.1121/1.4908235

Gaudrain, E., and Baskent, D. (2018). Discrimination of voice pitch and vocal-tract length in cochlear implant users. *Ear Hear.* 39, 226–237. doi: 10.1097/AUD.0000000000000480

Gfeller, K., Guthe, E., Driscoll, V., and Brown, C. J. (2015). A preliminary report of music-based training for adult cochlear implant users: rationales and development. *Cochlear Implants Int.* 16(Suppl. 3), S22–S31. doi: 10.1179/1467010015Z.000000000269

Gfeller, K., Knutson, J. F., Woodworth, G., Witt, S., and DeBus, B. (1998). Timbral recognition and appraisal by adult cochlear implant users and normal-hearing adults. *J. Am. Acad. Audiol.* 9, 1–19.

Gfeller, K., Turner, C., Mehr, M., Woodworth, G., Fearn, R., Knutson, J. F., et al. (2002). Recognition of familiar melodies by adult cochlear implant recipients and normal-hearing adults. *Cochlear Implants Int.* 3, 29–53. doi: 10.1179/cim.2002.3.1.29

Giguère, G. (2006). Collecting and analyzing data in multidimensional scaling experiments: A guide for psychologists using SPSS. *Tutor. Quant. Methods Psychol.* 2, 26–37.

Grey, J. M. (1977). Multidimensional perceptual scaling of musical timbres. *J. Acoust. Soc. Am.* 61, 1270–1277. doi: 10.1121/1.381428

Grey, J. M., and Gordon, J. W. (1978). Perceptual effects of spectral modification on musical timbres. *J. Acoust. Soc. Am.* 63, 1493–1500. doi: 10.1121/1.381843

Guzman, M., Lanas, A., Olavarria, C., Azocar, M. J., Muñoz, D., Madrid, S., et al. (2015). Laryngoscopic and spectral analysis of laryngeal and pharyngeal configuration i non-classical singing styles. *J. Voice* 29, .e21–.e28.

Hakes, J., Shipp, T., and Doherty, E. (1987). Acoustic properties of straight tone, vibrato, trill and trillo. *J. Voice* 1, 148–156. doi: 10.1016/s0892-1997(87)80038-3

Hallqvist, H., Lã, F. M., and Sundberg, J. (2017). Soul and musical therater: A comparison of two vocal styles. *J. Voice* 31, 229–235. doi: 10.1016/j.jvoice.2016.05.020

Hammarberg, B., Fritzel, L. B., Gauffin, J., Sundberg, J., and Wedin, L. (1980). Perceptual and acoustic correlates of abnormal voice qualities. *Acta Otolaryngol.* 90, 441–451. doi: 10.3109/00016488009131746

Handel, S., and Erickson, M. L. (2004). Sound source identification: The possible role of timbre transformations. *Music Percept.* 21, 587–610. doi: 10.1525/mp.2004.21.4.587

Hocking, R. R., and Pendelton, O. J. (1983). The regression dilemma. *Commun. Stat.* 12, 497–527.

Holden, L. K., Finely, C. C., Firszt, J. B., Holden, T. A., Brenner, C., Potts, L. G., et al. (2013). Factors affecting open-set word recognition in adults with cochlear implants. *Ear Hear.* 34, 342–360. doi: 10.1097/AUD.0b013e3182741aa7

Iverson, P., and Krumhansl, C. L. (1993). Isolating the dynamic attributes of musical timbre. *J. Acoust. Soc. Am.* 94, 2595–2603. doi: 10.1121/1.407371

Jiam, N. T., Caldwell, M. T., and Limb, C. J. (2017). What does music sound like for a cochlear implant user? *Otol. Neurotol.* 38, e240–e247. doi: 10.1097/MAO.0000000000001448

Johnson, A. M., and Kempster, G. (2011). Classification of the classical male singing voice using long-term average spectrum. *J. Voice* 25, 538–543. doi: 10.1016/j.jvoice.2010.05.009

Kang, R., Nimmons, G. L., Drennan, W., Longnion, J., Ruffin, C., Nie, K., et al. (2009). Development and validation of the University of Washington clinical assessment of music perception test. *Ear Hear.* 30, 411–418. doi: 10.1097/AUD.0b013e3181a61bc0

Kong, Y. Y., Mullangi, A., Marozeau, J. P., and Epstein, M. (2011). Temporal and spectral cues for musical timbre perception in electric hearing. *J. Speech Lang. Hear. Res.* 54, 981–994. doi: 10.1044/1092-4388(2010/10-0196)

Kovačić, D., and Balaban, E. (2009). Voice gender perception by cochler implantees. *J. Acoust. Soc. Am.* 126, 762–775. doi: 10.1121/1.3158855

Kramer, S., Vasil, K. J., Adunka, O. F., Pisoni, D. B., and Moberly, A. C. (2018). Cognitive functions in adult cochlear implant users, cochlear implant candidates, and normal-hearing listeners. *Laryngoscope Investig. Otolaryngol.* 3, 304–310. doi: 10.1002/lio2.172

Krimphoff, J., McAdams, S., and Winsberg, S. (1994). Caracterisation du timbre des sons complexes: II. Analyses acoustiques et quantification psychophysique [Characterization of the timbre of complex sounds. II. Acoustic analyses and psychophysical quantifications]. *J. Physiq.* 4, 625–628.

Krumhansl, C. L. (1989). "Why is musical timbre so hard to understand?," in *Structure and PERCEPTION of Electroacoustic Sound and MUSIC*, eds S. Nielzen, and O. Olsson (Amsterdam: Excerpta Medica), 43–53.

Kruskal, J. B. (1964). Multidimensional scaling by optimizing goodness-of-fit to a nonmetric hypothesis. *Psychometrika* 29, 1–28.

Kruskal, J. B., and Wish, M. (1978). *Multidimensional Scaling*. Beverly Hills, CA: Sage Publications.

Lakatos, S. (2000). A common perceptual space for harmonic and percussive timbres. *Percept. Psychphys.* 62, 1426–1439. doi: 10.3758/bf03212144

Limb, C. J., and Roy, A. T. (2014). Technological, biological, and acoustical constraints to music perception in cochlear implant users. *Hearing Res.* 308, 13–26. doi: 10.1016/j.heares.2013.04.009

Looi, V., McDermott, H. J., McKay, C., and Hickson, L. (2008). Music perception of cochlear implant users compared with that of hearing aid users. *Ear Hear.* 29, 421–434. doi: 10.1097/AUD.0b013e31816a0d0b

Macherey, O., and Delpeirre, A. (2013). Perception of musical timbre by cochlear implant listeners: A multidimensional scaling study. *Ear Hear.* 34, 426–436. doi: 10.1097/AUD.0b013e31827535f8

Mainka, A., Poznyakovskiy, A., Platzek, I., Fleischer, M., Sundberg, J., and Mürbe, D. (2015). Lower vocal tract morphologic adjustments are relevant for voice timbre in singing. *PLoS One* 10:e0132241. doi: 10.1371/journal.pone.0132241

Marozeau, J. P., De Cheveigné, A., McAdams, S., and Winsberg, S. (2003). The dependency of timbre on fundamental frequency. *J. Acoust. Soc. Am.* 114, 2946–2957.

Marozeau, J. P., and McKay, C. M. (2016). Perceptual spaces induced by cochlear implant all-polar stimulation mode. *Trends Hear.* 20, 1–9. doi: 10.1177/2331216516659251

Massida, Z., Marx, M., Belin, P., James, C., Fraysse, B., Barone, P., et al. (2013). Gender categorization in cochlear implant users. *J. Speech Lang. Hear. Res.* 56, 1389–1401. doi: 10.1044/1092-4388(2013/12-0132)

McAdams, S., and Rodet, X. (1988). "The role of FM-induced AM in dynamic spectral profile analysis," in *Basic Issues in Hearing*, eds H. Duifhius, J. W. Horst, and H. P. Wit (New York, NY: Academic Press), 359–367.

McAdams, S., Winsberg, S., Donnadieu, S., De Soete, G., and Krimphoff, J. (1995). Perceptual scaling of synthezised musical timbres: Common dimensions, specificities, and latent subject classes. *Psychol. Res.* 58, 177–192. doi: 10.1007/bf00419633

McDermott, H. J. (2004). Music perception wiht cochlear implants: A review. *Trends Amplif.* 8, 49–82. doi: 10.1177/108471380400800203

Migirov, L., Kronenberg, J., and Henkin, Y. (2009). Self-reported listening habits and enjoyment of music among adult cochlear implant recipients. *Ann. Otol. Rhinol. Laryngol.* 118, 350–355. doi: 10.1177/000348940911800506

Monsen, R. B., and Engebretson, A. M. (1983). The accuracy of formant frequency measurements: A comparison of spectrographic analysis and linear prediction. *J. Speech Hear. Res.* 26, 87–97.

Omori, K., Kacker, A., Carroll, L. M., Riley, D., and Blaugrund, S. M. (1996). Singing power ratio: Quantitative evaluation of singing voice qualilty. *J. Voice* 10, 228–235. doi: 10.1016/s0892-1997(96)80003-8

Peay, E. R. (1988). Multidimensional rotation and scaling of configurations to optimal agreement. *Psychometrika* 53, 199–208. doi: 10.1007/bf02294132

Petersen, B., Mortensen, M. V., Hansen, M., and Vuust, P. (2012). Singing in the key of life: A study on effects of musical ear training after cochlear implantation. *Psychomusic* 22, 134–151. doi: 10.1037/a0031140

Pfingst, B., Zhou, N., Colesa, D. J., Watts, M. M., Strahl, S. B., Garadat, S. N., et al. (2015). Importance of cochlear health for implant function. *Hear. Res.* 322, 77–88.

Roers, F., Mürbe, D., and Sundberg, J. (2009). Voice classification and vocal tract of singers: A study of x-ray images and morphology. *J. Acoust. Soc. Am.* 125, 503–512. doi: 10.1121/1.3026326

Roubeau, B., Henrich, N., and Castellengo, M. (2009). Laryngeal vibratory mechanisms: The notion of vocal register revisited. *J. Voice* 23, 425–438. doi: 10.1016/j.jvoice.2007.10.014

Sandell, G. J. (1995). Roles for spectral centroid and other factors in determining 'blended' instrument pairings in orchestration. *Music Percept.* 13, 209–246. doi: 10.2307/40285694

Schubert, E., Wolfe, J., and Tarnopolosky, A. (2004). "Spectral centroid and timbre in complex multiple instrumental textures," in *Proceedings of the 8th International Conference on Music Perception and Cognition*, eds S. D. Lipscomb, R. Ashley, R. O. Gjerdingen, and P. Webster (Evanston, IL: Northwestern University), 654–657.

Schulz, E., and Kerber, M. (1994). "Music perception with the Med-El Implants," in *Advances in Cochler Implants*, eds I. J. Hochmair-Desoyer, and E. S. Hochmair (Vienna: Manz).

Sjoberg, K. M., Driscoll, V. D., Gfeller, K., Welhaven, A. E., Kirk, K. I., and Prusick, L. (2017). The impact of electric hearing on children's timbre and pitch perception and talker discrimination. *Cochlear Implants Int.* 18, 36–48. doi: 10.1080/14670100.2016.1263406

Stone, R. E., Cleveland, T. F., Sundberg, J., and Prokop, J. (2003). Aerodynamic and acoustical measures of speech, operatic, and Broadway vocal styles in a professional female singer. *J. Voice* 17, 283–297. doi: 10.1067/s0892-1997(03)00074-2

Story, B. (2016). "The vocal tract in singing," in *The Oxford Handbook of Singing*, eds G. Welch, D. M. Howard, and J. Nix (Oxford: Oxford University Press).

Stropahl, M., Chen, L. C., and Debener, S. (2017). Cortical reorganization in postlingually deaf cochlear implant users: Intra-modal and cross-modal considerations. *Hear. Res.* 343, 128–137. doi: 10.1016/j.heares.2016.07.005

Sundberg, J. (1974). Articulatory interpretation of the "singing formant". *J. Acoust. Soc. Am.* 55, 838–844. doi: 10.1121/1.1914609

Sundberg, J. (1994). Perceptual aspects of singing. *J. Voice* 8, 106–122. doi: 10.1016/s0892-1997(05)80303-0

Sundberg, J. (2001). Level and center frequency of the singer's formant. *J. Voice* 15, 176–186. doi: 10.1016/s0892-1997(01)00019-4

Sundberg, J. (2013). "Perception of Singing," in *The Psychology of Music*, ed. D. Deutsch (San Diego, CA: Academic Press), 69–105. doi: 10.1016/b978-0-12-381460-9.00003-1

Sundberg, J., Cleveland, T. F., Stone, R. E., and Iwarsson, J. (1999). Voice source characteristics in six permier country singers. *J. Voice* 13, 168–183. doi: 10.1016/s0892-1997(99)80021-6

Sundberg, J., Gramming, P., and Lovetri, J. L. (1993). Comparisons of pharynx, source, formant, and pressure characteristics in operatic and musical theatre singing. *J. Voice* 7, 301–310. doi: 10.1016/s0892-1997(05)80118-3

Sundberg, J., and Högset, C. (2001). Voice source differences between falsetto and modal registers in counter tenors, tenors and baritones. *Log. Phon. Vocol.* 26, 26–36. doi: 10.1080/140154301300109107

Sundberg, J., and Kullberg, A. (1999). Voice source studies of register differences in untrailed female singing. *Log. Phon. Vocol.* 24, 76–83. doi: 10.1080/140154399435147

Sundberg, J., and Thalén, M. (2015). Respiratory and acoustical differences between belt and neutral style of singing. *J. Voice* 29, 418–425. doi: 10.1016/j.jvoice.2014.09.018

Sundberg, J., Thalén, M., Alku, P., and Vilkman, E. (2004). Estimating perceived phonatory pressedness in singing from flow glottgrams. *J. Voice* 18, 56–62. doi: 10.1016/j.jvoice.2003.05.006

Thalén, M., and Sundberg, J. (2001). Describing different styles of singing: A comparison of a female singer's voice source in "Classical", "Pop", "Jazz", and "Blues". *Log. Phon. Vocol.* 26, 82–93. doi: 10.1080/140154301753207458

Titze, I. R. (1994). *Principles of Voice Production*. Englewood Cliffs, NJ: Prentice Hall.

Vongphoe, M., and Feng, F. G. (2005). Speaker recognition with temporal cues in acoustic and electric hearing. *J. Acoust. Soc. Am.* 118, 1055–1061. doi: 10.1121/1.1944507

Watts, C., Barnes-Burroughs, K., Adrianopoulos, M., and Carr, M. (2003). Potential factors related to untrained singing talent: A survery of singing pedagogues. *J. Voice* 17, 298–307. doi: 10.1067/s0892-1997(03)00068-7

Windsor, W. L. (2004). "Data collection, experimental design, and statistics," in *Empirical Musicology: Aims, Methods, Prospects*, eds E. Clarke, and N. Cook (New York: Oxford University Press), 197–222. doi: 10.1093/acprof:oso/9780195167498.003.0009

Winn, M. B., Won, J. H., and Moon, I. J. (2016). Assessment of spectral and temporal resolution in cochlear implant users using psychoacoustic discrimination and speech cue categorization. *Ear Hear.* 37, e377–e390. doi: 10.1097/aud.0000000000000328

Yang, Y., Welch, G., Sundberg, J., and Himonides, E. (2015). Tuning features of Chinese folk song singing: A case study of Hua'er music. *J. Voice* 29, 426–432. doi: 10.1016/j.jvoice.2014.08.013

Zaltz, Y., Goldsworthy, R. L., Kishon-Rabin, L., and Eisenberg, L. S. (2018). Voice discrimination by adults with cochlear implants: The benefits of early implantation for vocal-tract length perception. *J. Assoc. Res. Otolaryngol.* 19, 193–209. doi: 10.1007/s10162-017-0653-5

7

Practices and Attitudes that Enhance Music Engagement of Adult Cochlear Implant Users

Kate Gfeller[1,2,3], Ruth MacMullen Mallalieu[4], Aleksander Mansouri[5], Gaelen McCormick[6], Renee Blue O'Connell[7], Jake Spinowitz[8] and Bettina Gellinek Turner[9]*

[1] *School of Music, College of Liberal Arts and Sciences, University of Iowa, Iowa City, IA, United States,* [2] *Department of Communication Sciences and Disorders, College of Liberal Arts and Sciences, University of Iowa, Iowa City, IA, United States,* [3] *Iowa Cochlear Implant Clinical Research Center, Department of Otolaryngology–Head and Neck Surgery, Carver College of Medicine, University of Iowa, Iowa City, IA, United States,* [4] *University Library, The University of Sheffield, Sheffield, United Kingdom,* [5] *Independent Scholar, Brighton, MA, United States,* [6] *Eastman School of Music, University of Rochester, Rochester, NY, United States,* [7] *Independent Scholar, Charlottesville, VA, United States,* [8] *Independent Scholar, San Francisco, CA, United States,* [9] *Independent Scholar, Newburyport, MA, United States*

***Correspondence:**
Kate Gfeller
kay-gfeller@uiowa.edu

Background: Cochlear implants (CIs) are auditory prostheses designed to support spoken communication in persons with severe to profound hearing loss. Many post-lingually deaf adult CI users achieve good speech recognition in quiet; unfortunately, CI technology conveys a degraded representation of pitch and timbre, essential components of music. Not surprisingly, most CI users achieve significantly poorer perception and enjoyment of music compared with normal hearing listeners. Anecdotal evidence indicates that this impacts music engagement, particularly singing and playing instruments requiring ongoing tuning to external pitches or producing intervallic ratios. Interestingly, a small cohort of adult CI users has shown remarkable success in recovering or developing musical skills, but their success is poorly understood. Greater understanding of their efforts and attitudes may suggest potential rehabilitative approaches for other CI users.

Purpose: This article documented personal characteristics and experiences perceived to contribute to high level musicianship. Research questions included: (1) What forms of practice/experience have most contributed to (re)establishing satisfying music making? (2) What situations or musical tasks are most frustrating or challenging? (3) What attitudes, motivational factors, or forms of support help CI users persist in working toward improved music engagement?

Methods: Qualitative and patient–engaged research methodologies were used. Our study involved a unique collaboration of six CI users engaged in high levels of musicianship and a researcher whose scholarship focuses on music and CIs. The CI recipients conveyed their experiences and attitudes regarding music and CIs through open-ended narratives. These narratives were analyzed using an integrative approach of inductive and deductive coding methods. The codes and themes that emerged through inductive methods were then organized within the Dynamic Problem Solving Model for Management of Music Listening Environments (Gfeller et al., 2019a).

Outcomes: This paper provides reflections of six CI users who successfully engage in active music making, including on-going tuning to external pitches and ensemble participation. Their perspectives emphasize the importance of pre-CI music instruction, extensive practice and immersion in music listening and playing, persistence and self-efficacy, and problem solving skills that optimize music engagement, and suggest possible strategies useful to other CI users interested in improving music experiences.

Keywords: cochlear implants, musicians, patient-engaged research, problem solving, music training, self-efficacy

INTRODUCTION

Cochlear implants (CIs) are auditory prostheses designed primarily to support persons with severe to profound hearing loss in spoken communication. Many post-lingually deaf adult CI recipients achieve good speech recognition in quiet (Looi et al., 2012). Unfortunately, most CI users achieve significantly poorer music perception and enjoyment than they possessed before hearing loss (Drennan et al., 2015), though there is considerable variability among CI users for music perception and engagement. Music perception typically does not improve significantly as a result of mere CI experience over time (for reviews, see Looi et al., 2012; Limb and Roy, 2014), though adult CI users may improve perception and enjoyment of some aspects of music as a result of focused listening and training programs (Gfeller et al., 2001; Fu and Galvin, 2007; Looi et al., 2012). Unfortunately, training programs designed for adult CI users are not readily available outside of selective research protocols (Gfeller et al., 2019a).

Most research on music and CIs focuses on enhanced perception and appreciation as measured in controlled laboratory environments, not production (for reviews, see Looi et al., 2012; Limb and Roy, 2014). A few pediatric studies indicate that some pediatric CI users do enjoy music making (e.g., Rocca, 2012; Gfeller et al., 2019b), but singing or playing in tune to an external pitch is problematic (Xu et al., 2009; Gfeller et al., 2012). These data are interesting, but cannot be generalized to adults whose auditory experiences included many years of normal hearing. The phenomenon of adult CI users who play music has received very limited attention to date within the CI literature.

While active music making may be thought of as a pleasant avocation, music making also has implications for (re)habilitation. Studies with normal hearing individuals document experience-based plasticity associated with longer-term music making (e.g., Kraus and Chandrasekaran, 2010; Herholz and Zatorre, 2012; Moreno and Bidelman, 2014; Patel, 2014). Music making involves several sensory systems (e.g., auditory, visual, tactile), the motor system, and makes demands on a variety of cognitive processes. Multimodal interactions that occur in longer-term instrumental playing can lead to stronger plastic changes in auditory processing than training in the auditory modality alone (Herholz and Zatorre, 2012). Music making is also associated with the reward system through direct feedback, pleasurable sounds, and social rewards in group music making (Herholz and Zatorre, 2012: Patel, 2014).

Due to reduced activation of regions that process spectrally complex sounds, the impact of music playing on experience-based plasticity likely differs from that of normal hearing adults (Strelnikov et al., 2015). More studies are needed to understand compensatory strategies used by the brain to decipher distorted input concerning music (Strelnikov et al., 2015). The phenomenon of music making among CI users is a topic currently under-represented in the literature and poorly understood. Factors such as residual hearing and the integration of non-auditory systems in experience-based plasticity may play an important role in music making. With regard to reward systems, despite the degraded signal, some adult CI users do find some forms of music enjoyable, and actively choose to listen to music (Looi et al., 2012; Gfeller et al., 2019a).

In addition to limited research on music making, the point of view of adult CI users, themselves, is greatly under-represented (Plant, 2015). CI recipients have typically been tested for perceptual accuracy or queried about music enjoyment through closed-ended items driven by researcher interests. Researcher-driven studies contribute extensively to our understanding of CIs and music, and research and development toward enhanced device technology remains an important goal for the CI field. Expanding our inquiries to explore the priorities and experiences of CI recipients, themselves, could shed new light on strategies for optimizing music, despite the current technology imperfect for conveying music (Limb and Roy, 2014). One possible approach is patient-engaged research.

A growing trend, patient-engaged (a.k.a. patient-centered) research, acknowledges that patients possess extensive knowledge and important insights into their own conditions as a result of lived experiences (Clancy and Collins, 2010). By ignoring the patient perspective, we lose a valuable source of information. Patient-engaged research calls for the involvement of patients at every stage in research planning, facilitation, and dissemination, though the extent of patient input varies dramatically from one study to the next (Bardes, 2012).

Qualitative research approaches are also considered effective in emphasizing patients' perspectives, exploring under-researched topics, and examining questions involving experiences in everyday life. This compliments research questions better suited toward controlled experiments (Bradley et al., 2007; Creswell, 2014; Mather et al., 2017).

A variety of approaches are acceptable in qualitative research (Creswell, 2014). In general qualitative research examines broad questions rather than *a priori* hypotheses through words rather than numbers. Analyses may include a combination of inductive and deductive methods. This involves line-by-line coding of meaningful units of text by one or more coders followed by more deductive processes in which the emerging codes are organized in relation to existing theories or models (Bradley et al., 2007). In qualitative research, large amounts of textual data are gathered, thus not all information can be included. Therefore, researchers aggregate data into a small number of themes (Savenye and Robinson, 1996; Creswell, 2014), which are reported in narratives, often within an organizing model, and with liberal reporting of the participants' own words (Bradley et al., 2007; Creswell, 2014).

The current study used qualitative and patient-engaged research methodologies to examine the phenomenon of adult CI recipients and music making. Rather than reporting on musical experiences of a broad cohort of "typical" adult CI users, it conveys the experiences of a select subsample of CI users who have achieved remarkable levels of musicianship. At present, high levels of music making by CI users is both rare and poorly understood. To better understand this phenomenon, the following research questions were examined:

(1) What forms of practice/experience have most contributed to (re)establishing satisfying music making?
(2) What sorts of situations or types of musical tasks are the most frustrating or challenging?
(3) What attitudes, motivational factors, or forms of support help CI users persist in working toward improved music engagement?

The life experiences of this group may offer insights regarding factors that contribute to extraordinary CI benefit.

MATERIALS AND METHODS

Approach

The overall approaches were qualitative and patient-engaged research methodology. The CI users were involved in the study conceptualization, selection of research questions, methodological choices, contribution of data, review of the analyses, and preparation of the manuscript.

Participant-Co-authors

The conceptualization of this paper evolved as a result of discussions at a symposium, The 2nd Music & Cochlear Implants Symposium, August 20–21, 2018, Montreal. The six musicians with CIs who collaborated on this paper discussed their musical experiences as part of a panel. These musicians were initially identified by the symposium organizing committee as possessing extraordinary musical skills. These skills were demonstrated at the symposium through videos or live performances, including improvization in a jazz ensemble. Their skill set includes singing or playing in tune on instruments (see **Table 1**) that do not have fixed pitches, which requires on-going tuning in solos and ensembles.

Consistent with qualitative methodology and case studies, this was a purposive sampling of individuals who possess characteristics relevant to the questions at hand. These individuals present a small "community" of shared life experiences: CI users who share a deep passion for music, whose daily lives involve many hours of engagement in music listening and playing, characteristics rare among CI users (Looi et al., 2012; Drennan et al., 2015).

Table 1 indicates a mix of professional musicians and musical avocation that requires considerable proficiency with tuning and production of pitch patterns well beyond the typical range of perceptual capabilities reported in the CI literature (for reviews, see Looi et al., 2012; Limb and Roy, 2014). Hearing history and musical background of the CI users appears in **Table 1**. As a group, they represent 182 years of musical training and production, and 52 years and 10 months of cochlear implant use.

Development of the Research Questions and Interview Items

Qualitative research utilizes broad questions which are oriented toward participant perspectives (Creswell, 2014). The three overarching research questions addressed in this study were selected by the 6 CI co-authors as priorities for exploration. The first author presented the group five possible broad questions based upon her 30 years of experience in the field, and also requested that the CI users propose additional questions for consideration. The CI users independently ranked the pool of questions by priority and the group's three top ranking questions were chosen; no additional research questions were suggested.

Consistent with qualitative methodology, the experiences of these CI users were gathered through open-ended inquiries, which tend to yield more detailed and personal perspectives than is typically yielded by quantitative studies using closed-ended items (Creswell, 2014). The co-authors, who live in 7 different locals, including 2 countries discussed via e-mail a protocol for gathering individual narratives followed by an interactive on-line focus group. The collaborators chose the first author to coordinate the research process, collect their narratives, to analyze the data, and to serve as "narrator" or primary writer of the study.

Data Collection

Following a review, the IRB committee of The University of Iowa waived the need for ethics committee approval of this study. However, in the spirit of fully informed consent, each CI recipient was also sent a formal invitation via e-mail to participate in the online questionnaire; the decision to complete the questionnaire constituted formal consent. Because the identity of the CI recipients is revealed in their capacity as co-authors, each co-author also signed and sent the first author a document indicating the desire to be listed as a co-author.

After formal consent was obtained from each CI user, the first author e-mailed each co-author the three research questions and instructions for completing the questions as a word document. On-line inquires rather than in-person focus groups were used because the group members lived in distant locations and because written responses also reduced the possibility of errors in transcribing oral accounts (Tates et al., 2009; Creswell, 2014). Responses were completed independently and each word document was returned to the first author for consolidation into a master document with the responses from all 6 participants; individual responses were identified by alphabetical letters. In a second round of data collection, each CI user independently reviewed the consolidated document and commented on all responses with corrections or additional thoughts. This process commonly used in qualitative research, called member checking,

TABLE 1 | Hearing profiles.

	AM	ROC	JS	BT	RM	GM
I play	Trombone	Guitar Flute/various wind Percussion	Guitar	Voice Piano Baroque recorder Fiddle/Ukulele	Clarinet	Double bass
Age	23	60	28	64	32	48
Gender	M	F	M	F	F	F
Status	Professional	Semi-professional	Amateur	Professional	Amateur	Professional
My musical training prior to implantation	Trombone lessons from middle school	High school percussion band and music theory. Private guitar lessons throughout twenties	None	Recorder, violin, piano lessons from age 7. University degree in music education. More than a decade of voice lessons; 45 years' experience of choral singing	Recorder lessons from age 6. Clarinet lessons from age 8, reaching ABRSM* Grade 6 and Grade 5 theory. Played in orchestra and wind bands	Classical music student from age 9. Undergraduate degree in music performance from Eastman School of Music. Masters degree in music performance from Carnegie Mellon University
My musical training post-implantation	Weekly trombone lessons from high school, played in band. Undergraduate degree in trombone performance, University of Delaware. Currently studying for a Master of Music at Boston University.	Private lessons for Galax dulcimer (wind instrument from Appalachian region). Folklife apprentice for the Virginia Foundation of Humanities. Private lessons for aural rehab purposes after CI activation, with focus on pitch and interval recognition, sight singing.	Started playing guitar after implantation. Regular composition and jamming sessions.	Weekly piano lessons and occasional voice coaching. Teach students in piano and recorder. Continue to sing in small choir.	Started regular lessons aged 30. Currently trying to finish ABRSM exams. Voice coaching and singing lessons for past year.	Continue to use knowledge and methods from prior training. Teach double bass students and collegiate music-related courses.
Hearing loss	Post-lingual, bilateral, severe. Caused by enlarged vestibular aqueduct. Left ear: sudden loss, around 5 years of age. Right ear: more gradual loss over some months, aged 12	Post-lingual, bilateral, progressive, likely from birth but detected in twenties. Glandular fever, aged 21, caused further deterioration	Prelingual, bilateral, severe/profound loss from birth. Residual hearing deteriorated sharply aged 15	Post-lingual, bilateral. Gradual, progressive loss from forties, from high to mid frequencies	Prelingual, bilateral, sensorineural profound loss from birth	Post-lingual, bilateral. Caused by Ménière's disease. Left ear: sudden onset deafness, aged 35, leading to profound loss by age 40. Right ear: Sudden onset Ménière's at age 43, leading to moderate to profound hearing loss by age 45
Age implanted	L: 13 R: 18	L: 50	R: 15	L: 63	R: 13 L: 23	L: 47
Cochlear implant make and model	Cochlear Nucleus 6 with long electrodes	Cochlear Nucleus 6 (electrode information not known)	Cochlear Nucleus 7 (electrode information not known)	Advanced Bionics CQ 90 EAS with HiFocus Slim – J electrode, full length	MED-EL Sonnet with COMBI 40 + with STANDARD electrode (R) and SONATA with FLEX SOFT electrode (L)	Advanced Bionics Naida Q90 (electrode information not known)
Additional devices used	N/A	R: ReSound hearing aid	L: ReSound hearing aid	R: Phonak Naida Link hearing aid	N/A	R: Widex, Beyond 440 hearing aid

**ABRSM, Associated Board of the Royal Schools of Music exams.*

allowed for verification and validation of data accuracy, and facilitated a more interactive component to data collection. The first author entered responses for the first and second rounds into a master word document for subsequent coding. All responses were downloaded into a password-protected database for analysis.

DATA ANALYSIS

The analysis involved an iterative and integrative approach, utilizing a combination of inductive and deductive coding (Bradley et al., 2007). The interview data were first read carefully multiple times by the first author to get a general sense of the data. Each participant's responses were analyzed independent of the three research questions because responses can apply to multiple questions. A line-by-line analysis was completed in which units of meaning (words, phrases, and sentences) were tagged or represented with an identifying code. The initial codes emerged inductively into like categories, with a total of 329 codes assigned to the narratives from the first two rounds of coding. Some sentences or paragraphs were assigned more than one code. Therefore, the percentage of codes that fit into categories exceeded 100%.

After the initial inductive coding, the codes were then grouped into more abstract, high level categories referred to as themes (Tates et al., 2009). Magnitude coding (frequency of codes), which can help determine the most prominent themes (Saldaña, 2013), was also used (see **Tables 2–4**).

Consistent with an integrative approach, the interaction of coding and themes that evolved from inductive coding were then examined deductively in relation to existing models and theories. The model chosen as the best fit was the Dynamic Problem Solving Model for the Management of Music Listening Environments (DPSM) which is described in detail in Gfeller et al. (2019a) (see **Figure 1**). This model was initially developed to conceptualize the music experiences of a broad range of adult CI users.

TABLE 2 | The frequencies of codes assigned to each theme/component of the DPSM model in rank order.

Theme within the DPSM	Frequency of items (+ or – if applicable*)	% of 329 total codes
Problem solving skills total	115	35%
Problem solving orientation	107 (86+, 21-)	32.5%
Music, Music and Speech	67	20%
Social context	54 (32+, 22-)	16.4%
Auditory profile	52	15.5%
Transfer of past knowledge	49 (42+, 7-)	15%
Change over time	34	10.3%
Domain specific knowledge	22	6.6%
Environment	11	3.0%

**+ refers to positive or helpful factors; – refers to factors that impair music listening.*

The DPSM guided the deductive stage of analysis for this study, which is described in the Results. The components of the DPSM is described more extensively in Gfeller et al. (2019a) (see **Figure 1**). Briefly, the outer elliptical components of the model (auditory profile, environment, music, music and speech, and social context) reflect the reciprocal processes associated with music listening responses. The listener's management of the music experiences appear within the ellipses: cognitive, affective and behavioral processes associated with self-efficacy, problem solving and self-management. Changes over Time emphasizes the dynamic and reciprocal nature of the music, listening environments, and listener attributes and actions (e.g., experience-based plasticity, changing attitudes and behaviors).

As part of verification and validation of the analyses associated with qualitative methods, 20% of the codes were reviewed by a second coder, a laboratory associate uninvolved in this study. Agreement between coders was 75%. Differences in coding choices were resolved through discussion. The results were then shared with the 6 CI users through member checking to validate that the themes reflected their responses (Creswell, 2014).

RESULTS

Table 2 presents in rank order the frequencies of codes assigned to each theme/component of the DPSM. Greater frequency, and thus larger proportion of the entire data set, suggests that an idea is more prevalent and important to the target group (Saldaña, 2013). Each of the themes represented in the DPSM is described in greater detail below in order of greatest to lowest frequency. While these themes and exemplars are presented as discrete categories, in real life, these factors often interact and overlap.

Problem Solving Skills

This theme includes specific strategies used for improving music experiences. A total of 115 out of 329 codes were assigned to this category. The precise and technical descriptions of strategies revealed a high level of technical knowledge regarding music theory and music pedagogy. Strategies differed somewhat as a function of the instrument played (e.g., relying on vibrotactile feedback from bass, guitar, or singing), prior background (e.g., formal theory instruction), and onset of hearing loss (e.g., internal representation of musical sounds developed through natural hearing).

Table 3 presents the skills or strategies in rank order of frequency. The strategies or methods used as part of training included accommodations (working around limitations), compensatory strategies (e.g., synergistic use of several sensorimotor inputs to compensate for degraded auditory input), and focused practice on music components (e.g., a semitone) that resulted in perceptual changes over time (e.g., being able to hear a semitone change, matching an external pitch).

Several individuals emphasized the benefit of multisensory input: "I believe that engaging all of the senses is very helpful to regain music perception." "Reading visual notation supports

TABLE 3 | Code frequency and examples for problem solving skills component.

Theme: skill or strategy	Frequency	Examples
Use of all senses	23	Visual, tactile, muscle memory, proprioception, movement
Top down processing	14	Using memory of musical sounds, imagination, internal sense of pitch
Selecting most accessible sounds	12	Latching on to most accessible sounds (e.g., best pitch range, best quality sound) as strategy for satisfaction or as jumping off point to extend skills
Focus and energy	11	It takes focus and energy to listen to music and improve; hard to do when tired
Music theory types of exercises	11	Many hours doing ear training exercises similar to what one learns in theory, such as interval training, using a fixed pitch, listening to sequences, listening for subtle pitches, applying pitches onto prior knowledge of songs
Extensive and focused listening to music	10	Taking many opportunities to listen to CDs, music on line, repeated listening for various layers of music
Extensive making of music	8	Practice a lot, playing in rehearsals, making music offers foundation for learning about music
Post-implant music lessons	6	Benefitted from guidance, motivation, specific exercises from theory or studio teachers
Social learning	5	Importance of input from other CI users at conferences, support groups, on line. More important than input from hearing professionals
Speech training exercises, listening to speech	5	Carry over of speech training to music, listening to different dialects, accents
Singing	4	Singing helps with intonation
Technology	4	Use of headphones, tuning apps, synergy of CI with HA

TABLE 4 | Code frequency and examples for problem solving orientation component.

Problem solving orientation	Frequency of codes	Examples of codes
Problems as an opportunity, a challenge	44	Enjoying a challenge, seeing problems as opportunities to learn more, seeing every music experience as a chance to learn more, hard work can be fun, life long learning, energy is important
Cognitive reframing	14	Being able to find the positive in a situation, such as realizing everyone hears differently, being realistic no one can do everything, focusing on what I can do, CI experiences resulting in an interesting life
Music as a passion and motivation to strive	9	Love of music, sense of identity, keeps one working, love of sound
Social component	7	There is a social component to striving; connecting with others at conferences, participating in research, networking with others, helping others
Positive expectancies	4	Belief things will come together over time, improvement with speech gave hope for improvement with music

perception of what I am hearing around me and informs me what sounds to expect." More accessible sounds were also chosen for practice or greater listening satisfaction: "In choosing pieces for myself, I avoid music that contains a lot of thick, complex chords." "Practicing with a fixed sound medium." Given current limitations of accessible music training materials that are designed for use by adult CI recipients (Gfeller et al., 2019a), the extensive codes in this category suggests a high level of personal ingenuity in finding resources.

While **Table 3** offers a rich menu of possible strategies for enhancing music, it is notable that many are based upon formal music theory or approaches that require reading notation or some level of music understanding.

> "I worked with a music teacher and did ear training/pitch recognition and sight singing exercises. My teacher would play two pitches either in succession or simultaneously and I would have to try and discern what interval she played. Things like major 3rd, perfect 4th, perfect 5th, octave, etc… Note that all of these exercises are done in basic music theory classes".

Some strategies required a commitment of time that could be considered excessive by some CI users: "It is not because we spent an occasional hour on a website aiming to improve our music perception post-CI. It is the immersion in musical pursuits that produces extraordinary results." This brings to mind another prevalent characteristic of these CI users: a strong problem solving orientation, which is the focus of the following section.

Problem Solving Orientation

A problem solving orientation includes personal characteristics such as viewing problems as opportunities, cognitive reframing (finding a positive interpretation to negative events), hardiness and persistence, enjoying challenges, and high sense of self-efficacy (confidence in accomplishing one's goals) (Hill-Briggs, 2003). Limited problem solving orientation includes seeing problems as uncontrollable, having negative expectations of outcomes, and low self-efficacy.

Problem solving orientation was the second highest (107) model component in coding frequency (see **Table 4**). The vast

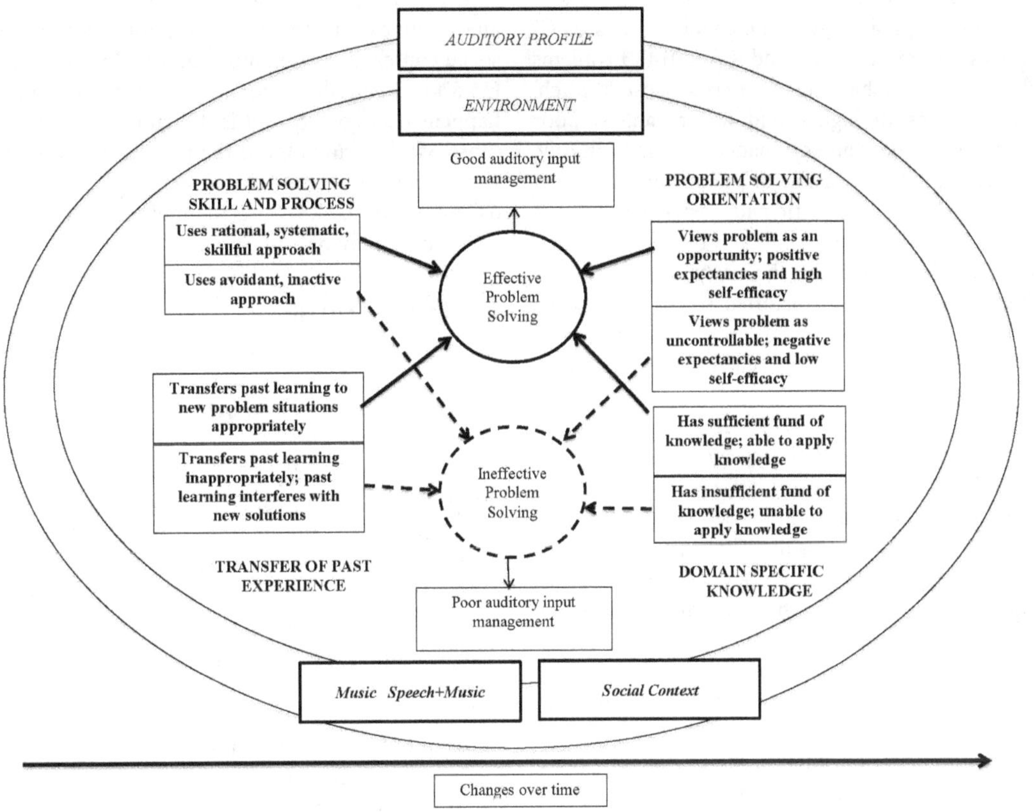

FIGURE 1 | Dynamic problem solving model for management of music listening environments.

majority (86) of the codes revealed a positive problem solving orientation. Several described themselves as a "lifelong learner" and emphasized persistence, hardiness and embracing challenges: "I challenge myself by listening to new music." "I believe that the key to improvement is within myself." "Be tenacious, persistent, curious, patient, understanding, open-minded, gentle and kind to yourself. Also have fun! Learning is fun and having a CI is a unique experience few get to have."

Examples of being able to focus on positive aspects (cognitive reframing) included: "I am trying to remain 'fascinated by the process'... and not get overwhelmed by the vast number of things I cannot hear anymore." "We must look for the good days rather than linger on the bad ones." "understanding that the rate at which you improve does not reflect whether you are a good person or 'good at music'."

Considering motivational factors that fueled a positive attitude, a strong passion for music was central to this attitude for several in this cohort: "Music has always been my greatest source of joy and I was determined to never give up on it or lose it." "The most important attitude component for helping with CI music perception is a personal passion for music and strong disposition to stick with music engagement even when the quality might not be satisfactory at the start." "I love sounds. Anything that can be heard is interesting to me, and hearing it better becomes my goal."

While all CI users showed a strong problem solving orientation, statements of frustration and lower self-efficacy tended to be expressed by the individuals with less than one year experience at the time of data collection. However, those CI users with greater length of device use also reflected back on difficulties they experienced in the early months following implantation. The first 6 months post-implant seemed particularly problematic. "For about 6 months, music sounded absolutely horrible and I was afraid I might never enjoy it again. But I persisted."

Among codes that reflected lack of control were frustration with chaotic and unpleasant sounds, feeling lack of control over sense of pitch, and needing to avoid some musical situations (singing with others, playing in large ensembles) because of difficulty and lack of emotional reward. One musician with less than one year's CI experience and some residual hearing noted "Listening to music is almost uniformly uncomfortable for me now, [with] the pitch distortion which makes all music sound chaotic." Avoidance as a strategy tended to occur more frequently in early months post-CI.

Music and Music and Speech

The third most frequent component (20%) addressed structural features of music or music in conjunction with speech. Perception of the structural features of music seemed to be particularly problematic during early CI use; 61% of the codes were contributed by CI users with less than one year's CI experience.

Within this category, difficulty with pitch made up 25% of all codes. This is not surprising given the characteristics of CI technology in relation to music (Limb and Roy, 2014). Problems regarding pitch included: establishing an internal sense of pitch, difficulty hearing pitches in higher and lower ranges, poor error detection, problems hearing key changes in the harmony, matching an external pitch, confusion of major and minor, or hearing a discrepancy between acoustic and electric stimulation (e.g., the pitches being a half step "off"). Problems with pitch seem to be particularly difficult in the early months of CI use, and resulted in a chaotic and distorted sound. As will be described later under "Changes over Time," several CI musicians experienced improved pitch perception, but this required many months of listening exercises.

Given the difficulties with pitch perception, it is unsurprising that multi-layered music (music with harmony or counterpoint) was a common subtheme (19%) of this category. Participants described separating out the parts of large vocal or instrumental ensembles as difficult or nearly impossible. This likely contributes to another sub-category of problem associated with music: playing or singing in ensembles with other musicians (9%). A participant with less than one year's experience stated, "It is very difficult for me to hear all voices and harmonies in a full ensemble, plus accompaniment if applicable. My experience can easily turn into what I call 'soundsoup.'"

Fifteen percent of the codes in this category described some instruments as more or less accessible and pleasant for CI recipients. One musician found using the piano in exercises to train pitch patterns and harmonies beneficial. Another described the resonance and wide frequency range of the clarinet as particularly helpful in accessing musical sounds. Most of this cohort plays instruments without fixed pitches: singing, playing guitar, bass, and trombone, which require ongoing tuning.

Other problem with music or speech included overall poor sound quality, unpleasant distribution of overtones, and an annoying overlay of noise in the CI signal. One musician described difficulty hearing the conductor's voice over the ensemble, and several described difficulty hearing music or speech against background noise, which is related to the social aspects of music making.

Social Context

Music making or listening to music often involves collaboration and shared learning. Music concerts and music-making often bring people together for aesthetic enrichment or entertainment (Hargreaves and North, 2010). In this dataset, social context comprised 16.4% of the total number of coded items. The most prominent sub-category (24% of items in this category) was encouragement and input from other CI users, especially those with musical background and interests. This cohort connected with other CI users on line, in support groups, and at conferences; these connections formed their most important source of motivation as well as information. Support of friends, family, and teachers were also noted: "having a supportive network of musicians is very helpful." "The people in my life. always encouraged me to pursue music." Good teachers were described as an important source of understanding, guidance, and motivation.

Even though the incidence of hearing loss is fairly common among musicians, the most common negative commentary on social context was stigmatization of CI users by other musicians (14.8%). "Being dismissed as a musician due to deafness or CI happens occasionally and is difficult to accept." "We stigmatize those with hearing loss in the pro music community, as if they were somehow at fault." Because of these social concerns, 3 of the 6 CI users now make efforts to inform others about CIs and music and to dispel myths.

Auditory Profile

This theme addresses hearing history (e.g., age of onset, residual hearing, CI or HA use, etc.) as well as music experiences that contributed to auditory development; it comprised 15.5% of all codes in the dataset.

The limitation of the CI for conveying musical structures was the primary sub-category (24 codes), including problem with sound quality and limitations for pitch and overtones: "Post-CI, my main issue has been a constant 'overlay of extra sounds' . . .." "The problems associated with the hearing loss, recovery, and day-to-day use of hearing aids, implants, or both are draining." Several commented that they need considerable energy to enjoy music through a CI.

Four of the participant co-authors use hearing aids to optimize residual hearing. A primary sub-category of this theme was the synergistic benefit of residual hearing (including bimodal hearing). "The bimodal set up (HA + CI) helped as I could still follow along with music reasonably well through the hearing aid even when the CI perception wasn't clear." As persons with technical knowledge of music, several were able to describe in precise terms inconsistencies between acoustic (residual hearing) and electric hearing, as well as resolution of those inputs over time. Music training before implantation (as part of hearing experiences) was described as an important foundation for learning music with the CI. One person utilized their memory of pitches from when they still had "natural hearing" before receiving the second implant as part of "relearning" correct pitches and intervals after receiving a second implant.

Transfer of Past Knowledge

This theme within the model makes up 15% of all the coded items. Five of the cohort had many years of formal music instruction before implantation, and 3 are professional musicians. Transfer of knowledge from prior vocal or instrumental music instruction (30.6%) included use of non-auditory cues (visual, tactile, proprioceptive), understanding the building blocks of music, work ethic, and discipline from taking lessons prior to hearing loss, being trained to listen for subtleties, and knowing strategies for collaborative music making. "In my formal music education, we sometimes talked about 'feeling the string' through the bow' contact with the hair on the string. I had taken that farther to feeling the string through my fingers contact of the bow."

This cohort transferred knowledge of theory or ear training strategies extensively toward optimizing CI use (28.5% of codes in this category). This included knowledge of pitch relationships, theory exercises, reading notation, and internal sense of pitch or timbre learned through natural hearing. Theoretical understanding of music provided a rich mental representation of music that fosters top-down processing, which contributed to the re-establishment of more normalize pitch percepts.

Several described a transfer of speech training to music. For example, "It was regular auditory training for baseline speech perception that formed the bedrock for my ability to appreciate music with the CI... once the vocals (lyrics) were formed as the baseline for what I could latch on to, other elements started to follow with time and persistence."

In some instances (14.3%), past knowledge did not carry over effectively to music making after implantation. For example, in collaborative music-making, the CI user could no longer rely on the overtones for creating sound quality. Given the degraded percepts of pitch and timbre, some described a period of exploration to find new strategies.

Changes Over Time

Changes over time were referred to directly in 10.3% of the coded responses. This included description of the first 6 months of CI use being especially bad, gradual improvement with time, or the many hours spent in practicing or listening. However, one can argue that passage of time is implied in most every aspect of the phenomenon of restoring musicality, and thus is an important addition to this model. Experience based plasticity, such as integration of multimodal input associated with ear training or music performance requires sufficient exposure to sound and repetition of tasks to support learning/plasticity; repetition occurs over time and neural changes take time (Herholz and Zatorre, 2012).

As one of the musicians described, "I chose to sit at a piano and play things [patterns of notes] until they sounded different. At first, the keys C and G, a perfect fifth interval, sounded the same." Over time, this musician was able to hear musical scale patterns, match pitches through singing, and eventually created correct pitches on trombone, which requires ongoing tuning.

Furthermore, music is a time-dependent art form; it involves combinations of pitch, timbre, rhythm, and amplitude that change rapidly over time. Changes such as hearing loss or implantation also may include a course of acceptance and adjustment that can affect problem-solving orientation (Gfeller et al., 2019a). As a more recently implanted participant noted, "I have not reached a level of 'satisfying music making'. but have reached a level of 'transitional acceptance,' which means I am still hoping for improvement."

Specific to this cohort of CI users, the most prevalent sub-theme was the amount of practice time required to achieve satisfactory outcomes (35.3%). Half of the CI users described themselves as life long learners, thus suggesting their musical quest does not have an end goal/destination. Another common theme was that music sounded really bad and chaotic at first (23.5% of codes), but as many (23.5%) codes indicated music gradually improved with time and effort.

Domain Specific Knowledge

This component of the model refers to knowledge of hearing loss, CIs, music, or combinations of those elements, and comprised only 6.6% of all coded comments. Despite the fact that 5 of the 6 CI users had many years of formal music training, there was limited reference to having specific knowledge in these areas. Musical knowledge was revealed indirectly through particular forms of knowledge, such as comments about distorted overtones in the CI signal. Twenty of the 22 codes referred to knowledge of music theory or understanding of the impact of hearing loss or CI use on music perception.

Environment

This theme represented within the model refers to issues such as poor room acoustics or competing noise in the environment – that is, the surrounding conditions in which music is heard. It made up a very small proportion (3.3%) of all codes for the CI users. Four of the CI users described problems of rehearsing in small rooms. "Playing in small venues is bad because the sound becomes one big mess during loud sections and directions are near impossible to hear." The acoustical environment and background noise also undermined enjoyment when attending concerts.

DISCUSSION

In considering the various themes represented in the DPSM, the strong problem solving orientation and ingenious approaches to problem solving are among the most notable characteristics of this group of CI users. Particularly impressive is the immersion and intensity with which these individuals have tackled the perceptual problems associated with accessing music through a CI. The capacity to persist with hours of listening and playing exercises despite annoying sound quality, no guarantees of eventual benefits, and very gradual improvement requires patience and fortitude.

While avoidance has been described in models of chronic illness as a less effective problem solving strategy (Hill-Briggs, 2003), avoidance may sometimes have adaptive value after initial hookup. More positive experiences were sometimes characterized as gradually "earned." Some started with the most accessible sound as a foundation for interpreting the signal, then eventually seeking more challenging situations. This might be likened to the behavioral technique of successive approximations, beginning with a simpler task that can be achieved and gradually building upon small successes. Thus, temporary avoidance may in fact be a realistic problem solving strategy in the first months after implantation. The problem solving orientation is likely a key to persisting from initial frustrations toward gradual improvement.

The experiences of this cohort is an interesting contrast to comments from a more diverse and "typical" group of 40 CI recipients described by Gfeller et al. (2019a), who represented a wide range of musical background (no musical training to college level instruction), interests and perceptual abilities. The "typical" group's average length of CI use was 12.25 years (2.44–28.07 years). In response to a question regarding potential interest in music training, the more "typical" group expressed a strong interest (90%) in music training as long as the training did not require more than 30 min a couple of times for a total length of 1 or 2 weeks. Because experience-based plasticity requires extensive repetitions or exposures, and CI technology is not inherently suitable for conveying fine structure, it is unrealistic that a CI user would be able to accomplish high-level musical skills as a result of a few hours of effort. However, prestige musicianship is also not a strong priority for all CI users.

This group of CI musicians offers an amazing profile of what can be accomplished despite a degraded signal. This group also shines a light on the impact of attitude and motivation as central to rehabilitation. Music is a passion and part of their identities. Thus, they are willing to invest immense effort and time to restore some musical enjoyment. Without this level of passion, such extensive effort is likely to be viewed as too time consuming or discouraging. This remarkable group does not represent the more typical profile of CI users on several factors, including age range, extent of residual hearing, extensive and formal musical training before or after implantation, and level of motivation; consequently, hearing professionals should make a strong effort to clearly understand the motivations, background, and aspirations of CI users before establishing unrealistic expectations for music enjoyment and rehabilitation. Nevertheless, these individuals demonstrate the impact of on-going focused training, and they offer possible strategies that might be used toward more modest levels of improvement.

In addition to immersion and motivation, the CI musicians also tended to focus on their internal capabilities for improving the sound and altering their auditory percepts to a greater extent than more typical CI users (Gfeller et al., 2019a). The CI musician group focused very little on technological options. As one user put it, "I think we can get too hung up on what we can hear – for example by mapping implants."

Only 3.3% of codes from this cohort addressed the problems of a noisy or acoustically difficult environment. The more diverse CI group reported by Gfeller et al. (2019a) tended to emphasize barriers to music enjoyment from the environment, situation, or CI technology. Their problem solving strategies tended to take the form of accommodations or avoidance of problematic sounds as opposed to rehabilitation or restoration. The more "typical" CI user, however, also does not possess the wellspring of musical training and resources of these musicians with CIs; consequently, accommodations or compensatory strategies may be a more realistic approach for less motivated CI users in managing complex listening situations.

How might the experiences of this unique group inform other CI users or their hearing professionals? A review of the problem solving skills listed in **Table 3** and problem solving orientation in **Table 4** offer some possible strategies, exercises, accommodations, and behavioral or attitudinal approaches that could act as a menu of options to consider if a CI user is interested in more satisfactory music involvement. As the DPSM indicates, a number of factors – auditory profile, type of music, environment, personal characteristics – can interact and change with time and circumstance. Thus, various options will be more suitable for some individuals than others, as well as for particular listening circumstances. Satisfactory engagement in music is likely to require some basic knowledge paired with flexible and dynamic problem solving.

In summary, the experiences of this cohort of CI musicians represents unusually high levels of domain-specific knowledge paired with a strong problem solving orientation and flexibility in applying problem solving skills. They have utilized accommodations, compensatory strategies, and training to enhance perception with end results that exceed expectations, based upon technical features of the device. These CI users might be referred to as auditory athletes, who like high-level athletes, push their capabilities to extreme levels. Comparisons come to mind with stroke patients who have pushed through months of painstaking rehabilitation, with no guarantees of outcomes, to restore motor or cognitive functions (Brown et al., 2014). While more typical CI recipients may have a less robust problem solving orientation and fewer resources upon which to build, this model nevertheless provides a framework for considering those factors needed for a given CI user to optimize their daily experiences with music listening or music making. These data also suggest some interesting avenues for future hypothesis testing to explore experience-based plasticity, compensatory strategies, motivation, and other internal factors that impact CI benefit.

ETHICS STATEMENT

Ethical review and approval was not required for the study on human participants in accordance with the local legislation and institutional requirements. The patients/participants provided their written informed consent to participate in this study. Written informed consent was obtained from the individual(s) for the publication of any potentially identifiable images or data included in this article. For further information, please see the author's correspondence with the IRB in the **Supplementary Material**.

AUTHOR CONTRIBUTIONS

KG coordinated data gathering, management, coding, and analyses. RM, AM, RO, JS, GM, and BGT contributed narratives regarding the music experiences of CI users. KG and RM addressed guidelines for IRB approval. RM gathered and analyzed the data for **Table 1**. KG served as primary writer for the manuscript, though all authors contributed to article content, and reviewed analyses of the data and article content. All authors contributed to the conceptualization of the manuscript and protocol for gathering information.

ACKNOWLEDGMENTS

We wish to acknowledge assistance from Virginia Driscoll with coding a portion of the dataset and assistance with manuscript preparation and submission.

REFERENCES

Bardes, C. L. (2012). Defining "patient-centered medicine". *N. Engl. J. Med.* 366, 782–783. doi: 10.1056/nejmp1200070

Bradley, E. H., Curry, L. A., and Devers, K. J. (2007). Qualitative data analysis for health services research: developing taxonomy, themes, and theory. *Health Serv. Res.* 42, 1758–1772. doi: 10.1111/j.1475-6773.2006.00684.x

Brown, M., Levak, W., McPherson, K. M., Dean, S. G., Reed, K., Weatherall, M., et al. (2014). Survival, momentum, and things that make me "me": patients' perceptions of goal setting after stroke. *Disabil. Rehabil.* 36, 1020–1026. doi: 10.3109/09638288.2013.825653

Clancy, C., and Collins, F. S. (2010). Patient-centered outcomes research institute: the intersection of science and health care. *Sci. Transl. Med.* 2, cm18–cm37.

Creswell, J. W. (2014). *A Concise Introduction to Mixed Methods Research* Thousand Oaks, CA: SAGE publications.

Drennan, W. R., Oleson, J. J., Gfeller, K., Crosson, J., Driscoll, V. D., Won, J. H., et al. (2015). Clinical evaluation of music perception, appraisal and experience in cochlear implant users. *Int. J. Audiol.* 54, 114–123. doi: 10.3109/14992027.2014.948219

Fu, Q., and Galvin, J. J. III (2007). Perceptual learning and auditory training in cochlear implant recipients. *Trends Appl.* 11, 193–205. doi: 10.1177/1084713807301379

Gfeller, K., Driscoll, V., and Schwalje, A. (2019a). Adult cochlear implant recipients' perspectives on experiences with music in everyday life: a mltifaceted and dynamic phenomenon. *Front. Neurosci.* 13:1229. doi: 10.3389/fnins.2019.01229

Gfeller, K., Driscoll, V., and Schwalje, A. (2019b). Beyond technology: the interaction of perceptual accuracy and experiential factors in pediatric music engagement. *Otol. Neurotol.* 40:e290. doi: 10.1097/MAO.0000000000002123

Gfeller, K., Driscoll, V., Smith, R., and Scheperle, C. (2012). The music experiences and attitudes of a first cohort of prelingually deaf adolescent and young adult cochlear implant recipients. *Semi. Hear.* 33, 346–360. doi: 10.1055/s-0032-1329224

Gfeller, K., Mehr, M., and Witt, S. (2001). Aural rehabilitation of music perception and enjoyment of adult cochlear implant users. *J. Acad. Rehabil. Audiol.* 34, 17–27.

Hargreaves, D. J., and North, A. C. (2010). "Experimental aesthetics and liking for music," in *Handbook of Music and Emotion: Theory, Research, Applications* eds P. N. Juslin, and J. A. Sloboda (Oxford: Oxford University Press), 515–546. doi: 10.1093/acprof:oso/9780199230143.003.0019

Herholz, S. C., and Zatorre, R. J. (2012). Musical training as a framework for brain plasticity: behavior, function, and structure. *Neuron* 76, 486–502. doi: 10.1016/j.neuron.2012.10.011

Hill-Briggs, F. (2003). Problem solving in diabetes self-management: a model of chronic illness self-management behavior. *Ann. Behav. Med.* 25, 182–193. doi: 10.1207/s15324796abm2503-04

Kraus, N., and Chandrasekaran, B. (2010). Music training for the development of auditory skills. *Nat. Neurosci.* 11, 599–605. doi: 10.1038/nrn2882

Limb, C. J., and Roy, A. T. (2014). Technological, biological, and acoustical constraints to music perception in cochlear implant users. *Hear. Res.* 308, 13–26. doi: 10.1016/j.heares.2013.04.009

Looi, V., Gfeller, K., and Driscoll, V. (2012). Music appreciation and training for cochlear implant recipients: a review. *Semi. Hear.* 33, 307–334. doi: 10.1055/s-0032-1329222

Mather, M. W., Hamilton, D., Robalino, S., and Rousseau, N. (2017). Going where other methods cannot: a systematic mapping review of 25 years of qualitative research in Otolaryngology. *Clin. Otolaryngol.* 43, 1443–1453. doi: 10.1111/coa.13200

Moreno, S., and Bidelman, G. M. (2014). Examining neural plasticity and cognitive benefit through the unique lens of musical training. *Hear. Res.* 308, 84–97. doi: 10.1016/j.heares.2013.09.012

Patel, A. D. (2014). Can nonlinguistic musical training change the way the brain processes speech? The expanded OPERA hypothesis. *Hear. Res.* 308, 98–108. doi: 10.1016/j.heares.2013.08.011

Plant, G. (2015). Musical FAVORS: Reintroducing music to adult cochlear implant users. *Cochlear Implants Int.* 16(Suppl. 3), S5–S12. doi: 10.1179/1467010015z.000000000271

Rocca, C. (2012). A different musical perspective: improving outcomes in music through habilitation, education, and training for children with cochlear implants. *Semi. Hear.* 33, 425–433. doi: 10.1055/s-0032-1329229

Saldaña, J. (2013). *The Coding Manual for Qualitative Researchers.* London: Sage.

Savenye, W. C., and Robinson, R. S. (1996). "Qualitative research issues and methods: an introduction for educational technologists," in *Handbook for Research for Educational Communication and Technology*, eds D. H. Jonassen and P. Harris (Mahwah, NJ: Lawrence Ehrlbaum Associates), 1171–1195.

Strelnikov, K., Marx, M., Lagleyre, S., Fraysee, B., Deguine, O., and Barone, P. (2015). PET-imagine of brain plasticity after cochlear implantation. *Hear. Res.* 322, 180–187. doi: 10.1016/j.heares.2014.10.001

Tates, K., Zwaanswijk, M., Otten, R., van Dulmen, S., Hoogerbrugge, P. M., Kamps, W. A., et al. (2009). Online focus groups as a tool to collect data in hard-to-include populations: examples from paediatric oncology. *BMC Med. Res. Methodol.* 9:15. doi: 10.1186/1471-2288-9-15

Xu, L., Zhou, N., Chen, X., Li, Y., Schultz, H. M., Zhao, X., et al. (2009). Vocal singing by prelingually-deafened children with cochlear implants. *Hear. Res.* 255, 129–134. doi: 10.1016/j.heares.2009.06.011

8

Perception of Musical Tension in Cochlear Implant Listeners

Steffen Spangmose, Jens Hjortkjær and Jeremy Marozeau*

Hearing Systems Group, Department of Health Technology, Technical University of Denmark, Lyngby, Denmark

***Correspondence:**
Jeremy Marozeau
jemaroz@dtu.dk

Despite the difficulties experienced by cochlear implant (CI) users in perceiving pitch and harmony, it is not uncommon to see CI users listening to music, or even playing an instrument. Listening to music is a complex process that relies not only on low-level percepts, such as pitch or timbre, but also on emotional reactions or the ability to perceive musical sequences as patterns of tension and release. CI users engaged in musical activities might experience some of these higher-level musical features. The goal of this study is to evaluate CI users' ability to perceive musical tension. Nine CI listeners (CIL) and nine normal-hearing listeners (NHL) were asked to rate musical tension on a continuous visual analog slider during music listening. The subjects listened to a 4 min recording of Mozart's Piano Sonata No. 4 (K282) performed by an experienced pianist. In addition to the original piece, four modified versions were also tested to identify which features might influence the responses to the music in the two groups. In each version, one musical feature of the piece was altered: tone pitch, intensity, rhythm, or tempo. Surprisingly, CIL and NHL rated overall musical tension in a very similar way in the original piece. However, the results from the different modifications revealed that while NHL ratings were strongly affected by music with random pitch tones (but preserved intensity and timing information), CIL ratings were not. Rating judgments of both groups were similarly affected by modifications of rhythm and tempo. Our study indicates that CI users can understand higher-level musical aspects as indexed by musical tension ratings. The results suggest that although most CI users have difficulties perceiving pitch, additional music cues, such as tempo and dynamics might contribute positively to their experience of music.

Keywords: cochlear implant, music perception, musical tension, hearing impairment, music enjoyment

INTRODUCTION

The perception and enjoyment of music can be challenging for hearing-impaired listeners. Apart from reducing sensitivity, hearing impairment can distort perceptual features important for music, including abnormal perception of loudness (Marozeau and Florentine, 2007), pitch (Moore and Carlyon, 2005) and timbre (Emiroglu and Kollmeier, 2008). Furthermore, hearing devices, such as hearing aids or cochlear implants (CI) typically alter the signal to improve speech perception rather than focusing on musical features (Fitz and McKinney, 2010; Marozeau et al., 2014). Specifically, studies have shown that CI users have difficulty perceiving pitch, identifying musical instruments, or segregating simultaneous melodies (for a review see McDermott, 2011). However, despite those limitations, it is not uncommon to find CI users engaged in musical activities, either listening at home, attending a concert, or actively playing an instrument (Gfeller et al., 2000; Migirov et al., 2009). Given many

CI users' engagement with musical activities, it is worthwhile investigating the musical features that might contribute to CI users' music perception. In this study, specifically, we will investigate how CI listeners (CIL) perceive musical tension.

The CI is a medical device dedicated to restoring speech perception in people with severe hearing impairment. It is composed of a sound processor, worn behind the ear, and a receiver located between the skin and the temporal bone. The receiver is connected to an array of 12–22 electrodes inserted in the scala tympani of the cochlea. Each electrode activates different regions of the auditory nerve. As the cochlea is organized tonotopically, the sound induced by an electrode should decrease in pitch as the electrode is inserted further into the cochlea. However, as those electrodes are limited in number and are not in direct contact with individual auditory nerve fibers, they cannot restore the frequency resolution needed to convey complex pitch information. Consequently, CI users have poor pitch discrimination, and most CI users cannot identify the direction of a pitch change for steps smaller than half an octave (Looi et al., 2004). This also prevents them from correctly identifying well-known melodies without additional lyrics and rhythm cues (Gfeller et al., 2002). Furthermore, CI users have greatly impaired perception of dissonance and consonance in chord changes (Caldwell et al., 2016) as well as impaired perception of timbre (Marozeau and Lamping, 2019). However, the CI device conveys precise temporal information. Studies using rhythm discrimination tasks show similar performance scores for CI and NH listeners (Kong et al., 2004).

Listening to music is an experience that arises from more than the sum of the sensations induced by its fundamental elements: pitch, timbre, rhythm. Listening to music is a pleasant experience that can evoke emotions or memories and can bring the listener to a specific mental state. If some CIL are still engaged in musical activities, it is likely because some of these more complex aspects of musical experiences are preserved. CI users can benefit from sung lyrics in music, allowing them to enjoy the content of the songs despite being unable to identify the melody. For music with a specific rhythm or groove, CIL might enjoy the rhythm and may, for instance, become motivated to dance (Au et al., 2012). They may also use tempo and rhythm cues to evaluate the emotional mood of the song (Vannson et al., 2015). However, it is still unknown to what extent they experience the complex cognitive structure that music enjoyment also relies on.

The experience of meaningful musical structure is often described as the experience of moments of tension and release (Schenker, 1935; Schoenberg, 1975; Lerdahl, 2001). Musical tension can be created by subtle musical cues that break the listener anticipation, for example, a dissonant chord or a delayed resolution. In tonal harmony, the resolution of a dominant chord on the tonic, for instance, is typically described as a release of tension. More formal descriptions of tension have been based on tonal music theory (Lerdahl and Jackendoff, 1983; Lerdahl, 2001; Lerdahl and Krumhansl, 2007) or psychological accounts of expectation (Narmour, 1990; Margulis, 2005). Hjortkjær (2011) proposed a parametric model that predicts continuous tension ratings of NHL from musical audio features. In this model, tension is predicted as a combination of low-level acoustic features including measures of intensity variation and distribution of spectral energy, as well as higher-level features related to changes in pitch class distribution and in tonality. Of these cues, CIL might be able to perceive intensity variations and coarse spectral changes (McKay, 2004) but are unlikely to have access to higher-level features that rely on accurate pitch processing. It is thus possible that CIL can use low-level cues related to loudness and spectral variation to judge musical tension. On the other hand, it is unlikely that they will have access to cues associated with the complex tonal structure of musical pieces that are thought to be central to the perception of musical tension in normal-hearing listeners.

The perception of musical tension is often linked to musical affect (Krumhansl, 1996), but tension does not necessarily directly predict musical preference or enjoyment. In a recent study, Vannson et al. (2015) asked CIL to rate their musical preferences on 24 different, unfamiliar piano pieces. The results were strongly correlated with the regularity of tempo and rhythm. CIL reported that they enjoyed musical compositions with faster tempi and more complex rhythms more than pieces with slower tempi and regular rhythms. Such results differed from the rating of NHL that enjoyed both fast and slow pieces.

In this study, we investigated musical tension and enjoyment ratings in CIL and normal-hearing listeners, NHL, controls. We examined the effects of selectively manipulating cues related to intensity, pitch, rhythm, and tempo that are each important for tension and enjoyment in NHL. We hypothesized that CIL would rely mostly on loudness and temporal cues in their tension ratings and that more regular rhythms would reduce the overall enjoyment of the music.

METHODS

Participants

Eighteen volunteers, divided into two groups, participated in this study. The first group consisted of 9 NHL (six males, three females, age range 23–31, mean age, 27) with audiometric threshold levels between −10 and 20 dB HL at octaves from 250 Hz to 8 kHz. The second group consisted of three bimodal and six bilateral CI recipients (six females, three males, age range 23–79, mean age 47.9). Seven of the CI participants were post-lingually deaf and 2 were pre-lingually deaf, all with more than 1 year of experience with the implant. They were all fitted with Cochlear Ltd devices (Freedom Contour Advance or newer, equipped with a CP800 or newer, fitted with ACE) except for one Medel user (Flex 24 with CP910) and one with Advanced Bionics (HiRes 90K with Naida CIQ70). One of the three bimodal users was fitted with a Phonak Naída hearing aid. All of the participants had none or <3 years of musical training. They provided informed consent before the study, and all experiments were approved by the Science-Ethics Committee for the Capital Region of Denmark (reference H-16036391).

Stimuli

The stimuli were based on W. A. Mozart's *Piano Sonata, No. 4 E♭ major, K282.* This piece has been used in several previous studies on musical tension in NHL wherein elaborate analyses of the musical structure exist (Krumhansl, 1996; Lerdahl, 1996, 2001; Narmour, 1996; Vega, 2003; Margulis, 2005; Hjortkjær, 2011). The piece was recorded by a trained pianist on an acoustic piano with 88-weighted keys (Roland V-piano), equipped with MIDI sensors that allow storing of all MIDI information: note-on event, note-off event, velocity, and foot controller activation. Audio files of the stimuli can be downloaded from the **Supplementary Material** section. Five stimuli were constructed: the baseline (original piece) and four modified versions: random notes melodies, fixed intensity, fixed tone duration, and increasing tempo changes. All versions were rendered based on the MIDI information using samples of a Steinway Grand Piano. In the four modified versions, specific musical features were altered on the MIDI information before the resynthesis. All the stimuli were 190 s in duration except condition 4, which had a duration of 275 s. All stimuli had a dynamic range of 30 dB except for condition 3 (fixed intensity), which had a dynamic range of 19 dB.

The four different stimulus manipulations were designed to examine the relative influence of various musical features on the tension ratings, including tonality, intensity, rhythm, and tempo. In the first manipulation, the pitch of each tone was randomized based on a uniform distribution within the melodic range of the original piece (Eb_1 to Bb_5). This manipulation removed both melody and tonal cues while preserving the original rhythm and intensity cues. In the second manipulation, each note onset was set to have equal intensity (MIDI velocity value 77 corresponding to mid-range intensity). Small local differences in perceived loudness could still persist due to potential loudness summation between simultaneous and overlapping notes and the dependency of loudness on frequency. Temporal irregularities of the baseline were removed by quantizing each note to the closest 1/16 note. In the third manipulation, the duration between tones was set to a fixed duration equivalent to a half-note (0.78 s at 154 bpm), and rest intervals were set to a constant of a 3/16 note (0.29 s). This manipulation disrupts temporal information and keeps the density of note events at a fixed level. Tone pitches were unaltered in this condition, but the manipulation of note onsets naturally also alters the perceived melody. The fourth and last manipulation artificially enhanced tempo variations relative to the original performed piece. Using the MIDI tempo track, the tempo was scaled so that the tempi of faster sections were further increased, and slower sections further decreased. This modification, therefore, exaggerated tempo changes.

Procedure

Participants were seated in a soundproof booth 1.5 m from a nearfield loudspeaker (Dynaudio Acoustics BM6) and presented with the different stimuli in random order. For each stimulus, participants were instructed to continuously rate the amount of perceived tension throughout the piece by adjusting the position of a vertical physical slider (Evolution MIDI controller, UC-33) placed in front of them. No explicit definition of musical tension was given to the participants to be consistent with previous studies and to avoid biases (Madsen and Fredrickson, 1993; Krumhansl, 1996; Hjortkjær, 2011). Previous work found that the instruction to rate tension yielded ratings that are consistent across listeners (Fredrickson, 1995; Lychner, 1998), and that more explicit definitions could bias the results (Hjortkjær, 2011). The slider was positioned at the lower extreme (low tension) at the onset of each piece. The experiment consisted of three blocks each comprising all the stimulus conditions presented in random order. So each stimulus was presented three times in total. After each stimulus, participants were told to rate the piece using another continuous vertical slider ranging from: "do not like at all" to "like very much." Overall the experiment lasted ~1 h, including a small break between blocks.

Bilateral CIL were instructed to turn off their processor on their least favorite hearing site. Bimodal CIL were fitted with an earplug to minimize the contribution of any residual hearing. All NHL were equipped with an ear-plug in their left ear. The CIL were told to use their preferred setting for music listening.

The experiment interface was designed in Pure Data (version 0.47.1), and the position of the slider was recorded every 200 ms with 7-bits precision integers.

The stimuli gain were set such that the $L_{Aeq,peak}$ through the total duration of the piece did not exceed 65 dB SPL measured with a sound level meter (B&K type 2250), repeated for all conditions. This level was selected because sounds at 65 dB SPL are mapped by default to the C-level (maximum possible current) of Cochlear Ltd devices.

Participants received no information about the different structure of the five different stimuli prior to the experiment.

Analysis

To compare continuous tension ratings across conditions that included different tempi, the rating values were interpolated per beat. In total, 128 sample values were used in the analysis corresponding to 32 measures with a 4/4 metric.

Non-parametric permutation tests were used to identify statistical differences in the tension ratings between conditions or between groups. For each time sample in the tension ratings, we randomly permuted the group or condition labels 100,000 times to generate a null distribution of group/condition differences. Differences in the tension ratings exceeding $p < 0.05$ of the null distribution were considered significant.

The correlation between tension ratings between groups was assessed with permutation-based statistics. To compare tension rating curves of the two groups, we first generated phase-scrambled versions of the ratings by randomizing the phase in the Fourier domain. This creates random data with the same frequency content as the original ratings. To generate a null distribution, we computed Pearson correlation coefficients between the true and phase-scrambled rating data 10,000 times. A p-value for the true correlation was then calculated as $(b + 1)/(m + 1)$ where b is the number of random correlation values that exceeds the true correlation, and m is the total number of random permutations (Phipson and Smyth, 2010). This approach generates an estimate of the strength of the correlation that is unbiased by the auto-correlated nature of the tension ratings.

Enjoyment ratings were compared with Student T-tests. Within each group, the baseline was compared with the other four conditions using a two-tail paired Student T-test.

Differences across groups in the baseline condition were compared with a two-sample Student *T*-test. To minimize the risk of *False Positive* due to multiple comparisons, *p*-values below 0.01 were considered significant (0.05 divided by the number of tests). Due to a technical problem, the enjoyment rating scores were saved for only 7 out of 9 CIL.

RESULTS

Condition 1: Baseline—The Unaltered Piece

In this condition, listeners rated the original piece without modifications. The piece was rendered from the recorded MIDI that includes information about note-on and -off events, the key signatures, velocity, and foot controller.

Consistency within groups of listeners was tested using a hierarchical cluster tree analysis. The analysis revealed that the ratings of one of the CI participants (CI4) was highly uncorrelated with the remaining CI participants. Furthermore, this listener also showed larger variability of rating across repetition of the same condition. Unlike the remaining participants, this listener had considerable difficulties understanding the task during the test. For these reasons, this listener was considered an outlier and was excluded from the rest of the analysis. The results from the other listeners were averaged within their groups and across repetitions.

Figure 1 shows the average tension rating as a function of time for both the NHL and CIL. A high degree of similarity between the groups in the overall contours of the rating curves is noticeable. In both groups, the ratings qualitatively follow the build-up and release of tension within the different musical segments. The ratings between CIL and NHL were found to be strongly correlated ($r = 0.92$, $p < 0.001$). The musical piece is composed of two main sections (A and B) that are repeated. The first part of section A gradually builds up to reach a climax (measures 6, 7), and then slowly resolves (measure 9). The section B starts with low tension (measure 10), then builds a first climax (measures 12, 13) that momentary resolves (measure 14), rebuilds a second climax (measures 15, 16) and resolves shortly after (measure 17). The piece then repeats, but with slightly different interpretation by the musician. The first presentation of the sections A and B will be named A1 and B2, their repetition A2 (measures 17 to 24) and B2 (from measure 25 to 32) (further detailed musical analysis can be found in Krumhansl, 1996; Narmour, 1996; Lerdahl, 2001). Aside from the resolution of the sections A (measures 9 and 24), CI users rated the piece overall as more tense, but the ratings were generally very similar. Non-parametric permutation tests were used to assess if specific sections were statistically different. Only the climaxes in the B sections were found to be significantly different between subject groups, as indicated by the red diamonds in **Figure 1**.

No significant difference of the enjoyment ratings was found between the two groups of listeners [mean enjoyment ratings NHL listeners: 63.43%; CIL: 50.39%, $t_{(13)} = 1.3835$, $p = 0.1898$].

The perhaps surprisingly high degree of similarity between the ratings of CIL and NHL indicate that CIL can relate musical sequences to ebbs and flow of musical tension. However, it is unclear which cues they are using as many of the musical features

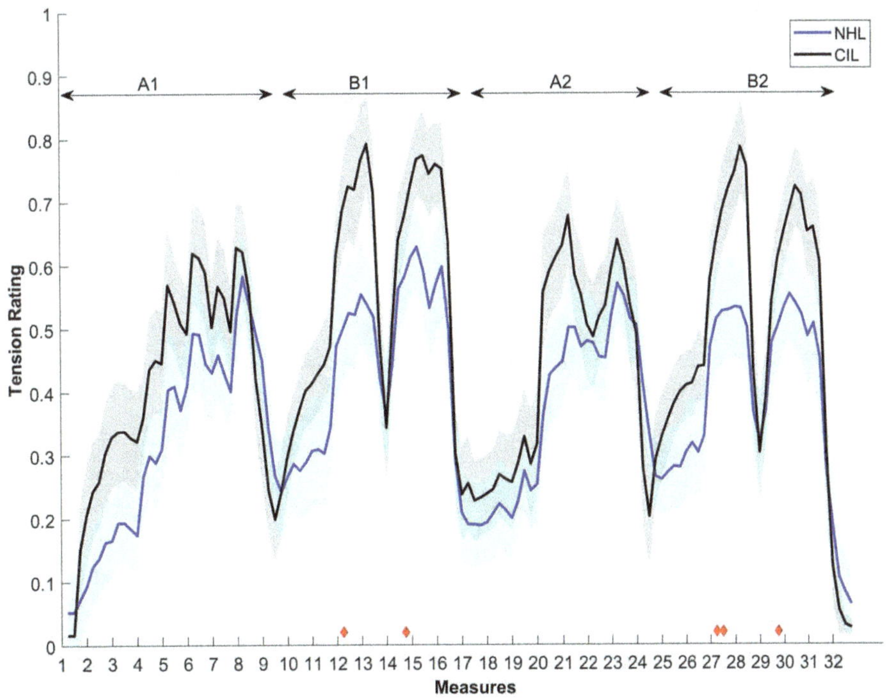

FIGURE 1 | Average tension ratings of 8 CIL (in black) and 9 NHL (in blue) as a function of the musical measures of the non-modified piece (baseline). Shaded areas represent standard errors. Red diamonds indicate the period in which the two ratings differ significantly. Horizontal double arrows outline the 4 parts of the piece (A1, B1, A2, B2).

that are predictive of tension ratings will covary. Therefore, the two groups could have based their judgment on different cues and still rated tension similarly. Therefore, other conditions were tested to assess the influence of different cues on the ratings.

Condition 2: Tonal Cues—Random Note Melodies

In this condition, the listeners were presented with a modified version of the original piece, where the pitch of each tone was set to a random value within the pitch range of the original piece. All other information, such as tone onset timing and intensity variations in the performance, were kept identical to the baseline.

Figure 2 shows the results for the NHL (upper panel) and the CIL (lower panel) in comparison to their group baseline. As can be observed, removing tonal information affected the ratings of the NHL significantly but affected the ratings of CIL to a lesser degree. Overall, tension ratings were higher in the random pitch condition in the NH group, which may relate to the higher degree of overall dissonance. For the NHL, significant differences were observed between the original and random pitch stimuli throughout the piece (as indicated by the red diamonds), except for the second part of section A. On the other hand, removing tonality from the original melody had a smaller effect on CIL ratings. With the random pitch, segments were judged to be more tense than the original mostly during the first part of section A, while the climax segments in the B sections were judged to be less tense than the original. The magnitude of the root-mean-square difference in ratings between stimulus conditions was evaluated for the NHL and CIL groups; values ranged from 0 (no difference at all) to 1 (maximal possible difference). The mean difference between stimulus conditions was more than twice as large for the NHL group (0.13) than for the CIL group (0.05).

This difference in rating between CIL and NHL can also be seen within their enjoyment rating. NHL' enjoyment rating dropped significantly from 63.43% in the baseline to 28.23% [$t_{(8)} = 3.9773, p = 0.0041$]. On the other hand CIL' ratings stayed at a similar level at 53.28% [$t_{(5)} = -0.9348, p = 0.3928$].

The results of this condition support the notion that the contribution of tonal cues is different for CIL and NHL. This outcome is expected, given the weak ability of CIL to discriminate pitch and poor melody recognition. Although the tension ratings for the NHL group were upwardly shifted with the random pitch, the overall baseline contour from the original was preserved with the random pitch. This also suggests that NHL can use other cues in their tension ratings that could possibly be processed by CIL. These could relate to loudness and timing cues that were assessed in the following conditions.

Condition 3: Loudness Cues—Fixed Intensity

The amplitude envelope of the signal can be a strong predictor of tension ratings (Hjortkjær, 2011), suggesting that intensity variation is an essential feature for musical tension. CIL should be able to perceive some form of intensity variations and may rely on them to judge musical tension. In this condition, all tones were set to the same onset velocity to remove intensity variations. Additionally, temporal irregularities of the baseline were removed by quantizing all notes at 1/16 note level. Overall, this manipulation creates artificial or "robotic" sounding stimuli, but where the tonal-rhythmic structure is preserved.

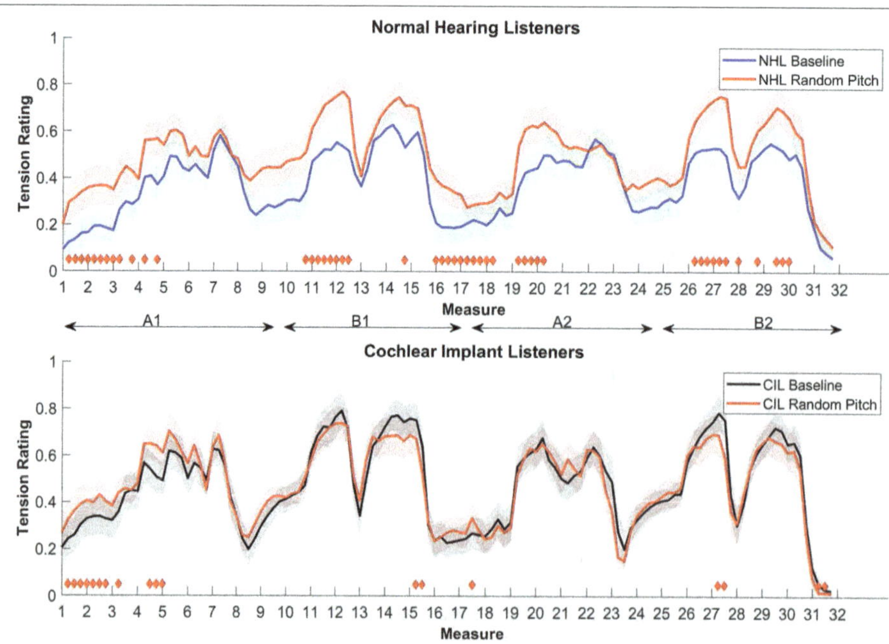

FIGURE 2 | Average tension ratings of 9 NHL **(top panel)** and 8 CIL **(bottom panel)** for the baseline and condition 2, random pitch (in red). See details in **Figure 1**.

Figure 3 shows the average rating for both groups. Both groups show different ratings compared to their baselines. However, this manipulation had a more pronounced effect on the ratings of the CIL (RMS difference to the baseline for CI = 0.14, NH = 0.09). For CIL, removing intensity cues had the effect of "neutralizing" the ratings with less overall variations. This result indicates an apparent impact of loudness cues on the ratings of CIL. For NHL, removing loudness cues also had a "neutralizing" effect, but the effect was less outspoken. The larger differences for the NHL can be seen in section B in which the climax is less efficient at creating a tense sensation and at the beginning of the A2 where the release is less pronounced.

NHL' enjoyment rating dropped significantly from 63.43 to 41.99% [$t_{(8)} = 4.1113, p = 0.0034$]. Enjoyment ratings of the CIL also drop from 50.39 to 42.38%, although this difference was not significant [$t_{(5)} = 0.9222, p = 0.3988$].

Condition 4: Temporal Cues—Fixed Tone Duration

As CIL can reliably discriminate rhythm and tempo, temporal cues might have an effect on the tension ratings. In this condition, the music stimulus was modified so that the duration of and between each note was fixed (to half-note length). This manipulation effectively removes tempo variations. Without access to tonal cues, fixed duration also removes rhythmic complexity.

Figure 4 shows the ratings for both groups. The change in temporal structure affected the ratings of both groups similarly. Mostly the climax of A and the second part of B were judged as less tense for both groups, while the transition between B1 and A2 were judged as more tense. Overall, NHL rated this condition less tense (23.62% of the time) or more tense (3.15% of the time) than baseline (RMS difference = 0.08). CIL judged this condition 22.05% of the time as less tense, and 5.51% of the time as more tense (rms of the difference 0.11). It is interesting to notice that the change in temporal cues had a similar effect on both groups, given that it has been showed that CIL have similar abilities as NHL in rhythm discrimination (Kong et al., 2004).

The enjoyment ratings were not significantly changed relative to the baseline for either group.

Condition 5: Increased Tempo Changes

This last condition was designed to test whether tension ratings can be influenced by tempo changes. Many styles of music allow for the tempo to vary quite dramatically, which can be used to convey tension or emotional content. In this condition, tempo variations of the baseline were artificially enhanced. The parts in which the performer slowed down were further reduced in tempo, and vice-versa. All other musical information was kept similar. **Figure 5** shows the tempo map of this condition in comparison to the baseline.

Figure 5 shows the average ratings for both groups. Overall, the differences in ratings were relatively small for both groups compared to their respective baselines. Nevertheless, some significant differences were observed. For the NHL, the modified tempo had the expected effect. A substantial increase of tempo during the section B1 induced a significant rise in tension (overall 7.09% more tense) and decreases in tempo between the measure 20 to 26 caused a significant lower tension rating (overall 3.15% less tense). The enhanced tempo variation also affected the ratings of the CIL but less so compared to the NHL (overall 4.72% more tense, and 1.57% less tense).

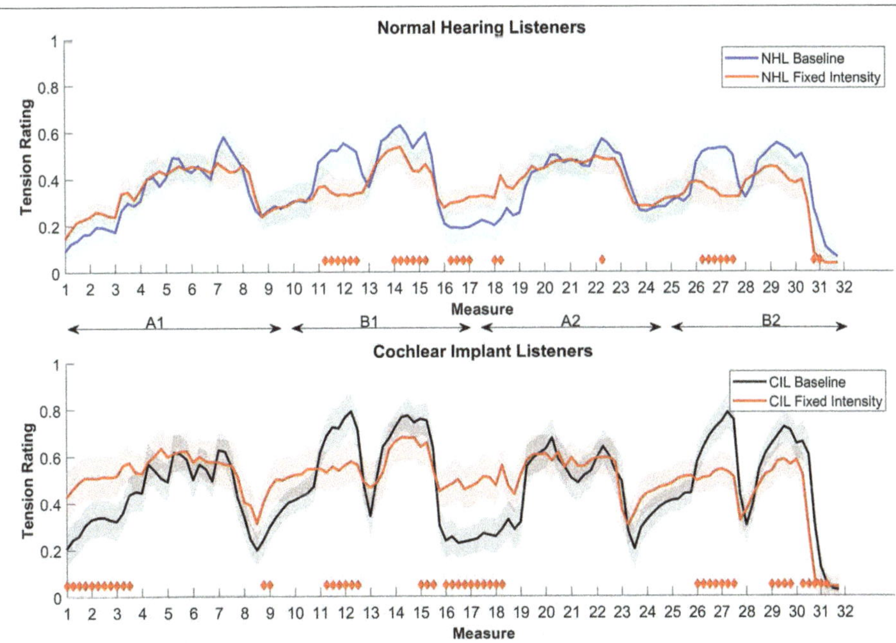

FIGURE 3 | Average tension ratings of 9 NHL **(top panel)** and 8 CIL **(bottom panel)** for the baseline and condition 3, fixed intensity (in red). See details in **Figure 1**.

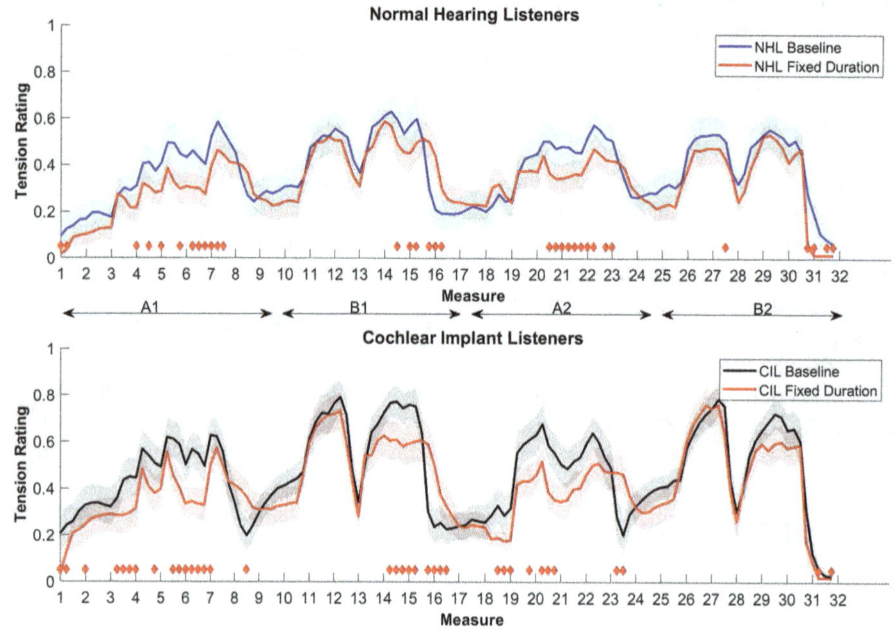

FIGURE 4 | Average tension ratings of 9 NHL **(top panel)** and 8 CIL **(bottom panel)** for the baseline and condition 4, fixed duration (in red). See details in **Figure 1**.

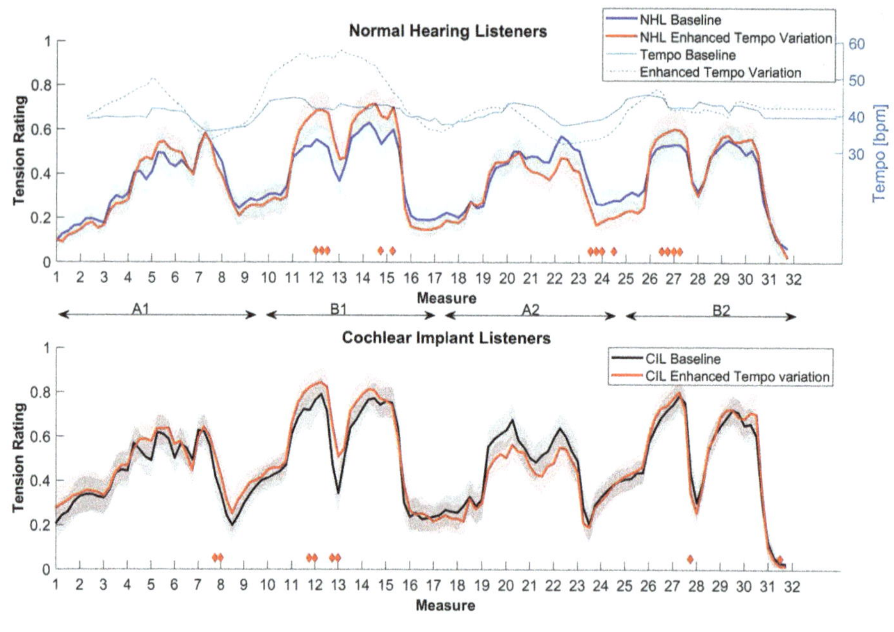

FIGURE 5 | Average tension ratings of 9 NHL **(top panel)** and 8 CIL **(bottom panel)** for the baseline and condition 5, enhanced tempo variation (in red). See details in **Figure 1**.

Enjoyment scores did not differ from the baseline for either group.

DISCUSSION

In this study, we compared continuous ratings of musical tension in CIL and NH controls to better understand what dimensions of musical experience might be preserved in CIL. In the unaltered baseline, the musical tension ratings of CIL were strikingly similar to those of NHL. The essential shape of the tension curves that define long-term ebbs and flow of tension throughout the musical piece was qualitatively similar in the two groups (**Figure 1**). This clearly suggests that CIL experience different levels of musical tension. This result is perhaps surprising, and is not, to the authors' knowledge, previously reported in the literature. Given the difficulty of CIL to perceive pitch and harmony, it would not have been surprising to find that CIL rate tension very differently from NHL. It worth noting that the notion of musical tension was not explicitly defined in any particular way to avoid biasing the participants. Therefore, it is possible that CIL and NHL interpreted the concept of tension differently despite similar ratings.

Although the average pattern of responses is very well-correlated with the one from NHL, **Figure 1** also shows that CIL rate the piece as more tense overall. This could potentially relate to their perception of the individual piano tones. It is not straightforward to evaluate how CIL perceive piano tones. However, a study on CI users with residual hearing suggested that they perceive a pulse train presented on a single electrode as an inharmonic sound (Lazard et al., 2012). It is, therefore, reasonable to assume that CIL will perceive single piano notes as inharmonic sounds as well. An overall more dissonant perception could potentially explain the overall increased tension ratings. In this case, the Random pitch condition should produce very similar patterns since NHL also lack tonal cues in that condition. **Figure 6** shows that the magnitudes of tension rated by the CIL during the baseline is indeed very similar to that of the NHL in the Random pitch condition, except for the measures linked to a release of tension after a climax (measures 8, 13, 16, 23, and 27).

We hypothesized that CIL would rely mostly on loudness variations and not on features that depend on the pitch in their tension ratings. The ratings of the musical stimulus with loudness variations reduced (**Figure 3**) support this showing a large difference from the ratings of the unaltered baseline piece. However, **Figure 2** shows that the ratings were also affected by the change in tonal cues. **Figure 7** summarizes the effect of the different conditions by showing the percentage of significant change for each condition. This indicates that removing loudness cues was the manipulation that had the largest impact on the tension ratings for the CIL and more than twice the effect of pitch cues. The trend is the opposite for the NHL where ratings were strongly affected by the removal of pitch cues and less so by removing loudness cues. The results indeed suggest that the perception of musical tension is dominated by loudness variations for the CIL, but also suggest a small impact of pitch variations. However, the effect of randomizing the pitch also affects the perception of overall loudness in the CIL. In the Cochlear device, the cut-off frequency of the lowest filter band is set by default to 188 Hz, which roughly correspond to $F_{\#3}$. Therefore, only the harmonics of the notes below that limit will be transmitted. Given that in condition 3, the notes were randomly assigned to a value between Eb_1 to Bb_5, it can be assumed that the loudness of many notes was altered.

Additionally, the small but significant effect of pitch that was observed in CIL might have been caused by the method that was used to randomize the notes. To generate random sequences, each note was picked randomly based on a uniform distribution within the original melodic range from Eb_1 to Bb_5. This introduces larger step intervals between consecutive notes compared to the distribution of step intervals in the original piece (and in tonal music in general). This might have introduced pitch changes that are more salient when perceived through the cochlear implant, which could have influenced the ratings of the CIL. It would have been possible instead to generate random sequences with a distribution of smaller step sizes which would still have destroyed the tonal cues. We would thus expect CIL ratings of random melodies with smaller pitch changes to be more similar to the baseline condition as CIL might not have perceived differences in pitch at all.

The sound level was set to optimize the perception of the dynamic range of the musical stimulus. We assigned a maximum level to 65 dB SPL since levels exceeding 65 dB are heavily compressed by the Cochlear device. At the other end, sounds at a level below 25 dB SPL are not transmitted. An acoustic

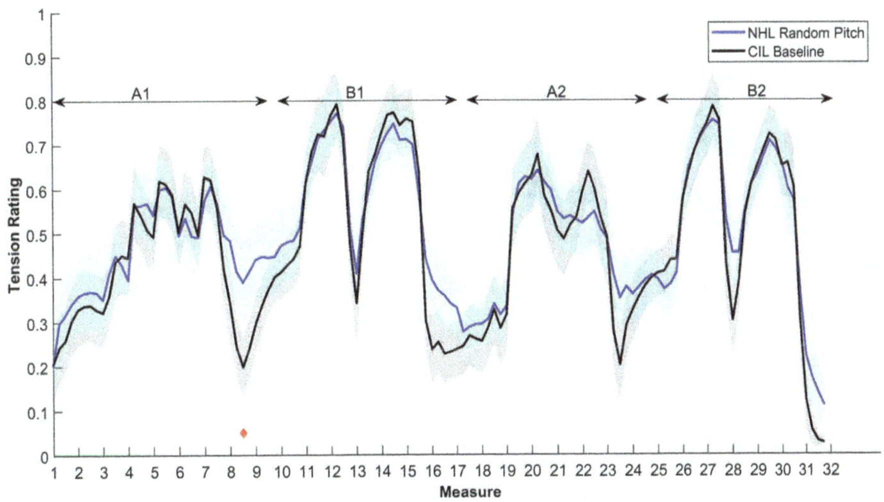

FIGURE 6 | Average tension ratings of 9 NHL for condition 2, random pitch (in blue), and 8 CIL for the baseline (in black). See details in **Figure 1**.

analysis of the baseline stimulus showed that the dynamic range of the piece was 30 dB, meaning that a maximum level of 65 dBA ensures that the soft parts can be clearly perceived. Since CIL appear to rely heavily on loudness cues, the level of presentation is likely to be very important. This study underlines the importance of presenting the music at an optimal level to optimize the perception of the musical dynamics. Additionally, it also suggests that compression stages should be considered with care, as they might alter this important cue.

Previous work by Vannson et al. (2015) indicated that CIL preferred music with faster tempi and more complex rhythm. Based on this, we investigated whether exaggerating tempo changes would enhance tension and enjoyment ratings in the CIL and whether removing rhythmic cues and tempo variations reduce them. However, removing or exaggerating tempo variations had only little effect on the ratings in either group. Tension ratings decreased in a similar way for NHL and CIL (**Figure 4**) in the fixed duration condition. However, artificially increasing tempo variations had disappointingly minor effects on either tension or enjoyment ratings, which were not significantly different from the baseline condition.

Overall, the different conditions had little effect on the enjoyment rating for CIL. **Figure 8** summarizes the average rating for each condition and group of listeners. The only statistical difference found was between the baseline and conditions 2 and 3 (tonal and intensity cues) for the NH group. However, a large variability can be observed in both groups. A large spread of music enjoyment ratings in CIL has already been reported in the literature (for example, see Migirov et al., 2009). **Figure 9** shows the individual enjoyment rating for each condition and group. Inside the CI group, the enjoyment rating of the baseline ranges from 12 to 71%. The different conditions did not affect those ratings except for two

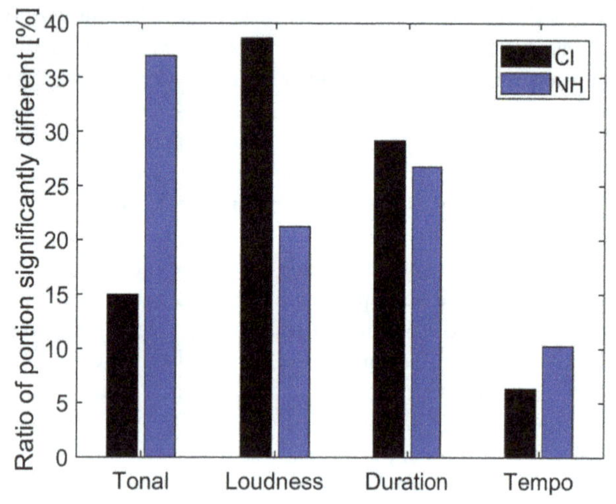

FIGURE 7 | Ratio of rating significantly different from the baseline for the four modified conditions: random pitch (Tonal), fixed intensity (Loudness), fixed duration (Duration) and enhanced tempo variation (Tempo).

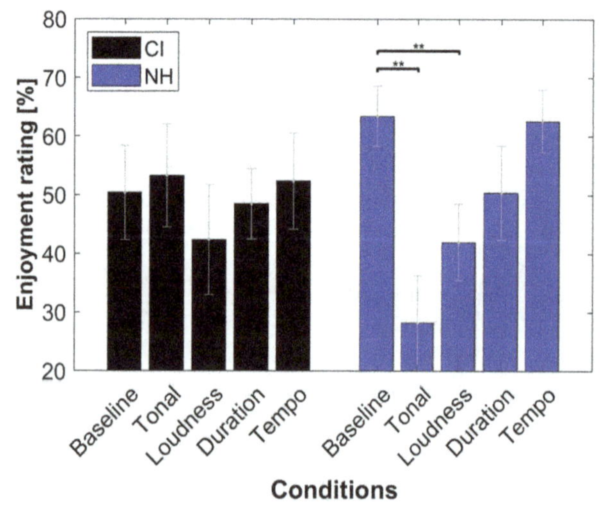

FIGURE 8 | Average enjoyment ratings for each condition of 6 CIL (in black) and 9 NHL (in blue). Horizontal lines and asterisks indicate significant differences ($p < 0.01$). See details in **Figure 7**.

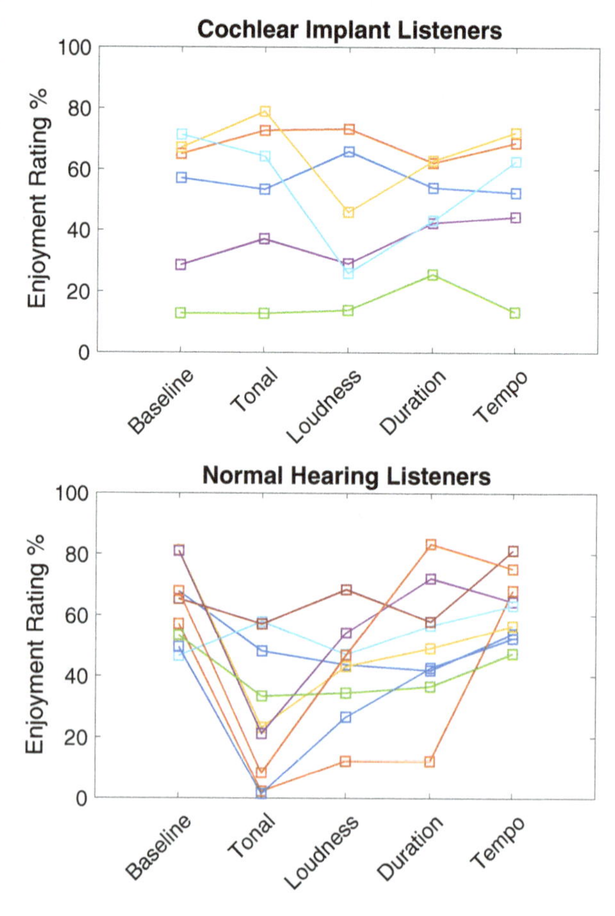

FIGURE 9 | Individual enjoyment ratings for each participant (represented by different colors). See details in **Figure 7**.

CIL that showed a large decrease of enjoyment for condition 3 (Loudness fixed). On the other hand, condition 2 (Tonal cues) was rated as dramatically less enjoyable for half of the NHL, while remaining stable for the other half. It is possible that this difference in ratings could be related to the listeners' familiarity with contemporary music.

If a musical piece is viewed as a mixture of the structure written by the composer and the interpretation of the musician, condition 3 (fixed intensity) can be seen as keeping only the effect of the composer (same tones and rhythm) and removing the effect of the musician. On the other hand, condition 2 (random notes) can be seen as keeping only the effect of the musician, while stripping away the work of the composer. This study shows that NHL rely on both aspects to enjoy and the experience music. Since the performance follows the dynamical structure of the composed music, features, such as loudness and tempo variations also convey the tension and release patterns of the music. CIL appear to be able to perceive the tension-release structure via such cues even without access to the tonal structure of the music. This might explain why CIL often enjoy music listening despite their poor perception of pitch.

CONCLUSIONS

Despite a poor perception of pitch and harmony, many cochlear implant, CI, users enjoy music. In this study, we show that CI users rate musical tension in a very similar way as normal-hearing listeners. By modifying the music on different dimensions, our results indicate that CI users rely mostly on rhythm and intensity cues to judge musical tension. This suggests that the perception of music can be conveyed by other features than the tone pitch itself. The importance of intensity variations for CI listeners also underlines the importance of listening to music at an appropriate level and without excessive compression.

ETHICS STATEMENT

The studies involving human participants were reviewed and approved by Science-Ethics Committee for the Capital Region of Denmark (reference H-16036391). The patients/participants provided their written informed consent to participate in this study.

AUTHOR CONTRIBUTIONS

JM initiated the project. SS designed the experimental interface, recruited the participant, and collected the data. This experiment was performed during SS master's final research project supervised by JM. All the authors have contributed toward the experimental design, the analysis, and the writing of the paper.

ACKNOWLEDGMENTS

The authors would like to thanks the participants for their time and effort, and Maxime Bru for performing the piece on the piano.

REFERENCES

Au, A., Marozeau, J., Innes-Brown, H., Schubert, E., and Stevens, C. (2012). Music for the cochlear implant: audience response to six commissioned compositions. *Semin. Hear.* 33, 335–345. doi: 10.1055/s-0032-1329223

Caldwell, M., Jadejvong, P., and Limb, C. (2016). Impaired perception of sensory consonance and dissonance in cochlear implant users. *Otol. Neurotol.* 37, 229–234. doi: 10.1097/MAO.0000000000000960

Emiroglu, S., and Kollmeier, B. (2008). Timbre discrimination in normal-hearing and hearing-impaired listeners under different noise conditions. *Brain Res.* 1220, 199–207. doi: 10.1016/j.brainres.2007.08.067

Fitz, K., and McKinney, M. (2010). Music through hearing aids: perception and modeling. *J. Acoust. Soc. Am.* 127:1951. doi: 10.1121/1.3384933

Fredrickson, W. E. (1995). A comparison of perceived musical tension and aesthetic response. *Psychol. Music* 23, 81–87. doi: 10.1177/0305735695231006

Gfeller, K., Christ, A., Knutson, J., Witt, S., Murray, K., and Tyler, R. (2000). Musical backgrounds, listening habits, and aesthetic enjoyment of adult cochlear implant recipients. *J. Am. Acad. Audiol.* 11, 390–406.

Gfeller, K., Turner, C., Mehr, M., Woodworth, G., Fearn, R., Knutson, J., et al. (2002). Recognition of familiar melodies by adult cochlear implant recipients and normal-hearing adults. *Cochlear Implants Int.* 3, 29–53. doi: 10.1179/cim.2002.3.1.29

Hjortkjær, J. (2011). *Toward a cognitive theory of musical tension* (PhD thesis), Copenhagen University, Copenhagen, Denmark.

Kong, Y. Y., Cruz, R., Ackland Jones, J., and Zeng, F. G. (2004). Music perception with temporal cues in acoustic and electric hearing. *Ear Hear.* 25, 173–185. doi: 10.1097/01.AUD.0000120365.97792.2F

Krumhansl, C. L. (1996). A perceptual analysis of Mozart's Piano Sonata K. 282: segmentation, tension, and musical ideas. *Music Percept.* 13, 401–32. doi: 10.2307/40286177

Lazard, D. S., Marozeau, J., and McDermott, H. J. (2012). The sound sensation of apical electric stimulation in cochlear implant recipients with contralateral residual hearing. *PLoS ONE* 7:e38687. doi: 10.1371/journal.pone.0038687

Lerdahl, F. (1996). Calculating tonal tension. *Music Percept.* 13, 319–363. doi: 10.2307/40286174

Lerdahl, F. (2001). *Tonal Pitch Space*. New York, NY: Oxford University Press.

Lerdahl, F., and Jackendoff, R. (1983). *A Generative Theory of Tonal Music.* Cambridge, MA: MIT Press.

Lerdahl, F., and Krumhansl, C. L. (2007). Modeling tonal tension. *Music Percept.* 24, 329–366. doi: 10.1525/mp.2007.24.4.329

Looi, V., McDermott, H. J., McKay, C. M., and Hickson, L. (2004). Pitch discrimination and melody recognition by cochlear implant users. *Int. Congr. Series* 1273, 197–200. doi: 10.1016/j.ics.2004.08.038

Lychner, J. A. (1998). An empirical study concerning terminology relating to aesthetic response to music. *J. Res. Music Educ.* 46, 303–319. doi: 10.2307/3345630

Madsen, C. K., and Fredrickson, W. E. (1993). The experience of musical tension: a replication of Nielsen's research using the continuous response digital interface. *J. Music Ther.* 30, 46–63. doi: 10.1093/jmt/30.1.46

Margulis, E. H. (2005). A model of melodic expectation. *Music Percept.* 22, 663–714. doi: 10.1525/mp.2005.22.4.663

Marozeau, J., and Florentine, M. (2007). Loudness growth in individual listeners with hearing losses: a review. *J. Acoust. Soc. Am.* 122, 81–87. doi: 10.1121/1.2761924

Marozeau, J., and Lamping, W. (2019). "Timbre perception with cochlear implants," in *Timbre: Acoustics, Perception, and Cognition*, eds K. Siedenburg, C. Saitis, S. McAdams, A. Popper, and R. Fay (Cham: Springer), 273–293.

Marozeau, J., Simon, N., and Innes-brown, H. (2014). Cochlear implants can talk but cannot sing in tune. *Acoust. Aust.* 42, 131–135.

McDermott, H. J. (2011). "Music perception," in *Auditory Prostheses: New Horizons*, eds A. N. Popper, F.-G. Zeng, and R. R. Fay (New York, NY: Springer), 305–339.

McKay, C. M. (2004). "Psychophysics and electrical stimulation," in *Cochlear Implants. Auditory Prosthesis and Electric Hearing*, eds F.-G. Zeng, A. N. Popper, and R. R. Fray (New York, NY: Springer-Verlag), 286–333.

Migirov, L., Kronenberg, J., and Henkin, Y. (2009). Self-reported listening habits and enjoyment of music among adult cochlear implant recipients. *Ann. Otol. Rhinol. Laryngol.* 118, 350–355. doi: 10.1177/000348940911800506

Moore, B. C., and Carlyon, R. P. (2005). "Perception of pitch by people with cochlear hearing loss and by cochlear implant users," in *Pitch Coding and Perception*, eds R. R. Fay, A. J. Oxenham, A. N. Popper (New York, NY: Springer), 234–277.

Narmour, E. (1990). *The Analysis and Cognition of Basic Melodic Structures: The Implication-Realization Model.* Chicago, IL: University of Chicago Press.

Narmour, E. (1996). Analyzing form and measuring perceptual content in Mozart's Sonata K. 282: a new theory of parametric analogues. *Music Percept.* 13, 265–318. doi: 10.2307/40286173

Phipson, B., and Smyth, G. (2010). Permutation *p*-values should never be zero: calculating exact *p*-values when permutations are randomly drawn. *Stat. Appl. Genet. Mol. Biol.* 9:39. doi: 10.2202/1544-6115.1585

Schenker, H. (1935). *Free Composition*, ed T. E. Oster (New York, NY: Longman).

Schoenberg, A. (1975). *Style and Idea.* New York, NY: St. Martins Press.

Vannson, N., Innes-Brown, H., and Marozeau, J. (2015). Dichotic listening can improve perceived clarity of music in cochlear implant users. *Trends Hear.* 19, 1–10. doi: 10.1177/2331216515598971

Vega, D. (2003). A perceptual experiment on harmonic tension and melodic attraction in Lerdahl's *Tonal Pitch Space*. *Music. Sci.* 7, 35–55. doi: 10.1177/102986490300700103

9

The CI MuMuFe – A New MMN Paradigm for Measuring Music Discrimination in Electric Hearing

Bjørn Petersen[1*†], Anne Sofie Friis Andersen[1†], Niels Trusbak Haumann[1], Andreas Højlund[2], Martin J. Dietz[2], Franck Michel[3], Søren Kamaric Riis[4], Elvira Brattico[1] and Peter Vuust[1]

[1] Center for Music in the Brain, Department of Clinical Medicine, Aarhus University and The Royal Academy of Music, Aarhus/Aalborg, Aarhus, Denmark, [2] Center of Functionally Integrative Neuroscience, Aarhus University, Aarhus, Denmark, [3] Audiological Clinic, Department of Otorhinolaryngology, Head and Neck Surgery, Aarhus University Hospital, Aarhus, Denmark, [4] Oticon Medical, Smørum, Denmark

***Correspondence:**
Bjørn Petersen
bpe@musikkons.dk

† These authors share first authorship

Cochlear implants (CIs) allow good perception of speech while music listening is unsatisfactory, leading to reduced music enjoyment. Hence, a number of ongoing efforts aim to improve music perception with a CI. Regardless of the nature of these efforts, effect measurements must be valid and reliable. While auditory skills are typically examined by behavioral methods, recording of the mismatch negativity (MMN) response, using electroencephalography (EEG), has recently been applied successfully as a supplementary objective measure. Eleven adult CI users and 14 normally hearing (NH) controls took part in the present study. To measure their detailed discrimination of fundamental features of music we applied a new multifeature MMN-paradigm which presented four music deviants at four levels of magnitude, incorporating a novel "no-standard" approach to be tested with CI users for the first time. A supplementary test measured behavioral discrimination of the same deviants and levels. The MMN-paradigm elicited significant MMN responses to all levels of deviants in both groups. Furthermore, the CI-users' MMN amplitudes and latencies were not significantly different from those of NH controls. Both groups showed MMN strength that was in overall alignment with the deviation magnitude. In CI users, however, discrimination of pitch levels remained undifferentiated. On average, CI users' behavioral performance was significantly below that of the NH group, mainly due to poor pitch discrimination. Although no significant effects were found, CI users' behavioral results tended to be in accordance with deviation magnitude, most prominently manifested in discrimination of the rhythm deviant. In summary, the study indicates that CI users may be able to discriminate subtle changes in basic musical features both in terms of automatic neural responses and of attended behavioral detection. Despite high complexity, the new CI MuMuFe paradigm and the "no-standard" approach provided reliable results, suggesting that it may serve as a relevant tool in future CI research. For clinical use, future studies should investigate the possibility of applying the paradigm with the purpose of assessing discrimination skills not only at the group level but also at the individual level.

Keywords: cochlear implants, mismatch negativity, auditory discrimination, music perception, multi-feature paradigm

INTRODUCTION

The cochlear implant (CI) represents a major breakthrough in the history of medicine and has meant a tremendous difference in the lives of thousands of people. After receiving this auditory prosthesis, patients with moderate to profound hearing loss are able to gain or regain the sense of hearing, allowing not only postlingually deafened adults to reestablish speech comprehension but also children with profound congenital hearing loss to acquire spoken language (Limb and Rubinstein, 2012). Moreover, recent technological refinements and a general rise in bilateral implantation have further improved implant outcomes over the last decades. Correspondingly, there has been a dramatic rise in the number of CI surgeries, and today >500,000 CI recipients worldwide use the device in their daily communication (source: EuroCIU).

Despite the success of CIs, some problems remain unsolved. Lack of temporal fine-structure, low spectral resolution, and a limited dynamic range in the CI signal are the cause of poor perception of pitch, timbre, and intensity (Drennan and Rubinstein, 2008). As a consequence, CI users experience challenges with perception of prosody (Peng et al., 2008) and emotional prosody (Hopyan-Misakyan et al., 2009; Nakata et al., 2012). Due to the complex temporal and tonal features of music, music listening is particularly challenging. This is indicated by reduced levels of music enjoyment (Gfeller et al., 2000; Lassaletta et al., 2008; Looi and She, 2010; Moran et al., 2016; Dritsakis et al., 2017a), poor perception of pitch (Gfeller et al., 2007; Zeng et al., 2014), impaired recognition of melodic contour (Galvin et al., 2007) and difficulties in identifying musical instruments (Driscoll, 2012; Kim et al., 2015; for a review see Jiam, 2017). Since improved perception of music represents a strong desire and could improve quality of life in CI users (Drennan and Rubinstein, 2008; Dritsakis et al., 2017b), a number of ongoing efforts aim to improve music perception with a CI (Petersen et al., 2012, 2014; Gfeller et al., 2015; Bedoin et al., 2018; Fuller et al., 2018; Jiam et al., 2019). Regardless of whether these efforts are of a rehabilitative or technological nature, it is imperative that measurements of the effect are valid and reliable.

In clinical context as well as in research, CI-users' auditory perception skills are typically measured by behavioral methods. In recent years, however, electroencephalographic (EEG) methods have been successfully applied as a supplementary measure. EEG offers the opportunity to investigate auditory function with a high temporal resolution by recording event-related brain potentials (ERPs). Especially one ERP, the mismatch negativity (MMN) response, has proven to be a reliable and objective marker for CI users' ability to accurately discriminate auditory stimuli (for a review see Näätänen et al., 2017). The MMN is a neural response elicited when a sensory input does not match the predicted pattern. Thus, the MMN indexes an error in the predictive coding of the environment, e.g., when a deviation in pitch, timbre, or rhythm occurs in a regular pattern of standard stimuli. The MMN is characterized by a greater negativity and it usually peaks 100–250 ms after deviation onset (Näätänen et al., 2001). Moreover, the MMN is an automatic response which means that it can be studied independently of the participant's attention (Näätänen et al., 1978; Alho, 1992; Paavilainen et al., 1993). As such, recording of the MMN is particularly relevant in small children who are unable to provide subjective responses.

In normally hearing (NH) individuals, the amplitude and the latency of the MMN response are in general related to the deviation magnitude, such that large deviations yield larger MMN amplitudes with shorter latencies and vice versa (Kujala, 2007; Vuust et al., 2011). In CI users, MMN responses typically show trends of smaller amplitudes and longer latencies compared to NH controls (Titterington et al., 2003; Kelly, 2005; Roman, 2005; Timm et al., 2014). It should be emphasized, however, that some studies have been unable to demonstrate reliable MMN responses in CI users which may be attributed to reduced recruitment of the auditory cortex as a consequence of prelingual hearing loss and/or long duration of deafness (Zhang, 2011; Petersen et al., 2013; Näätänen et al., 2017).

Historically, the MMN has been recorded with oddball paradigms in which an occasional deviant is randomly introduced into sequences of standards (Näätänen, 1992), typically at a ratio of 2:8. Recently, multi-feature paradigms have been introduced in which the standards alternate with several types of deviants, thus allowing for recording of MMNs to several features. An early version of a multi-feature paradigm, "Optimum 1" (Näätänen et al., 2004; Pakarinen et al., 2007), was first used with adult CI-listeners by Sandmann et al. (2010). In their configuration, identical synthesized clarinet tones alternated with deviants in either pitch, intensity, or duration at one of four levels of deviation magnitude. The authors found that CI users produced smaller MMN amplitudes for frequency and intensity deviations compared to NH listeners and failed to show any magnitude-of-deviance effect. According to the authors, these difficulties in discriminating small changes in the acoustic properties of musical sounds could to some extent account for CI users' poor perception and enjoyment of music.

With the purpose of creating a more complex and musically rich stimulation Vuust et al. (2011) introduced the "Musical Multi-feature" (MuMuFe) paradigm which instead of repeating notes presents arpeggiated triads in alternating keys. In two previous studies, we successfully adapted a version of the MuMuFe paradigm to investigate music discrimination skills in postlingually deaf adult and prelingually deaf adolescent CI users (Petersen et al., 2014; Timm et al., 2014). Both studies showed robust MMN responses to deviations in timbre and intensity in CI users. However, while the adult group failed to show robust MMN responses to rhythm, the adolescents failed to show robust MMN responses to pitch. Except for two magnitudes of the pitch deviant, these paradigms only contained one level of deviation which excluded assessment of discrimination thresholds. Recently, Hahne et al. (2016) carried out two experiments using modified versions of the MuMuFe, each presenting a different level of deviation magnitude. The authors reported marked effects of deviation magnitude on MMN amplitude across CI and NH groups. Furthermore, they found strong between-group differences attributed to CI users' lower MMN responses to intensity, rhythm, and pitch. Interestingly, while postlingually deaf participants showed larger

MMN responses than prelingually deaf participants, only the pitch condition showed a significant between-group difference.

The present study aimed to investigate CI users' discrimination accuracy for changes in salient musical features at a high level of detail. For this purpose, we adapted a version of the MuMuFe MMN paradigm which presented four deviants at four levels of magnitude. Furthermore, to reduce recording time and at the same time increase the speed with which deviants are presented, we applied a "no-standard" approach (Pakarinen et al., 2010) to be tested with CI users for the first time. Unlike the original version of the paradigm in which every other pattern included a "standard" note, every pattern in the no-standard version presents one type of deviant, thus omitting the standards (Kliuchko et al., 2016). As a complementary measure, we applied a behavioral test which examined attentive discrimination of the same features and levels also presented in the MMN-paradigm.

We hypothesized that despite a high complexity, the MMN-paradigm would elicit significant MMN responses in CI users as well as NH controls. Furthermore, by presenting deviants at different levels, we hypothesized that MMN-amplitudes and behavioral measures would reflect deviation magnitude and thus, by extension, reflect the paradigm's potential to estimate the resolution threshold at which CI-users are able to accurately discriminate different musical sounds. For potential validation of the paradigm's viability in CI-research and possible revision, a key aim was to test whether an effect of level on the MMN strength was present for each feature in each group. Extending previous findings, we expected that CI-users' overall MMN-responses would be significantly smaller in amplitude and longer in latency than those of NH controls.

MATERIALS AND METHODS

Participants

Eleven experienced CI users (M^{age}: 56.1 years; range 34–77 years; nine women) were recruited for the study through the Danish CI users' organization and their online platform. The CI users had an average duration of deafness prior to CI of 24 years (range 0.5–56 years) and their mean experience with the CI was 7 years (range 1–14 years) Two CI users were bilaterally implanted and four used a hearing aid on the side contralateral to their CI. Nine participants reported ability to speak on the phone, indicating a high level of CI outcome (see **Table 1** for details).

Fourteen older adults with normal hearing (M^{age}: 63.4 years; range 56–77 years; seven women) were included for reference and validation of the paradigm, recruited via social media. Comparison of age by means of a t-test showed that the mean age did not differ significantly between the two groups (p = 0.079). Normality of hearing was assured by passing of an online hearing test which adaptively estimated a threshold for perception of words and numbers in background noise[1].

All participants in both groups met criteria for being non-musicians, i.e., <5 years of formal singing or instrument training and no or only moderate formal knowledge of music. All participants received oral and written information about the study before giving consent to participate. The study was conducted in accordance with the Helsinki declaration and approved by the Research Ethics Committee of the Central Denmark Region. No monetary compensation was provided.

The study is part of a broader project which also investigates the neural plasticity underlying adaptation to the CI in naive implantees and the potential beneficial effects of a novel sound compression strategy in the Oticon Medical Neuro CI system (VoiceGuard) on the music perception of CI users. In addition to the MuMuFe, the participants were also presented with a free-listening EEG-paradigm, presenting real music to be reported in a separate paper.

Stimuli

The CI MuMuFe MMN-paradigm is adapted from the musical multifeature paradigm developed by Vuust et al. (2011) and integrates the no-standards approach from Kliuchko et al. (2016). Four different deviants, representing basic parameters of music, are embedded in an Alberti bass configuration, a four-tone arpeggiated accompaniment pattern, typically used in classical music. Deviants are presented randomly at four levels of magnitude: small (S), medium (M), large (L), and extra-large (XL), adding to a total of 16 variants. In all cases, the deviants occur at the place of the third note in the pattern.

The paradigm incorporates the following deviants and levels: (1) An intensity deviant created by decreasing the intensity of the regular note with 3, 6, 9, or 12 decibel (dB). (2) A pitch deviant created by lowering the regular note with either one, two, three, or eight semitones. (3) A timbre deviant created by exchanging the regular piano sound with either a bright piano sound, a blues piano sound, a trumpet sound, or a guitar sound. (4) A rhythm deviant created by shortening the second note by 26, 52, 103, or 155 ms while at the same time lengthening the third note accordingly to avoid a silent gap. The four displacements of the third note equivalates a 64th-, a 32nd-, a 16th-, and a dotted 16th-note, respectively, at a tempo of 146 BPM (**Figure 1**).

Piano sounds were created using the virtual piano Alicia's Keys (Native Instruments). The four deviant sounds were taken from the sample library of the software sampler Halion SE in Cubase Pro 8 (version 8.0.30). The sounds were exported in mono with a sampling frequency of 44.100 Hz and subsequently modified with an 18 ms rise and fall and amplitude normalized in Adobe Audition (2015.0 Release). Modification of the intensity and rhythm deviants was performed similarly.

Each tone was 200 ms long and was presented with an interstimulus interval (ISI) of 5 ms. Following three repetitions of each deviant, a change of key occurred. Notes were kept in the middle register of the piano going from Ab3 (208) to E5 (659 Hz). The order of the four possible keys (C, Eb, Gb, and A) and of deviants was pseudorandomized using Matlab (R2016a).

The paradigm was presented using the Presentation software (Neurobehavioral systems) and presented each deviant level 96 times incorporating a total of 6144 (4 * 4 * 4 * 96) stimuli. The stimuli were presented in four blocks lasting 8 min with a pause of approximately 1 min between blocks, adding to a total recording time of approximately 35 min.

[1] www.beltonehearingtest.com/dk1/

TABLE 1 | Demographic and clinical characteristics of the 11 CI users.

Group ID	Age at project start (years)	Duration of deafness prior to CI (years)	CI experience (years)	Number of implants	Side of implant used for tests	Hearing aid	Telephone ability
CI01	65–70	32	7	1	L	x	x
CI02	45–50	36	10	1	L	–	x
CI03	50–55	20	5	1	R	–	x
CI04	55–60	17	9	2	R	–	x
CI05	60–65	56	4	1	L	–	x
CI06	60–65	10	14	2	L	–	x
CI07	45–50	17	7	1	R	x	x
CI08	65–70	55	8	1	R	–	–
CI09	75–80	8	4	1	L	–	–
CI10	35–40	9	1	1	R	x	x
CI11	35–40	0	8	1	L	x	x
Mean	56	24	7				

Hearing aid: the participant wears a hearing aid on the ear contralateral to the implanted ear. Telephone ability: the participant reports ability to communicate via telephone via CI or CI + HA.

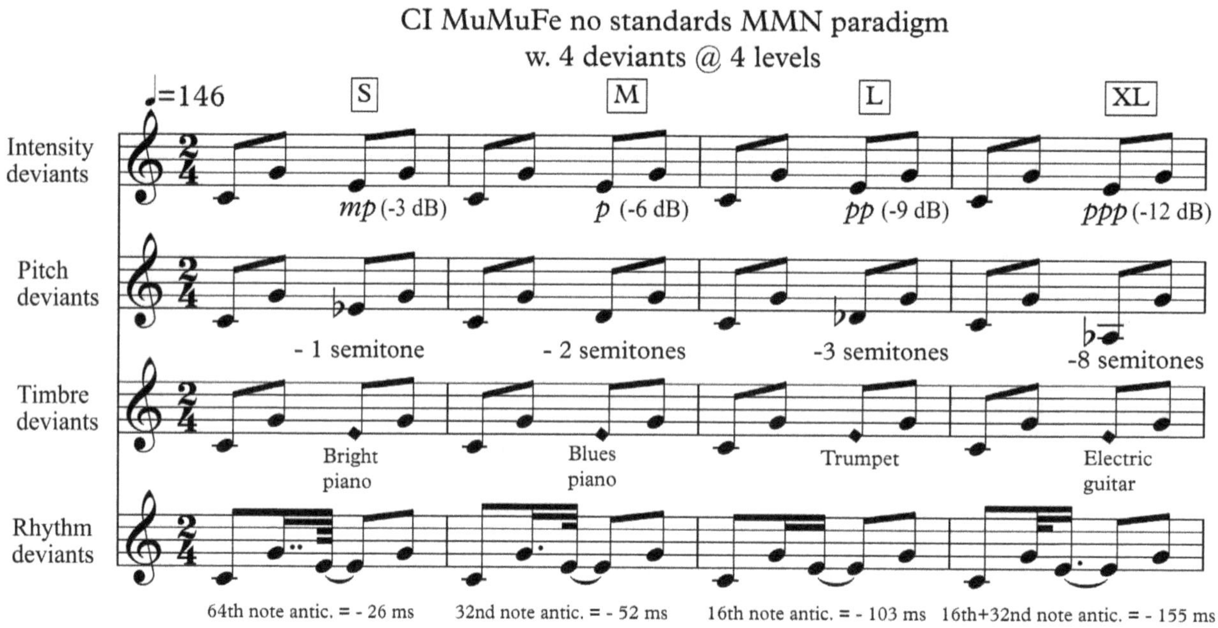

FIGURE 1 | The CI MuMuFe no standards 4 deviants/4 levels MMN paradigm. The paradigm is randomly presented in four keys: C, Eb, Gb, and A major. Lowest note is Ab3 (208 Hz), highest note is E5 (659 Hz). S, small; M, medium; L, large; XL, extra-large.

Procedure

Electroencephalography was recorded at the MINDLab EEG facility of Danish Neuroscience Center, Aarhus, Denmark, using a BrainAmp amplifier system (Brain Products, Gilching, Germany) with a 32-electrode cap with electrodes placed according to the international 10/20 system. Electrode numbers 28 and 32 were placed beside and over the left eye to record the electrooculogram (EOG). For CI users, some parietal channels could not be used because of interference with the CI transmitter coil. Data were recorded with a sampling rate of 1000 Hz using the position FCz as reference. Electrode impedances were maintained <25 kΩ prior to data acquisition.

During EEG recordings participants sat in an electrically and acoustically shielded room and were instructed to ignore the auditory stimuli and focus on a movie in which the audio was muted. For all participants, the sound level was individually adjusted to a comfortable level from a defined starting point of 65 dB SPL. NH participants received sound bilaterally through in-ear Shure headphones. To ensure comparable test conditions, CI users received sound monaurally. Bilateral CI users were asked to use their preferred implant; bimodally aided participants were asked to remove their hearing aid. To rule out any residual hearing, CI users received the stimuli directly in their implant via audio cable with microphones muted. CI users used their everyday processor settings during the EEG session. In cases in which the CI speech processor lacked a direct audio input, a spare processor was programmed with the participant's settings and used instead.

EEG Data Analysis and Statistics

The EEG data were preprocessed with the FieldTrip Toolbox for Matlab (Oostenveld et al., 2011). The data were first downsampled to 250 Hz and bandpass filtered between 1 and 25 Hz. Unused channels and other bad channels were replaced by interpolation of neighboring channels for CI users (mean: 2.5; range: 1–3 electrodes) and for NH controls (mean: 0.1; range: 0–1 electrode). This was achieved with the FieldTrip *ft_channelrepair* function applying the default interpolation based on an average weighted by the distance of neighboring channels. Eye movement and CI artifact components were isolated with the infomax independent component analysis (ICA) algorithm for EEG (Makeig et al., 1996; Delorme et al., 2007). A clear vertical eye movement component was visually observed and removed in all CI users and all except one of the NH controls. A salient horizontal eye movement component was visually identified and removed in 9 of 11 CI users and 10 of the 14 NH. For each CI user, one to eight CI artifact components were visually identified and removed, based on whether their topographical centroids were located above the implant site (Viola et al., 2011; Näätänen et al., 2017) and their waveforms were distinguishable from ordinary auditory evoked responses and neurophysiological oscillations.

Following the approach of previous MMN studies with CI-users in which consistent mastoid signals could not be obtained (Bishop and Hardiman, 2010; Sandmann et al., 2010; Zhang, 2011) data were re-referenced to the mean across all channels. Subsequently, trials were extracted using a 100 ms baseline corrected pre-stimulus window and a 400 ms post-stimulus time window. An exception was the responses to the rhythm deviants, where the baseline was corrected from −100 to 0 ms in relation to the onset of the preceding note (i.e., the second note). We implemented this measure in order to avoid the possibility that the temporal variance would affect the baseline. Any undetected noisy trials with amplitudes exceeding $\pm 100\ \mu V$ were automatically detected and removed (0.2% of all trials). As in the previous no-standard MuMuFe studies (Haumann et al., 2016; Kliuchko et al., 2016; Bonetti et al., 2017, 2018), the ERPs to notes 1, 2, and 4 were applied as the best option for standards (see **Supplementary Material**). The trials were averaged, and the standard responses subtracted from the deviant responses to identify potential MMN responses.

Statistical analysis on the MMN difference waves was conducted by following the clinical conventions of obtaining the average Fz electrode amplitude (Duncan et al., 2009; Näätänen et al., 2017) across a 30 ms time window centered on the feature-specific negative peak in the grand average ERP waveform (Näätänen et al., 2017). With the current stimulus paradigm and population samples, similar but slightly differing feature-specific MMN peak latencies were measured for each feature across groups: 148 ms for intensity, 156 ms for pitch, 132 ms for rhythm, and 152 ms for timbre MMN. For latency analysis, individual participants' peaks were identified as the most negative peak in the difference wave between 100 and 250 ms.

The statistical results for the MMN amplitudes and latencies were obtained using a three-way mixed effects ANOVA model using the IBM SPSS v25 software package. The tested between-subject factor was Group (NH controls, CI users) and within-subject factors were deviant Feature (Intensity, Pitch, Timbre, Rhythm) and Level (S, M, L, XL). Since Mauchly's test of sphericity showed violation of the sphericity assumption for the Feature factor ($p = 0.004$) with respect to MMN amplitude, the Greenhouse–Geisser correction for non-sphericity was applied for the Feature factor. According to our *a priori* hypotheses, we were interested in the potential main effect of Group and Level, the potential interaction between Group and Feature, as well as the three-way interaction between Group, Feature, and Level. We therefore focused our statistical analyses on these four terms, and thus adjusted the alpha level for the ANOVA by a factor of four to account for the four terms tested ($\alpha = 0.05/4 = 0.0125$).

Furthermore, to first test for significant MMN responses for all types of deviants, we conducted one-sample t-tests for the MMN amplitudes against 0 μV for each Level and Feature in each Group, applying Bonferroni-correction of the alpha-level [$\alpha = 0.05/(4*4) = 0.0031$]. In order to fully investigate the discrimination resolution of the paradigm, we carried out planned comparisons of the Level factor for each Feature and each Group on the MMN amplitudes, i.e., six Level contrasts ($3 + 2 + 1$) for each of the four Features, using paired-samples t-tests with Bonferroni-correction of the significance level for multiple comparisons [$\alpha = 0.05/(6*4) = 0.0021$].

Behavioral Test

In addition to the EEG measurements, all participants completed a three-alternative forced choice (3-AFC) test to obtain a behavioral measurement of the same music parameters and levels of magnitude as presented in the MMN paradigm.

A four-tone musical pattern, like the one presented in the MMN paradigm, was presented twice in the standard and once in the deviant condition [$p(\text{deviant}) = 0.33$]. The participants were hereafter instructed to manually choose the deviant pattern based on a pictorial representation on the computer screen. The deviant could occur in either the first, second, or third pattern in a randomized order. Each of the 16 deviants were presented six times adding up to a total of 96 trials. The scores were converted to percent correct hit rates for each deviant condition.

The 3-AFC data did not meet the criteria for normal distribution (NH: Shapiro–Wilk, $p = 0.10^{-6}$–0.131; CI: Shapiro–Wilk, $p = 0.10^{-7}$–0.535). Consequently, to test whether hit rates differed significantly from chance level, one-sample Wilcoxon signed rank-tests against the value 33.3% were conducted. Again, we focused our statistical analyses on the potential main effects of Group and Level, as well as the potential interactions between Group and Feature and Group, Feature and Level. NH and CI hit rates were compared with a Mann–Whitney U-test, and effects of Level (S, M, L, XL) on hit rates were tested with Friedman's ANOVA, both with a Bonferroni-corrected alpha level of factor two ($\alpha = 0.05/2 = 0.025$). Given that the standard Friedman's ANOVA does not include tests of interaction effects, we report

Bonferroni-corrected comparisons for the potential Group by Feature interaction ($\alpha = 0.05/4 = 0.0125$) together with the other *post hoc* comparisons. Finally, the potential three-way interaction was implicitly tested as part of our planned comparisons of the Level factor for each feature and each group which was tested with Wilcoxon signed rank tests with Bonferroni-corrected significance levels [$\alpha = 0.05/(6 * 4) = 0.0021$].

Correlation Analysis

To identify possible predictive factors and relationships, we performed a multiple regression analysis of the CI users' MMN amplitudes, behavioral hit rates, clinical data, and music appreciation data. Clinical factors were age, age at hearing loss, age at implantation, duration of hearing loss prior to CI, and duration of CI experience. Music appreciation data included music listening habits (hours/week), level of music enjoyment (1–7), and rating of quality of music with CI (mean VAS score across seven bipolar adjective descriptors). The latter were extracted from responses given in a revised version of the IOWA musical background questionnaire on the online platform SurveyXact.

RESULTS

Overall MMN Responses

All deviant types and levels elicited statistically significant MMN responses in both the NH group ($p < 10^{-4}$) and in the CI group ($p < 0.001$) (**Table 2** and **Supplementary Figure 1**). For both groups, the Bonferroni-corrected alpha level of $\alpha = 0.05/(4 * 4) = 0.0031$ was used.

Effects of Level and Group on MMN Amplitude

Main Effects

There was no main effect of Group on MMN amplitude (mean CI users = −1.02 μV, SD = 0.30; mean NH controls = −1.19 μV, SD = 0.34), suggesting that the overall MMN across levels and features did not differ significantly between CI users and NH listeners (**Table 2**). There was a statistically significant main effect of Level on MMN amplitudes ($S = -0.97$ μV, SD = 0.31; $M = -0.89$ μV, SD = 0.31; $L = -1.22$ μV, SD = 0.50; XL = −1.36 μV, SD = 0.40) [$F(3,69) = 21.33$, $p < 10^{-9}$, $\eta_p^2 = 0.48$) (**Figure 2** and **Table 3**). *Post hoc* comparisons confirmed that the effect was driven by a significantly higher MMN amplitude to the XL and L compared to the M and S levels (**Table 4**).

Interactions

Neither the two-way interaction between Group and Feature nor the 3-way interaction between Feature, Level, and Group passed the Bonferroni-corrected threshold $\alpha = 0.05/4 = 0.0125$ (**Table 3**).

Planned Comparisons

In accordance with our planned comparisons, we here report results of paired samples *t*-tests comparing all levels for each feature within each group. Only results meeting the Bonferroni-corrected significance level at $\alpha = 0.05/(4 * (3 + 2 + 1)) = 0.05/(4 * 6) = 0.0021$ are reported here. For full reporting, all results, including trending results at $p < 0.05$ without correction for multiple comparisons, are shown in **Table 4**. Plots showing difference waves for all deviants and levels are provided in **Figures 3, 4**.

TABLE 2 | MMN amplitudes.

Feature	Level	NH Controls				CI users			
		Latency in ms (SD)	Amplitude in μV (SD)	*t*	*P*	Latency in ms (SD)	Amplitude in μV (SD)	*t*	*p*
Intensity	S	161 (50)	−0.63 (0.34)	−6.94	$<10^{-4}$**	151 (24)	−0.87 (0.57)	−5.12	<0.001**
	M	175 (47)	−0.72 (0.44)	−6.00	$<10^{-4}$**	164 (53)	−0.84 (0.53)	−5.31	<0.001**
	L	169 (39)	−0.89 (0.55)	−6.03	$<10^{-4}$**	162 (35)	−1.03 (0.54)	−6.35	$<10^{-4}$**
	XL	173 (32)	−1.11 (0.49)	−9.25	$<10^{-6}$**	150 (30)	−1.38 (0.70)	−6.54	$<10^{-4}$**
Pitch	S	154 (32)	−1.33 (0.69)	−7.16	$<10^{-4}$**	181 (32)	−0.98 (0.46)	−7.12	$<10^{-4}$**
	M	171 (41)	−1.12 (0.65)	−6.48	$<10^{-4}$**	176 (40)	−0.90 (0.31)	−9.64	$<10^{-5}$**
	L	182 (47)	−1.18 (0.72)	−6.10	$<10^{-4}$**	173 (32)	−0.91 (0.69)	−4.39	0.001**
	XL	151 (17)	−1.83 (0.87)	−7.90	$<10^{-5}$**	174 (36)	−0.92 (0.47)	−6.51	$<10^{-4}$**
Timbre	S	158 (41)	−1.04 (0.54)	−7.21	$<10^{-4}$**	148 (12)	−1.43 (0.35)	−13.67	$<10^{-7}$**
	M	174 (40)	−0.82 (0.47)	−6.49	$<10^{-4}$**	192 (40)	−0.50 (0.41)	−4.05	0.002**
	L	175 (39)	−1.46 (0.70)	−7.74	$<10^{-5}$**	165 (28)	−1.24 (0.60)	−6.88	$<10^{-4}$**
	XL	145 (31)	−1.47 (0.72)	−7.61	$<10^{-5}$**	157 (36)	−1.57 (0.78)	−6.72	$<10^{-4}$**
Rhythm	S	161 (42)	−0.84 (0.36)	−8.59	$<10^{-5}$**	203 (30)	−0.63 (0.53)	−3.93	0.003**
	M	143 (32)	−1.34 (0.64)	−7.76	$<10^{-5}$**	164 (41)	−0.84 (0.54)	−5.10	<0.001**
	L	150 (39)	−1.55 (0.81)	−7.13	$<10^{-5}$**	166 (46)	−1.48 (0.82)	−5.99	<0.001**
	XL	149 (48)	−1.65 (0.88)	−7.05	$<10^{-5}$**	151 (45)	−0.95 (0.65)	−4.83	<0.001**

*Results of one-sample t-tests comparing MMN amplitudes against the signal level at baseline 0 μV at the Fz electrode. Showing mean peak latencies and mean amplitudes with standard deviations (SD). Degrees of freedom (df) for the NH controls = 13; df for CI users = 10. Cases where MMN amplitude diverged significantly from the baseline after Bonferroni-correction (p < 0.003) are marked with **.*

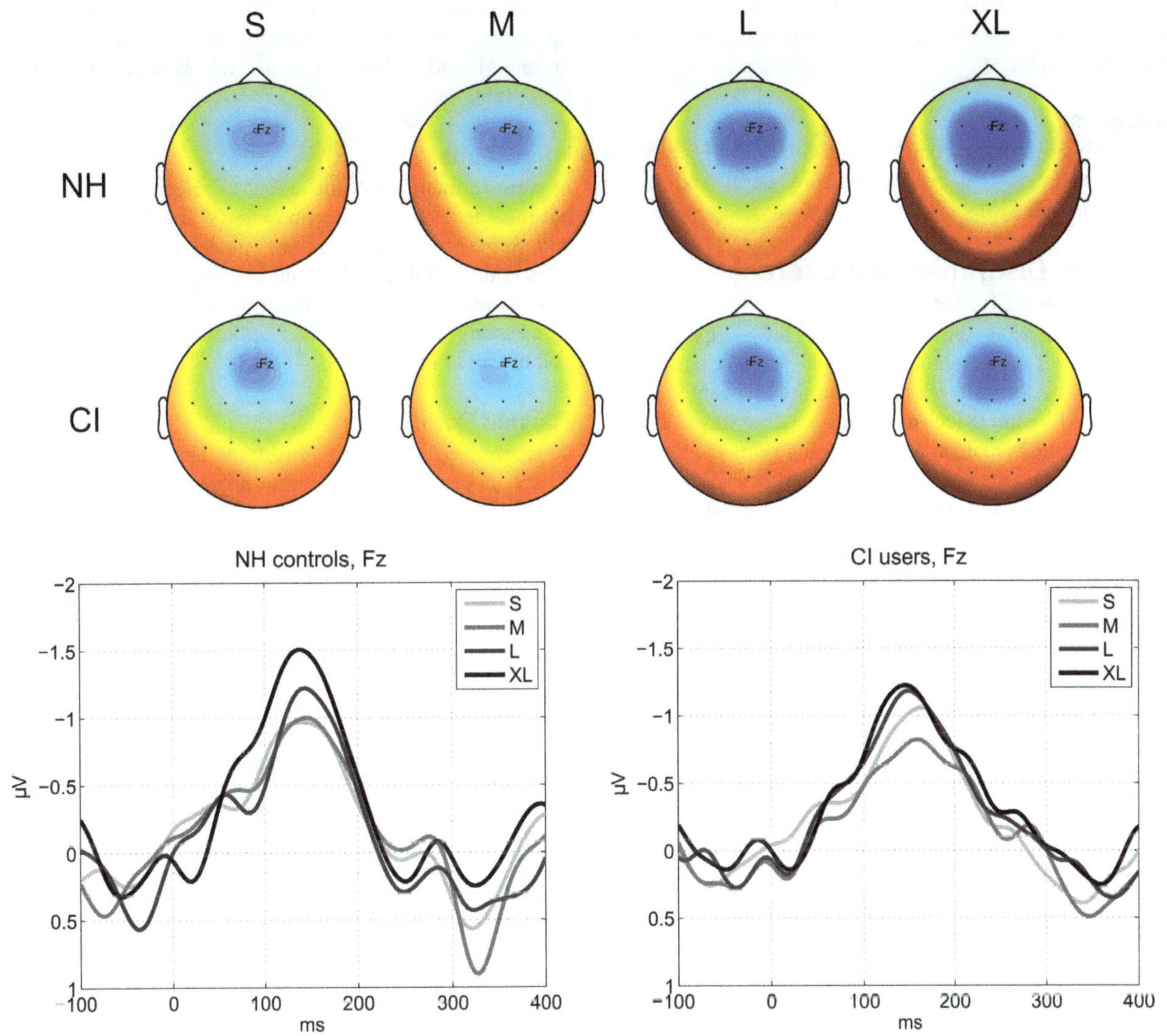

FIGURE 2 | MMN responses to deviant levels. **(Top)** Average MMN scalp topographies measured in a 30 ms time window centered on the global peak in the grand-average waveform at a latency of 147 ms. The colors are scaled from −2 μV (blue) to +2 μV (red). **(Bottom)** Average MMN waveforms for each deviant level and group measured at the Fz electrode.

Intensity

Normally hearing listeners showed no differentiation between any levels of the Intensity deviant. In CI users, there was a significantly larger MMN amplitude to the XL compared to the M intensity deviants.

Pitch

In NH listeners the MMN amplitude to the XL deviant was significantly larger than that of the L, M, and S deviants. The CI users did not show any significant differences in their MMN amplitudes between pitch levels.

Timbre

In the NH group, no significant differences were found between any levels of the Timbre deviant. CI users demonstrated a significantly higher MMN amplitude to the XL compared to the M deviant. By contrast, CI users' MMN amplitude to the S deviant was significantly higher than that elicited by the M deviant.

Rhythm

Normally hearing listeners' MMN amplitudes to rhythm deviants were significantly larger for the XL and L deviants compared to S deviants. In CI users, the MMN amplitude was significantly higher to the L deviant than to M and S deviants.

Effects of Level, Feature, and Group on MMN Latency

Main Effects

There was no main effect of Group on MMN latency (mean CI users = 168 ms, SD = 11; mean NH controls = 162 ms, SD = 14), suggesting that the overall MMN latency across levels and deviants did not differ significantly between CI users and NH listeners (**Table 3**). Also, there was no main effect of Level on MMN latency (**Table 3**).

Interactions

Neither the two-way interaction between Group and Feature nor the three-way interaction between Feature, Level, and Group were significant for MMN latency.

Behavioral Discrimination Scores

Performance vs. Chance

One-sample Wilcoxon signed rank tests showed that for NH controls hit rates were significantly higher than chance level (33%) for all features and levels, except for the Intensity S and M, Timbre S, and Rhythm S deviants (**Table 5**). CI users exhibited a high degree of individual variability, scoring significantly above chance level only for the Rhythm XL, L, and M deviants as well as the Timbre L and XL deviants (Bonferroni-corrected threshold: $\alpha = 0.05/16 = 0.003$) (**Table 5**).

Main Effects

The Mann–Whitney U-test comparing the group scores across Features and Levels revealed an overall significant difference between groups, with lower hit rates for the CI-users (median: 75%) than the NH controls (median: 100%) [$U(25) = 34.50$, $p = 0.015$, $r = 0.49$]. Furthermore, the Friedman's ANOVA showed a main effect of Level [$\chi^2(25) = 49.53$, $p < 10^{-9}$, $r = 0.69$] (**Table 3**). *Post hoc* comparisons confirmed that the effect was driven by significantly higher hit rates for the XL and L compared to the M and S levels and for the M compared to the S level (**Table 4**).

TABLE 3 | Analysis of variance.

Effect on MMN amplitude	df	df error	F	p	η_p^2
Level	3	69	21.33	$<10^{-9**}$	0.48
Group	1	23	1.43	0.244	0.06
Level × Group	3	69	2.27	0.088	0.09
Level × Group × Feature	9	207	1.94	0.048*	0.08
Effect on MMN latency	**df**	**df error**	F	p	η_p^2
Level	3	69	2.71	0.052	0.11
Group	1	23	1.25	0.276	0.05
Level × Group	3	69	0.84	0.476	0.04
Level × Group × Feature	9	207	0.98	0.461	0.04
Effect on behavioral hit rates					
	df	n	χ^2	p	
Level	3	25	49.54	$<10^{-9**}$	
	df	n	U	p	
Group	1	25	34.50	0.015**	

*First is shown the effects of Level, Group, Group by Feature, and Group by Feature by Level on MMN amplitude and latency (tested with mixed-effects ANOVA). Finally, the effects of Level (tested with Friedman's ANOVA) and Group (investigated with the Mann–Whitney U-test) on behavioral hit rates are reported. ** indicates significant differences; * marks trends at p < 0.05 without correction for multiple comparisons.*

Interactions

As already mentioned, the standard Friedman's ANOVA does not include tests of interaction effects, and we therefore report *post hoc* comparisons for the potential Group by Feature interaction in **Table 4**. They indicated that the group difference was mainly driven by significantly lower hit rates in the CI group compared to the NH group for the pitch deviants (**Table 4** and **Figure 5**).

Planned Comparisons

In accordance with our planned comparisons, we here report results of one-sample Wilcoxon signed rank tests comparing all levels for each feature within each group. We only report results passing the Bonferroni-corrected significance level at $p = 05/(6 * 4) = 0.0021$ here. All results, including trending results at $p < 0.05$ without correction for multiple comparisons, are shown in **Table 4** for full reporting. Violin plots illustrating the behavioral results are provided in **Figure 5**.

Intensity

In the NH group, the intensity XL and L deviants resulted in significantly larger hit rates compared to the S deviant. No significant differences between any levels were observed in CI users.

Pitch

The NH group showed a ceiling effect with no significant difference between any levels. In CI users, no significant differences in hit rates were observed.

Timbre

For timbre, none of the two groups showed any significant differentiation of any of the deviant levels.

Rhythm

Normally hearing participants showed significantly higher hit rates for the XL, L, and M compared to the S rhythm deviant. CI users did not show any significant differentiation in terms of hit rates.

Correlation Between MMN Amplitude, Behavioral Scores, and Clinical and Music Appreciation Factors

We found no statistically significant effects of any clinical or music appreciation factors on neither the CI users' MMN responses nor their behavioral hit rates. A weak positive relationship was found between age at hearing loss and strength of MMN amplitudes for the rhythm ($p = 0.026$, uncorrected) and timbre ($p = 0.071$, uncorrected) deviants, indicating that a larger MMN was associated with later age at hearing loss.

TABLE 4 | *Post hoc* comparisons.

MMN amplitude					Behavioral hit rates				
Feature	**Level**	**XL**	**L**	**M**	**Feature**	**Level**	**XL**	**L**	**M**
Planned comparisons for each Group, Feature, and Level by Level (corrected α = 0.05/24 = 0.0021)									
Normal hearing (*n* = 14)									
Intensity	L	0.186			Intensity	L	0.014*		
	M	0.008*	0.231			M	0.004*	0.038*	
	S	0.011*	0.125	0.540		S	<0.001**	0.001**	0.008*
Pitch	L	<0.001**			Pitch	L	0.317		
	M	<0.001**	0.764			M	0.039*	0.024*	
	S	<0.001**	0.422	0.198		S	0.024*	0.024*	0.886
Timbre	L	0.961			Timbre	L	0.317		
	M	0.014*	0.005*			M	0.040*	0.017*	
	S	0.019*	0.043*	0.243		S	0.005*	0.003*	0.065
Rhythm	L	0.636			Rhythm	L	0.285		
	M	0.132	0.147			M	0.141	0.066	
	S	0.002**	<0.001**	0.003*		S	0.001**	0.001**	0.002**
CI users (*n* = 11)									
Intensity	L	0.068			Intensity	L	0.865		
	M	0.002**	0.245			M	0.139	0.153	
	S	0.016*	0.406	0.849		S	0.028*	0.038*	0.344
Pitch	L	0.942			Pitch	L	0.068		
	M	0.915	0.971			M	0.206	0.175	
	S	0.697	0.754	0.677		S	0.943	0.015*	0.235
Timbre	L	0.186			Timbre	L	0.599		
	M	<0.001**	0.005*			M	0.122	0.191	
	S	0.463	0.402	<0.001**		S	0.011*	0.028*	0.812
Rhythm	L	0.037*			Rhythm	L	0.414		
	M	0.618	<0.001**			M	0.038*	0.157	
	S	0.225	<0.001**	0.235		S	0.007*	0.010*	0.011*

MMN amplitude				Behavioral hit rate			
Level	**XL**	**L**	**M**	**Level**	**XL**	**L**	**M**
***Post hoc* comparisons for main effect of Level (corrected α = 0.05/6 = 0.0083)**							
All participants (*n* = 25)							
L	0.043*			L	0.576		
M	$<10^{-6}$**	0.001**		M	0.003**	0.002**	
S	$<10^{-5}$**	<0.001**	0.175	S	$<10^{-4}$**	$<10^{-4}$**	$<10^{-4}$**

MMN amplitude					Behavioral hit rate				
Feature	**Intensity**	**Pitch**	**Timbre**	**Rhythm**	**Feature**	**Intensity**	**Pitch**	**Timbre**	**Rhythm**
***Post hoc* comparisons for Group by Feature (corrected α = 0.05/4 = 0.0125)**									
All participants (*n* = 25)									
CI–NH					CI–NH	0.015*	<0.001**	0.058	0.434

*p-values for (1) the planned comparisons for each Group, Feature, and Level tested by comparing the deviant levels, (2) the main effect of Level, and (3) the potential interaction between Group and Feature. Mean MMN amplitudes for Level differences are compared with paired-samples t-tests. For behavioral hit rates, Level and Feature differences are compared using Wilcoxon signed rank tests. ** indicates significant differences; * marks trends at p < 0.05 without correction for multiple comparisons.*

DISCUSSION

This experiment assessed the cortical and behavioral discrimination of musical features in adult CI users and NH controls. The electrophysiological measurements were performed using a multifeature MMN-paradigm presenting four musical features at four levels of deviation magnitude in a "no-standard"-design. In accordance with our hypothesis, the paradigm elicited robust MMN responses to all deviation levels in both NH controls and CI users. Furthermore, across participants, the results showed an overall relationship between MMN strength and deviation magnitude; the larger the deviation, the stronger the MMN response. Finally, contrary to our hypothesis, neither the overall MMN amplitudes nor latencies of the CI users were significantly different from those of the NH group. The findings extend previous multi-feature MMN

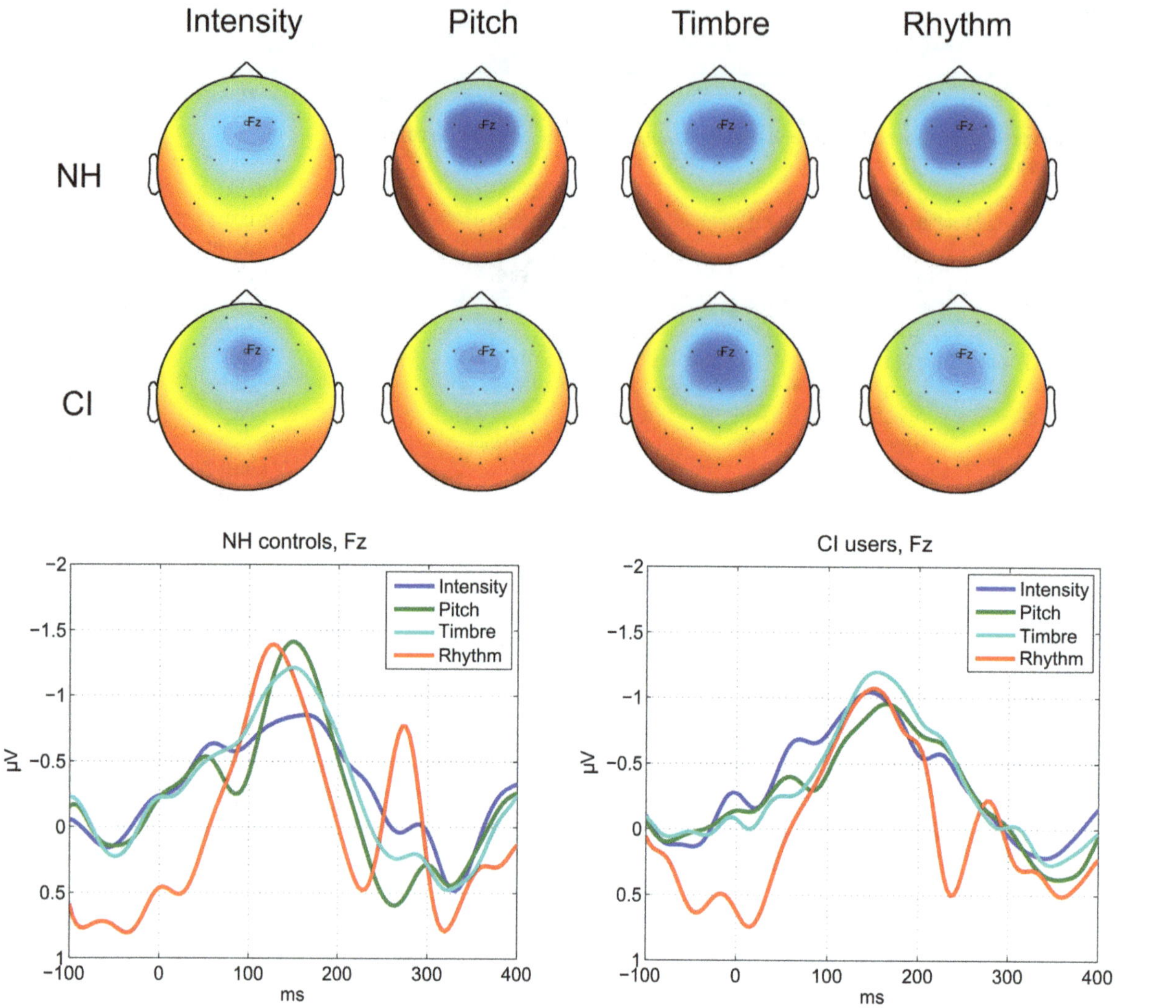

FIGURE 3 | MMN responses to deviants in each auditory feature. **(Top)** Average MMN scalp topographies measured in a 30 ms time window centered on the peaks for each feature. The colors are scaled from −2 μV (blue) to +2 μV (red). NH, normal hearing controls; CI, adult cochlear implant users. **(Bottom)** Average MMN waveforms for each feature and group measured at the Fz electrode.

studies indicating that CI-recipients using present-day speech processing technology may be capable of detailed discrimination of musical sounds even when presented in a complex context (Sandmann et al., 2010; Torppa et al., 2012; Petersen et al., 2014; Timm et al., 2014; Hahne et al., 2016).

The CI-MuMuFe MMN-paradigm constitutes an unprecedented level of complexity in MMN research of CI-users. Nevertheless, our results indicate that the paradigm is both accurate and feasible and may provide strong evidence of CI users' musical discrimination abilities and thresholds as a tool for objective measurements of music discrimination. The use of the paradigm could be of clinical relevance, because it allows for detailed measurement of auditory discrimination abilities in CI patients within a time frame sufficiently short to avoid fatigue and demotivation (Näätänen et al., 2004). Furthermore, in a clinical context, the CI MuMuFe-paradigm could be used as an objective tool for assessment of auditory rehabilitation after CI, e.g., auditory verbal therapy (Sandmann et al., 2010; Rahne et al., 2014) or music training. Especially in the case of young children who receive implants before language acquisition and in whom subjective responses are difficult to interpret, MMN responses might provide useful information regarding the development of auditory functions (Sharma, 2006). To fully qualify for clinical use, however, it is important to improve the analytical methodologies such that MMN measures can be estimated not only at the group level but also in individuals (Bishop and Hardiman, 2010). This is further substantiated by the high degree of variance in the individual MMN traces shown in **Supplementary Figure 2**.

Behavioral Measurements

On average, the CI users scored significantly below the NH listeners in the behavioral discrimination of the four types of music deviants. This was particularly true for Pitch and Intensity,

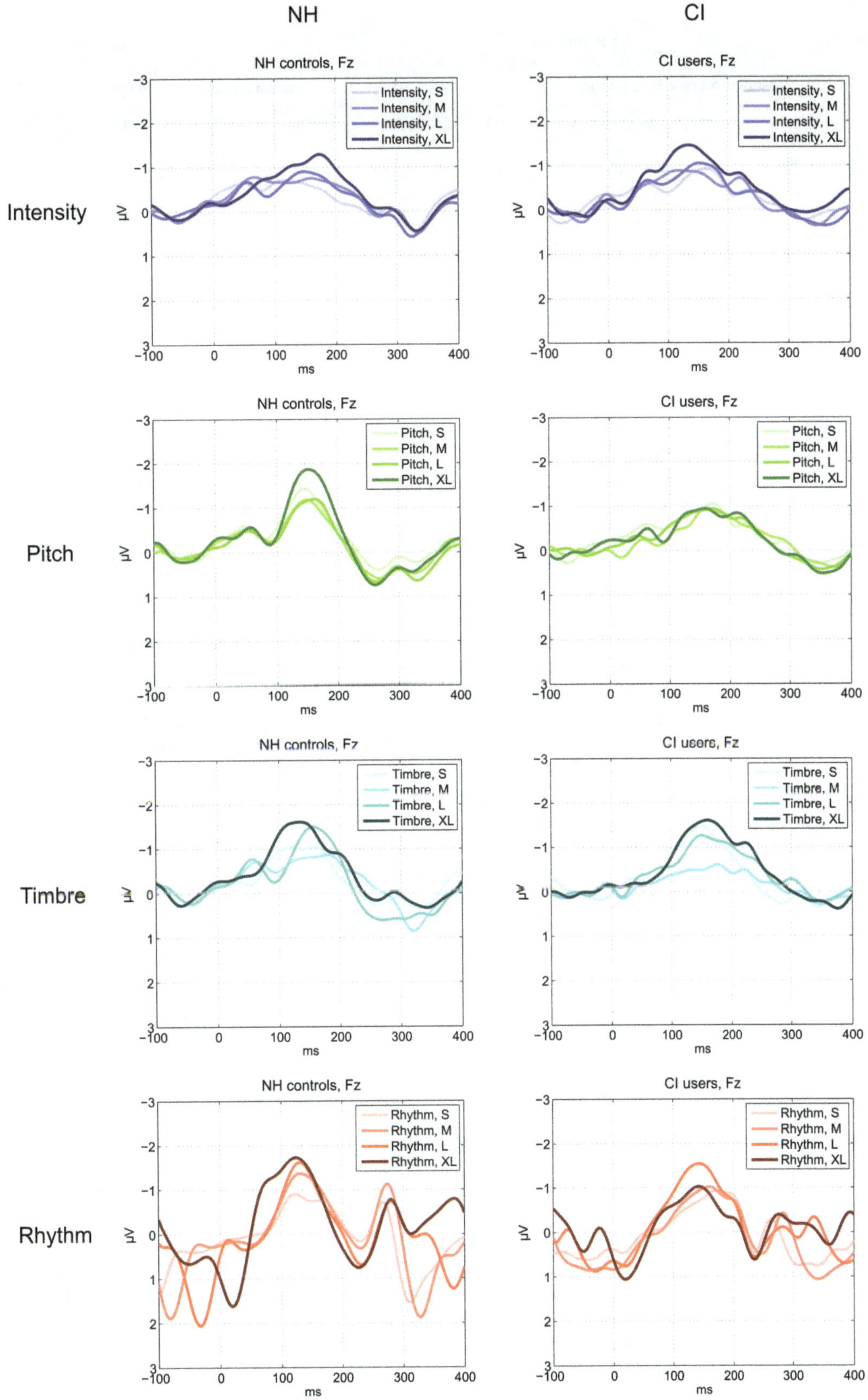

FIGURE 4 | MMN responses to deviants for each feature, level, and group measured at the Fz electrode.

TABLE 5 | Behavioral hit rates.

Feature	Level	NH controls			CI users		
		Median hit rate in % (range)	*z*	*p*	Median hit rate in % (range)	*z*	*p*
Intensity	S	33.0 (17 – 50)	1.05	0.293	33.0 (0 – 67)	−0.54	0.592
	M	58.5 (17 – 83)	2.69	0.007*	33.0 (0 – 83)	−0.27	0.789
	L	75.0 (33 – 100)	3.12	0.002**	50.0 (17 – 83)	2.05	0.040*
	XL	100.0 (50 – 100)	3.37	$<10^{-3}$**	50.0 (0 – 100)	1.78	0.075
Pitch	S	100.0 (50 – 100)	3.37	$<10^{-3}$**	66.7 (17 – 100)	2.41	0.016*
	M	100.0 (50 – 100)	3.37	$<10^{-3}$**	83.0 (17 – 100)	2.68	0.007*
	L	100.0 (67 – 100)	3.64	$<10^{-3}$**	100.0 (33 – 100)	2.93	0.003*
	XL	100.0 (67 – 100)	3.56	$<10^{-3}$**	67.0 (0 – 100)	2.43	0.015*
Timbre	S	83.0 (17 – 100)	2.94	0.003*	66.7 (33 – 100)	2.86	0.004*
	M	91.7 (33 – 100)	3.28	0.001**	66.7 (17 – 100)	2.69	0.007*
	L	100.0 (100 – 100)	3.74	$<10^{-3}$**	83.0 (50 – 100)	2.97	0.003**
	XL	100.0 (83 – 100)	3.64	$<10^{-3}$**	100.0 (50 – 100)	2.99	0.003**
Rhythm	S	50.0 (17 – 100)	2.38	0.017*	50.0 (17 – 100)	2.42	0.016*
	M	100.0 (50 – 100)	3.40	$<10^{-3}$**	83.0 (50 – 100)	2.98	0.003**
	L	100.0 (83 – 100)	3.56	$<10^{-3}$**	100.0 (33 – 100)	3.03	0.002**
	XL	100.0 (50 – 100)	3.56	$<10^{-3}$**	100.0 (83 – 100)	3.21	0.001**

*Behavioral hit rates exceeding the chance level for correct answers at 33.3%. Median hit rates are depicted with ranges (min–max). Degrees of freedom (df) for the NH controls = 13; df for CI users = 10. Hit rates significantly greater than chance level after Bonferroni-correction ($p < 0.003$) are marked with **; those significant without correction ($p < 0.05$) are marked with *.*

whereas the CI users' detection of changes in Rhythm was not significantly different from that of their NH counterparts (**Table 4**). This confirms previous reports, showing that CI users score significantly below NH controls in pitch-related tasks such as melodic contour recognition but usually perform at nearly comparable levels on rhythmic tasks (Gfeller et al., 2007; Drennan and Rubinstein, 2008; Jiam, 2017). As for MMN, the behavioral results showed a significant effect of level across groups. The effect was most prominent in the NH listeners' detection of changes in Intensity and Rhythm while the CI group showed no significant effect of level for any features. However, as also suggested in the violin plots in **Figure 5**, the CI-users in general showed trends toward scoring more accurately when presented with larger changes of the different features.

Individual Variation

As already noted, the CI users' behavioral performance was characterized by a large amount of variation. While some CI users scored at or below chance, others were able to achieve 100% correct scores for all deviant levels except the two lowest levels of the Intensity deviant. This gross variability in performance is a well-known phenomenon in CI-research and may reflect differences in the patients' history of hearing loss (Blamey et al., 2013) and, in this case, musical background. However, our correlation analyses did not identify any significant clinical or music-related factors predictive of either neurophysiological or behavioral performance. The only exception was age at hearing loss which tended to be positively associated with MMN amplitude, indicating that loss of hearing at a young age may hamper the development of fine-tuned auditory processing.

Another potential source of variation is age. However, despite a wide span of age (35–80 years) among the CI-users, age showed no significant relation with any outcome measures. The difference in mean age between the two groups with NH controls being slightly (albeit non-significantly) older than the CI users might represent a possible limitation. As aging can affect the MMN negatively (Schiff et al., 2008), it is fair to speculate that this might to some degree contribute to the lack of difference in MMN amplitude between the two groups. We will in a subsequent article report on the potential effect of aging on the MMN as measured with the CI-MuMuFe paradigm from a separate study involving also a group of NH young adults.

MMN and Behavior Relationship

So why were CI users' behavioral performances poorer than NH listeners' when their MMNs were not significantly different? The presence of significant MMNs indicates that at the early pre-attentive stages of sound processing, the brain is able to detect the subtle sound differences. However, in the active attended listening task, other factors than perceptual sensitivity might influence the performance (Bishop, 2007; Bishop and Hardiman, 2010). For CI users, making meaning of complex sounds constitutes a great demand for cognitive resources and listening effort (Giraud et al., 2000; Hughes et al., 2018). Thus, in a task involving unfamiliar sounds and with the absence of visual cues, some degree of fatigue or unsustained attention may explain this inconsistency between neurophysiology and behavior.

It is also important to point out that MMN and behavioral testing performance often fail to correspond in a strict one-to-one fashion; strong MMNs are not necessarily associated with higher scores (Bishop and Hardiman, 2010; Ortmann et al., 2017). This is also indicated in this study by the lack of significant correlations between MMN amplitudes and hit rates, which thus lends further support to the notion that a group difference at the behavioral

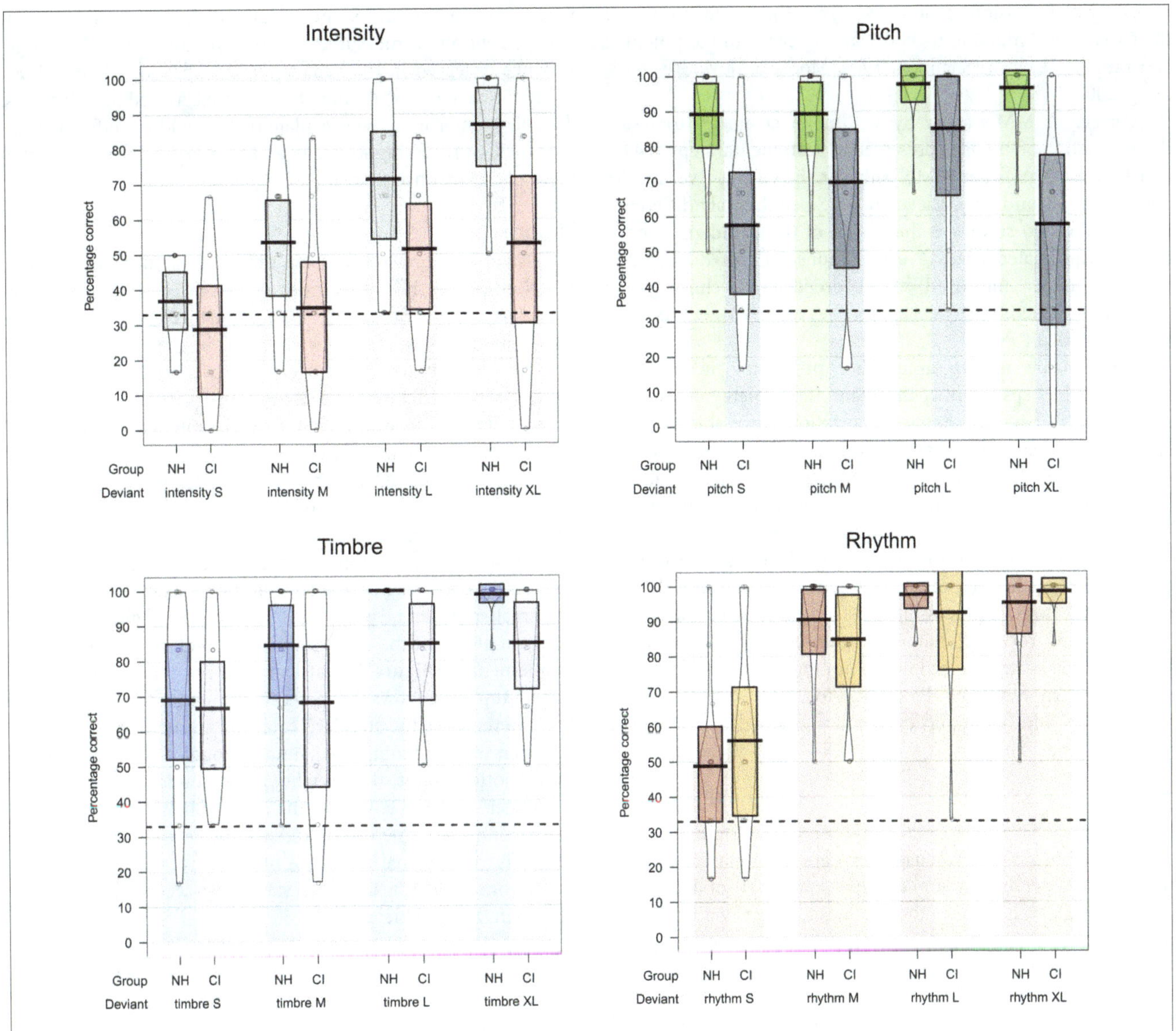

FIGURE 5 | Violin plots showing behavioral hit rates for each feature, level, and group. Dotted line indicates chance level.

level may not necessarily correspond to a group difference at the neurophysiological level.

Discrimination vs. Music Appreciation

On average, the CI users were able to detect some of the subtle changes incorporated in the paradigm, albeit more so at the neural than at the behavioral level. It should be emphasized, however, that this does not necessarily warrant music appreciation. As also suggested by the lack of a relationship between self-reported music appreciation and discrimination skills, other factors may play a significant role in the degree to which CI users tend to like music. Whereas many CI users experience reduced music enjoyment after implantation (Mirza et al., 2003), some studies show that for some CI users enjoyment of music is not hindered despite lack of ability to perceive pitch and timbre (Looi et al., 2012), and that especially rhythm and lyrics are important components of enjoyment (for a review see Riley et al., 2018). It is beyond the scope of this study to deal with this interesting research avenue in further detail. However, future research could potentially employ the CI-MuMuFe paradigm to further elucidate the role of different musical features in CI users' music appreciation.

Features

Intensity

Intensity (or loudness) contributes to the experience of dynamics and is an important prerequisite for the full extent of music enjoyment. In the present experiment, the changes in intensity were quite subtle, as reflected both in the very low hit rates and the relatively weak MMN responses observed in the NH listeners. Nevertheless, CI users exhibited cortical responses that reflected the level hierarchy. This was quite surprising, since, because of necessary compression of the sound signal, the dynamic range of the CI is often limited to 6–30 dB, as compared to the potential NH range of 120 dB (Shannon, 1983; Moore and Moore, 2003; Zeng, 2004).

A previous MMN-study by Sandmann et al. (2010) tested discrimination of intensity presented in decremental steps of 4 dB and found a significant MMN only for the largest level in NH and for the second largest level in CI. Since the only difference between the two studies is the design of the paradigm - odd-ball vs. arpeggiated triads - explanations for this discrepancy could be either improved sound processing technology or differences in methodological approaches related to recording or analysis of the ERPs.

It would be fair to argue that presenting intensity in decremental steps only paints an incomplete picture of perception of dynamic changes. The rationale for this one-way approach, however, is to avoid exceeding the sound level of 65 dB and the potential risk of distortion at the higher levels. In their study with CI children, Torppa et al. (2012) presented both decremental and incremental intensity deviants but found MMN responses only for the decremental deviants. The authors speculated that the lack of response could be linked either to CI-listeners' limited processing of stronger loudness levels or to the sound processor's automatic gain control. This possible limitation will be further explored in our ongoing investigation of CI users' neurophysiological responses to a new "Free-listening"-paradigm in which the participants are exposed to real music (Poikonen et al., 2016).

Pitch

Pitch perception is crucial for identifying melodic contour both in relation to music and to language. Several studies have concluded that CI users' perception of pitch is poor and that some CI users may need intervals of several semitones to identify a change of pitch (Looi et al., 2012; Limb and Roy, 2014). Interestingly, the CI users in the present study showed a robust MMN response not only to the larger but also to the smallest pitch change of one semitone. This is consistent with Hahne et al. (2016) who found that whereas a pitch deviant of +1 semitone elicited a "good MMN potential", a −24 ct (a quarter of a semitone mistuning) did not. The authors concluded that "the real performance optimum of pitch discrimination of the CI stimulation might be still somewhat below 1 semitone." In that perspective, taking also the CI users' undifferentiated neural discrimination of levels of pitch change into account, it may be worth considering including a quarter-tone (half semitone) pitch deviant in a future revision of the CI-MuMuFe. Such an adjustment might also to some extent reduce the ceiling effect found in the NH controls' behavioral performance.

The CI users' behavioral discrimination of the pitch deviant showed a large variability, failing to reach a within-group consistent above-chance level. Nevertheless, whereas the MMN responses did not reflect effects-of-magnitude, tendencies in the behavioral results suggested that CI-users might obtain higher discrimination accuracy for the L compared to the S and M deviation levels (**Figure 5** and **Table 5**). This may reflect the difference between the early pre-attended change detection represented by the MMN and the attended, conscious detection and perception as measured in the behavioral task. The large variance observed in the behavioral identification of the XL 8-semitone-change, exhibiting floor as well as ceiling effects, is difficult to interpret. We speculate that individual differences in both the CI-processing strategies and auditory profiles may be the cause of this inconsistency.

Timbre

Consistent with previous reports, timbre deviants elicited robust MMN responses in both groups (Petersen et al., 2014; Timm et al., 2014; Hahne et al., 2016). Furthermore, the neural discrimination of the four deviant levels in general reflected the deviation magnitude. In CI users, however, the small "bright" piano variation elicited an MMN response that was significantly larger than the medium "blues" variation. This unexpected difference in automatic detection could be due to extraction of envelopes triggered by the richer representation of higher frequencies in the activation of electrodes, as also illustrated in **Supplementary Figure 5**.

While the selection of the trumpet and electric guitar deviants was based on experience gained from previous experiments, the two smaller deviants were created from the logic of making slight variations of the standard piano sound. As can be seen in **Supplementary Figure 5**, that logic was not totally wrong. The bar plot top right shows the increasing amount of spectral energy that differentiates the standard sound from the deviant sounds. However, when running the sounds through a CI simulator, as shown bottom right, the "bright" piano sound clearly exhibits a stronger spectral envelope than the "blues" variation. The phenomenon is a fine exemplification of how different electric hearing is from normal hearing. A future revision of the paradigm should consider taking this observation into account by reversing the two in the level hierarchy.

Of interest in this context is a study on timbre perception in adult CI users using behavioral performance as a model for individually adapted MMN stimuli (Rahne et al., 2014). Instead of instrument sounds, the paradigm presented synthesized tones with varying relationship between the fundamental and a spectrum of harmonics. The authors concluded that MMN responses reflected the individual threshold for automatic detection of timbre changes.

Even though the CI users here exhibited differentiated neural detection of changes in timbre, it is important to note that this may not necessarily reflect ability to distinguish or recognize instruments. This task is notoriously challenging for CI users (Heng, 2011; Looi et al., 2012; Limb and Roy, 2014), although effects of training have been reported (Driscoll, 2012; Petersen et al., 2012; Jiam et al., 2019). What we show is the neurophysiological and behavioral capability to identify subtle changes in the "color" of a sound which is a prerequisite for possible further training of this skill.

Rhythm

Whereas the spectral resolution of the CI signal is low, the temporal resolution is high as reflected in near normal rhythm discrimination reported in behavioral studies (Limb et al., 2010),

MMN studies (Petersen et al., 2014; Hahne et al., 2016), as well as in effect of targeted rhythm training (Petersen et al., 2012). Our results confirm this, showing CI performance that is not significantly different from that of the NH group and significantly better for rhythm than for the other three deviants (**Table 4** and **Figure 5**).

The four rhythm deviants in the paradigm follow the logic of beat subdivision, such that the 26 ms anticipation in a musicological concept is a 64th note syncopation whereas the largest deviant equals a dotted 16th-note syncopation (**Figure 1**). Both NH and CI listeners' discrimination of the rhythm deviants tended to follow this musical logic: the shorter the displacement of the third note the more difficult the detection.

As a single exception, the CI users showed the strongest MMN response to the second largest rhythm deviant and not the largest (**Table 2**). This could be explained by the very short distance (50 ms) between the second and third note which may be perceived as a merging of the two notes. So, even though the two notes are three semitones apart, they may be perceived as the same note because of the CI's poor representation of pitch. By contrast, in their attended behavioral detection of the rhythm deviants, the CI group detected the largest deviant most accurately (**Figure 5**). However, in that task the requirement is to detect which of three patterns is different. Thus, the largest rhythm deviant is clearly identifiable because of the omission of the third tone at the expected position.

Methodological Considerations

The Standard Response

In the original paradigm from Vuust et al. (2011), a standard pattern was played in between every deviant pattern. Thus, the ERP elicited from the third tone in the standard configuration could be subtracted directly from the response to the third tone in the deviant pattern, eliciting the MMN response. In the no-standards paradigm from Kliuchko et al. (2016) the standard pattern was omitted which meant that the third tone was never a standard. Consequently, no direct comparison between the standard and deviant response was possible. Instead, the standard response was defined as the response to the first, second, and fourth tone of the Alberti bass pattern, because these tones never occurred as deviants. An average between the first, second, and fourth tone is a compromise between several other less ideal standard responses in an attempt to mimic the relatively stable and neutral response to the third tone obtained in the original paradigm. The less ideal standard responses (the first, the second, or the fourth tone, respectively) are all confounded by the MMN response or by N1 enhancement in their baseline or in their post-stimulus time window, which is visualized in **Supplementary Figure 3**. For clarity it is important to point out that since the same standard response is subtracted from each of the compared 16 deviants, the statistical differences observed for the within-subject factors of Level and Feature could not have been affected by the choice of standard response.

See the **Supplementary Material** for a more in-depth discussion of the different scenarios for selecting an appropriate standard response.

The Rhythm Deviant and Its Baseline Correction

The rhythm deviant is different from the other deviants as it actually consists of two deviants in one. First, it is a duration deviant because the second note in a rhythm deviant sequence is shortened 26, 52, 103, and 155 ms, respectively. Second, it is a rhythm deviant since the third note is thereby presented earlier than expected. The fourth note, however, is unchanged and occurs at the usual time because the third note of the rhythm deviant sequence is prolonged accordingly.

The epochs are centered around the prolonged third note to best capture the mismatch response to the rhythm deviant and thereby compare the individual rhythm deviants. However, as the second note becomes shorter, the P50 response occurs closer to the onset of the third note, and in the case of the XL deviant, the P50 response to the shortened note actually begins when the third note has its onset. This presents a challenge with regard to baseline correction because the conventional 100 ms baseline window preceding the third note is hereby contaminated with P50 responses to the preceding note to varying degrees depending on the extent of the shortening, and thus especially so for the L and XL deviants as illustrated in **Supplementary Figure 4**.

The contamination of the conventional baseline window thus co-varies with the four levels of the rhythm deviants, which constitute a factor in the statistical analyses. Therefore, we opted for the 100 ms period preceding the shortened second note as baseline correction window for the rhythm deviants. The ongoing activity in this time window was unaffected by the varying overlap between P50 responses and baseline windows caused by the shortening of the second note, and thus served as a good estimate of the ongoing background activity prior to the rhythm deviants (see the **Supplementary Material** for more details on the choice of baseline window for the rhythm deviants).

Speaker vs. Cable

In the present study, CI users were presented with the sound stimuli through a direct audio input cable rather than listening via loudspeakers. This allows for control of which sound inputs are presented to the participants and eliminate confounding factors such as residual hearing. Some challenges, however, are associated with this method. First, present-day CIs are quite small, leaving no room for an audio input port. Thus, for most of the CI users, a spare processor had to be programmed with their personal mappings. This obviously may be the source of some experimental uncertainty as well as participant concern. The newest generation of CI processors, however, provide a fast, wireless connection which may eventually eliminate this problem.

Some of the CI users had bilateral CIs and were forced to choose their best performing ear for the tests. Both for them and for the bimodal listeners, the monaural stimulation represented a listening situation that was less satisfactory and quite far from what they were used to. We can only speculate the degree to which this affected their performance. We would argue that even though there is a trade-off when presenting the stimuli directly it represents the most optimal basis for a fair comparison and standardizes one factor in a population already characterized by a multitude of profiles.

Sound Intensity

Due to quite varying degrees of tolerance of the volume of the stimuli, we were unable to maintain a perfect match in the sound intensity between CI-participants. This may introduce a possible variance in the recorded EEG data. However, because the participants had to listen to the stimuli for 32 min and were asked not to focus on the sound, we considered it most important that the sound level was tolerable for the individual participant. The MMN is affected by attention, which means that if an individual was disturbed by the stimuli, this might affect the results. Because the perceived loudness with a CI depends on both the chosen program and the individual settings, a direct comparison of sound levels between CI users is virtually impossible. Thus, we conclude that the individual comfortable level is the most optimal way to set the intensity level. Measuring the intensity of the sound coming into the CI is possible by connecting the implant to a software system for visual inspection. However, one thing is what can be seen objectively on a screen, another thing is what is subjectively perceived by the participant.

SUMMARY AND CONCLUSION

Our findings confirm and expand previous reporting on adult CI-users' music perception abilities. Despite degraded representation of spectral fine structure in the CI-signal, CI-users exhibited MMN-responses to changes in basic features of music that were significant and not significantly different from those of NH controls. Both groups showed MMN strength that was in alignment with the deviation magnitude. In CI users, however, discrimination of pitch levels remained undifferentiated. CI users' behavioral performance was significantly below that of the NH group, mainly due to poor pitch discrimination. Although no significant effects were found, CI users' behavioral results tended to be in accordance with deviation magnitude, most prominently manifested in discrimination of the rhythm deviant.

The findings indicate that the new MuMuFe paradigm can effectively estimate musical discrimination abilities and thresholds in CI users. Furthermore, the large heterogeneity of the CI-users tested in the present study suggests that the paradigm has a promising potential for assessing a wide range of perceptual profiles. Thus, the paradigm may be a valuable tool in measurements of the effect of training or in studies which examine neural plasticity following CI. Furthermore, the CI MuMuFe may have clinical relevance with a potential of evaluating thresholds and limits in follow-up procedures, e.g., in young children for whom subjective measurements are difficult to interpret. Future studies should investigate the possibility of applying the paradigm with the purpose of assessing discrimination skills not only at the group level but also at the individual level.

ETHICS STATEMENT

This study was carried out in accordance with the recommendations of the Research Ethics Committee of the Central Denmark Region. All subjects gave written informed consent in accordance with the Declaration of Helsinki. The protocol was approved by the Research Ethics Committee of the Central Denmark Region.

AUTHOR CONTRIBUTIONS

BP, PV, EB, and SR contributed to the conception and design of the study. BP and AA conceived the paradigm and the behavioral test and created all stimuli, and wrote the first draft of the manuscript. AA organized and carried out the recruitment and tests. NH, AH, and MD processed the EEG and behavioral data and performed the statistical analyses. FM provided the technical assistance with programming of spare processors and information about CI participants. NH and AH wrote the sections of the manuscript. All authors contributed to the manuscript revision, and read and approved the submitted version of the manuscript.

ACKNOWLEDGMENTS

The authors wish to thank all the participants for their unrestricted commitment. The authors thank MD Hanne Owen and CI coordinator Minna Sandahl from the Clinic of Audiology at Aarhus University Hospital and the Danish CI organization for assistance with recruitment. Special thanks to Dora Grauballe, Center for Functionally Integrative Neuroscience, for invaluable and unconditioned help with bookings and management of laboratory facilities. A final thanks to Dr., MD, Therese Ovesen for her great role in the initial phase of the project.

REFERENCES

Alho, K. (1992). Selective attention in auditory processing as reflected by event-related brain potentials. *Psychophysiology* 29, 247–263. doi: 10.1111/j.1469-8986.1992.tb01695.x

Bedoin, N., Besombes, A. M., Escande, E., Dumont, A., Lalitte, P., and Tillmann, B. (2018). Boosting syntax training with temporally regular musical primes in children with cochlear implants. *Ann. Phys. Rehabil. Med.* 61, 365–371. doi: 10.1016/j.rehab.2017.03.004

Bishop, D. V. (2007). Using mismatch negativity to study central auditory processing in developmental language and literacy impairments: where are we, and where should we be going? *Psychol. Bull.* 133, 651–672. doi: 10.1037/0033-2909.133.4.651

Bishop, D. V. M., and Hardiman, M. J. (2010). Measurement of mismatch negativity in individuals: a study using single-trial analysis. *Psychophysiology* 47, 697–705. doi: 10.1111/j.1469-8986.2009.00970.x

Blamey, P., Artieres, F., Başkent, D., Bergeron, F., Beynon, A., Burke, E., et al. (2013). Factors affecting auditory performance of postlinguistically deaf adults using cochlear implants: an update with 2251 patients. *Audiol. Neurotol.* 18, 36–47. doi: 10.1159/000343189

Bonetti, L., Haumann, N. T., Brattico, E., Kliuchko, M., Vuust, P., Sarkamo, T., et al. (2018). Auditory sensory memory and working memory skills: association between frontal MMN and performance scores. *Brain Res.* 1700, 86–98. doi: 10.1016/j.brainres.2018.06.034

Bonetti, L., Haumann, N. T., Vuust, P., Kliuchko, M., and Brattico, E. (2017). Risk of depression enhances auditory Pitch discrimination in the brain as indexed by the mismatch negativity. *Clin. Neurophysiol.* 128, 1923–1936. doi: 10.1016/j.clinph.2017.07.004

Delorme, A., Plamer, J., Oostenveld, R., Onton, J., and Makeig, S. (2007). *Comparing Results of Algorithms Implementing Blind Source Separation of EEG Data.* Boston: Swartz Foundation and NIH Grant.

Drennan, W. R., and Rubinstein, J. T. (2008). Music perception in cochlear implant users and its relationship with psychophysical capabilities. *J. Rehabil. Res. Dev.* 45, 779–789.

Driscoll, V. D. (2012). The effects of training on recognition of musical instruments by adults with cochlear implants. *Semin. Hear.* 33, 410–418. doi: 10.1055/s-0032-1329230

Dritsakis, G., van Besouw, R. M., Kitterick, P., and Verschuur, C. A. (2017a). A music-related quality of life measure to guide music rehabilitation for adult cochlear implant users. *Am. J. Audiol.* 26, 268–282. doi: 10.1044/2017_AJA-16-0120

Dritsakis, G., van Besouw, R. M., and O'Meara, A. (2017b). Impact of music on the quality of life of cochlear implant users: a focus group study. *Cochl. Implants Int.* 18, 207–215. doi: 10.1080/14670100.2017.1303892

Duncan, C. C., Barry, R. J., Connolly, J. F., Fischer, C., Michie, P. T., Näätänen, R., et al. (2009). Event-related potentials in clinical research: guidelines for eliciting, recording, and quantifying mismatch negativity. P300, and N400. *Clin. Neurophysiol.* 120, 1883–1908. doi: 10.1016/j.clinph.2009.07.045

Fuller, C. D., Galvin, J. J., Maat, B., Başkent, D., and Free, R. H. (2018). Comparison of two music training approaches on music and speech perception in cochlear implant users. *Trends Hear.* 22:2331216518765379. doi: 10.1177/2331216518765379

Galvin, J. J., Fu, Q. J., and Nogaki, G. (2007). Melodic contour identification by cochlear implant listeners. *Ear Hear.* 28, 302–319. doi: 10.1097/01.aud.0000261689.35445.20

Gfeller, K., Christ, A., Knutson, J. F., Witt, S., Murray, K. T., and Tyler, R. S. (2000). Musical backgrounds, listening habits, and aesthetic enjoyment of adult cochlear implant recipients. *J. Am. Acad. Audiol.* 11, 390–406.

Gfeller, K., Guthe, E., Driscoll, V., and Brown, C. J. (2015). A preliminary report of music-based training for adult cochlear implant users: rationales and development. *Cochl. Implants Int.* 16(Suppl.3), S22–S31. doi: 10.1179/1467010015Z.000000000269

Gfeller, K., Turner, C., Oleson, J., Zhang, X., Gantz, B., Froman, R., et al. (2007). Accuracy of cochlear implant recipients on pitch perception, melody recognition, and speech reception in noise. *Ear. Hear.* 28, 412–423. doi: 10.1097/aud.0b013e3180479318

Giraud, A. L., Truy, E., Frackowiak, R. S., Gregoire, M. C., Pujol, J. F., and Collet, L. (2000). Differential recruitment of the speech processing system in healthy subjects and rehabilitated cochlear implant patients. *Brain* 123(Pt 7), 1391–1402. doi: 10.1093/brain/123.7.1391

Hahne, A., Mainka, A., Leuner, A., and Murbe, D. (2016). Adult Cochlear implant users are able to discriminate basic tonal features in musical patterns: evidence from event-related potentials. *Otol. Neurotol.* 37, e360–e368. doi: 10.1097/MAO.0000000000001067

Haumann, N. T., Parkkonen, L., Kliuchko, M., Vuust, P., and Brattico, E. (2016). Comparing the performance of popular MEG/EEG artifact correction methods in an evoked-response study. *Comput. Intell. Neurosci.* 2016:7489108. doi: 10.1155/2016/7489108

Heng, J. (2011). Impaired perception of temporal fine structure and musical timbre in cochlear implant users. *Hear. Res.* 280, 192–200. doi: 10.1016/j.heares.2011.05.017

Hopyan-Misakyan, T. M., Gordon, K. A., Dennis, M., and Papsin, B. C. (2009). Recognition of affective speech prosody and facial affect in deaf children with unilateral right cochlear implants. *Child Neuropsychol.* 15, 136–146. doi: 10.1080/09297040802403682

Hughes, S. E., Hutchings, H. A., Rapport, F. L., McMahon, C. M., and Boisvert, I. (2018). Social connectedness and perceived listening effort in adult cochlear implant users: a grounded theory to establish content validity for a new patient-reported outcome measure. *Ear. Hear.* 39, 922–934. doi: 10.1097/AUD.0000000000000553

Jiam, N. T. (2017). What does music sound like for a cochlear implant user? *Otol. Neurotol.* 38, e240–e247. doi: 10.1097/MAO.0000000000001448

Jiam, N. T., Deroche, M. L., Jiradejvong, P., and Limb, C. (2019). A randomized controlled crossover study of the impact of online music training on pitch and timbre perception in cochlear implant users. *J. Assoc. Res. Otolaryngol.* 20, 247–262. doi: 10.1007/s10162-018-00704-700

Kelly, A. S. (2005). Electrophysiological and speech perception measures of auditory processing in experienced adult cochlear implant users. *Clin. Neurophysiol.* 116, 1235–1246. doi: 10.1016/j.clinph.2005.02.011

Kim, S. J., Cho, Y. S., Kim, E. Y., and Yoo, G. E. (2015). Can young adolescents with cochlear implants perceive different timbral cues? *Cochlear Implants Int.* 16, 61–68. doi: 10.1179/1754762814Y.0000000083

Kliuchko, M., Heinonen-Guzejev, M., Vuust, P., Tervaniemi, M., and Brattico, E. (2016). A window into the brain mechanisms associated with noise sensitivity. *Sci. Rep.* 6:39236. doi: 10.1038/srep39236

Kujala, T. T. (2007). The mismatch negativity in cognitive and clinical neuroscience: theoretical and methodological considerations. *Biol. Psychol.* 74, 1–19. doi: 10.1016/j.biopsycho.2006.06.001

Lassaletta, L., Castro, A., Bastarrica, M., Perez-Mora, R., Herran, B., Sanz, L., et al. (2008). Changes in listening habits and quality of musical sound after cochlear implantation. *Otolaryngol. Head Neck Surg.* 138, 363–367. doi: 10.1016/j.otohns.2007.11.028

Limb, C. J., Molloy, A. T., Jiradejvong, P., and Braun, A. R. (2010). Auditory cortical activity during cochlear implant-mediated perception of spoken language, melody, and rhythm. *JARO* 11, 133–143. doi: 10.1007/s10162-009-0184-9

Limb, C. J., and Roy, A. T. (2014). Technological, biological, and acoustical constraints to music perception in cochlear implant users. *Hear. Res.* 308, 13–26. doi: 10.1016/j.heares.2013.04.009

Limb, C. J., and Rubinstein, J. T. (2012). Current research on music perception in cochlear implant users. *Otolaryngol. Clin. North Am.* 45, 129–140. doi: 10.1016/j.otc.2011.08.021

Looi, V., Gfeller, K., and Driscoll, V. (2012). Music appreciation and training for cochlear implant recipients: a review. *Semin. Hear* 33, 307–334. doi: 10.1055/s-0032-1329222

Looi, V., and She, J. (2010). Music perception of cochlear implant users: a questionnaire, and its implications for a music training program. *Int. J. Audiol.* 49, 116–128. doi: 10.3109/14992020903405987

Makeig, S., Bell, A. J., Jung, T.-P., and Sejnowski, T. J. (1996). "Independent component analysis of electroencephalographic data," in *Advances in Neural information Processing Systems*, eds M. C. Mozer, M. I. Jordan, and T. Petsche, (Cambridge, MA: MIT Press), 145–151.

Mirza, S., Douglas, S. A., Lindsey, P., Hildreth, T., and Hawthorne, M. (2003). Appreciation of music in adult patients with cochlear implants: a patient questionnaire. *Cochlear. Implants. Int.* 4, 85–95. doi: 10.1179/cim.2003.4.2.85

Moore, B. C., and Moore, G. A. (2003). "Discrimination of the fundamental frequency of complex tones with fixed and shifting spectral envelopes by normally hearing and hearing-impaired subjects," in *Proceedings of the Hearing Research 39th Workshop on Inner Ear Biology*, Liege.

Moran, M., Rousset, A., and Looi, V. (2016). Music appreciation and music listening in prelingual and postlingually deaf adult cochlear implant recipients. *Int. J. Audiol.* 55(Suppl. 2), S57–S63. doi: 10.3109/14992027.2016.1157630

Näätänen, R. (1992). *Attention and Brain Function.* London: LawrenceErlbaumAss.

Näätänen, R., Gaillard, A. W., and Mantysalo, S. (1978). Early selective-attention effect on evoked potential reinterpreted. *Acta Psychol.* 42, 313–329. doi: 10.1016/0001-6918(78)90006-9

Näätänen, R., Pakarinen, S., Rinne, T., and Takegata, R. (2004). The mismatch negativity (MMN): towards the optimal paradigm. *Clin. Neurophysiol.* 115, 140–144. doi: 10.1016/j.clinph.2003.04.001

Näätänen, R., Petersen, B., Torppa, R., Lonka, E., and Vuust, P. (2017). The MMN as a viable and objective marker of auditory development in CI users. *Hear. Res.* 353, 57–75. doi: 10.1016/j.heares.2017.07.007

Näätänen, R., Tervaniemi, M., Sussman, E., Paavilainen, P., and Winkler, I. (2001). "Primitive intelligence" in the auditory cortex. *Trends Neurosci.* 24, 283–288. doi: 10.1016/s0166-2236(00)01790-2

Nakata, T., Trehub, S. E., and Kanda, Y. (2012). Effect of cochlear implants on children's perception and production of speech prosody. *J. Acoust. Soc. Am.* 131, 1307–1314. doi: 10.1121/1.3672697

Oostenveld, R., Fries, P., Maris, E., and Schoffelen, J. M. (2011). FieldTrip: open source software for advanced analysis of MEG, EEG, and invasive electrophysiological data. *Comput. Intell. Neurosci.* 2011:156869. doi: 10.1155/2011/156869

Ortmann, M., Zwitserlood, P., Knief, A., Baare, J., Brinkheetker, S., Am Zehnhoff-Dinnesen, A., et al. (2017). When hearing is tricky: speech processing strategies in prelingually deafened children and adolescents with cochlear implants having good and poor speech performance. *PLoS One* 12:e0168655. doi: 10.1371/journal.pone.0168655

Paavilainen, P., Tiitinen, H., Alho, K., and Näätänen, R. (1993). Mismatch negativity to slight pitch changes outside strong attentional focus. *Biol. Psychol.* 37, 23–41. doi: 10.1016/0301-0511(93)90025-4

Pakarinen, S., Huotilainen, M., and Naatanen, R. (2010). The mismatch negativity (MMN) with no standard stimulus. *Clin. Neurophysiol.* 121, 1043–1050. doi: 10.1016/j.clinph.2010.02.009

Pakarinen, S., Takegata, R., Rinne, T., Huotilainen, M., and Näätänen, R. (2007). Measurement of extensive auditory discrimination profiles using the mismatch negativity (MMN) of the auditory event-related potential (ERP). *Clin. Neurophysiol.* 118, 177–185. doi: 10.1016/j.clinph.2006.09.001

Peng, S. C., Tomblin, J. B., and Turner, C. W. (2008). Production and perception of speech intonation in pediatric cochlear implant recipients and individuals with normal hearing. *Ear. Hear.* 29, 336–351. doi: 10.1097/AUD.0b013e318168d94d

Petersen, B., Gjedde, A., Wallentin, M., and Vuust, P. (2013). Cortical plasticity after cochlear implantation. *Neural Plast.* 2013:11. doi: 10.1155/2013/318521

Petersen, B., Mortensen, M. V., Hansen, M., and Vuust, P. (2012). Singing in the key of life: a study on effects of musical ear training after cochlear implantation. *Psychomusicology* 22, 134–151. doi: 10.1111/j.1749-6632.2009.04796.x

Petersen, B., Weed, E., Sandmann, P., Brattico, E., Hansen, M., Derdau, S., et al. (2014). Brain responses to musical feature changes in adolescent cochlear implant users. *Front. Hum. Neurosci.* 9:7. doi: 10.3389/fnhum.2015.00007

Poikonen, H., Alluri, V., Brattico, E., Lartillot, O., Tervaniemi, M., and Huotilainen, M. (2016). Event-related brain responses while listening to entire pieces of music. *Neuroscience* 312, 58–73. doi: 10.1016/j.neuroscience.2015.10.061

Rahne, T., Plontke, S. K., and Wagner, L. (2014). Mismatch negativity (MMN) objectively reflects timbre discrimination thresholds in normal-hearing listeners and cochlear implant users. *Brain Res.* 1586, 143–151. doi: 10.1016/j.brainres.2014.08.045

Riley, P. E., Ruhl, D. S., Camacho, M., and Tolisano, A. M. (2018). Music appreciation after cochlear implantation in adult patients: a systematic review. *Otolaryngol. Head Neck Surg.* 158, 1002–1010. doi: 10.1177/0194599818760559

Roman, S. (2005). Mismatch negativity and tone discrimination in cochlear-implanted patients. *Cochl. Implants Int.* 6(Suppl. 1), 53–55. doi: 10.1179/cim.2005.6.supplement-1.53

Sandmann, P., Kegel, A., Eichele, T., Dillier, N., Lai, W., Bendixen, A., et al. (2010). Neurophysiological evidence of impaired musical sound perception in cochlear-implant users. *Clin. Neurophysiol.* 121, 2070–2082. doi: 10.1016/j.clinph.2010.04.032

Schiff, S., Valenti, P., Andrea, P., Lot, M., Bisiacchi, P., Gatta, A., et al. (2008). The effect of aging on auditory components of event-related brain potentials. *Clin. Neurophysiol.* 119, 1795–1802. doi: 10.1016/j.clinph.2008.04.007

Shannon, R. V. (1983). Multichannel electrical stimulation of the auditory nerve in man. I. Basic psychophysics. *Hear. Res* 11, 157–189. doi: 10.1016/0378-5955(83)90077-1

Sharma, A. (2006). Central auditory development in children with cochlear implants: clinical implications. *Adv. Oto Rhino Laryngol.* 64, 66–88. doi: 10.1159/000094646

Timm, L., Vuust, P., Brattico, E., Agrawal, D., Debener, S., Buchner, A., et al. (2014). Residual neural processing of musical sound features in adult cochlear implant users. *Front. Hum. Neurosci.* 8:181. doi: 10.3389/fnhum.2014.00181

Titterington, J., Watson, D., Toner, J., and Henry, A. (2003). "What can the mismatch negativity (MMN) tell us about short-term auditory sensory memory function in cochlear implanted children? *Cochl. Implants Int.* 4(Suppl. 1), 70–72. doi: 10.1002/cii.114

Torppa, R., Salo, E., Makkonen, T., Loimo, H., Pykäläinen, J., Lipsanen, J., et al. (2012). Cortical processing of musical sounds in children with Cochlear Implants. *Clin. Neurophysiol.* 123, 1966–1979. doi: 10.1016/j.clinph.2012.03.008

Viola, F. C., Thorne, J. D., Bleeck, S., Eyles, J., and Debener, S. (2011). Uncovering auditory evoked potentials from cochlear implant users with independent component analysis. *Psychophysiology* 48, 1470–1480. doi: 10.1111/j.1469-8986.2011.01224.x

Vuust, P., Brattico, E., Glerean, E., Seppanen, M., Pakarinen, S., Tervaniemi, M., et al. (2011). New fast mismatch negativity paradigm for determining the neural prerequisites for musical ability. *Cortex* 47, 1091–1098. doi: 10.1016/j.cortex.2011.04.026

Zeng, F. G. (2004). Trends in cochlear implants. *Trends Amplif.* 8, 1–34. doi: 10.1177/108471380400800102

Zeng, F.-G., Tang, Q., and Lu, T. (2014). Abnormal pitch perception produced by cochlear implant stimulation. *PLoS One* 9:e88662. doi: 10.1371/journal.pone.0088662

Zhang, F. (2011). Mismatch negativity and adaptation measures of the late auditory evoked potential in cochlear implant users. *Hear. Res.* 275, 17–29. doi: 10.1016/j.heares.2010.11.007

10

Pleasantness Ratings for Harmonic Intervals with Acoustic and Electric Hearing in Unilaterally Deaf Cochlear Implant Patients

Emily R. Spitzer[1], David M. Landsberger[1], David R. Friedmann[1] and John J. Galvin III[2]*

[1] Department of Otolaryngology–Head and Neck Surgery, New York University School of Medicine, New York, NY, United States, [2] House Ear Institute, Los Angeles, CA, United States

Correspondence:
Emily R. Spitzer
emily.spitzer@nyulangone.org

Background: Harmony is an important part of tonal music that conveys context, form and emotion. Two notes sounded simultaneously form a harmonic interval. In normal-hearing (NH) listeners, some harmonic intervals (e.g., minor 2nd, tritone, major 7th) typically sound more dissonant than others (e.g., octave, major 3rd, 4th). Because of the limited spectro-temporal resolution afforded by cochlear implants (CIs), music perception is generally poor. However, CI users may still be sensitive to relative dissonance across intervals. In this study, dissonance ratings for harmonic intervals were measured in 11 unilaterally deaf CI patients, in whom ratings from the CI could be compared to those from the normal ear.

Methods: Stimuli consisted of pairs of equal amplitude MIDI piano tones. Intervals spanned a range of two octaves relative to two root notes (F3 or C4). Dissonance was assessed in terms of subjective pleasantness ratings for intervals presented to the NH ear alone, the CI ear alone, and both ears together (NH + CI). Ratings were collected for both root notes for within- and across-octave intervals (1–12 and 13–24 semitones). Participants rated the pleasantness of each interval by clicking on a line anchored with "least pleasant" and "most pleasant." A follow-up experiment repeated the task with a smaller stimulus set.

Results: With NH-only listening, within-octave intervals minor 2nd, major 2nd, and major 7th were rated least pleasant; major 3rd, 5th, and octave were rated most pleasant. Across-octave counterparts were similarly rated. With CI-only listening, ratings were consistently lower and showed a reduced range. Mean ratings were highly correlated between NH-only and CI-only listening (r = 0.845, p < 0.001). Ratings were similar between NH-only and NH + CI listening, with no significant binaural enhancement/interference. The follow-up tests showed that ratings were reliable for the least and most pleasant intervals.

Discussion: Although pleasantness ratings were less differentiated for the CI ear than the NH ear, there were similarities between the two listening modes. Given the lack of spectro-temporal detail needed for harmonicity-based distinctions, temporal envelope interactions (within and across channels) associated with a perception of roughness may contribute to dissonance perception for harmonic intervals with CI-only listening.

Keywords: cochlear implant, music perception, single-sided deafness, dissonance, harmonic intervals

INTRODUCTION

Along with language, music is a near-universal part of the human experience. Although cochlear implants (CIs) can enable those with severe hearing loss to understand speech with high levels of intelligibility, these devices are extremely poor at conveying most tonal aspects of music (e.g., melody and harmony) that are crucial for music perception and appreciation. The coarse spectro-temporal resolution provided by a CI is adequate for speech recognition, due to the availability of low-frequency temporal envelope cues. However, this coarse resolution is not sufficient for music perception, especially perception of pitch, timbre, harmonicity, etc. (e.g., Smith et al., 2002; Shannon et al., 2004). The limited number of implanted electrodes, the broad acoustic-to-electric frequency allocation, the strong channel interaction among the implanted electrodes, and patient-related idiosyncrasies in terms of the position of the electrodes in relation to healthy neural populations (the "electrode-neural interface") all contribute to distorted perception of musical intervals, relative to acoustic hearing (e.g., McDermott, 2004; Galvin et al., 2007, 2009a; Gfeller et al., 2007; Nimmons et al., 2008; Kang et al., 2009; Cousineau et al., 2010; Limb and Roy, 2014). Distorted perception of melodic (i.e., sequential) intervals contributes to CI users' poor melody perception, especially when rhythm cues are unavailable (e.g., Gfeller et al., 2002, 2007; Kong et al., 2004; Vongpaisal et al., 2006). With polyphonic music (multiple instruments or voices), CI users' melodic pitch perception worsens further (e.g., Galvin et al., 2009b, 2012; Penninger et al., 2013, 2014; Crew et al., 2015). While perception of melodic intervals has been extensively studied, relatively little is known about CI users' perception of harmonic (i.e., simultaneous) intervals.

Simultaneous presentation of musical intervals forms the basis of harmony and is used to build musical chords. Depending on the component notes, harmonic intervals may be perceived as having different degrees of consonance or dissonance, sounding complementary, pleasant, unpleasant or neutral (e.g., Dowling and Harwood, 1986; Deutsch, 2007; Bidelman and Krishnan, 2009). With normal hearing (NH), some harmonic intervals may sound harsh or dissonant (e.g., minor 2nd, tritone), while others may sound more pleasing (e.g., major 3rd, 5th). When notes are combined, the harmonic spectra and temporal properties of each component note are also combined. As such, the degree of "harmonicity" in the combined spectrum (which relates to the spacing of the harmonics) may contribute to perceived consonance (e.g., Tramo et al., 2001; McDermott et al., 2010). Temporal beating or roughness may also contribute to perceived dissonance for harmonic intervals (e.g., Plomp and Levelt, 1965; Tramo et al., 2001). Individual preferences for consonance may also be influenced by musical training (McDermott et al., 2010) and experience with Western musical structure (McDermott et al., 2016). Perception of dissonance contributes strongly to emotional responses to music (Fritz et al., 2009), as does the perception of harmonic "syntax" (how harmonic intervals and chords relate to each other in a piece of music; e.g., Patel, 2003).

It is unclear whether CI users are able to perceive dissonance for harmonic intervals with electric hearing. Brockmeier et al. (2011) reported that CI users were able to discriminate musical chords, but that discrimination was poorer than that of NH listeners. Caldwell et al. (2016) altered the accompanying chords to a melody to be overtly consonant or dissonant; pleasantness ratings decreased as the degree of dissonance in the accompaniment increased for NH listeners, but not for CI listeners. Knobloch et al. (2018) reported that CI users were able to discriminate chords, and that chord preference ratings (from top to bottom: major, minor, suspended 4th, augmented, diminished, and diminished 5th) were generally similar to those of NH listeners. These studies suggest that some differentiation among harmonic intervals is possible with electric hearing, but perception of dissonance for specific intervals has yet to be reported.

Arguably, the greatest benefit for CI users' music perception has been the inclusion of acoustic hearing (where possible) in the ear contralateral or ipsilateral to the CI ear. CI indications have expanded to allow for increasing amounts of acoustic hearing in the contralateral ear. Preservation of residual low-frequency acoustic hearing in the implanted ear is becoming more frequent due to advanced electrode designs and surgical techniques (Santa Maria et al., 2014; Causon et al., 2015; Wanna et al., 2015; Sierra et al., 2019). Many studies have shown significant benefits for music perception with combined acoustic and electric hearing over CI-only performance (e.g., Kong et al., 2005; Dorman et al., 2008; Vermeire et al., 2008; Sucher and McDermott, 2009; Cullington and Zeng, 2011; Crew et al., 2015; Cheng et al., 2018). Depending on the listening task, binaural enhancement over acoustic hearing may be limited. For example, Crew et al. (2015, 2016) found no significant binaural enhancement over acoustic hearing alone for melodic contour identification; some participants even exhibited binaural interference relative to acoustic hearing alone, suggesting that acoustic and electric stimulation patterns were not optimally combined. The data also suggested that for melodic pitch perception, the CI contributed very little to bimodal perception, due to the availability of temporal fine-structure (TFS) cues with acoustic hearing that are important for melodic pitch perception.

Over the last decade, increasing numbers of patients with single-sided deafness (SSD) have undergone cochlear implantation. SSD-CI patients have normal or near-normal acoustic hearing in one ear and a CI in the other ear. Many studies have shown significant benefits of cochlear implantation for SSD patients in terms of reduced tinnitus severity, as well as improved localization, speech understanding and quality of life (e.g., Van de Heyning et al., 2008; Vermeire et al., 2008; Vermeire and Van de Heyning, 2009; Firszt et al., 2012; Mertens et al., 2015; Friedmann et al., 2016; Arndt et al., 2017; Dillon et al., 2017a,b; Galvin et al., 2018). Landsberger et al. (2019) reported significantly higher musical sound quality ratings when SSD-CI participants listened with acoustic and electric hearing than with acoustic hearing alone. SSD-CI patients represent a unique patient population with which to compare auditory perception between acoustic and electric hearing within participants [e.g., inter-aural pitch matching (Vermeire et al., 2008, 2015; Goupell et al., 2019); sound quality differences between acoustic and electric hearing (Vermeire et al., 2013; Dorman et al., 2017); melodic interval distortion (Todd et al., 2017)]. SSD-CI patients would be similarly valuable for comparing harmonic interval perception between acoustic and electric hearing. Pleasantness ratings for different intervals obtained with acoustic hearing can provide an accurate reference for ratings obtained with electric hearing in the same listener (rather than across NH and CI listeners, as in most previous studies).

In the present study, pleasantness ratings were obtained for harmonic intervals in SSD-CI participants with the NH ear alone, the CI ear alone, and with both ears. We expected that ratings with the NH ear would be similar to those found for NH listeners in previous studies (McDermott et al., 2010; Cousineau et al., 2012). However, we hypothesized that due to the poor spectro-temporal resolution with the CI (which would not support harmonicity cues that are important to consonance perception), pleasantness ratings would be generally poor with electric hearing and would not correspond to ratings with acoustic hearing. Despite the expected poor ratings with the CI, we hypothesized significant binaural enhancement over the NH ear alone, similar to Landsberger et al. (2019) and in agreement with anecdotal reports from SSD-CI patients that music sounds better with combined acoustic and electric hearing than with acoustic hearing alone.

EXPERIMENT 1: HARMONIC INTERVAL PERCEPTION

Methods

Participants

Eleven SSD-CI patients (5 males, 6 females) participated in the study. All participants were adults with post-lingual SSD, with profound hearing loss in one ear and normal or near-normal hearing in the contralateral ear. Six participants used Cochlear Ltd. Devices (codes begin with "N"), four used MED-EL devices (codes begin with "M"), and one used an Advanced Bionics (AB) device (code begins with "C"). Two participants (N10 and C1) reported extensive formal music education, one reported informal musical education (N6), and the other eight reported no music training. Average age was 53.91 years (range: 27–70 years). Further demographic information can be found in **Table 1**. All participants were paid for their participation and provided written informed consent in accordance with the Institutional Review Board Procedures of New York University (IRB #S14-00809 and #S14-00435) and in accordance with the Declaration of Helsinki.

Stimuli

Stimuli were equally tempered MIDI piano notes generated using Matlab and a MIDI library by Ken Schutte[1]. Each note was 1s in duration. For a given interval, both notes were normalized to have the same root-mean-square (RMS) amplitude (−26.9 dBFS) and then mixed together. Stimuli were ramped on and off to eliminate sharp onsets and offsets. All samples were recorded with a 44.1 kHz sampling rate at 16-bit depth. Harmonic interval stimuli are shown in **Table 2**. Each interval was comprised of one of two "root notes" [F3 (≈175 Hz) or C4 (≈262 Hz)] presented simultaneously with a second note. In this study, "root note" is defined as the lower note in the interval. It was important to test two different root notes to avoid entrainment to a particular frequency, and to accommodate potential differences across SSD-CI patients in terms of frequency allocation and the electrode-neural interface. Given these potential differences, ratings might differ across root notes for particular subjects. Two "interval spans" were also tested: 1–12 semitones ("within-octave") and 13–24 semitones ("across-octave"). For NH listeners, there is some evidence that harmonic intervals separated by an octave or more are perceived to be more consonant than the same interval presented within an octave (Plomp and Levelt, 1965; Kameoka and Kuriyagawa, 1969). While it was unclear if this relationship would hold for CI listeners, we hypothesized that many of the within-octave intervals would be represented on the same channel (due to the clinical CI frequency allocation). This would result in some amount of within-channel temporal beating. Even for larger within-octave intervals, channel interactions may cause both notes to be represented by overlapping neural populations. Including a set of intervals presented across-octave allows for component notes to be delivered to different electrode locations and increases the likelihood that notes will be encoded by separate neural populations. Thus, pleasantness ratings for a given interval could be compared within or across channels. The interval span conditions may also shed light on the importance of place cues for dissonance perception. **Table 2** shows the within- and across-octave intervals. Overall, there were 24 stimuli per root note, for a total of 48 test intervals.

Stimuli were presented using custom software via audio device (Tascam US-322), and were routed to the NH ear via circumaural headphone (Sony MDR-7506) and to the CI ear via isolated direct audio input (DAI). Three listening conditions were tested: NH-only (monaural), CI-only (monaural), and NH + CI (diotic binaural). For MED-EL users, the "red" DAI cable was connected between the audio device and the CI processor, which

[1] http://kenschutte.com/midi

TABLE 1 | Demographic information for SSD-CI subjects.

Participant	Lab code	Dur deaf (yrs)	CI exp (yrs)	Etiology	Device	Strategy	CI ear	Non-CI ear PTA (dB HL)	CI ear CNC % correct
C1	SSD-C1	2.6	3.01	Idiopathic SSHL	AB HiRes90k Mid Scala	HiRes Optima-P	R	8.3	30
M2	SSD-M1	0.3	1	Cochlear Schwannoma/NF2	MED-EL Synchrony Flex 28	FS4-P	R	25.0	4
M3	SSD-M2	1.3	0.31	Idiopathic progressive	MED-EL Synchrony Flex 28	FS4-P	L	11.7	30
M4	SSD-M3	0.9	2.45	Idiopathic SSHL	MED-EL Synchrony Flex 28	FS4-P	L	26.7	44
M5	SSD-M4	6.6	1.07	Idiopathic SSHL	MED-EL Synchrony Flex 28	FS4-P	L	5.0	DNT
N6	SSD-N1	4.2	8.26	Idiopathic SSHL	Cochlear N512 CI512	ACE	R	43.3	70
N7	SSD-N6	2.4	3.3	Idiopathic SSHL	Cochlear Profile CI512	ACE	R	3.3	84
N8	SSD-N7	0.4	4.21	Idiopathic SSHL	Cochlear Profile CI512	ACE	R	15.0	48
N9	SSD-N8	1.1	1.56	Genetic	Cochlear Profile CI532	ACE	L	8.3	92
N10	SSD-N9	9	0.79	Temporal bone fracture	Cochlear Profile CI512	ACE	L	16.7	66
N11	SSD-N10	3.2	1.95	Idiopathic SSHL	Cochlear Profile CI532	ACE	R	26.7	70

For simplicity, subjects are referred to in this manuscript by subject code (i.e., C1-N11). The letter before the number refers to the manufacturer of the device ("C": Advanced Bionics; "M": MED-EL, and "N": Cochlear). The internal lab code for each subject is also provided for comparison purposes to other publications. Dur deaf = duration of deafness. CI exp = cochlear implant experience. AB = Advanced Bionics. ACE = Advanced Combination Encoder. PTA = pure-tone average thresholds across 500, 1000, and 2000 Hz. DNT = did not test. For all subjects except for C1, M3, and M5, CNC scores with the CI-only were obtained after 1 year of CI experience. For C1 and M3, scores were obtained after 3 months of CI experience; no scores were available for M5.

TABLE 2 | Test intervals for Exp. 1.

Within-octave		**Interval:**	**Minor 2nd**	**Major 2nd**	**Minor 3rd**	**Major 3rd**	**4th**	**Tritone**	**5th**	**Minor 6th**	**Major 6th**	**Minor 7th**	**Major 7th**	**Octave**
		Semitones:	**1**	**2**	**3**	**4**	**5**	**6**	**7**	**8**	**9**	**10**	**11**	**12**
	F3	Note: F3 +	F#3	G3	G#3	A3	A#3	B3	C4	C#4	D4	D#4	E4	F4
		MIDI note: 53 +	54	55	56	57	58	59	60	61	62	63	64	65
		Frequency: 175 Hz +	185	196	208	220	233	247	262	277	294	311	330	349
	C4	Note: C4 +	C#4	D4	D#4	E4	F4	F#4	G4	G#4	A4	A#4	B4	C5
		MIDI note: 60 +	61	62	63	64	65	66	67	68	69	70	71	72
		Frequency: 262 Hz +	277	294	311	330	349	370	392	415	440	466	494	523
Across-octave		**Interval:**	**Minor 9th**	**Major 9th**	**Minor 10th**	**Major 10th**	**11th**	**Diminished 12th**	**12th**	**Minor 13th**	**Major 13th**	**Minor 14th**	**Major 14th**	**Double Octave**
		Semitones:	**13**	**14**	**15**	**16**	**17**	**18**	**19**	**20**	**21**	**22**	**23**	**24**
	F3	Note: F3 +	F#4	G4	G#4	A4	A#4	B4	C5	C#5	D5	D#5	E5	F5
		MIDI note: 53 +	66	67	68	69	70	71	72	73	74	75	76	77
		Frequency: 175 Hz +	370	392	415	440	466	494	523	554	587	622	659	698
	C4	Note: C4 +	C#5	D5	D#5	E5	F5	F#5	G5	G#5	A5	A#5	B5	C6
		MIDI note: 60 +	73	74	75	76	77	78	79	80	81	82	83	84
		Frequency: 262 Hz +	554	587	622	659	698	740	784	831	880	932	988	1047

The top section shows within-octave intervals (1–12 semitones) and the bottom section shows across-octave intervals (13–24 semitones). Two root notes (F3 and C4) were tested for each interval; the different rows show the notes in terms of musical notation, MIDI notation, and frequency. The columns show the name, symbol, and semitone distance from the root note.

provided a mix of 90% audio input and 10% microphone input. Participants were tested with their clinical settings. For Cochlear users, participants' clinical maps were programed onto loaner N6 (CP910) processors configured for DAI input only. Similarly, for the AB user, the clinical map was programed onto a loaner Harmony processor; the map was configured for DAI input only.

Procedure

Before testing began, all participants were asked to set the loudness of the stimuli presented to the NH and CI ear to an equally loud most-comfortable level. A musical interval was played alternately between the CI ear and the NH ear, and the participant adjusted the output volume of each channel of the audio device until both channels were equally loud and at the most-comfortable listening level. After these initial adjustments, participants were not allowed to adjust the volume of either output for the remainder of the experiment.

All three listening conditions and all 48 intervals were presented within each test block (144 stimuli in total). Listening conditions and intervals were randomized within each test block.

A total of five blocks (i.e., five repetitions of each interval) were tested for each participant; the test blocks were administered during a single session lasting approximately 3 hours. During testing, a stimulus was randomly selected from the stimulus set and presented to the participant, who was asked to rate the pleasantness by clicking on a continuous bar with the anchors "least pleasant" and "most pleasant" at either end (no other scaling of the range was provided). A short practice session was given prior to starting the experiment to familiarize participants with the stimuli and test procedure. Participants were allowed to repeat each stimulus as many times as they wanted. Pleasantness ratings were averaged for each interval, root note, and listening conditions across the five repetitions from each test block.

Results

Pleasantness ratings were scaled from 0 to 10 according to where participants clicked on the rating bar. **Figure 1** shows group (n = 11) mean pleasantness ratings for the NH-only, CI-only and NH + CI listening conditions as a function of interval size. Consistent with McDermott et al. (2010), for NH-only listening, some intervals were consistently rated least pleasant (minor 2nd, tritone, and major 7th), while others were consistently rated most pleasant (major 3rd, 5th, and octave). Ratings with CI-only listening were much poorer than with NH-only or NH + CI listening. Ratings were similar between NH-only and NH + CI listening. A four-way repeated measures analysis of variance (RM ANOVA) was performed with listening condition (NH, CI, NH + CI), interval span (within-octave, across-octave), root note (F3, C4) and interval size (12 levels: 1–12 semitones) as within-subject factors. Significant main effects were observed only for listening condition [$F(1,10) = 18.115$, $p < 0.001$] and interval size [$F(11,110) = 14.95$, $p < 0.001$]. A summary of the analysis is shown in **Supplementary Appendix 1**. We also analyzed the data using a 3-way RM ANOVA, removing the factor of interval span and thus considering intervals from 1 to 24 semitones. Results were nearly identical to those from the above the 4-way RM ANOVA, with the exception of an interaction between listening condition, interval size, and root note [$F(46, 460) = 1.48$, $p = 0.027$].

Post hoc analyses were conducted to compare the NH-only and NH + CI listening conditions. To observe whether there was any binaural enhancement for individual participants, paired t-tests were conducted on individual participants' NH-only and NH + CI data. Because the four-way RM ANOVA showed no significant effect of interval span or root note, data were combined for a total of 48 comparisons between the NH-only and NH + CI listening conditions within each participant. Complete results are shown in **Supplementary Appendix 2**. Results showed no significant difference between NH-only and NH + CI ratings for 7 of the 11 participants ($p > 0.05$ in all cases). For two participants, there was significant binaural enhancement [N7: $t(47) = -30.96$, $p < 0.001$; N9: $t(47) = -19.54$, $p < 0.001$]. For another two participants, there was significant binaural interference [C1: $t(47) = 2.54$, $p = 0.015$; M2: $t(47) = 13.91$, $p < 0.001$]. Pearson correlation analysis showed no significant relationship between the degree of binaural enhancement (NH + CI – NH-only) and the difference between NH and CI ratings ($r = -0.04$, $p = 0.901$).

Figure 2 shows individual pleasantness ratings as a function of interval size for the F3 root note (within-octave interval) with NH-only (black line, left ordinate) and CI-only listening (red line, right ordinate). While the range is much larger with NH-only than with CI-only listening, the rating patterns are somewhat similar between acoustic and electric hearing, especially for some participants (e.g., C1, N8). Most participants rated minor 2nd lowest, whether with acoustic or electric hearing. With NH-only listening, major 3rd, 4th, 5th, and octave were generally rated highest. With CI-only listening, octave was often rated highest; other intervals that also produced relatively high ratings varied across participants. Visual examination of the data showed that some participants exhibited minimal variation in ratings with the CI ear (e.g., M2, M3, M4, M5, N11) while others exhibited minimal variation with the NH ear (M2, N7).

Figure 3 shows mean CI-only pleasantness ratings for each interval as a function of NH-only ratings for the different root note and interval span conditions. Linear regressions were fit to the data in each panel; r- and p-values for each regression are shown at the bottom left in each panel. Strong correlations were observed for all root note and interval span conditions. Across all root notes and interval span conditions, correlations were highly significant between NH-only and CI-only listening ($r = 0.845$, $p < 0.001$), and between NH-only and NH + CI listening ($r = 0.995$, $p < 0.001$). Because of the strong correlations at the group level, additional correlational analyses were performed within individual participants (**Supplementary Appendix 3**). For NH-only versus CI-only listening, significant correlations ($p < 0.05$) were observed only for participants C1 (F3 within-octave and F3 across-octave), N6 (F3 within-octave and C4 within-octave), and N8 (F3 across-octave). For NH-only versus NH + CI listening, significant correlations ($p < 0.05$) were observed in most cases, with the exceptions of M2 (F3 within-octave, C4 within-octave, C4 across-octave), M5 (F3 within-octave, C4 within-octave, F3 across-octave), and N7 (F3 within-octave). Additional correlational analyses were performed to compare mean ratings across interval span and/or root note for the different listening conditions (**Supplementary Appendix 4**). For the F3 root note, significant correlations ($p < 0.01$) were observed between within- and across-octave interval ratings for NH-only, CI-only, and NH + CI listening. For C4, significant correlations ($p < 0.01$) were observed between within- and across-octave ratings for NH-only and NH + CI listening, but not for CI-only listening. For both within- and across-octave intervals, significant correlations were observed between F3 and C4 ($p < 0.015$ in all cases). For all root note and interval span conditions, significant correlations were also observed between NH-only and NH + CI listening ($p < 0.028$ in all cases).

Experiment 1 Discussion

With the NH ear, pleasantness ratings were comparable to those for the NH controls in Cousineau et al. (2012). To compare more directly the pattern of results between studies, the present ratings were converted to z-scores, as in Cousineau et al. (2012). **Figure 4** shows z-scores for SSD-CI ratings with NH-only and CI-only

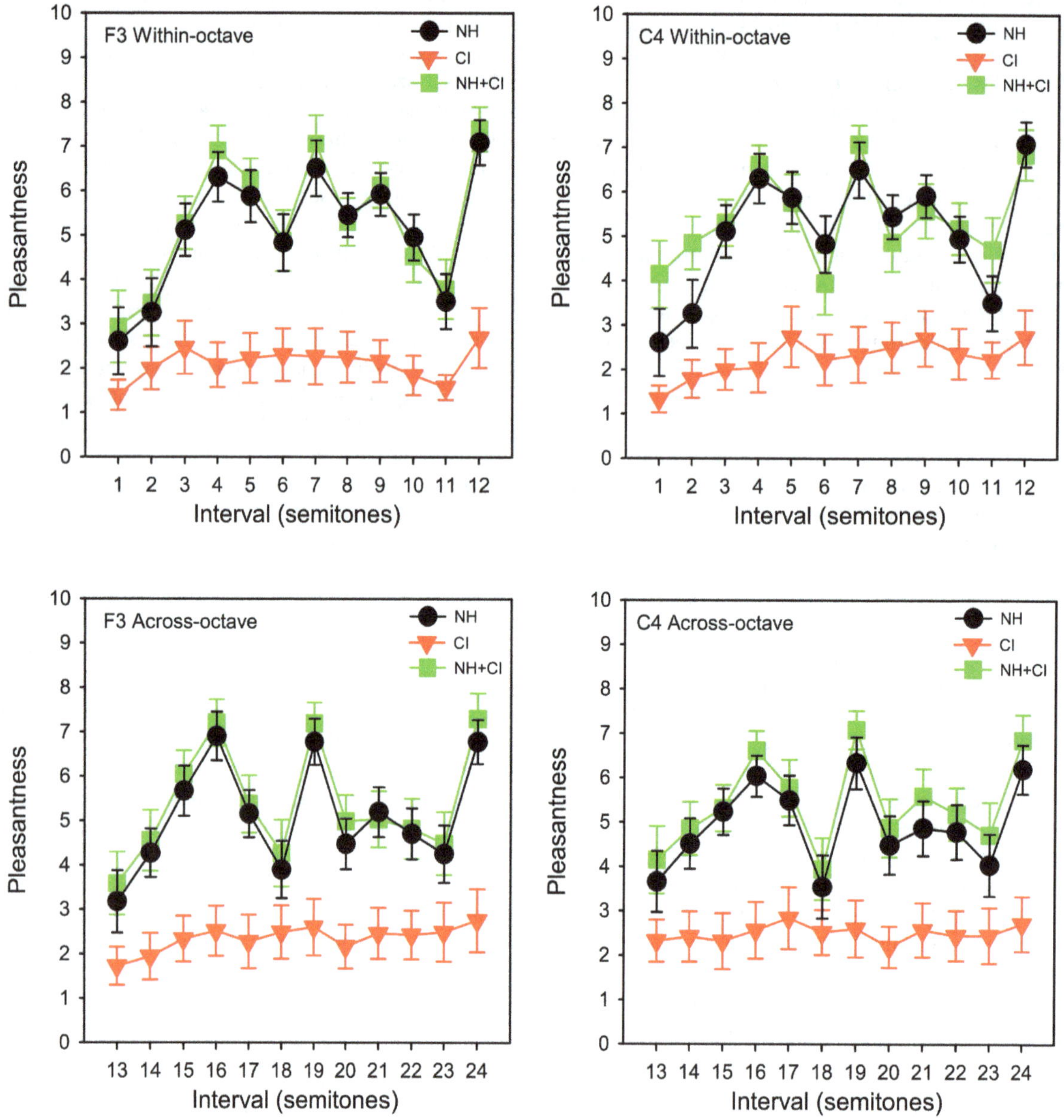

FIGURE 1 | Mean pleasantness ratings for SSD-CI participants (n = 11) with NH-only (black), CI-only (red), and NH + CI (green) listening as a function of interval size. Interval size in semitones is shown on the abscissa. Data for the F3 and C4 root notes are shown in the right and left columns, respectively. Data for within- and across-octave intervals are shown in the top and bottom rows, respectively. The error bars show the standard error.

listening for within-octave intervals with the F3 root note; z-score data for NH controls and amusics were extracted from **Figure 2** from Cousineau et al. (2012). Note that the instruments and note ranges used in the experiments differed. NH-only SSD-CI scores were quite similar to the NH control scores from Cousineau et al. (2012). However, CI-only SSD-CI scores were markedly different from amusic scores, especially for minor 2nd and major 7th. Except for major 3rd, tritone, and 5th, SSD-CI z-scores were generally similar between NH-only and CI-only listening. This suggests that beating or roughness may have been a similarly strong cue for both listening conditions. As reported by Cousineau et al. (2012), ratings were markedly different between the NH controls and amusics, especially for minor 2nd and major 7th. Interestingly, the amusics in Cousineau et al. (2012) were able to discriminate between beating and non-beating stimuli, suggesting that the presence of beating may not have driven ratings for minor 2nd and major 7th. The SSD-CI participants in the present study had a normal periphery in one ear, presumably normal central perception of the harmonic intervals (based on the NH-only scores), and a degraded periphery in the other ear. For amusics, the periphery was normal in both ears, discrimination of beating was similar to NH controls, but pleasantness ratings were not consistent with the NH controls, especially for minor 2nd and major 7th, where beating might be a strong cue.

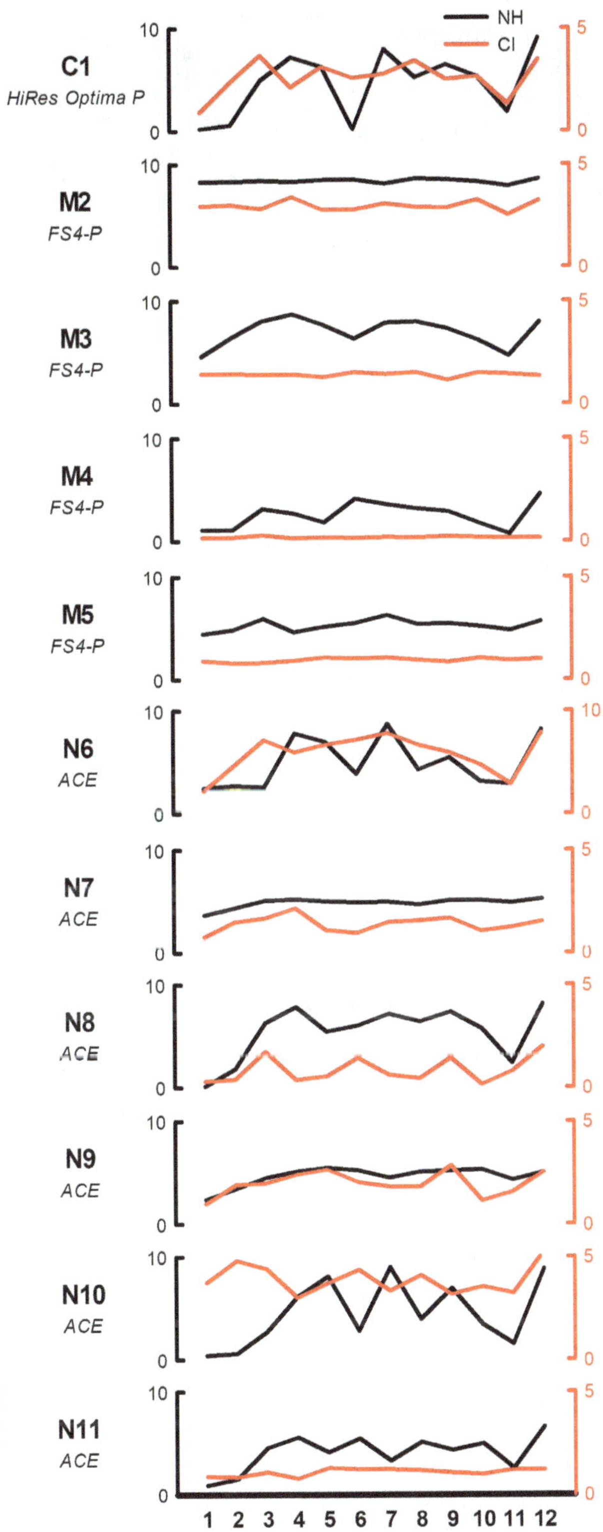

FIGURE 2 | Pleasantness ratings for individual SSD-CI participants with NH-only (black, left ordinate) and CI-only listening (red, right ordinate), for the F3 root note (within-octave) as a function of interval size. Note that the scale for CI-only ratings is half of that for NH-only ratings for all participants except N6. The clinical CI signal processing strategy is listed under each subject's code.

Cousineau et al. (2012) suggested that a disordered perception of harmonicity may have given rise to the ambiguous pleasantness ratings in amusics.

As expected, overall ratings were much higher with NH-only than with CI-only listening. Somewhat surprisingly, there was no significant difference between NH + CI and NH-only ratings at the group level. This pattern of results is not consistent with the binaural enhancement observed for the music sound quality ratings (CI-MUSHRA) in SSD-CI participants reported by Landsberger et al. (2019). In that study with SSD-CI listeners, binaural (NH + CI) quality ratings were substantially and significantly higher than with the NH ear alone. Many factors may have contributed to the different patterns of results. First, in Landsberger et al. (2019), two excerpts of musical recordings ("Ring of Fire" and "Rhapsody in Blue") were used to obtain sound quality ratings. These excerpts were much longer (9–15 s) than the stimuli used in the present study (1 s), and consisted of multiple instruments and/or vocals (versus the piano samples used in the present study). The longer duration and more complex musical sounds may have contributed to the binaural enhancement found in Landsberger et al. (2019). While participants were asked to rate the pleasantness of the stimuli in both studies, participants may have focused attention on different aspects of the stimuli. For the musical intervals presented in the present study, listeners may have attended to the roughness or beating within the stimuli to judge dissonance. The longer duration of the stimuli in Landsberger et al. (2019) may have allowed some qualitative benefit for adding the CI that was not observed in the present study. Note that in Landsberger et al. (2019), the binaural enhancement for SSD-CI users, while substantial, was much less than for NH participants, suggesting that electric hearing was not able to fully restore binaural sound quality for music.

In the present study, binaural ratings for harmonic intervals were clearly dominated by the NH ear, with little contribution from the CI ear. Although one participant (N6) exhibited substantial binaural enhancement, there was no clear factor that appeared to limit binaural enhancement. Previous speech perception studies with bimodal and bilateral CI listeners showed that the degree of binaural enhancement may depend on the degree of performance difference across ears, with binaural enhancement improving as across-ear asymmetry in performance was reduced (Yoon et al., 2011, 2015). Here, there was no significant relationship between the degree of rating asymmetry across ears and the amount of binaural enhancement. It is possible that the general across-ear asymmetry was so large that the relatively minor variability among participants had no effect. In this sense, the present data are consistent with the Yoon et al. studies, in that no binaural enhancement was observed for the highly asymmetrical ratings across ears. Note that in the Yoon et al. studies, speech performance asymmetry was in terms of percent correct; it is unclear whether the pattern of results would have been similar if listeners were asked to rate the quality of speech.

With NH-only or NH + CI listening, the pattern of results for simple intervals was similar to those reported for NH listeners in McDermott et al. (2010) and Cousineau et al. (2012), with

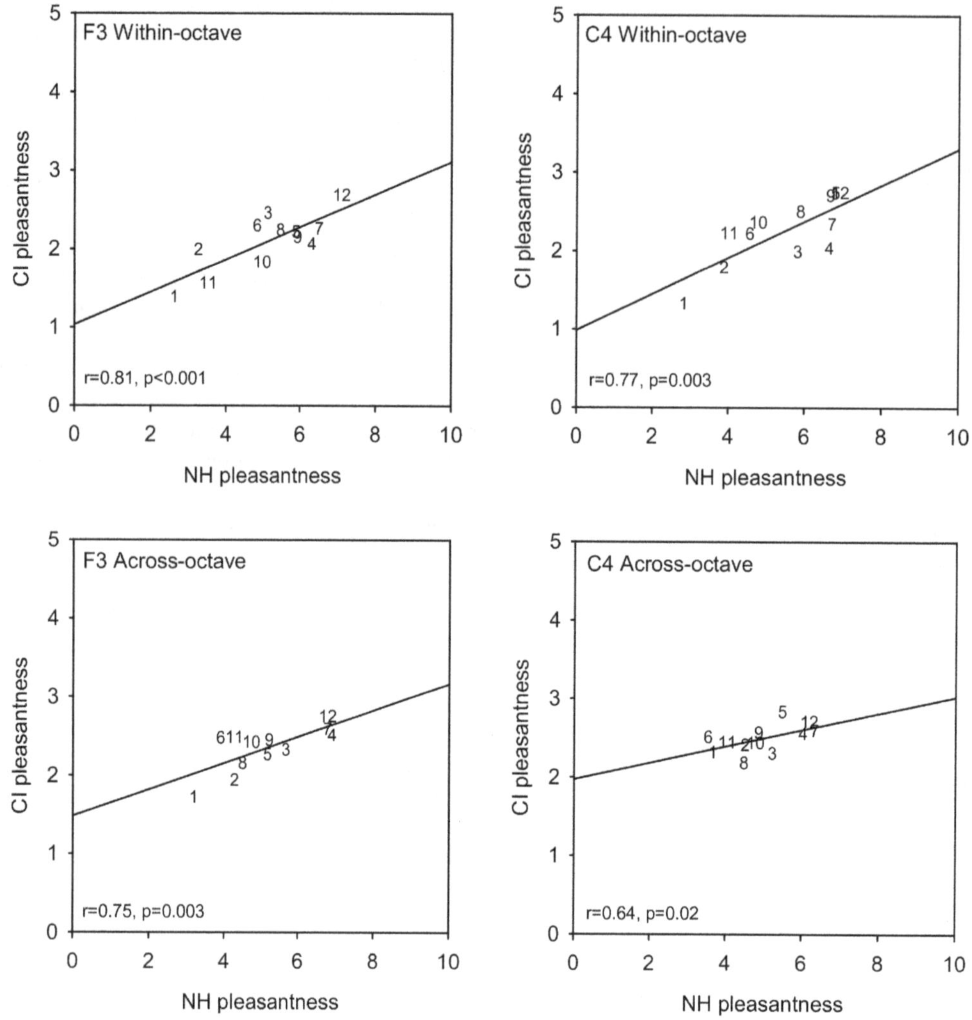

FIGURE 3 | Mean CI-only pleasantness ratings (across subjects) as a function of mean NH-only ratings. Data for the F3 and C4 root notes are shown in the right and left columns, respectively. Data for within- and across-octave intervals are shown in the top and bottom rows, respectively. Note that the range for the CI-only ratings in half of that for the NH-only ratings. Interval size is indicated as numbers in each panel. The diagonal lines show linear regression fits to the data; *r*- and *p*-values are shown for each regression.

minor 2nd, tritone, and major 7th consistently rated lowest, and major 3rd, 4th, 5th, and octave consistently rated highest (top panels of **Figure 1**). With the CI alone, minor 2nd and major 7th were generally rated lowest and major 3rd, 4th, and octave were generally rated highest. With CI-only listening, there was little sensitivity to the dissonance of the tritone observed with NH-only or NH + CI listening, although some participants (N7, N8, N9, N10) exhibited a dip in ratings in the vicinity of the tritone (red traces in **Figure 2**). It is possible that due to differences in the electrode-neural interface, the dip in ratings near the tritone may have been slightly shifted across participants. For all three listening conditions, similar rating patterns were observed between within- and across-octave intervals and for both root notes. Statistical analyses showed no significant effects of root note or interval span. The lack of effect of root note suggests differences in frequency allocation were either inconsequential for harmonic interval perception or were varied enough among subjects to wash out any effect of greater dissonance (i.e., temporal beating) for one root note versus the other.

With CI-only listening, participants were likely able to discriminate between an interval presented within or across octaves (e.g., minor 2nd vs. minor 9th) due to differences in the spectral pattern; however, these stimuli were consistently and similarly rated lowest in terms of pleasantness. With CI-only listening, the octave and double octave were generally rated as most pleasant, possibly because of highly periodic temporal envelope cues. However, the place of stimulation for the two component notes did not likely correspond to octave place in the cochlea (Landsberger et al., 2015), given the frequency allocation, electrode neural interface, etc. Thus, while CI users may have perceived the lack of temporal beating in the octave and double octave, they most likely did not receive spectral (harmonicity) cues that would have been available in the NH ear. It is unclear whether the present SSD-CI users perceived

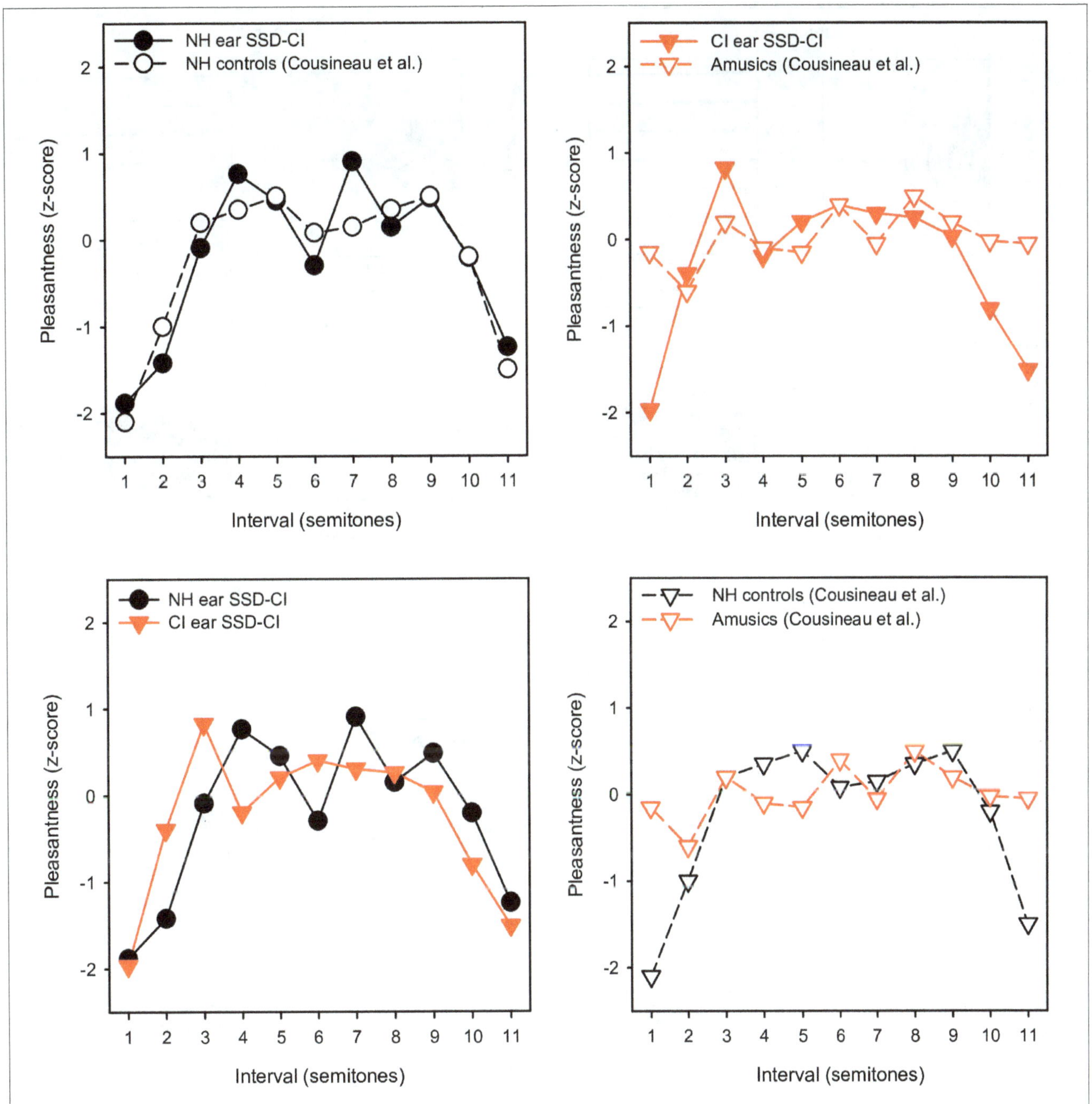

FIGURE 4 | Mean pleasantness ratings (converted to *z*-scores) for SSD-CI participants in the present study (within-octave intervals with F3 root note) and NH controls and amusics from Cousineau et al. (2012). In the **top left panel**, the present SSD-CI NH-only data are plotted alongside the NH control data from Cousineau et al. (2012). In the **top right panel**, the present SSD-CI CI-only data are plotted alongside the amusic data from Cousineau et al. (2012). In the **bottom left panel**, the present SSD-CI NH-only data are plotted alongside the present SSD-CI CI-only data. In the **bottom right panel**, the NH control data from Cousineau et al. (2012) are plotted alongside the amusic data from Cousineau et al. (2012).

octaves similarly between acoustic and electric hearing; however, octaves were most pleasant relative to other intervals with either listening mode.

The lack of effect of interval span for CI listening led us to re-analyze the data using a 3-way RM ANOVA by removing the factor of interval span and considered interval size as a continuous range from 1 to 24. Results were nearly identical to the 4-way RM ANOVA reported above. Therefore, we chose to leave interval span as a factor in order to be consistent with the original study design.

In the present study, harmonic intervals were presented acoustically to the NH ear via headphone and to the CI ear via DAI. For acoustic hearing, listeners could access both temporal envelope interactions between each component interval as well

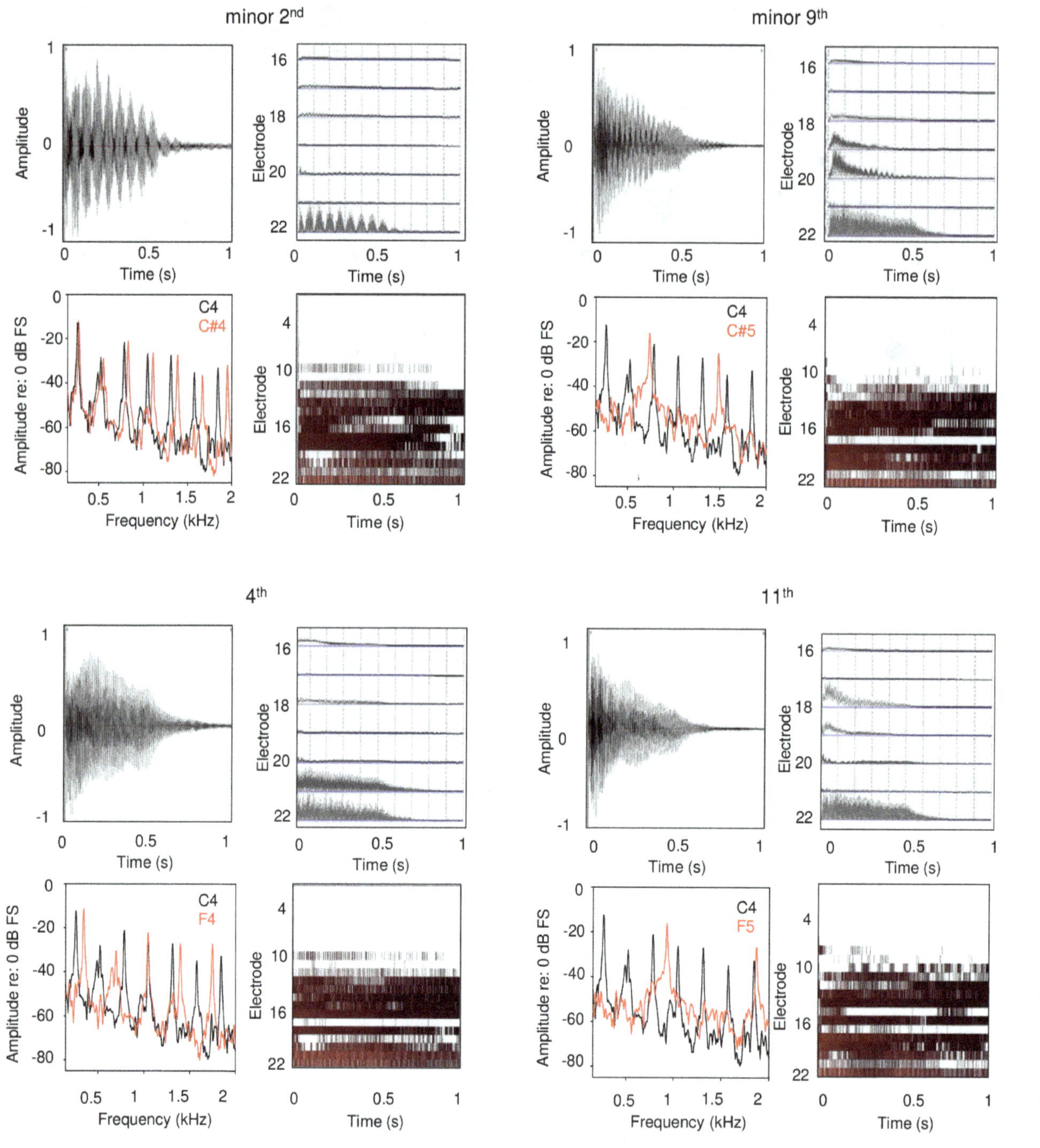

FIGURE 5 | Waveforms, frequency analyses, extracted temporal envelopes, and electrodograms for example dissonant (top panels) and consonant intervals (bottom panels); the left and right panels show within- and across-octave intervals, respectively. The root note for all intervals was C4. Each panel shows (in clockwise order from the top left): waveform, temporal envelopes extracted from each CI signal processor analysis band, electrodogram, and frequency analysis. The extracted temporal envelopes and electrodograms were generated using custom software and using default parameters for Cochlear devices (e.g., ACE strategy, 8 maxima, 900 pulses/second stimulation rate, input frequency range 188–7938 Hz, etc.).

as the degree of "harmonicity" for the combined intervals. For electric hearing, due to the limited spectro-temporal resolution, harmonicity cues would have largely been unavailable; this most likely underlies the overall poor ratings with the CI. As such, temporal envelope interactions (perceived as the degree of roughness or beating in the interval) may have driven differences in ratings across intervals.

Each panel in **Figure 5** shows waveforms and spectra for an acoustic interval, as well as the extracted temporal envelopes for low-frequency channels and electrodograms across all channels for the default CI processor settings for Cochlear devices. For minor 2nd with the C4 root note (top left panel), low-frequency envelope modulation can be observed in the waveform, and the spectra for low-frequency components are slightly offset; these two features would likely give rise to a strong dissonant perception with acoustic hearing. The extracted temporal envelopes exhibit similar beating, especially for the most apical channel (electrode 22). For the electrodogram, there is no clear pattern that would suggest harmonicity or inharmonicity. For minor 9th (top right panel), another typically dissonant interval, the roughness/beating of the temporal envelope can be observed in the waveform, as well as some degree of inharmonicity in the spectra. The roughness/beating can also be observed in the extracted temporal envelope for the CI, especially for electrode 20. For the 4th and 11th intervals (typically rated as consonant), the beating is less apparent in the waveform, and the spectra are more evenly spaced and/or overlapping (greater harmonicity). Overt low-frequency beating is not apparent in electrodograms. While the electrodograms are somewhat different across the minor 2nd, minor 9th, 4th, and 11th intervals, there is no clear pattern that would differentiate any degree of harmonicity among the stimuli. Note that these electrodograms and extracted temporal envelopes specifically apply to Cochlear devices.

Although the temporal and spectral patterns may differ with AB or MED-EL devices, the envelope cues and coarse spectral resolution are likely to be similar for any CI device that represents temporal information by amplitude modulation. In designing the experimental conditions, the different root notes and interval spans were used to accommodate differences among participants' CI frequency allocations and electrode-neural interfaces (i.e., spectral cues). These accommodations did not appear to affect the general pattern of results, as there were no significant effects of either root note or interval span on CI ratings. For electric hearing, temporal envelope interactions appear to be the dominant cue for the relative dissonance ratings with the CI. This is consistent with Lu et al. (2014), who found that CI users were able to tune a guitar with electric hearing largely by listening to temporal envelope beating. Interestingly, one of the SSD-CI participants in Lu et al. (2014) showed better tuning with acoustic than with electric hearing, possibly due to better access to both harmonicity and temporal beat cues.

To our knowledge, there has been relatively few reports of perception of widely spaced harmonic intervals by NH listeners, outside of early studies by Plomp and Levelt (1965) and Kameoka and Kuriyagawa (1969). These studies suggest greater consonance when notes were separated by an octave or more, possibly because of a greater reliance on spectral than on temporal cues as the notes became more widely separated. Our NH-only data suggest that consonance and dissonance ratings were very similar for the within- and across- octave conditions (e.g., the highly significant correlation between with- and across-octave rating with the NH ear alone in **Supplementary Appendix 4**, the lack of significant effect of interval span in the RM ANOVA). With CI-only listening, relative dissonance ratings were largely maintained within and across octaves. This suggests that the chroma of the harmonic intervals were largely maintained between acoustic and electric hearing, despite the large differences in sound quality between listening modes.

EXPERIMENT 2: REPLICATION OF RATINGS FOR A REDUCED SET OF INTERVALS

The data from Exp. 1 showed a significant correlation at the group level for pleasantness ratings between acoustic and electric hearing. However, significant correlations were observed for only a few individual participants. The specific intervals that produced maximum and minimum ratings with the CI may have differed across participants, due to differences in frequency allocation, electrode neural interface, etc. The large number of stimuli tested may have increased the potential for Type 1 error (i.e., finding a significant effect where none exists). It may also have reduced contrasts between strongly consonant and dissonant stimuli. Finally, it was important that the ratings from Exp. 1 be validated for both acoustic and electric hearing to ensure that participants were capable of the task, given that the majority of participants had no musical training. In Exp. 2, pleasantness ratings were obtained for subsets of stimuli that produced the maximum and minimum pleasantness ratings within each listening condition for Exp. 1.

Methods

Participants

The same 11 participants from Exp. 1 also participated in Exp. 2.

Stimuli

Test stimuli were generally the same as for Exp. 1, except that only a subset of intervals (i.e., four lowest and four highest rated intervals within each listening condition from Exp. 1) was used for Exp. 2. Note that the lowest and highest four intervals somewhat differed across subjects, especially for CI-only listening. To determine the subset of stimuli for each participant in Exp. 2, the median rating across the five test blocks of Exp. 1 was calculated for each interval within each listening condition. For each participant, ratings were then sorted from low to high within each listening condition; note that stimuli were combined across root note and interval span before sorting. After sorting, the four lowest-rated and the four highest-rated stimuli were identified for each participant for each listening condition from Exp. 1. Thus, for each participant, an optimized stimulus set was created that consisted of the four lowest-rated and the four highest-rated intervals for each listening condition, for a total of 24 stimuli in the stimulus set.

Procedures

Test procedures were identical to those in Exp. 1, except that pleasantness ratings were obtained for the stimulus set optimized for each participant and listening condition. As in Exp. 1, five test blocks were administered, and ratings were averaged across the five blocks. Exp. 2 was conducted during the same test session as for Exp. 1, and lasted 30 min. The intervals and listening conditions were randomized within each test block.

TABLE 3 | Results of linear regressions between Exp. 1 and Exp. 2 rating data.

	NH-only			CI-only			NH + CI		
Subject	**Slope**	***r***	***p***	**Slope**	***r***	***p***	**Slope**	***r***	***p***
C1	0.98	0.99	<0.001*	1.71	0.93	<0.001*	0.96	0.99	<0.001*
M2	0.01	0.05	0.899	0.36	0.16	0.708	0.04	0.42	0.303
M3	0.81	0.95	<0.001*	0.15	0.57	0.137	0.62	0.97	<0.001*
M4	0.70	0.84	0.008*	−0.02	0.07	0.864	1.03	0.97	<0.001*
M5	1.02	0.96	<0.001*	−0.09	0.22	0.595	0.90	0.83	0.011*
N6	0.97	0.98	<0.001*	0.97	0.99	<0.001*	1.05	0.99	<0.001*
N7	0.10	0.77	0.025*	0.57	0.81	0.014*	0.29	0.92	0.001*
N8	0.86	0.99	<0.001*	0.71	0.84	0.010*	0.92	0.99	<0.001*
N9	0.97	0.92	0.001*	0.56	0.88	0.004*	1.37	0.85	0.007*
N10	0.95	0.99	<0.001*	0.56	0.86	0.006*	0.99	0.99	<0.001*
N11	0.85	0.99	<0.001*	0.38	0.91	0.002*	0.86	0.98	<0.001*

Pleasantness ratings for the four lowest rated and four highest rated stimuli (across root notes and interval spans) in Exp. 1 were re-measured in Exp. 2. Linear regressions were fit to these data for each participant. The asterisks indicate significant correlations between Exp. 1 and Exp. 2 data. The shaded cells indicate instances where participants were unable to replicate the data from Exp. 1.

Results

Table 3 shows slopes, r- and p-values for linear regressions fit between Exp. 1 and Exp. 2 ratings for the optimized stimuli, for each participant and listening condition. Significant positive slopes indicate good replication between Exp. 1 and Exp. 2. Slopes > 1 indicate an expanded range of ratings for Exp. 2 relative to Exp. 1, and slopes < 1 indicate a compressed range of ratings for Exp. 2 relative to Exp. 1. With NH-only listening, significant correlations were observed for all participants (except for M2), with generally high r-values ($r \geq 0.77$). Slopes for these correlations ranged from 0.10 to 1.02. With CI-only listening, significant correlations were observed for all but the MED-EL participants (M2, M3, M4, and M5). Among the significant correlations, r-values were generally high ($r \geq 0.81$). Slopes for these correlations ranged from 0.38 to 1.71. With NH + CI listening, significant correlations were observed for all participants except for M2. Slopes ranged from 0.29 to 1.37. The high number of significant correlations suggest that for most participants, the results from Exp. 1 were replicated in Exp. 2. Note that the slopes for most of the correlation functions were < 1, indicating that the range of ratings for Exp. 2 were compressed relative to Exp. 1.

Experiment 2 Discussion

Given the significant correlations between Exp. 1 and Exp. 2 for NH-only listening, the replication data suggest that 10 of the 11 participants were able to reliably rate relative dissonance with the present stimuli and methods. The same pattern of results was found for NH + CI listening. It is unclear why participant M2 was unable to replicate the data from Exp. 1. For M2, the range of ratings (across all stimuli) was 7.9–8.7; for the remaining participants, the range was 1.9–4.5. It is unclear why there was so little differentiation in NH-only ratings for M2. It is possible that all intervals sounded pleasant in general, or that the typical distinctions between consonant and dissonant stimuli were not perceived as different.

Too few patients were tested to compare results across devices fairly. Nevertheless, it seems noteworthy that while AB and Cochlear users were able to replicate the CI ratings from Exp. 1, none of the MED-EL users were able to do so. Excluding M2 (who was unable to reliably perform the task with NH-only listening), the range of ratings (across all stimuli) with CI-only listening for the remaining three MED-EL participants was 0.1–1.9, and the mean rating was 0.9. For the AB and Cochlear participants, the range of ratings was 0.1–8.6, and the mean rating was 2.8. Thus, the three MED-EL participants exhibited a smaller range and lower mean ratings than did the AB and Cochlear participants. It is possible that the differences in ratings among the devices may be due to differences in encoding temporal information across CI signal processing strategies. The AB and Cochlear participants used Optima and ACE processing, respectively. These strategies represent temporal information extracted from frequency analysis channels by modulating fixed-rate pulse trains delivered to the appropriate electrodes. MED-EL's FS4-p processing similarly modulates fixed-rate pulse trains delivered to electrodes 5–12 (which typically represent 710 – 8500 Hz). However, on the most apical electrodes (1–4, which typically represent 100–710 Hz), modulation is applied to variable rate pulse trains that correspond to the zero-crossings in each channel. As such, the F0s for the component notes for most intervals would have been delivered to "fine-structure" (FS) channels 1–4; harmonic information above 710 Hz would have been delivered to the fixed-rate channels 5–12. With the FS channels, frequency is primarily encoded by rate of stimulation and temporal beating would be encoded by a temporal jitter rather than amplitude modulation (AM) beating. It is therefore possible that perception of temporal beating (especially for minor 2nd and major 7th) may have differed for FS4-P and the envelope-based strategies. Again, this pattern of results may have been due to the interaction between the relatively low root notes and the frequency allocation for the FS channels in MED-EL users. With higher root notes (e.g., A5, or 880 Hz), the fixed-rate channels 5–12 would have been stimulated and the pattern of results may have been more comparable to those of the present AB and Cochlear users.

For most participants, the slopes between Exp. 1 and Exp. 2 ratings were close to 1 for NH-only and NH + CI listening, suggesting that ratings for these stimuli were largely the same when presented as a subset of the larger group tested in Exp. 1. For most of the participants who replicated the Exp. 1 data with CI-only listening, slopes were considerably less than 1 suggesting that with the reduced stimulus set in Exp. 2 produced a smaller range of ratings. This suggests that with the smaller stimulus set in Exp. 2, relative dissonance was less pronounced than with the larger stimulus set from Exp. 1.

GENERAL DISCUSSION

The SSD-CI participants tested in the present study represent a unique patient population with which to explore perception of harmonic intervals. Pleasantness ratings with the NH ear provided an estimate of participants' abilities to perceive relative dissonance; ratings were similar to those for NH listeners in previous studies (e.g., McDermott et al., 2010; Cousineau et al., 2012). Via DAI, ratings were also obtained with CI-only listening. With combined acoustic and electric hearing, the relative contributions of the NH and CI ears could be observed. Thus, the data set with SSD-CI listeners provides direct comparison of pleasantness rating for very different peripheral representations within the same participant. The generally low CI-only ratings are consistent with previous studies that show difficulties in CI users' perception of polyphonic music (e.g., Donnelly et al., 2009; Galvin et al., 2009b, 2012; Penninger et al., 2013, 2014; Crew et al., 2015; Chari et al., 2019). The present pattern of results with CI-only listening is also generally consistent with Knobloch et al. (2018), who found that adult post-lingually deaf CI users rated major chords as sounding more pleasant than minor augmented, suspended, and diminished chords. Similar to previous studies with bimodal CI listeners (e.g., Crew et al., 2015, 2016), the NH ear appeared to drive binaural quality ratings, with the CI ear contributing little to binaural ratings.

Despite the large difference in absolute ratings between NH-only and CI-only listening (**Figure 1**), perception of relative dissonance was largely similar between acoustic and electric hearing (**Figures 1–3**). This suggests that while CI-only ratings were generally poor, some intervals consistently sounded less pleasant than others. This finding was not fully in agreement with our hypothesis that CI-only ratings would be poor, with little relation to the pattern of ratings with NH-only listening. The CI-only data suggest that participants were mostly sensitive to dissonance (roughness, perceived for minor 2nd, major 7th, and minor 9th), with some sensitivity to consonance ("harmonicity," perceived for the octave); for the remaining intervals, pleasantness ratings were largely similar. The transitions in ratings from minor 2nd to major 3rd and from major 6th to major 7th were generally similar between acoustic and electric hearing (at least for the F3 root note). Ratings were highly correlated across root notes and interval spans (**Supplementary Appendix 4**), suggesting that the spectral pattern did not contribute strongly to relative dissonance ratings. The electrodograms in **Figure 5** also do not indicate any useful distinctions that might underlie ratings. Given that differences in spectral patterns did not seem to contribute to CI-only ratings, it is likely that temporal envelope cues were responsible for the relative dissonance ratings in Exp. 1. Note that 3 of the 10 participants who were able to replicate Exp. 1 ratings in Exp. 2 with NH-only listening were unable to do so with CI-only listening. As discussed previously, these participants were all MED-EL users, and interactions between the root notes tested and the FS4-p processing may have contributed to the pattern of results. If so, this would suggest that it is important to accurately preserve temporal envelope cues across all channels to perceive dissonance with electric hearing.

Interestingly, the present CI-only data suggest that while stimuli sounded generally inharmonic (due to poor spectral resolution), relative pleasantness ratings hewed close to NH-only ratings. This suggests that beating, rather than perception of inharmonicity played a stronger role in relative ratings with CI-only listening. The similarity between the NH-only and CI-only data further suggest that temporal information (e.g., beating) may play a strong role in dissonance perception, and that the degree of underlying harmonicity may not affect contrasts between consonant and dissonant intervals. This is not to say that harmonicity is not important when rating the pleasantness of a sound. Clearly, CI-only ratings were generally poor, and were lower than the least-pleasant NH-only ratings (**Figure 1**). However, when data were compared across listening modes (**Figure 3**) the pattern of ratings was quite similar, despite the large differences in spectral resolution across ears.

Several studies have shown that CI users are susceptible to temporal modulation interference, even when temporal envelope information is spatially distant (e.g., Chatterjee, 2003; Kreft et al., 2013; Chatterjee and Kulkarni, 2018). In such modulation detection interference (MDI) studies, CI users were asked to detect an amplitude-modulated (AM) probe stimulus in the presence of masking AM stimuli with similar or different AM rates as the probe; the electrode positions of the masker and probe stimuli were varied to be spatially proximate (which would produce the most energetic masking and perhaps the greatest interference) or spatially remote (which would produce less energetic masking and perhaps less interference). After accounting for energetic masking, significant amounts of "modulation masking" were observed even when electrodes were spatially remote. Modulation masking may have been due to the broad current spread associated with electric stimulation and/or to more central processing of temporal envelope information (e.g., Dau et al., 1997). In MDI studies, masker and probe AM rates are typically selected to avoid low-frequency beating and/or harmonically related AM rates.

In the present study, the harmonic intervals would be expected to produce different degrees of beating and harmonically related temporally envelope information. These musical intervals are used to compose Western music and are therefore commonly experienced. Different from MDI studies that suggest that modulation masking may limit perception of important temporal envelope cues, the present data suggest that CI users may use temporal envelope interaction cues to make qualitative judgments about a stimulus in ways that are similar to acoustic hearing. While the underlying mechanisms may be similar between MDI and harmonic interval perception, the listening task may give rise to different percepts (detection of a masked AM stimulus versus rating the pleasantness of combined temporal envelope information). Although the across-octave intervals in the present study did not offer the same degree of electrode separation as in some MDI CI studies, pleasantness ratings were very similar for within- and across-octave intervals. It is unclear whether this was due to the broad current spread associated with electric stimulation or to central processing of temporal envelope cues. As shown in **Figure 5**, the temporal envelope information associated with dissonant intervals (due to beating) was largely preserved by CI signal processing. One advantage in CI research is the ability to separate temporal (AM, stimulation rate) and spectral cues (electrode location), which has been exploited in

MDI studies. In future CI research, it would be worthwhile to study how dissonance ratings are affected by both temporal envelope interactions and electrode interactions. Finally, the generally low CI ratings may be due in part to temporal envelope interactions across all electrodes. The MDI data from previous studies suggest strong temporal envelope interactions even when electrodes are spatially separated. For the present harmonic intervals, such widespread temporal envelope interactions may reduce overall sound quality.

Contrary to our hypothesis, we did not find significant binaural enhancement for interval ratings for the present SSD-CI listeners. This finding is also not consistent with MUSHRA ratings from SSD-CI listeners in Landsberger et al. (2019) or from SSD-CI questionnaire data that suggest better overall sound quality for binaural listening after cochlear implantation (e.g., Távora-Vieira et al., 2013; Friedmann et al., 2016; Dillon et al., 2017b; Galvin et al., 2018). The short stimulus duration and other methodological factors may have limited binaural enhancement in the present study. Longer musical excerpts (as used in Landsberger et al., 2019) may be necessary to perceive a qualitative binaural advantage over NH-only listening. Similarly, longer-term experience with binaural listening (along with SSD-CI patients' anecdotal reports) may give rise to a stronger sense of binaural enhancement. It is worth noting that in many of these SSD-CI studies, there are typically small benefits for binaural speech understanding when speech and noise are co-located, despite subjective data that suggest strong binaural enhancement. Indeed, SSD-CI users are often surprised by the poor sound quality and intelligibility with CI-only compared to NH + CI listening. The NH ear seems to capture the quality of binaural listening somehow, despite the likely asymmetry in quality across ears. As such, the source of binaural enhancement is unclear. It may be that some gross binaural restoration improves sound quality over monaural, NH-only listening. However, these potentially strong top-down effects may not provide useful information toward improving CI sound quality, which is important to improve binaural sound quality. The present harmonic interval perception data may provide insights into the limited contribution of the CI to combined acoustic-electric sound quality. Ideally, both absolute and relative dissonance patterns observed with the NH ear should be preserved with the CI ear. Understanding the limits of the CI ear may guide future CI signal processing and technology to improve CI quality for music perception, thereby improving binaural enhancement for SSD-CI (and possibly, bimodal and bilateral CI) patients.

Note that only pleasantness ratings were measured in the present study. It is unclear how discriminable these intervals were, especially with the CI ear alone. The relationship between interval discrimination and pleasantness is unclear. With the NH ear alone, it is likely that all intervals would be reliably discriminated, but some intervals would have been similarly rated (e.g., major 3rd, 5th, major 10th, 12th). With the CI ear alone, it is unclear how discriminable some intervals were. For example, the dip in ratings for the tritone with the NH ear alone was not observed with the CI ear alone. It is possible that CI users may not have been able to discriminate among the 4th, tritone, and 5th. However, they are likely to have been able to discriminate between a minor 2nd and a minor 9th on the basis of the spectral patterns; yet these stimuli were rated similarly unpleasant for the F3 root note. In future studies, it may be useful to measure discrimination as well as similarity ratings (using multi-dimensional scaling) for harmonic intervals with acoustic and electric hearing.

Testing with SSD-CI users allowed us to verify whether the pattern of dissonance ratings observed with CI-only listening was related to the pattern with the NH ear (which was presumably and decidedly similar to that of NH listeners in general). The strong correlations between the NH-only and CI-only ratings, as well as the replication of ratings in Exp. 2 further support the relationship between acoustic and electric hearing for relative dissonance ratings for harmonic intervals. However, it is important to note that SSD-CI users most likely do not rely on their implant in the same way as bilaterally deaf CI users, which may influence their perception of sound through the device and in this case, the dissonance of harmonic intervals. Therefore, while using the SSD-CI population allowed for assurance of task understanding, especially in a group with very little formal musical training, it may be difficult to generalize these results to bilaterally or asymmetrically deaf CI users. In particular, considering that very few participants showed correlations between ratings in the NH-only and CI-only conditions, it may not be expected that each individual has access to the perception of dissonance through the CI.

The present study sheds new light on CI users' difficulty with consonance perception for harmonic intervals. Many previous studies have shown that CI users have great difficulty with melodic interval perception (e.g., Gfeller and Lansing, 1991; Gfeller et al., 2002, 2007; Galvin et al., 2007, 2009a; Looi et al., 2008; Nimmons et al., 2008). Distortions to interval size (due to frequency allocation, the limited number of electrodes, and the electrode-neural interface) result in distortions to melody. While factors that underlie poor melodic interval perception may have contributed to the overall poor ratings in harmonic interval perception, the present results suggest that some aspects of harmonic interval perception observed with acoustic hearing were preserved with electric hearing. Note that the present methodology was restricted to acute pleasantness ratings for isolated "vertical" intervals. In ongoing polyphonic music, there are horizontal and vertical dimensions that can be analyzed independently and synthesized together. Although CI users may be able to analyze some aspects of harmony, they have difficulty synthesizing harmony and melody. In Knobloch et al. (2018), CI users' chord preferences were generally similar to those of NH listeners. Unlike NH listeners, CI users were unable to perceive "authentic cadences" at the end of a musical excerpt, indicating difficulties in perceiving harmonic "syntax." Thus, relative dissonance perception was not helpful in perceiving the resolution of a polyphonic melody. Given the limits of current CI technology, it may not be possible to achieve the necessary spectral resolution to support good polyphonic music perception. Optimizing combined acoustic and electric hearing (e.g., reducing interaural frequency mismatch, reducing CI channel interaction, etc.) may be the most promising approach toward improving music perception in CI users.

CONCLUSION

In the present study, pleasantness ratings for harmonic intervals were measured in adult, unilaterally deaf CI users while listening with the CI ear alone, the NH ear alone, and with both ears (NH + CI). The root note and interval span (within- or across-octave) were varied to accommodate differences across participants in terms of the acoustic-to-electric frequency allocation and electrode-neural interface. Findings include:

1. Overall ratings were much poorer with the CI than with NH. There was no significant binaural enhancement with NH + CI over NH-only listening.
2. Despite the large asymmetry in overall ratings across ears, significant correlations were observed between NH-only and CI-only ratings, suggesting that relative dissonance was similar between acoustic and electric hearing.
3. All but one of the SSD-CI participants were able to replicate relatively low and high ratings with NH-only listening with a smaller, high-contrast stimulus set. Only some participants were able to replicate ratings with CI-only listening.
4. There was no significant effect of root note or interval span on ratings for any of the listening conditions, suggesting that spectral cues did not contribute strongly to CI-only interval ratings. More likely, temporal envelope interactions (beating, roughness) contributed to relative dissonance perception with electric hearing.

ETHICS STATEMENT

All participants were paid for their participation and provided written informed consent in accordance with the study protocols reviewed and approved by Institutional Review Board at New York University (IRB #S14-00809 and #S14-00435).

AUTHOR CONTRIBUTIONS

ES, DL, and JG contributed to the study design, creation of stimuli, statistical analyses, and writing of the manuscript. ES contributed to the participant recruitment and data collection. DL wrote the software used to run the experiments and collect the data. DF contributed to the study design and writing of the manuscript. All authors read and approved the final submitted version.

ACKNOWLEDGMENTS

We are grateful to the SSD CI users for participating in this study.

REFERENCES

Arndt, S., Laszig, R., Aschendorff, A., Hassepass, F., Beck, R., and Wesarg, T. (2017). Cochlear implant treatment of patients with single-sided deafness or asymmetric hearing loss. *HNO* 65, 98–108. doi: 10.1007/s00106-016-0297-295

Bidelman, G. M., and Krishnan, A. (2009). Neural correlates of consonance, dissonance, and the hierarchy of musical pitch in the human brainstem. *J. Neurosci.* 29, 13165–13171. doi: 10.1523/JNEUROSCI.3900-09.2009

Brockmeier, S. J., Fitzgerald, D., Searle, O., Fitzgerald, H., Grasmeder, M., Hilbig, S., et al. (2011). The MuSIC perception test: a novel battery for testing music perception of cochlear implant users. *Cochlear Implants Int.* 12, 10–20. doi: 10.1179/146701010X12677899497236

Caldwell, M. T., Jiradejvong, P., and Limb, C. J. (2016). Impaired perception of sensory consonance and dissonance in cochlear implant users. *Otol. Neurotol.* 37, 229–234. doi: 10.1097/MAO.0000000000000960

Causon, A., Verschuur, C., and Newman, T. A. (2015). A retrospective analysis of the contribution of reported factors in cochlear implantation on hearing preservation outcomes. *Otol. Neurotol.* 36, 1137–1145. doi: 10.1097/MAO.0000000000000753

Chari, D. A., Jiradejvong, P., and Limb, C. J. (2019). Tripolar stimulation improves polyphonic pitch detection in cochlear implant users. *Otol. Neurotol.* 40, 38–46. doi: 10.1097/MAO.0000000000002061

Chatterjee, M. (2003). Modulation masking in cochlear implant listeners: envelope versus tonotopic components. *J. Acoust. Soc. Am.* 113, 2042–2053. doi: 10.1121/1.1555613

Chatterjee, M., and Kulkarni, A. M. (2018). Modulation detection interference in cochlear implant listeners under forward masking conditions. *J. Acoust. Soc. Am.* 143, 1117–1127. doi: 10.1121/1.5025059

Cheng, X., Liu, Y., Wang, B., Yuan, Y., Galvin, J. J. III, Fu, Q.-J., et al. (2018). The benefits of residual hair cell function for speech and music perception in pediatric bimodal cochlear implant listeners. *Neural Plast.* 2018, 1–10. doi: 10.1155/2018/4610592

Cousineau, M., Demany, L., Meyer, B., and Pressnitzer, D. (2010). What breaks a melody: perceiving F0 and intensity sequences with a cochlear implant. *Hear. Res.* 269, 34–41. doi: 10.1016/j.heares.2010.07.007

Cousineau, M., McDermott, J. H., and Peretz, I. (2012). The basis of musical consonance as revealed by congenital amusia. *Proc. Natl. Acad. Sci. U.S.A.* 109, 19858–19863. doi: 10.1073/pnas.1207989109

Crew, J. D., Galvin, J. J. III, and Fu, Q.-J. (2016). Perception of sung speech in bimodal cochlear implant users. *Trends Hear.* 20:2331216516669329. doi: 10.1177/2331216516669329

Crew, J. D., Galvin, J. J. III, Landsberger, D. M., and Fu, Q.-J. (2015). Contributions of electric and acoustic hearing to bimodal speech and music perception. *PLoS One* 20:e0120279. doi: 10.1371/journal.pone.0120279

Cullington, H. E., and Zeng, F.-G. (2011). Comparison of bimodal and bilateral cochlear implant users on speech recognition with competing talker, music perception, affective prosody discrimination, and talker identification. *Ear Hear.* 1, 16–30. doi: 10.1097/AUD.0b013e3181edfbd2

Dau, T., Kollmeier, B., and Kohlrausch, A. (1997). Modeling auditory processing of amplitude modulation. I. Detection and masking with narrow-band carriers. *J. Acoust. Soc. Am.* 102, 2892–2905. doi: 10.1121/1.420344

Deutsch, D. (2007). Music perception. *Front. Biosci.* 12:4473–4482. doi: 10.2741/2402

Dillon, M. T., Buss, E., Anderson, M. L., King, E. R., Deres, E. J., Buchman, C. A., et al. (2017a). Cochlear implantation in cases of unilateral hearing loss: initial localization abilities. *Ear Hear.* 38, 611–619. doi: 10.1097/AUD.0000000000000430

Dillon, M. T., Buss, E., Rooth, M. A., King, E. R., Deres, E. J., Buchman, C. A., et al. (2017b). Effect of cochlear implantation on quality of life in adults with unilateral hearing loss. *Audiol. Neurootol.* 22, 259–271. doi: 10.1159/000484079

Donnelly, P. J., Guo, B. Z., and Limb, C. J. (2009). Perceptual fusion of polyphonic pitch in cochlear implant users. *J. Acoust. Soc. Am.* 126, 128–133. doi: 10.1121/1.3239464

Dorman, M. F., Gifford, R. H., Spahr, A. J., and McKarns, S. A. (2008). The benefits of combining acoustic and electric stimulation for the recognition of speech, voice and melodies. *Audiol. Neurotol.* 13, 105–112. doi: 10.1159/000111782

Dorman, M. F., Natale, S. C., Butts, A. M., Zeitler, D. M., and Carlson, M. L. (2017). The sound quality of cochlear implants: studies with single-sided deaf patients. *Otol. Neurotol.* 38, 268–273. doi: 10.1097/MAO.0000000000001449

Dowling, W. J., and Harwood, J. L. (1986). *Music Cognition*, 1st Edn. Orlando, FL: Academic Press.

Firszt, J. B., Holden, L. K., Reeder, R. M., Waltzman, S. B., and Arndt, S. (2012). Auditory abilities after cochlear implantation in adults with unilateral deafness: a pilot study. *Otol. Neurotol.* 33, 1339–1346. doi: 10.1097/MAO.0b013e318268d52d

Friedmann, D. R., Ahmed, O. H., McMenomey, S. O., Shapiro, W. H., Waltzman, S. B., and Roland, J. T. (2016). Single-sided deafness cochlear implantation: candidacy, evaluation, and outcomes in children and adults. *Otol. Neurotol.* 37, 154–160. doi: 10.1097/MAO.0000000000000951

Fritz, T., Jentschke, S., Gosselin, N., Sammler, D., Peretz, I., Turner, R., et al. (2009). Universal recognition of three basic emotions in music. *Curr. Biol.* 19, 573–576. doi: 10.1016/j.cub.2009.02.058

Galvin, J. J. III, Eskridge, E., Oba, S., and Fu, Q.-J. (2012). Melodic contour identification training in cochlear implant users with and without a competing instrument. *Semin. Hear.* 33, 399–409. doi: 10.1055/s-0032-1329227

Galvin, J. J. III, Fu, Q.-J., and Oba, S. I. (2009b). Effect of a competing instrument on melodic contour identification by cochlear implant users. *J. Acoust. Soc. Am.* 125, 98–103. doi: 10.1121/1.3062148

Galvin, J. J. III, Fu, Q.-J., and Shannon, R. V. (2009a). Melodic contour identification and music perception by cochlear implant users. *Ann. N. Y. Acad. Sci.* 1169, 518–533. doi: 10.1111/j.1749-6632.2009.04551.x

Galvin, J. J. III, Fu, Q.-J., Wilkinson, E. P., Mills, D., Hagan, S. C., Lupo, J. E., et al. (2018). Benefits of cochlear implantation for single-sided deafness: data from the House Clinic-University of Southern California-University of California, Los Angeles clinical trial. *Ear Hear.* 40, 766–781. doi: 10.1097/AUD.0000000000000671

Galvin, J. J. III, Fu, Q.-J., and Nogaki, G. (2007). Melodic contour identification by cochlear implant listeners. *Ear Hear.* 28, 302–319. doi: 10.1097/01.aud.0000261689.35445.20

Gfeller, K., and Lansing, C. R. (1991). Melodic, rhythmic, and timbral perception of adult cochlear implant users. *J. Speech. Hear. Res.* 34, 916–920. doi: 10.1044/jshr.3404.916

Gfeller, K., Turner, C., Mehr, M., Woodworth, G., Fearn, R., Knutson, J. F., et al. (2002). Recognition of familiar melodies by adult cochlear implant recipients and normal-hearing adults. *Cochlear Implants Int.* 3, 29–53. doi: 10.1179/cim.2002.3.1.29

Gfeller, K., Turner, C., Oleson, J., Zhang, X., Gantz, B., Froman, R., et al. (2007). Accuracy of cochlear implant recipients on pitch perception, melody recognition, and speech reception in noise. *Ear Hear.* 28, 412–423. doi: 10.1097/AUD.0b013e3180479318

Goupell, M. J., Cosentino, S., Stakhovskaya, O. A., and Bernstein, J. G. W. (2019). Interaural pitch-discrimination range effects for bilateral and single-sided-deafness cochlear-implant users. *J. Assoc. Res. Otolaryngol.* 20, 187–203. doi: 10.1007/s10162-018-00707-x

Kameoka, A., and Kuriyagawa, M. (1969). Consonance theory part I: consonance of dyads. *J. Acoust. Soc. Am.* 45, 1451–1459. doi: 10.1121/1.1911623

Kang, R., Nimmons, G. L., Drennan, W., Longnion, J., Ruffin, C., Nie, K., et al. (2009). Development and validation of the University of Washington clinical assessment of music perception test. *Ear Hear.* 30, 411–418. doi: 10.1097/AUD.0b013e3181a61bc0

Knobloch, M., Verhey, J. L., Ziese, M., Nitschmann, M., Arens, C., and Böckmann-Barthel, M. (2018). Musical harmony in electric hearing. *Music Percept.* 36, 40–52. doi: 10.1525/mp.2018.36.1.40

Kong, Y. Y., Cruz, R., Jones, J. A., and Zeng, F.-G. (2004). Music perception with temporal cues in acoustic and electric hearing. *Ear Hear.* 25, 173–185. doi: 10.1097/01.AUD.0000120365.97792.2F

Kong, Y. Y., Stickney, G. S., and Zeng, F.-G. (2005). Speech and melody recognition in binaurally combined acoustic and electric hearing. *J. Acoust. Soc. Am.* 117, 1351–1361. doi: 10.1121/1.1857526

Kreft, H. A., Nelson, D. A., and Oxenham, A. J. (2013). Modulation frequency discrimination with modulated and unmodulated interference in normal hearing and in cochlear-implant users. *J. Assoc. Res. Otolaryngol.* 14, 591–601. doi: 10.1007/s10162-013-0391-392

Landsberger, D. M., Svrakic, M., Roland, J. T., and Svirsky, M. (2015). The relationship between insertion angles, default frequency allocations, and spiral ganglion place pitch in cochlear implants. *Ear Hear.* 36, e207–e213. doi: 10.1097/AUD.0000000000000163

Landsberger, D. M., Vermeire, K., Stupak, N., Lavender, A., Neukam, J., Van de Heyning, P., et al. (2019). Music is more enjoyable with two ears, even if the second one receives a degraded signal provided by a cochlear implant. *Ear Hear.* [Preprint].

Limb, C. J., and Roy, A. T. (2014). Technological, biological, and acoustical constraints to music perception in cochlear implant users. *Hear. Res.* 308, 13–26. doi: 10.1016/j.heares.2013.04.009

Looi, V., McDermott, H., McKay, C., and Hickson, L. (2008). Music perception of cochlear implant users compared with that of hearing aid users. *Ear Hear.* 29, 421–434. doi: 10.1097/AUD.0b013e31816a0d0b

Lu, T., Huang, J., and Zeng, F.-G. (2014). Accurate guitar tuning by cochlear implant musicians. *PLoS One* 9:e92454. doi: 10.1371/journal.pone.0092454

McDermott, J. H. (2004). Music perception with cochlear implants: a review. *Trends Amplif.* 8, 49–82. doi: 10.1177/108471380400800203

McDermott, J. H., Lehr, A. J., and Oxenham, A. J. (2010). Individual differences reveal the basis of consonance. *Curr. Biol.* 20, 1035–1041. doi: 10.1016/j.cub.2010.04.019

McDermott, J. H., Schultz, A. F., Undurraga, E. A., and Godoy, R. A. (2016). Indifference to dissonance in native Amazonians reveals cultural variation in music perception. *Nature* 535, 547–550. doi: 10.1038/nature18635

Mertens, G., Kleine Punte, A., De Bodt, M., and Van de Heyning, P. (2015). Binaural auditory outcomes in patients with postlingual profound unilateral hearing loss: 3 years after cochlear implantation. *Audiol. Neurootol.* 20(Suppl. 1), 67–72. doi: 10.1159/000380751

Nimmons, G. L., Kang, R. S., Drennan, W. R., Longnion, J., Ruffin, C., Worman, T., et al. (2008). Clinical assessment of music perception in cochlear implant listeners. *Otol. Neurotol.* 29, 149–155. doi: 10.1097/mao.0b013e31812f7244

Patel, A. D. (2003). Language, music, syntax and the brain. *Nat. Neurosci.* 6, 674–681. doi: 10.1038/nn1082

Penninger, R. T., Kludt, E., Limb, C. J., Leman, M., Dhooge, I., and Buechner, A. (2014). Perception of polyphony with cochlear implants for 2 and 3 simultaneous pitches. *Otol. Neurotol.* 35, 431–436. doi: 10.1097/MAO.0000000000000255

Penninger, R. T., Limb, C. J., Vermeire, K., Leman, M., and Dhooge, I. (2013). Experimental assessment of polyphonic tones with cochlear implants. *Otol. Neurotol.* 34, 1267–1271. doi: 10.1097/MAO.0b013e3182923f04

Plomp, R., and Levelt, W. J. (1965). Tonal consonance and critical bandwidth. *J. Acoust. Soc. Am.* 38, 548–560. doi: 10.1121/1.1909741

Santa Maria, P. L., Gluth, M. B., Yuan, Y., Atlas, M. D., and Blevins, N. H. (2014). Hearing preservation surgery for cochlear implantation: a meta-analysis. *Otol. Neurotol.* 35, 256–269. doi: 10.1097/MAO.0000000000000561

Shannon, R. V., Fu, Q.-J., and Galvin, J. J. III (2004). The number of spectral channels required for speech recognition depends on the difficulty of the listening situation. *Acta Otolaryngol. Suppl.* 552, 50–54. doi: 10.1080/03655230410017562

Sierra, C., Calderón, M., Bárcena, E., Tisaire, A., and Raboso, E. (2019). Preservation of residual hearing after cochlear implant surgery with deep insertion electrode arrays. *Otol. Neurotol.* 40, 373–380. doi: 10.1097/MAO.0000000000002170

Smith, Z. M., Delgutte, B., and Oxenham, A. J. (2002). Chimaeric sounds reveal dichotomies in auditory perception. *Nature* 416, 87–90. doi: 10.1038/416087a

Sucher, C. M., and McDermott, H. J. (2009). Bimodal stimulation: benefits for music perception and sound quality. *Cochlear Implants Int.* 10, 96–99. doi: 10.1179/cim.2009.10.Supplement-1.96

Távora-Vieira, D., Marino, R., Krishnaswamy, J., Kuthbutheen, J., and Rajan, G. P. (2013). Cochlear implantation for unilateral deafness with and without tinnitus: a case series. *Laryngoscope* 123, 1251–1255. doi: 10.1002/lary.23764

Todd, A. E., Mertens, G., Van de Heyning, P., and Landsberger, D. M. (2017). Encoding a melody using only temporal information for cochlear-implant and normal-hearing listeners. *Trends Hear.* 21:2331216517739745. doi: 10.1177/2331216517739745

Tramo, M. J., Cariani, P. A., Delgutte, B., and Braida, L. D. (2001). Neurobiological foundations for the theory of harmony in western tonal music. *Ann. N.Y. Acad. Sci.* 930, 92–116. doi: 10.1111/j.1749-6632.2001.tb05727.x

Van de Heyning, P., Vermeire, K., Deibl, M., Nopp, P., Anderson, I., and De Ridder, D. (2008). Incapacitating unilateral tinnitus in single-sided deafness treated by cochlear implantation. *Ann. Otol. Rhinol. Laryngol.* 117, 645–652. doi: 10.1177/000348940811700903

Vermeire, K., Landsberger, D. M., Schleich, P., and Van de Heyning, P. H. (2013). Multidimensional scaling between acoustic and contralateral electric stimuli predicts speech understanding in CI users with contralateral hearing. *Hear. Res.* 306, 29–36. doi: 10.1016/j.hearres.2013.09.004

Vermeire, K., Landsberger, D. M., Van de Heyning, P. H., Voormolen, M., Kleine Punte, A., Schatzer, R., et al. (2015). Frequency-place map for electrical stimulation in cochlear implants: change over time. *Hear. Res.* 326, 8–14. doi: 10.1016/j.heares.2015.03.011

Vermeire, K., Nobbe, A., Schleich, P., Nopp, P., and Van de Heyning, P. H. (2008). Neural tonotopy in cochlear implants: an evaluation in unilateral cochlear implant patients with unilateral deafness and tinnitus. *Hear. Res.* 245, 98–106. doi: 10.1016/j.hearres.2008.09.003

Vermeire, K., and Van de Heyning, P. H. (2009). Binaural hearing after cochlear implantation in subjects with unilateral sensorineural deafness and tinnitus. *Audiol. Neurootol.* 14, 163–171. doi: 10.1159/000171478

Vongpaisal, T., Trehub, S. E., and Schellenberg, E. G. (2006). Song recognition by children and adolescents with cochlear implants. *J. Speech Lang. Hear. Res.* 49, 1091–1103. doi: 10.1044/1092-4388(2006/078)

Wanna, G. B., Noble, J. H., Gifford, R. H., Dietrich, M. S., Sweeney, A. D., Zhang, D., et al. (2015). Impact of intrascalar electrode location, electrode type, and angular insertion depth on residual hearing in cochlear implant patients: preliminary results. *Otol. Neurotol.* 36, 1343–1348. doi: 10.1097/MAO.0000000000000829

Yoon, Y., Li, Y., Kang, H.-Y., and Fu, Q.-J. (2011). The relationship between binaural benefit and difference in unilateral speech recognition performance for bilateral cochlear implant users. *Int. J. Audiol.* 50, 554–565. doi: 10.3109/14992027.2011.580785

Yoon, Y. S., Shin, Y.-R., Gho, J.-S., and Fu, Q.-J. (2015). Bimodal benefit depends on the performance difference between a cochlear implant and a hearing aid. *Cochlear Implants Int.* 16, 159–167. doi: 10.1179/1754762814Y.0000000101

11

Musical Sound Quality as a Function of the Number of Channels in Modern Cochlear Implant Recipients

Katelyn Berg[1], Jack Noble[1,2,3], Benoit Dawant[2,3], Robert Dwyer[1], Robert Labadie[2,3], Virginia Richards[4] and René Gifford[1,3]*

[1] Department of Hearing and Speech Sciences, Vanderbilt University Medical Center, Nashville, TN, United States, [2] Department of Electrical Engineering and Computer Science, Vanderbilt University, Nashville, TN, United States, [3] Department of Otolaryngology, Vanderbilt University Medical Center, Nashville, TN, United States, [4] Department of Cognitive Science, University of California, Irvine, Irvine, CA, United States

***Correspondence:**
René Gifford
rene.gifford@Vanderbilt.edu

Objectives: This study examined musical sound quality (SQ) in adult cochlear implant (CI) recipients. The study goals were to determine: the number of channels needed for high levels of musical SQ overall and by musical genre; the impact of device and patient factors on musical SQ ratings; and the relationship between musical SQ, speech recognition, and speech SQ to relate these findings to measures frequently used in clinical protocols.

Methods: Twenty-one post-lingually deafened adult CI recipients participated in this study. Electrode placement, including scalar location, average electrode-to-modiolus distance ($\overline{M}$), and angular insertion depth were determined by CT imaging using validated CI position analysis algorithms (e.g., Noble et al., 2013; Zhao et al., 2018, 2019). CI programs were created using 4–22 electrodes with equal spatial distribution of active electrodes across the array. Speech recognition, speech SQ, music perception via a frequency discrimination task, and musical SQ were acutely assessed for all electrode conditions. Musical SQ was assessed using pre-selected musical excerpts from a variety of musical genres.

Results: CI recipients demonstrated continuous improvement in qualitative judgments of musical SQ with up to 10 active electrodes. Participants with straight electrodes placed in scala tympani (ST) and pre-curved electrodes with higher $\overline{M}$ variance reported higher levels of musical SQ; however, this relationship is believed to be driven by levels of musical experience as well as the potential for preoperative bias in device selection. Participants reported significant increases in musical SQ beyond four channels for all musical genres examined in the current study except for Hip Hop/Rap. After musical experience outliers were removed, there was no relationship between musical experience or frequency discrimination ability and musical SQ ratings. There was a weak, but significant correlation between qualitative ratings for speech stimuli presented in quiet and in noise and musical SQ.

Conclusion: Modern CI recipients may need more channels for musical SQ than even required for asymptotic speech recognition or speech SQ. These findings may be used to provide clinical guidance for personalized expectations management of music appreciation depending on individual device and patient factors.

Keywords: cochlear implant, music, sound quality, channels, electrode placement

INTRODUCTION

The cochlear implant (CI) is the most successful sensory prosthetic device to date, yielding significant improvements in speech understanding (e.g., Holden et al., 2013) and quality of life (e.g., McRackan et al., 2017) for the majority of recipients. Despite its success for restoration of auditory detection and speech recognition, music perception and appreciation remain major challenges for most CI recipients, due to a number of factors including poor pitch and timbre perception as well as reduced spectral resolution (e.g., Kang et al., 2009; Jung et al., 2012) as well as potential for poor auditory neural health. Focusing on the latter, the classic literature concluded that CI recipients have limited access to spectral cues due to channel interaction (spread of electrical excitation). A discrete number of 5–10 independent channels may be available to these recipients for various speech and auditory measures, despite having up to 12–22 intracochlear electrodes (Fishman et al., 1997; Friesen et al., 2001, 2005). These previous studies were completed using older-generation speech coding strategies with patients implanted using more traumatic surgical approaches, unknown electrode placement, and stricter candidacy criteria. Patients in these earlier studies also had less residual hearing, poorer speech understanding, and longer durations of deafness compared to modern CI recipients (e.g., Holder et al., 2018b). Several factors limit the precision of intracochlear electrical stimulation and negatively affect spectral resolution, including: (1) channel interaction, which has been shown to span one-third or more of the array (e.g., Hughes et al., 2013; Padilla and Landsberger, 2016); (2) the amount of viable spiral ganglion cells along the length of the cochlear duct, which is currently unable to be quantified; and (3) electrode placement within the cochlea, which is unknown for the majority of patients due to a lack of postoperative imaging. Electrode placement is especially critical as multiple studies have documented that the electrode–neural interface is rarely uniform along the array with distances ranging from 0 to 2 mm from the closest modiolar location (Davis et al., 2016) and 13% of implanted devices have extracochlear electrodes not referenced in the operative report (Holder et al., 2018a).

More recent studies have re-examined speech recognition and spectral resolution abilities for CI recipients implanted under current expanded criteria, using atraumatic electrode design and surgical approaches as well as speech coding strategies used in today's clinic. These latest reports suggest that modern-day CI recipients with pre-curved electrode arrays may have greater channel independence than previous generation recipients. Croghan et al. (2017) investigated channel independence for newer generation adult CI recipients with Nucleus devices. For sentence recognition at various signal-to-noise ratios (SNRs), they reported better performance using 22 active electrodes with 8 maxima versus 12 active electrodes with 8 maxima. However, they kept the number of maxima constant in an n-of-m strategy irrespective of the number of active electrodes. Another limitation of the Croghan et al.'s (2017) study was the lack of image-based confirmation of electrode location for the nine pre-curved electrode recipients: an electrode documented to result in translocation (ST–SV) in up to 42% of cases (Wanna et al., 2014). Berg et al. (2019) investigated channel independence for a group of 11 adult recipients with Nucleus pre-curved arrays, verified by postoperative imaging to be completely in the scala tympani (ST). They reported significant increases in speech recognition in noise with increasing channels up to 22 channels with 16 maxima (16-of-22), compared to continuous interleaved sampling (CIS) maps with 4–10 channels; considering CIS alone, 16-channel CIS provided significantly higher speech recognition in quiet than even 10-channel CIS. Berg et al. (2019) also reported significantly higher speech recognition in quiet and noise with 16 maxima (16-of-22) compared to 8 maxima (8-of-22) – an effect significantly correlated with mean electrode-to-modiolus distance along the implanted array. Because lower electrode-to-modiolus distances – associated with well-placed pre-curved electrodes that evenly hug the modiolar wall – require less charge for upper stimulation levels (e.g., Davis et al., 2016), CI recipients with pre-curved electrodes in ST may experience less channel interaction (e.g., Chatterjee and Shannon, 1998), affording better spectral resolution. Given recent evidence for greater channel independence for adult CI recipients in the speech domain, the current study wanted to investigate the effect of channels and channel independence on the largely unexplored music domain.

Poor spectral resolution has also contributed to poor pitch discrimination, as well as melody and timbre identification for CI recipients (e.g., McDermott, 2004; Moore and Carlyon, 2005; Drennan and Rubinstein, 2008; Won et al., 2010). Nimmons et al. (2008) found that nearly all of their participants had F0 discrimination ability between 1 and 6 semitones, but varied significantly more with complex-tone pitch discrimination, ranging from less than 1 semitone up to 12 semitones. However, few studies have focused on assessing musical SQ with CIs, even though CI recipients report significant musical SQ impairments following implantation, and musical SQ is rated as the most significant factor responsible for music listening enjoyment (Lassaletta et al., 2008a,b; Roy et al., 2012). This is problematic because no clear relationship exists between music perceptual accuracy and the perceived SQ of music (Gfeller et al., 2008; Looi et al., 2011). While music perception or musical SQ are rarely assessed in the Audiology clinic, speech recognition and speech SQ are addressed through regular evaluations and programming adjustments. It is unknown if a relationship exists between speech recognition performance and SQ, and musical SQ; and if speech measures can suffice for addressing musical SQ impairments.

The purpose of this study was to assess musical SQ in adult CI recipients implanted under expanded criteria and current technology to determine: (a) the number of channels needed to achieve the highest level of overall musical SQ; (b) the impact of device factors, such as electrode type, electrode scalar location, mean electrode-to-modiolus distance, variance in electrode-to-modiolus distance, insertion depth of the electrode array, surgeon, and implant manufacturer on these ratings; (c) the impact of musical genre on the number of channels needed to achieve asymptotic ratings of musical SQ; (d) the impact of patient factors, such as musical experience, music perception abilities via a frequency discrimination task, duration of CI use (since activation), and pre-operative hearing thresholds; and (e) the relationship between musical SQ, speech recognition, and speech SQ to understand how these findings relate to measures frequently used in clinical protocols.

Given that music is spectrally complex, we hypothesized that lower electrode-to-modiolus distance would lead to increased ratings of musical SQ due to less channel interaction. While older studies were limited by the existing technology, modern advances in electrode design, surgical technique, candidacy criteria, and imaging have increased the potential for greater channel independence (e.g., Croghan et al., 2017; Berg et al., 2019). Due to these advances, the current study was able to assess subjective musical SQ over a wider range of participants and devices than previous work. Specifically, our hypotheses were that: (1) musical SQ ratings would continue to increase with more available independent channels; (2) pre-curved electrodes positioned in the ST would show increased ratings in musical SQ compared to straight or translocated (ST–SV) pre-curved and straight electrodes; (3) participants with more musical experience, better frequency discrimination ability, and longer device use would rate musical SQ higher than participants with less experience and ability; and (4) CI recipients with better speech recognition performance and speech SQ ratings would also rate musical SQ as better than poorer-performing CI recipients.

MATERIALS AND METHODS

Study Participants

Twenty-one postlingually deafened adult CI recipients (range = 34–80 years; mean age = 58.8 ± 13.5 years) participated. Each of the three FDA-approved CI manufacturers were represented with seven Advanced Bionics (AB), seven Cochlear, and seven MED-EL recipients. Of the participants with AB devices, there was one 1J recipient, three Mid-Scala, and three SlimJ electrodes. Of the participants with cochlear devices, there were three CI512, two CI532, and two CI522 electrodes. Of the Med-El participants, there was one Standard and six Flex28 electrodes. Surgeries were performed by five different surgeons at the authors' current institution and four surgeons at outside institutions. The type of surgical approach (i.e., cochleostomy, round window, extended round window) was not reported or available for all of our participants, so this was not included in the current study. Of the 21 participants, 5 were unilateral CI recipients without contralateral amplification, 8 were bimodal CI recipients indicating a CI on the tested ear and a contralateral hearing aid, 5 were bilateral CI recipients, and 3 used electric-acoustic stimulation (EAS) and a contralateral hearing aid. See **Figure 1** for participant pre-operative hearing thresholds. Participants using EAS in their clinical map were converted to full bandwidth programs and acoustic stimulation was deactivated. All testing was completed in the CI-alone condition. Participants with residual hearing in the contralateral ear were occluded using an E.A.R plug in addition to a circum-aural ear muff. Inclusion criteria required at least 6 months of CI experience and at least 14, 18, and 10 active electrodes in use for AB, Cochlear, and MED-EL, respectively. Participants also needed to score at least 20% correct on AzBio sentences in +5 dB SNR with their clinical map to avoid floor effects. **Table 1** provides demographic information.

Conditions and Materials

All experimental activities were completed in accordance with IRB approved protocols at the Vanderbilt University and the Vanderbilt University Medical Center. Electrode placement, including scalar location, mean and variance of electrode-to-modiolus distance, and angular insertion depth were all determined by CT imaging using validated CI position analysis algorithms (Noble et al., 2013; Zhao et al., 2018, 2019). These algorithms were created using a statistical shape model of 10 cadaver temporal bone microCT images. The statistical shape model was then built onto each participant's pre-operative clinical CT scan to determine the scala divisions within the cochlea. The participant's post-implantation CT scan was then fit onto their pre-operative CT to enable calculating the exact location of each individual electrode with respect to scalar location and the distance to the nearest modiolar surface. The average electrode to modiolus distance ($\overline{M}$) and variance across the arrays were then calculated from these measurements.

Cochlear implant programs were created for electrode counts ranging from 4 to 22 with equal spatial distribution of active

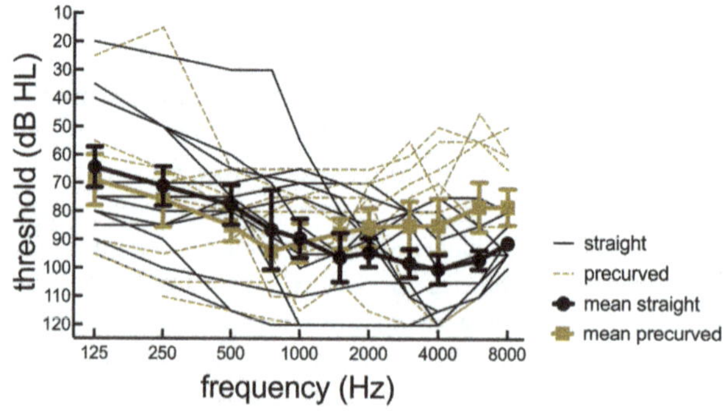

FIGURE 1 | Participant preoperative hearing thresholds. Individual thresholds (dB HL) as a function of pure tone frequency (Hz) for 21 cochlear implant listeners. Straight electrode recipients are plotted in dotted lines and pre-curved recipients are plotted in solid black lines.

TABLE 1 | Demographic information.

ID	Implant manufacturer	Channel stimulation rate	Number of active channels	Electrode type	Electrode	Ear implanted	Scalar location	Insertion depth	$\overline{M}$	CI experience (months)	Frequency discriminatory. threshold (semitones)	Ollen index	LF Pre-op PTA (0.25, 0.5, 0.75 kHz)	Pre-op PTA (0.5, 1, 2, 4 kHz)
S1	AB	1547	16	Pre-curved	Mid-Scala	R	ST	354.28	0.51	46	1.5	18	78.3	106.3
S2	MED-EL	1207	12	Straight	Standard	L	ST	446.83	1.26	29	1.4	118	102.5	110
S3	Cochlear	900	20(1–2)	Pre-curved	CI512	R	ST	356.09	0.44	12	0.4	218	105	86.3
S4	AB	2855	15(16)	Pre-curved	Mid-Scala	R	ST	392.41	0.53	11	1.4	31	88.3	90
S5	Cochlear	900	21(1)	Pre-curved	CI512	R	ST-SV	396.56	0.59	23	0.5	87	40	73.8
S6	MED-EL	1237	12	Straight	Flex28	R	ST	499.72	1.12	46	0.4	273	78.3	85
S7	MED-EL	1247	11(12)	Straight	Flex28	R	ST-SV	466.56	1.47	34	0.5	18	80	73.8
S8	AB	3535	14(15–16)	Pre-curved	Mid-Scala	R	ST	439.98	0.58	26	0.4	261	73.3	70
S9	MED-EL	1389	12	Straight	Flex28	R	ST	509.82	1.37	34	1.7	102	80	92.5
S10	MED-EL	1207	11(2)	Straight	Flex28	L	ST	406.38	1.30	67	1.4	104	57.5	82.5
S11	AB	1547	15(16)	Pre-curved	Mid-Scala	R	ST	326.23	0.59	23	0.4	162	77.5	76.3
S12	MED-EL	1210	11(12)	Straight	Flex28	R	ST	305.85	1.24	57	3.5	33	82.5	88.8
S13	MED-EL	1207	12	Straight	Flex28	R	ST	584.04	1.18	70	1.8	132	70	75
S14	AB	3712	15(16)	Straight	SlimJ	R	ST	508.34	1.13	13	0.4	304	75	107.5
S15	Cochlear	900	22	Pre-curved	CI512	L	ST-SV	375.21	0.59	129	1.8	71	110	118.8
S16	AB	3712	14(15–16)	Straight	SlimJ	R	ST	339.87	1.17	11	0.4	779	28.3	68.8
S17	Cochlear	900	21(1)	Straight	CI522	L	ST	481.26	1.09	23	6.5	275	108.3	118.8
S18	Cochlear	900	20(1–2)	Pre-curved	CI532	L	ST	401.75	0.44	29	0.5	31	67.5	61.3
S19	Cochlear	900	19(1–3)	Pre-curved	CI532	L	ST	430.49	0.39	19	0.8	98	88.3	87.5
S20	AB	2184	14(9,16)	Straight	1J	L	ST-SV	322.47	1.18	187	0.6	94	113.3	118.8
S21	Cochlear	900	22	Straight	CI522	R	ST	351.61	0.96	18	0.5	719	60	76.3
Mean										43.2	1.3	187.1	79.2	88.9
SD										42.9	1.4	207.5	21.9	17.8

Channel stimulation rate was set from the clinical map and kept constant throughout all conditions. Number of active channels in the clinical map are listed; the clinically deactived channels are listed in parentheses. Insertion depth is represented in degrees. Average electrode to modiolus distance ($\overline{M}$) is represented in millimeters. Cochlear implant experience is represented in months since date of activation for tested ear Hearing thresholds displayed in dB HL.

electrodes across the array to follow the electrode deactivation methods of Friesen et al. (2001). For all conditions, the frequency map was automatically re-allocated based on the number of active electrodes to simulate a clinical manipulation. It is possible that SQ ratings were affected by these acute manipulations due to the participant's lack of experience listening to music with the maps used in this study. Refer to **Table 2** for specific electrodes activated to achieve the spatially selective maps. Note the bandwidths of the 16-channel map and the clinical map for AB participants differed slightly due to the difference in stimulation type (CIS versus current steering strategies). For participants with electrodes deactivated clinically, the adjacent electrode was activated if the electrode condition required an electrode to be active that had been clinically deactivated. All experimental programs used a classic CIS (Wilson et al., 1991) stimulation strategy except for the participants' clinical maps. The participants' clinical maps all used iterations of CIS including Optima-S, Advanced Combination Encoder (or n-of-m), and FS4 for AB, Cochlear, and MED-EL, respectively. All of the clinical maps used the highest number of active electrodes possible for that participant (**Table 1**).

Channel stimulation rate and pulse duration were kept constant across all conditions, but manufacturer dependent (**Table 1**). Threshold levels were not adjusted from the participant's own map; however, aided detection thresholds were verified to be within 15–30 dB HL from 250 to 6000 Hz before the participant began the study. Upper stimulation levels were globally adjusted using the participants' own maps to achieve equivalent loudness across all experimental maps. All front-end processing features were deactivated, with the exception of Autosensitivity Control (ASC) and Adaptive Dynamic Range Optimization (ADRO) for cochlear participants as all participants were longtime users of ASC and ADRO.

Electrode condition and measure assessment order were both randomized using a Latin Square design. All testing was completed acutely. Each of the conditions was tested using a loudspeaker at 0-degrees azimuth and 1 m from the participant in a single walled sound booth using: CNC monosyllabic words (Peterson and Lehiste, 1962) and AzBio sentences (Spahr et al., 2012) in +5 SNR using 20-talker babble noise. One list of CNC words and AzBio sentences in +5 dB SNR was presented for each channel condition; lists were only used once per participant. Target speech stimuli were presented at a calibrated level of 60 dB SPL. Subjective SQ judgments were assessed using a visually presented 10-point scale (1 = very poor; 10 = very good), in which the participant rated the overall SQ of the list of CNC words and AzBio sentences in +5 dB SNR for each condition. Prior to statistical analyses, all speech recognition scores were converted to rationalized arcsine units (RAUs) (Studebaker, 1985) and all speech SQ ratings were converted to z-scores.

Musical SQ was assessed using a randomly selected subset of 15 30-s song clips from a group of 30 possible songs, all from various genres and styles. The clips were presented at a comfortable listening level, kept constant for all conditions, and the participant was asked to make subjective SQ judgments immediately after they listened to the clip. Participants were given verbal instructions prior to beginning the musical SQ task, asking them to select their rating for each musical excerpt based on the clarity, richness, and pleasantness of the voices and instruments and not how much they liked or were familiar with the excerpt. The participant typed in their rating on a keypad after each clip using a 10-point scale (0 = very poor; 9 = very good) presented on a touch-screen computer. Prior to analyses, all of the musical SQ ratings were converted to z-scores. The transformed z-scores for mean overall musical SQ ratings of all 15 clips for each condition as well as the mean musical SQ rating for each genre for each condition were used for analyses. The musical genres were determined by the record label's description of each song. The musical genres used for analyses included Alternative, Hip Hop and Rap, Jazz, Popular, Rhythm and Blues (R&B), and Rock n Roll. Within each condition, an individual participant could potentially listen to up to six songs from the same genre. Participants listened to at least one sample from each genre for every condition.

A measure of frequency discrimination was also assessed for each condition via the frequency discrimination test in Angel Sound[1]. An adaptive, three-alternative forced-choice (3AFC) procedure was used to determine the frequency change threshold. In each trial, the participant would listen to a series of three pure tones, two reference tones (440 Hz), and the target tone. The target tone varied in the number of semitones it differed from the reference tone, always ascending. The order of reference and target stimuli was randomized. The participant was asked to select the target (which one is different from the other two tones) by tapping one of three boxes on a touchscreen computer and without feedback. The step size adjusted according to a two-down one-up staircase technique based on the participants' response. The transformed up-down staircase technique was used to track the 79% correct point on the psychometric function. Important to note, a score of less than a 0.5 semitone threshold was not possible due to the set-up of the task (Zhang et al., 2019).

Participants also completed the Ollen Musical Sophistication Index (OMSI) as part of the study to help classify them as more or less musically sophisticated (Ollen, 2006). Musical sophistication includes the participant's knowledge about music; her ability to play a musical instrument or sing; and to understand, respond to, and create music. The OMSI is a 10-item questionnaire that yields a numerical score indicating the probability (in percent times 10) that a music expert would categorize the participant as "more musically sophisticated." Participants with scores greater than 500 are considered "more musically sophisticated," while participants with scores less than 500 are considered "less musically sophisticated." See **Table 1** for individual participant Ollen scores.

RESULTS

Number of Channels Needed for Musical Sound Quality and Impact of Device Factors

A linear mixed model was completed with the number of channels, scalar location, and electrode type as independent

[1] http://angelsound.tigerspeech.com/

TABLE 2 | Active electrodes by condition and manufacturer.

Advanced bionics channel conditions

16 active electrodes using Optima-S (clinic default)

1-2	2-3	3-4	4-5	5-6	6-7	7-8	8-9	9-10	10-11	11-12	12-13	13-14	14-15	15-16

238 442 578 646 782 918 1054 1257 1529 1801 2141 2549 3025 3568 4248 8054

16 active electrodes using HiRes-S

1	2	3	4	5	6	7	8	9	10	11	12	13	14	15	16

238 442 510 646 714 850 986 1189 1393 1597 1937 2277 2617 3093 3704 4316 8054

12 active electrodes using HiRes-S

1	2	3	6	6	7	9	10	11	13	14	15

238 510 646 714 918 1121 1393 1733 2141 2617 3229 4044 8054

10 active electrodes using HiRes-S

1	3	4	6	7	9	10	12	13	15

238 510 646 850 1054 1393 1801 2277 2957 3772 8054

8 active electrodes using Hi-Res-S

1	3	5	7	9	11	13	15

238 578 782 1054 1393 1869 2549 3500 8054

4 active electrodes using HiRes-S

1	6	11	16

238 782 1393 2481 8054

Cochlear channel conditions

22 active electrodes with 8 maxima using ACE (clinic default)

1	2	3	4	5	6	7	8	9	10	11	12	13	14	15	16	17	18	19	20	21	22

188 313 438 563 688 813 938 1063 1188 1313 1563 1813 2063 2313 2688 3063 3563 4063 4688 5313 6063 6938 7938

16 active electrodes with 16 maxima using ACE

1	3	4	5	7	8	9	11	12	13	15	16	17	19	20	21

188 313 438 563 688 813 938 1188 1438 1813 2188 2688 3313 4063 5063 6313 7938

12 active electrodes with 12 maxima using ACE

1	3	5	7	9	11	13	15	17	19	21	22

188 313 438 563 813 1063 1438 1938 2563 3438 4563 6063 7938

10 active electrodes with 10 maxima using ACE

3	5	7	9	11	13	15	17	19	21

188 313 438 688 938 1313 1938 2813 3938 5563 7938

8 active electrodes with 8 maxima using ACE

1	4	7	10	13	16	19	22

188 313 438 688 1063 1813 2938 4813 7938

4 active electrodes with 4 maxima using ACE

2	8	14	20

188 438 1188 3063 7938

Model channel conditions

12 active electrodes using FS4 (clinic default)

1	2	3	4	5	6	7	8	9	10	11	12

250 335 450 604 810 1087 1458 1956 2624 3520 4723 6336 8500

12 active electrodes using HDCIS

1	2	3	4	5	6	7	8	9	10	11	12

250 335 450 604 810 1087 1458 1956 2624 3520 4723 6336 8500

10 active electrodes using HDCIS

1	2	3	4	5	7	8	9	11	12

250 356 506 720 1025 1458 2074 2951 4199 5974 8500

8 active electrodes using HDCIS

1	2	3	5	7	9	11	12

250 388 604 938 1458 2265 3520 5470 8500

4 active electrodes using HDCIS

1	4	8	12

250 604 1458 3520 8500

Frequency tables for all channel conditions tested each cochlear implant manufacturer. Large numbers within cells indicate the electrode number that is active for that condition. Small numbers underneath cells indicate bandwidths of channels in Hertz (Hz).

variables and musical SQ ratings as the dependent variable. *Post hoc* analyses were completed using a Sidak adjustment with all-pairwise, multiple comparisons. For overall musical SQ ratings, there was a significant main effect of number of channels [$F_{(5,31)} = 5.007$, $p = 0.002$], electrode type [$F_{(1,108)} = 17.363$, $p < 0.001$], and electrode scalar location [$F_{(1,108)} = 5.747$, $p = 0.018$]. There was no significant interaction between electrode type and scalar location for this sample [$F_{(1,109)} = 2.286$, $p = 0.133$].The raw data for these comparisons are displayed in **Figure 2** with panels A and B displaying mean and individual data, respectively. *Post hoc* analyses revealed significant performance differences between 4 and 10 channels ($p = 0.035$), 4 and 12 channels ($p = 0.001$), 4 and 16 channels ($p = 0.026$), and 4 channels and the clinic map ($p = 0.023$). No other channel comparisons were statistically significant for this sample.

Straight electrode recipients (mean = 4.727, $SD = 0.234$) demonstrated significantly higher overall musical SQ ratings compared to pre-curved electrode recipients (mean = 3.543, $SD = 0.237$, $t_{19} = 14.53$, $p < 0.001$), though on average, all recipients reported generally neutral to poor musical SQ ratings. Participants with electrodes completely in the ST (mean = 4.567, $SD = 0.165$) demonstrated significantly higher overall musical SQ ratings compared to patients with translocated electrodes (mean = 3.703, $SD = 0.328$, $p = 0.019$). **Figure 2B** displays linear regression fits for the pre-curved (solid line), straight (dashed line), and translocated (dotted line) electrode recipients. Regression analysis revealed that the regression slope coefficient was significantly different from zero for pre-curved recipients only [$F_{(1,4)} = 9.0$, $p = 0.04$]. For both straight electrode [$F_{(1,4)} = 5.1$, $p = 0.09$] and translocated electrode recipients [$F_{(1,4)} = 0.29$,

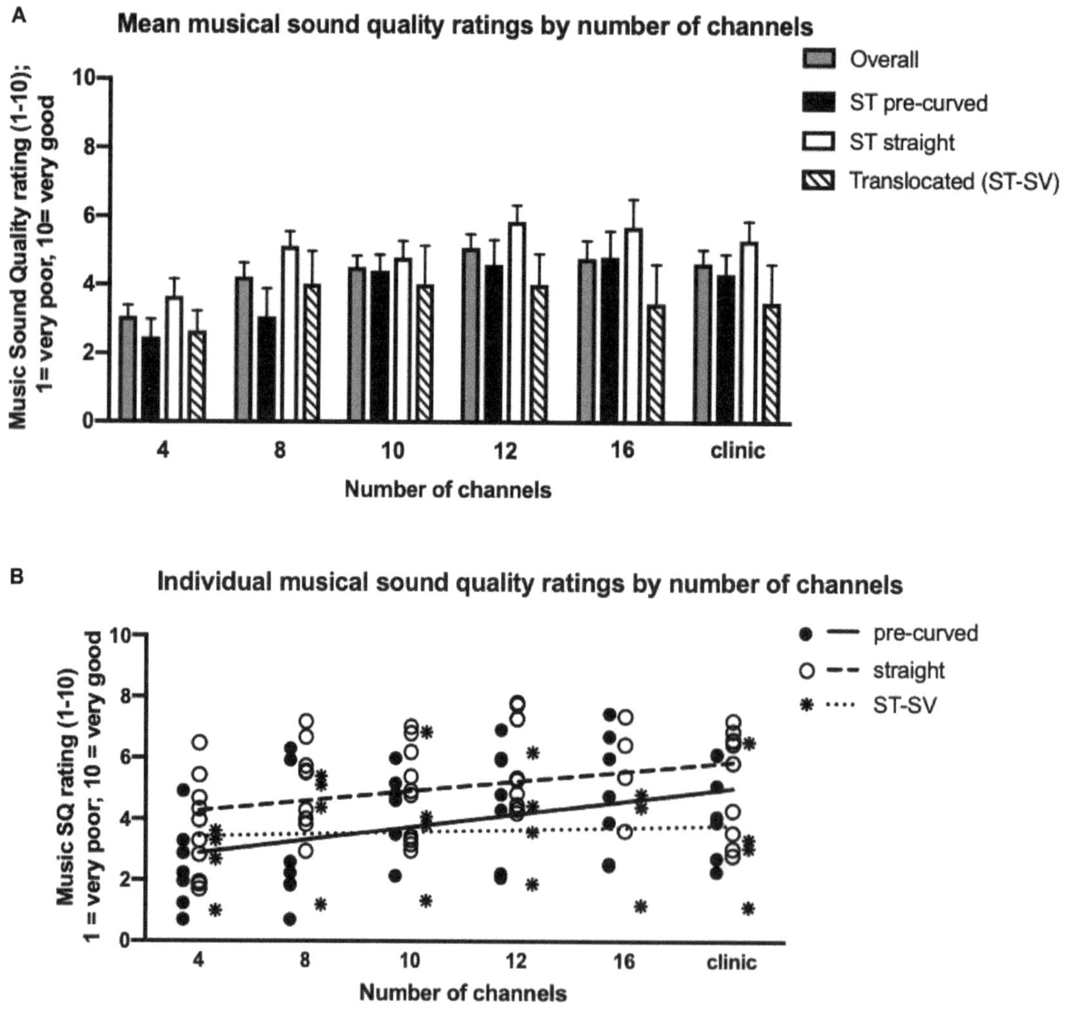

FIGURE 2 | Musical sound quality ratings as a function of the number of channels by electrode type and scalar location. Mean **(A)** and individual **(B)** musical sound quality ratings for 21 cochlear implant listeners across all tested channel conditions. In panel **A**, mean data for all listeners combined (solid gray), ST pre-curved (solid black), ST straight (solid white), and ST-SV electrode recipients (diagonal black stripes) are shown. Error bars are +1 SEM. In panel **B**, individual data for ST pre-curved electrode recipients (solid black circles) with the group mean shown (solid line), ST straight electrode recipients (solid white circles) with the group mean shown (dashed line), and ST–SV electrode recipients (black stars) with the group mean shown (dotted line).

$p = 0.58$], the regression slope coefficient was not significantly different from zero.

The effect of manufacturer on overall musical SQ ratings was examined using a one-way ANOVA was completed with CI manufacturer as the independent variable and overall musical SQ ratings using the clinical map was the dependent variable. There was no significant effect of manufacturer on overall musical SQ ratings of this sample [$F_{(2,18)} = 0.78$, $p = 0.473$]. The effect of surgeon on overall musical SQ ratings was also examined using a one-way ANOVA with surgeon as the independent variable and overall musical SQ rating using the clinical map as the dependent variable. There was no significant effect of surgeon for this sample [$F_{(5,15)} = 1.493$, $p = 0.250$].

Pearson correlations were used to examine the relationship between overall musical SQ ratings using the clinical map and average electrode-to-modiolus distance, the variance in electrode-to-modiolus distance across the array, and electrode insertion depth in degrees. There was a significant positive correlation between mean electrode-to-modiolus distance ($\overline{M}$, in mm) and overall musical SQ ratings ($r = 0.28, p = 0.002$), meaning higher $\overline{M}$ was associated with better musical SQ ratings. $\overline{M}$ was further examined by electrode type and a significant positive correlation was found between $\overline{M}$ of pre-curved electrodes and overall musical SQ ratings ($r = 0.71, p = 0.01$). $\overline{M}$ as a function of overall musical SQ ratings (raw data) is displayed in **Figure 3**. There was no significant relationship between $\overline{M}$ of straight electrodes and overall musical SQ ratings ($r = 0.05$, $p = 0.43$), likely due to the relative homogeneity of $\overline{M}$ values for the straight electrode recipients (**Table 1**). To better understand why a higher $\overline{M}$ value would lead to higher overall musical SQ ratings, the variance in electrode-to-modiolus distances across the array was also examined. There was a positive significant relationship between greater $\overline{M}$ variance and higher musical SQ ratings for those electrodes completely in ST ($r = 0.51, p = 0.03$), but not for those in ST–SV ($r = 0.77, p = 0.22$). By electrode type, there was a positive significant relationship between greater $\overline{M}$ variance and higher musical SQ ratings for pre-curved electrodes ($r = 0.95$, $p = 0.001$), but not for straight electrodes ($r = 0.25$, $p = 0.47$). There was no significant relationship between insertion depth of the electrode measured in degrees and overall musical SQ ratings ($r = 0.03, p = 0.768$).

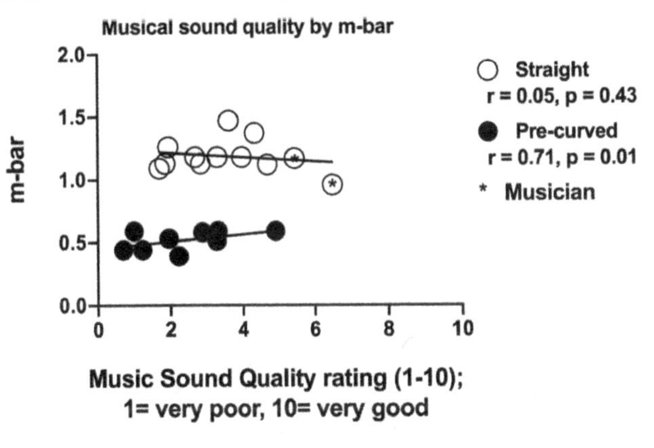

FIGURE 3 | Impact of average electrode to modiolus distance ($\overline{M}$) and variance of $\overline{M}$ on musical sound quality ratings with clinical map by electrode type. Individual average electrode to modiolus distance ($\overline{M}$) values and variance of $\overline{M}$ across the array (y-axis) as a function of musical sound quality ratings using the participant's clinical map (x-axis). Black circles represent pre-curved electrodes and white circles represent straight electrodes. Of note, variability of $\overline{M}$ for the pre-curved electrode sample is smaller than the general clinical population. Of note, the two white circles farthest to the right are the two musicians.

Impact of Musical Genre on Number of Channels Needed for Musical Sound Quality Ratings

The effect of musical genre on the number of channels as a function of musical SQ was examined using a linear mixed model with number of channels as the independent variable and musical SQ ratings by genre (Alternative, Hip Hop and Rap, Jazz, Popular, R&Bs, and Rock n Roll) as the dependent variable. **Figure 4** shows this analysis using the raw data for musical SQ ratings. *Post hoc* analyses included paired t-tests between channel conditions for each musical genre. For Alternative music, there was a significant main effect of number of channels [$F_{(5,30)} = 3.38$, $p = 0.016$]. *Post hoc* analyses revealed significant performance differences between 4 and 10 channels ($t = -4.594$, $p < 0.001$) and 4 and 12 channels ($t = -5.692$, $p < 0.001$). None of the other channel comparisons were significantly different for alternative music. For Hip Hop and Rap, there was no significant main effect of number of channels [$F_{(5,36)} = 2.292$, $p = 0.06$]. For Jazz, there was a significant main effect of number of channels [$F_{(5,30)} = 2.676$, $p = 0.041$]. *Post hoc* analyses for Jazz revealed significant performance differences between 4 and 12 channels ($t = -4.893$, $p < 0.001$). None of the other channel comparisons were significantly different for jazz music SQ ratings. For Popular music, there was a significant main effect of number of channels [$F_{(5,36)} = 3.592, p = 0.010$]. *Post hoc* analyses revealed significant performance differences between 4 and 8 channels ($t = -4.478$, $p < 0.001$) and 4 and 12 channels ($t = -4.972, p < 0.001$). None of the other channel comparisons were significantly different for popular music. For R&Bs, there was a significant main effect of number of channels [$F_{(5,38)} = 3.744$, $p = 0.007$]. *Post hoc* analyses revealed significant performance differences between 4 and 12 channels ($t = -4.123$, $p = 0.001$). None of the other channel comparisons were significantly different for R&B. For Rock n Roll, there was a significant main effect of number of channels [$F_{(5,33)} = 6.229, p < 0.001$]. *Post hoc* analyses revealed significant performance differences between 4 and 10 channels ($t = -4.468, p < 0.001$), 4 and 12 channels ($t = -5.317, p < 0.001$), as well as 4 and the clinical map with all active electrodes ($t = -4.798, p < 0.001$). None of the other channel comparisons were significantly different for Rock n Roll.

Impact of Patient Factors on Musical Sound Quality

Pearson correlations were used to examine the relationship between musical experience as measured by the Ollen index,

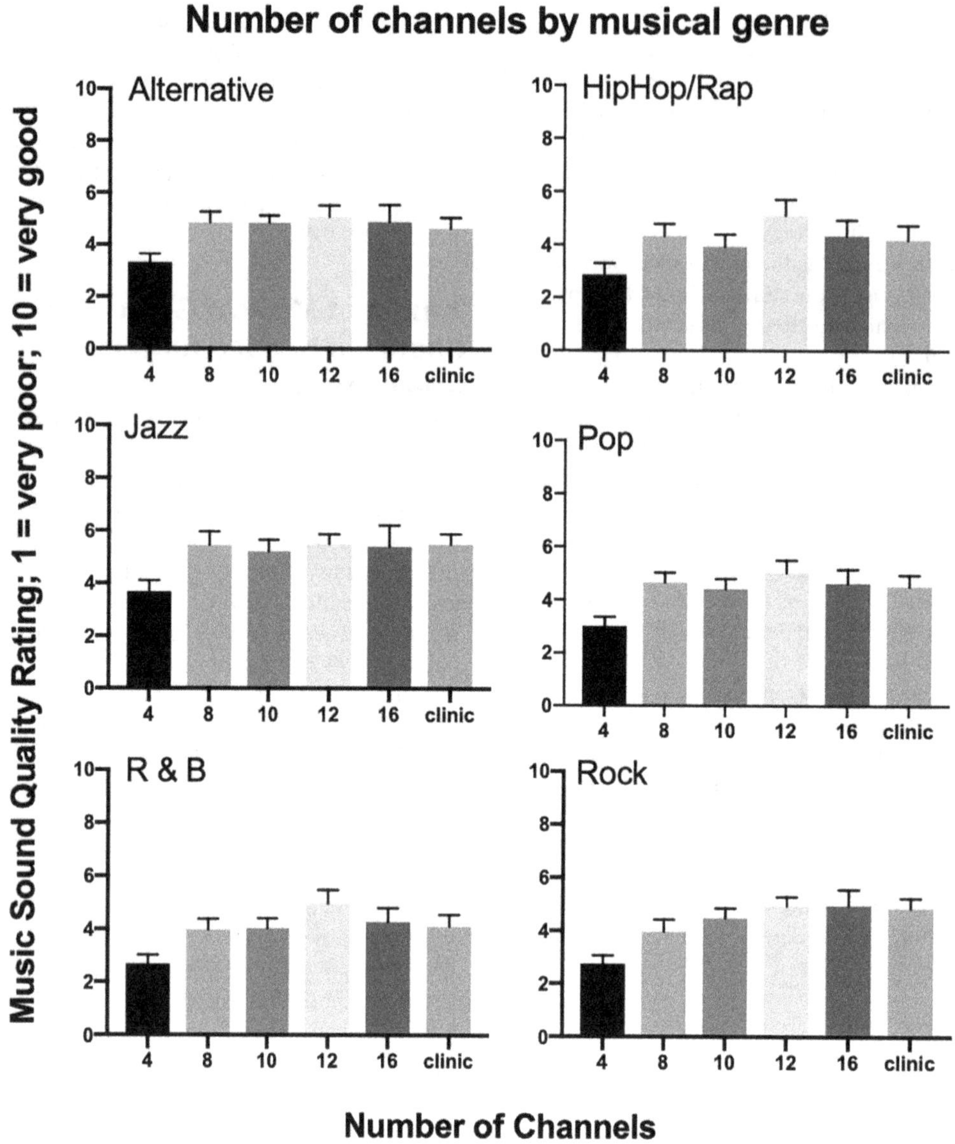

FIGURE 4 | Number of channels by musical genre. Mean musical sound quality ratings for six musical genres, including Alternative, Hip Hop/Rap, Jazz, Pop, Rhythm and Blues (R&B), and Rock for 21 cochlear implant listeners across all tested channel conditions. Error bars are +1 SEM.

pre-operative hearing thresholds, measured at the CI work-up appointment, music perception ability via frequency discrimination thresholds, and CI experience, in months, since activation. See **Table 1** for Ollen scores, pre-operative pure tone averages, frequency discrimination thresholds, and duration of CI experience by participant. Musical SQ ratings with the clinical map were used for these analyses. There was a significant positive correlation between Ollen index of Musical Sophistication scores and overall musical SQ ratings ($r = 0.40, t = -10.086, p < 0.001$); that is, individuals with more musical experience rated musical SQ higher than individuals with less musical experience, as shown in **Figure 5** using the raw data for musical SQ ratings. When the impact of musical experience is further broken down by electrode type, there is a significant positive correlation between musical experience and musical SQ ratings for straight electrodes ($r = 0.67$, $p = 0.03$), but there was no significant relationship between musical experience and musical SQ ratings for pre-curved electrodes ($r = 0.19, p = 0.67$). However, when the two outliers with greater Ollen scores are removed, the positive correlation is no longer significant ($r = 0.11$, $p = 0.80$). The relationship between pre-operative hearing thresholds, using both a low-frequency pure tone average (LFPTA) (250,500, and 750 Hz) and a standard four frequency pure tone average (500, 1000, 2000, and 4000 Hz), and overall musical SQ ratings was examined in an attempt to understand why straight electrode recipients rated musical SQ better than pre-curved recipients. Pre-operative hearing thresholds are shown in **Figure 1**. However, there was no significant relationship between overall

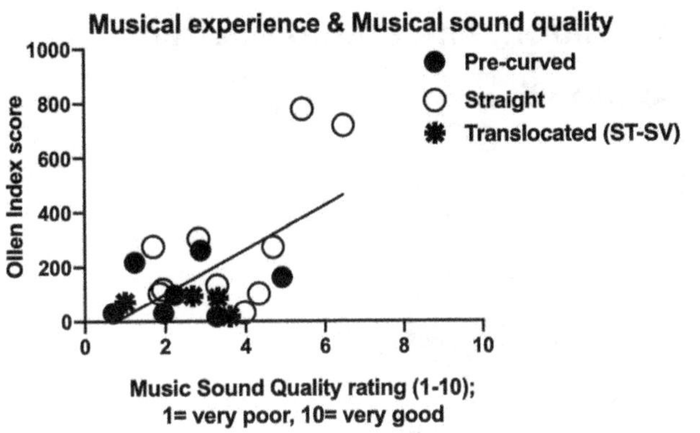

FIGURE 5 | Impact of patient musical experience on musical sound quality ratings with clinical map. Individual Ollen Index of Musical Sophistication scores (*y*-axis) as a function of musical sound quality ratings using the clinical map (*x*-axis). Higher Ollen Index scores indicate more musical experience. Black circles represent pre-curved electrodes and white circles represent straight electrodes. Translocated electrodes that include two pre-curved and two straight electrode recipients are represented by the black stars.

musical SQ ratings and LFPTA ($r = 0.22$, $p = 0.35$) or using the standard pure tone average ($r = 0.06$, $p = 0.79$). There was also no significant relationship between music perception ability measured via the AngelSound frequency discrimination task ($r = -0.23$, $p = 0.50$) or CI experience and overall musical SQ ratings ($r = -0.116$, $p = 0.21$).

Relationship Between Musical Sound Quality, Speech Recognition, and Speech Sound Quality

Pearson correlation analyses were completed for z-transformed scores of overall musical SQ ratings and speech recognition scores in RAU (CNC words and AzBio sentences at +5 dB), as well as speech SQ ratings. However, for easier translation to the Audiology clinic, **Figure 6** displays speech recognition scores in percent correct along with the raw SQ ratings. Musical SQ ratings using the clinical map were used for these analyses. For measures of speech recognition, there was a significant, but weak positive correlation between CNC word recognition in RAU and overall musical SQ ratings ($r = 0.20$, $t = -27.636$, $p = 0.027$). Similarly, there was a significant, but weak positive correlation between AzBio sentence recognition in noise in RAU and overall musical SQ ratings ($r = 0.22$, $t = -7.268$, $p = 0.017$). For transformed z-scores of speech SQ, there was a significant positive correlation between CNC SQ ratings and overall musical SQ ratings ($r = 0.51$, $t = -26.492$, $p < 0.001$), as well as a significant positive correlation between SQ ratings for AzBio in noise and overall musical SQ ratings ($r = 0.33$, $t = -12.622$, $p < 0.001$).

DISCUSSION

Hypothesis 1: *Musical SQ ratings will continue to increase with more available independent channels for pre-curved electrodes positioned in ST compared to straight or translocated (ST–SV) electrodes.*

Consistent with our primary hypothesis, adult CI recipients demonstrated continuous gains in musical SQ ratings with 10–22 channels compared with four channels. Regression analysis revealed that the increases in music SQ with number of channels was significant for pre-curved electrode recipients, but not for straight or translocated electrode recipients (**Figure 2B**). This finding is consistent with recent studies evaluating the number of channels needed for speech recognition with modern CI recipients (e.g., Croghan et al., 2017; Berg et al., 2019) suggesting that a greater number of independent channels may be both available and necessary than previously thought for asymptotic speech recognition and musical SQ, particularly for pre-curved electrode recipients. Also consistent with our primary hypothesis, participants with electrodes completely in ST reported significantly higher overall ratings for musical SQ than those with translocated arrays, emphasizing the importance of electrode insertion and resultant scalar location. Of note, this sample did have lower translocation rates for pre-curved electrodes (2/9 = 22%) and slightly higher translocation rates for straight electrodes (2/12 = 16.7%) than is reported in the literature (e.g., Wanna et al., 2014).

Contrary to our primary hypothesis and recent evidence, however, straight electrode recipients reported higher overall musical SQ ratings than pre-curved electrode recipients. In fact, the strong positive correlation between mean electrode-to-modiolus distance ($\overline{M}$) and overall musical SQ ratings suggest that arrays farther away from the modiolus (i.e., straight arrays) may yield higher musical SQ. The straight electrode recipients had greater musical experience than the other participants in this sample (see below) which is a likely explanation; however, further work is needed to better understand this preliminary finding. A potential limitation of the current study was that many electrode conditions did not use the most basal or apical contact resulting in a downshift or upshift in frequencies compared to the participants' clinical maps. Changing the number of electrodes invariably changed the spiral ganglion cells being stimulated in response to different frequencies, which could have potentially had an effect on music perception and subjective musical SQ ratings. Further, the strong positive correlation between greater variance in $\overline{M}$ for ST pre-curved electrodes, but not for ST straight electrodes also supports the idea that greater electrode-to-modiolus distance is advantageous for musical SQ. Of note, the straight electrode recipients did have greater musical experience than the other participants in this sample (see below), which is a likely contributor; however, further work is needed to better understand these preliminary findings.

Another related consideration is that the straight and pre-curved electrode recipients may have had different levels of underlying neural health which could impact perceptual quality. Specifically, it is quite possible that participants with straight electrodes were those with better preoperative hearing given that acoustic hearing preservation rates are generally higher for straight electrode arrays. We did not complete any measurements thought to reflect underlying neural health, such as multipulse

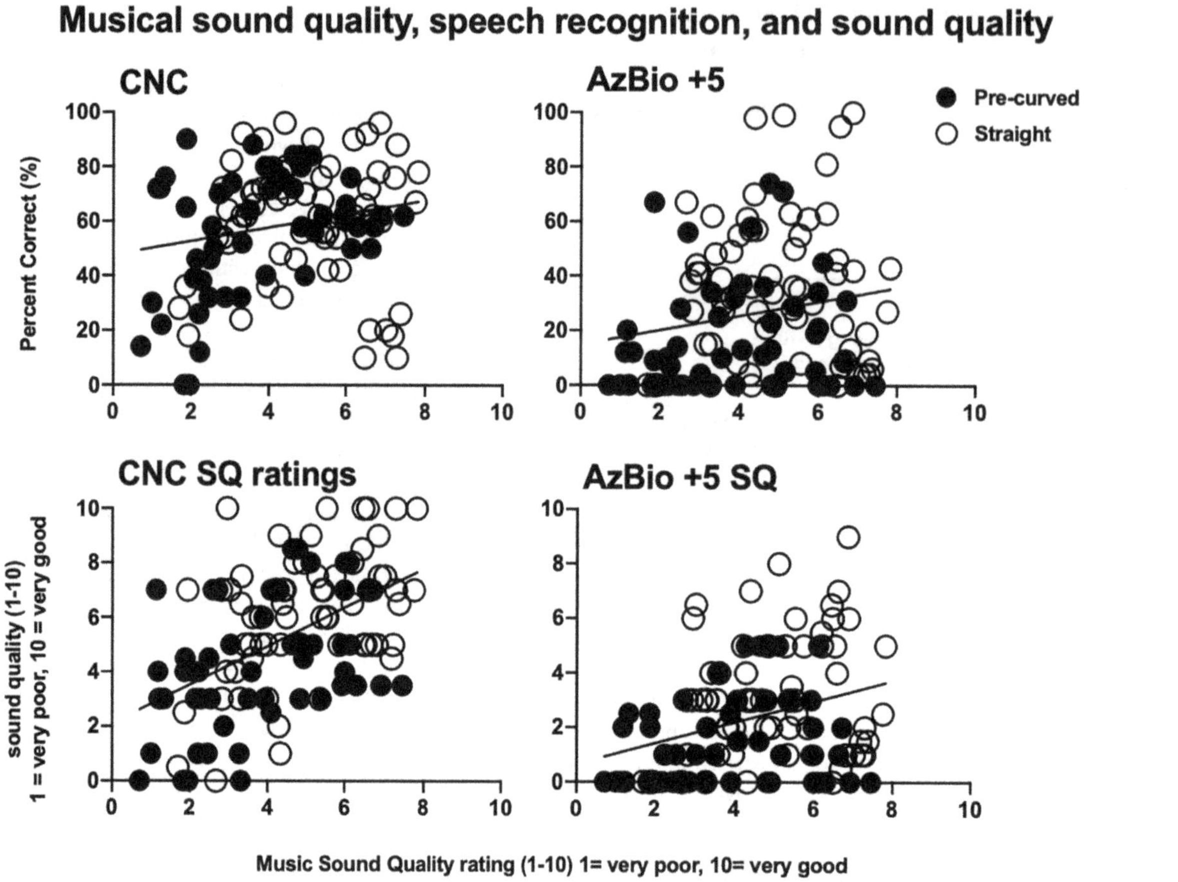

FIGURE 6 | Musical sound quality ratings compared to speech recognition scores and sound quality ratings. Individual speech recognition for CNC monosyllabic words in quiet and AzBio sentences at +5 dB SNR **(top row)** in percent correct and speech sound quality for CNC monosyllabic words in quiet and AzBio sentences at +5 dB SNR **(bottom row)** as a function of musical sound quality ratings (*x*-axes). Black circles represent pre-curved electrodes and white circles represent straight electrodes.

integration (Zhou and Dong, 2017; Zhou et al., 2018), polarity sensitivity (e.g., Macherey et al., 2017; Hughes et al., 2018; Jahn and Arenberg, 2019), or amplitude growth functions for electrically evoked compound action potentials (e.g., Schvartz-Leyzac and Pfingst, 2016; He et al., 2018; Hughes et al., 2018). We did, however, complete two-tailed *t*-tests comparing preoperative audiometric thresholds for the CI ear in the straight and pre-curved electrode groups for LFPTA (125, 250, and 500 Hz), traditional PTA (500, 1000, and 2000 Hz), and high-frequency PTA (2000, 4000, and 8000 Hz). These analyses revealed no significant differences between preoperative audiometric thresholds in the CI ear across groups for LFPTA (t_{19} = −0.504, p = 0.62), PTA (t_{19} = 0.255, p = 0.80), or HFPTA (t_{19} = 2.07, p = 0.053). Nevertheless, we recognize that audiometric thresholds cannot necessarily serve as a surrogate for underlying neural health and as such, additional investigation into this relationship is warranted. Furthermore, given that our recipient recruitment did not control for musical experience nor was electrode group assignment completed randomly, we believe that the relationship between electrode array type and overall music ratings is confounded by both musical experience as well as the potential for preoperative device selection bias. We plan to investigate this relationship further in future investigations.

Another potential limitation of this study may be that the current measures are not sensitive enough to accurately measure spectral resolution because these results potentially suggest that greater channel interaction may be related to higher musical SQ ratings. Future studies should investigate more direct measures of spectral resolution, such as using the Quick Spectral Modulation Detection (QSMD) task (Gifford et al., 2014). Furthermore, many electrode conditions did not use the most basal or apical contact resulting in a downshift or upshift in frequencies compared to the participants' clinical maps when the frequency tables were reallocated. Changing the number of electrodes invariably changed the spiral ganglion cells being stimulated in response to different frequencies, which could have potentially had an effect on music perception and subjective musical SQ ratings.

> Hypothesis 2: *Participants with more musical experience, better frequency discrimination ability, and longer device use would rate musical SQ higher than participants with less experience and ability.*

As described above, participants with straight electrodes rated musical SQ to be significantly higher than participants with pre-curved arrays. Rather than concluding that greater $\overline{M}$ values are more desirable for musical SQ, we believe that patient factors may explain this result. Specifically, our sample of straight electrode recipients had significantly greater musical experience, as measured by the Ollen Index of Musical Sophistication, than our sample of pre-curved electrode recipients. This was driven primarily by S16 and S21, who were both serious amateur musicians. These two subjects also had more pre-operative hearing than traditional CI candidates which likely influenced surgeon selection of a straight electrode array. In their everyday settings, both subjects use EAS stimulation, which could influence their perception and appreciation of music differently than CI recipients who use electric stimulation for the full bandwidth (though the acoustic earhook was not used for the current study). After removing data from these two musicians, the positive correlation between musical experience and overall musical SQ ratings is greatly reduced and becomes non-significant.

These results contraindicated our hypothesis that participants with more musical experience would demonstrate higher overall musical SQ ratings. In the broader data set, there was no relationship found between pre-operative hearing thresholds and overall musical SQ and there was no difference in pre-operative hearing thresholds between electrode types. Using behavioral hearing thresholds as a correlate for greater neural survival, this suggests that greater neural survival did not significantly influence musical SQ ratings. However, this finding is very preliminary and the impact of neural survival on musical SQ should be investigated further in future studies.

While the Ollen scores of straight electrodes were significantly and positively correlated with overall musical SQ ratings, there was no significant relationship between these two measures for pre-curved electrode recipients. Again, when the data for the two musicians in our sample were removed, the positive correlation between straight electrode recipient Ollen scores and overall musical SQ ratings is greatly reduced and also becomes non-significant. The non-significant relationship between music perceptual accuracy and perceived musical SQ ratings found in this study is in keeping with previous studies (Gfeller et al., 2008; Looi et al., 2011) and suggests that music appreciation and SQ ratings cannot be predicted by measuring music perception abilities. Currently, music perception is rarely measured in the clinic, but measures of musical SQ are almost never included in CI clinical protocols. This is hugely problematic because CI recipients consistently report musical SQ impairments following implantation, and musical SQ is rated as the most significant factor responsible for music listening enjoyment (Lassaletta et al., 2008a,b; Roy et al., 2012). Future work should consider clinically feasible measures of musical SQ to address this gap in our battery of clinical assessments.

Although CI surgeons have traditionally selected straight electrodes for patients with greater pre-operative audiometric thresholds due to their lower rates of translocation compared to pre-curved arrays (e.g., O'Connell et al., 2016), this was not the case for our sample. Our results indicated no difference in pre-operative standard and LFPTAs between recipients with straight electrodes and those with pre-curved arrays. We also did not see an effect of surgeon, suggesting that surgical technique did not impact musical SQ ratings for this sample. Although it was not the aim of the current study, it is possible that the straight electrode recipients in this sample had shorter durations of deafness, better neural survival, or some combination of these factors compared to the participants with pre-curved electrodes. Future studies should more rigorously assess these factors as they relate to musical SQ and channel independence.

> Hypothesis 3: *CI recipients with higher speech recognition performance and speech SQ ratings will rate musical SQ higher than poorer performing CI recipients.*

Speech recognition and speech SQ tasks were found to be significantly and positively correlated with musical SQ ratings. These positive relationships between speech recognition, speech SQ, and musical SQ may be useful for managing realistic expectations for patients in the Audiology clinic. Those patients who perform better on speech recognition tasks may also experience better perceptual SQ for speech and music stimuli. While previous literature has found a positive relationship between speech recognition performance and music perception abilities (Gfeller et al., 2003), the relationship between speech recognition and musical SQ, as well as speech SQ and musical SQ have not been explored prior to the current study. These relationships should continue to be explored in future studies to better individualize expectations management for music appreciation with a CI, as well as to potentially develop music-based intervention. This positive relationship between speech recognition and musical SQ also emphasizes the importance of including a measure of musical SQ in the clinical test battery, even for patients who do not consider music appreciation of high importance in their quality of life.

Musical Genre Effects

All musical genres examined in the current study demonstrated significant increases in musical SQ ratings beyond four channels except for Hip Hop and Rap, perhaps due to the emphasis on rhythmic features and spoken lyrics often present in this genre. However, there was considerable variability both within and across genres for this relatively small population. While previous research has looked at CI recipients' preference for less complex genres of music (Gfeller et al., 2003), no published studies have specifically investigated musical SQ ratings of various musical genres in an acute setting or as a function of the number of channels. Even though participants were instructed not to include music familiarity or preference in the selection of SQ ratings, it was not possible to eliminate the potential for participant bias in the present study. This potential bias should be considered in future studies, perhaps by limiting all samples to original/unfamiliar music or individualized music selections.

SUMMARY

The findings of this study are summarized as follows:

- Musical SQ ratings significantly increased from 4 to 10 independent channels.
    - Regression slope coefficient for music SQ versus number of channels was significantly different from zero for pre-curved electrode recipients, but not for straight electrode nor translocated electrode recipients.
- Musical SQ ratings were significantly higher for adult CI recipients with:
    - Electrodes localized to ST compared to those with translocated arrays.
    - Pre-curved electrodes that had more variability in electrode-to-modiolus distance across the array.
- Musical experience was not correlated with higher musical SQ ratings after controlling for two participants with significantly greater musical experience than the rest of the sample.
    - Control of patient variables including musical experience and music selection familiarity is recommended for future studies.
- There was no relationship between CI experience and musical SQ ratings.
- Musical SQ ratings were significantly and positively correlated with both speech recognition scores, in RAU, and speech SQ ratings.
- Musical SQ ratings significantly increased beyond four channels for all genres except Hip Hop and Rap.
    - There was considerable within- and between-genre variability in SQ ratings.
    - Future investigation into genre effects may prove useful for identifying recommended music listening progression for auditory training of newly implanted patients.

ETHICS STATEMENT

The studies involving human participants were reviewed and approved by Vanderbilt University Institutional Review Board. The patients/participants provided their written informed consent to participate in this study.

AUTHOR CONTRIBUTIONS

KB and RG contributed to the conception and design of the study. JN, BD, RL, and RD contributed to collect the imaging data and perform the imaging analysis. KB recruited the potential subjects and conducted the experiments, and wrote the first draft of the manuscript with significant input from RG, RD, and VR. VR helped with the data analysis. All authors contributed to the manuscript revisions, and read and approved the submitted version of the manuscript.

REFERENCES

Berg, K. A., Noble, J. H., Dawant, B. M., Dwyer, R. T., Labadie, R. F., and Gifford, R. H. (2019). Speech recognition as a function of the number of channels in perimodiolar electrode recipients. *J. Acoust. Soc. Am.* 145, 1556–1564. doi: 10.1121/1.5092350

Chatterjee, M., and Shannon, R. V. (1998). Forward masked excitation patterns in multielectrode electrical stimulation. *J. Acoust. Soc. Am.* 103, 2565–2572. doi: 10.1121/1.422777

Croghan, N. B. H., Duran, S. I., and Smith, Z. M. (2017). Re-examining the relationship between number of cochlear implant channels and maximal speech intelligibility. *J. Acoust. Soc. Am.* 142:EL537. doi: 10.1121/1.5016044

Davis, T. J., Zhang, D., Gifford, R. H., Dawant, B. M., Labadie, R. F., and Noble, J. H. (2016). Relationship between electrode-to-modiolus distance and current levels for adults with cochlear implants. *Otol. Neurotol.* 37, 31–37. doi: 10.1097/MAO.0000000000000896

Drennan, W. R., and Rubinstein, J. T. (2008). Music perception in cochlear implant users and its relationship with psychophysical capabilities. *J. Rehabil. Res. Dev.* 45, 779–789. doi: 10.1682/JRRD.2007.08.0118

Gifford, R. H., Hedley-Williams, A., and Spahr, A. J. (2014). Clinical assessment of spectral modulation detection for adult cochlear implant recipients: a non-language based measure of performance outcomes. *Int. J. Audiol.* 53, 159–164. doi: 10.3109/14992027.2013.851800

Fishman, K. E., Shannon, R. V., and Slattery, W. H. (1997). Speech recognition as a function of the number of electrodes used in the SPEAK cochlear implant speech processor. *J. Speech. Lang. Hear. Res.* 40, 1201–1215. doi: 10.1044/jslhr.4005.1201

Friesen, L. M., Shannon, R. V., Baskent, D., and Wang, X. (2001). Speech recognition in noise as a function of the number of spectral channels: comparison of acoustic hearing and cochlear implants. *J. Acoust. Soc. Am.* 110, 1150–1163. doi: 10.1121/1.1381538

Friesen, L. M., Shannon, R. V., and Cruz, R. J. (2005). Effects of stimulation rate on speech recognition with cochlear implants. *Audiol. Neurootol.* 10, 169–184. doi: 10.1159/000084027

Gfeller, K., Christ, A., Knutson, J., Witt, S., and Mehr, M. (2003). The effects of familiarity and complexity on appraisal of complex songs by cochlear implant recipients and normal hearing adults. *J. Music Ther.* 40, 78–112. doi: 10.1093/jmt/40.2.78

Gfeller, K., Oleson, J., Knutson, J. F., Breheny, P., Driscoll, V., and Olszewski, C. (2008). Multivariate predictors of music perception and appraisal by adult cochlear implant users. *J. Am. Acad. Audiol.* 19, 120–134. doi: 10.3766/jaaa.19.2.3

He, S., Shahsavarani, B. S., McFayden, T. C., Wang, H., Gill, K. E., Xu, L., et al. (2018). Responsiveness of the electrically stimulated cochlear nerve in children with cochlear nerve deficiency. *Ear Hear.* 39, 238–250. doi: 10.1097/AUD.0000000000000467

Holden, L. K., Finley, C. C., Firszt, J. B., Holden, T. A., Brenner, C., Potts, L. G., et al. (2013). Factors affecting open-set word recognition in adults with cochlear implants. *Ear Hear.* 34, 342–360. doi: 10.1097/AUD.0b013e3182741aa7

Holder, J. T., Kessler, D. M., Noble, J. H., Gifford, R. H., and Labadie, R. F. (2018a). Prevalence of extracochlear electrodes. *Otol. Neurotol.* 39:e325. doi: 10.1097/MAO.0000000000001818

Holder, J. T., Reynolds, S. M., Sunderhaus, L. W., and Gifford, R. H. (2018b). Current profile of adults presenting for preoperative cochlear implant evaluation. *Trends Hear.* 22:233121651875528. doi: 10.1177/2331216518755288

Hughes, M. L., Choi, S., and Glickman, E. (2018). What can stimulus polarity and interphase gap tell us about auditory nerve function in cochlear-implant recipients? *Hear Res.* 359, 50–63. doi: 10.1016/j.heares.2017.12.015

Hughes, M. L., Stille, L. J., Baudhuin, J. L., and Goehring, J. L. (2013). ECAP spread of excitation with virtual channels and physical electrodes. *Hear. Res.* 306, 93–103. doi: 10.1016/j.heares.2013.09.014

Jahn, K. N., and Arenberg, J. G. (2019). Evaluating psychophysical polarity sensitivity as an indirect estimate of neural status in cochlear implant listeners. *J. Assoc. Res. Otolaryngol.* 20, 415–430. doi: 10.1007/s10162-019-00718-712

Jung, K. H., Won, J. H., Drennan, W. R., Jameyson, E., Miyasaki, G., Norton, S. J., et al. (2012). Psychoacoustic performance and music and speech perception in prelingually deafened children with cochlear implants. *Audiol. Neurootol.* 17, 189–197. doi: 10.1159/000336407

Kang, R., Nimmons, G. L., Drennan, W., Longnion, J., Ruffin, C., Nie, K., et al. (2009). Development and validation of the university of washington clinical assessment of music perception test. *Ear Hear.* 30, 411–418. doi: 10.1097/AUD.0b013e3181a61bc0

Lassaletta, L., Castro, A., Bastarrica, M., Perez-Mora, R., Herran, B., Sanz, L., et al. (2008a). Changes in listening habits and quality of musical sound after cochlear implantation. *Otolaryngol. Head. Neck Surg.* 138, 363–367. doi: 10.1016/j.otohns.2007.11.028

Lassaletta, L., Castro, A., Bastarrica, M., Perez-Mora, R., Herran, B., Sanz, L., et al. (2008b). Musical perception and enjoyment in post-lingual patients with cochlear implants. *Acta Otorrinolaringol. Esp.* 59, 228–234. doi: 10.1016/s2173-5735(08)70228-x

Looi, V., Winter, P., Anderson, I., and Sucher, C. (2011). A music quality rating test battery for cochlear implant users to compare the FSP and HDCIS strategies for music appreciation. *Int. J. Audiol.* 50, 503–518. doi: 10.3109/14992027.2011.562246

Macherey, O., Carlyon, R. P., Chatron, J., and Roman, S. (2017). Effect of pulse polarity on thresholds and on non-monotonic loudness growth in cochlear implant users. *J. Assoc. Res. Otolaryngol.* 18, 513–527. doi: 10.1007/s10162-016-0614-614

McDermott, H. J. (2004). Music perception with cochlear implants: a review. *Trends Amplif.* 8, 49–82. doi: 10.1177/108471380400800203

McRackan, T. R., Bauschard, M., Hatch, J. L., Franko-Tobin, E., Droghini, H. R., Nguyen, S. A., et al. (2017). Meta-analysis of quality-of-life improvement after cochlear implantation and associations with speech recognition abilities. *Laryngoscope* 128, 982–990. doi: 10.1002/lary.26738

Moore, B. C. J., and Carlyon, R. P. (2005). "Perception of Pitch by People with Cochlear Hearing Loss and by Cochlear Implant Users," in *Springer Handbook of Auditory Research Pitch, eds C. J. Plack, R. R. Fay, A. J. Oxenham, and A. N. P. Popper* New York, NY: Springer.

Nimmons, G. L., Kang, R. S., Drennanm, W. R., Longnion, J., Ruffin, C., Worman, T., et al. (2008). Clinical assessment of music perception in cochlear implant listeners. *Otol. Nerotol.* 29, 149–155. doi: 10.1097/mao.0b013e31812f7244

Noble, J. H., Labadie, R. F., Gifford, R. H., and Dawant, B. M. (2013). Image-guidance enables new methods for customizing cochlear implant stimulation strategies. *IEEE Trans. Neural Syst. Rehabil. Eng.* 21, 820–829. doi: 10.1109/TNSRE.2013.2253333

O'Connell, B. P., Hunter, J. B., and Wanna, G. B. (2016). The importance of electrode location in cochlear implantation. *Laryngoscope Investig. Otolaryngol.* 1, 169–174. doi: 10.1002/lio2.42

Ollen, J. E. (2006). *A Criterion-Related Validity Test of Selected Indicators of Musical Sophistication using Expert Ratings.* Available at: http://marcs-survey.uws.edu.au/OMSI/ (accessed May 22, 2019).

Padilla, M., and Landsberger, D. M. (2016). Reduction in spread of excitation from current focusing at multiple cochlear locations in cochlear implant users. *Hear. Res.* 333, 98–107. doi: 10.1016/j.heares.2016.01.002

Peterson, G. E., and Lehiste, I. (1962). Revised CNC lists for auditory tests. *J. Speech Hear. Disord.* 27, 62–70. doi: 10.1044/jshd.2701.62

Roy, A. T., Jiradejvong, P., Carver, C., and Limb, C. J. (2012). Assessment of sound quality perception in cochlear implant users during music listening. *Otol. Neurotol.* 33, 319–327. doi: 10.1097/MAO.0b013e31824296a9

Schvartz-Leyzac, K. C., and Pfingst, B. E. (2016). Across-site patterns of electrically evoked compound action potential amplitude-growth functions in multichannel cochlear implant recipients and the effects of the interphase gap. *Hear. Res.* 341, 50–65. doi: 10.1016/j.heares.2016.08.002

Spahr, A. J., Dorman, M. F., Litvak, L. M., Van Wie, S., Gifford, R. H., Loizou, P. C., et al. (2012). Development and validation of the AzBio sentence lists. *Ear Hear.* 33, 112–117. doi: 10.1097/AUD.0b013e31822c2549

Studebaker, G. A. (1985). A "rationalized" arcsine transform. *J. Speech Hear. Res.* 28, 455–462. doi: 10.1044/jshr.2803.455

Wanna, G. B., Noble, J. H., Carlson, M. L., Gifford, R. H., Dietrich, M. S., Haynes, D. S., et al. (2014). Impact of electrode design and surgical approach on scalar location and cochlear implant outcomes. *Laryngoscope* 124(Suppl. 6), S1–S7. doi: 10.1002/lary.24728

Wilson, B. S., Finley, C. C., Lawson, D. T., Wolford, R. D., Eddington, D. K., and Rabinowitz, W. M. (1991). Better speech recognition with cochlear implants. *Nature* 352, 236–238. doi: 10.1038/352236a0

Won, J. H., Drennan, W. R., Kang, R. S., and Rubinstein, J. T. (2010). Psychoacoustic abilities associated with music perception in cochlear implant users. *Ear Hear.* 31, 796–805. doi: 10.1097/AUD.0b013e3181e8b7bd

Zhang, F., Underwood, G., McGuire, K., Liang, C., Moore, D. R., and Fu, Q.-J. (2019). Frequency change detection and speech perception in cochlear implant users. *Hear. Res.* 379, 12–20. doi: 10.1016/J.HEARES.2019.04.007

Zhao, Y., Chakravorti, S., Labadie, R. F., Dawant, B. M., and Noble, J. H. (2019). Automatic graph-based method for localization of cochlear implant electrode arrays in clinical CT with sub-voxel accuracy. *Med. Image Anal.* 52, 1–12. doi: 10.1016/j.media.2018.11.005

Zhao, Y., Dawant, B. M., Labadie, R. F., and Noble, J. H. (2018). Automatic localization of closely spaced cochlear implant electrode arrays in clinical CTs. *Med. Phys.* 45, 5030–5040. doi: 10.1002/mp.13185

Zhou, N., and Dong, L. (2017). Evaluating multipulse integration as a neural-health correlate in human cochlear-implant users: relationship to psychometric functions for detection. *Trends. Hear.* 21, 1–12. doi: 10.1177/2331216517690108

Zhou, N., Dong, L., and Hang, M. (2018). Evaluating multipulse integration as a neural-health correlate in human cochlear implant users: effects of stimulation mode. *J. Assoc. Res. Otolaryngol.* 19, 99–111. doi: 10.1007/s10162-017-0643-647

12

Musical Emotion Perception in Bimodal Patients: Relative Weighting of Musical Mode and Tempo Cues

Kristen L. D'Onofrio[1]*, Meredith Caldwell[2], Charles Limb[3], Spencer Smith[4], David M. Kessler[1] and René H. Gifford[1]

[1] Cochlear Implant Research Laboratory, Department of Hearing and Speech Sciences, Vanderbilt University, Nashville, TN, United States, [2] Vanderbilt University Medical Center, Nashville, TN, United States, [3] Department of Otolaryngology–Head and Neck Surgery, University of California, San Francisco, San Francisco, CA, United States, [4] Department of Communication Sciences and Disorders, The University of Texas at Austin, Austin, TX, United States

***Correspondence:**
Kristen L. D'Onofrio
kristen.l.donofrio@vanderbilt.edu

Several cues are used to convey musical emotion, the two primary being musical mode and musical tempo. Specifically, major and minor modes tend to be associated with positive and negative valence, respectively, and songs at fast tempi have been associated with more positive valence compared to songs at slow tempi (Balkwill and Thompson, 1999; Webster and Weir, 2005). In Experiment I, we examined the relative weighting of musical tempo and musical mode among adult cochlear implant (CI) users combining electric and contralateral acoustic stimulation, or "bimodal" hearing. Our primary hypothesis was that bimodal listeners would utilize both tempo and mode cues in their musical emotion judgments in a manner similar to normal-hearing listeners. Our secondary hypothesis was that low-frequency (LF) spectral resolution in the non-implanted ear, as quantified via psychophysical tuning curves (PTCs) at 262 and 440 Hz, would be significantly correlated with degree of bimodal benefit for musical emotion perception. In Experiment II, we investigated across-channel spectral resolution using a spectral modulation detection (SMD) task and neural representation of temporal fine structure via the frequency following response (FFR) for a 170-ms /da/ stimulus. Results indicate that CI-alone performance was driven almost exclusively by tempo cues, whereas bimodal listening demonstrated use of both tempo and mode. Additionally, bimodal benefit for musical emotion perception may be correlated with spectral resolution in the non-implanted ear via SMD, as well as neural representation of *F*0 amplitude via FFR – though further study with a larger sample size is warranted. Thus, contralateral acoustic hearing can offer significant benefit for musical emotion perception, and the degree of benefit may be dependent upon spectral resolution of the non-implanted ear.

Keywords: cochlear implant, bimodal, music perception, musical emotion, hearing loss, frequency following response, spectral modulation detection, psychophysical tuning curve

INTRODUCTION

Cochlear implant (CI) technology has improved significantly over the past 30 years, enabling CI users to achieve high levels of speech understanding in quiet listening environments (e.g., average AzBio sentence recognition ranging from 60 to over 80%, even in the absence of visual cues) (Gifford et al., 2018; Gifford and Dorman, 2018; Sladen et al., 2018); however, processing of more complex inputs remains a significant challenge for most CI users (e.g., Hsiao and Gfeller, 2012).

At present, most modern CI processing use an envelope-based strategy in which a fixed pulse rate is amplitude modulated by the envelope of the signal. During this process, the temporal fine structure of the input is discarded. Additional processing limitations include a restricted overall bandwidth (approximately 100–8500 Hz), electrode place mismatch, and spectral smearing. Spectral smearing is particularly problematic and can result from several factors, including a discrete number of electrodes that serve to replace the function of thousands of hair cells, channel interaction due to the inevitable spread of electrical current in a fluid-filled cavity, variable neural survival/degeneration of nerve fibers, and the lack of stochastic neural firing behavior with electrical stimulation. The lack of spectro-temporal detail provided by most CI processing strategies prevents complex signals from being transmitted with accuracy, especially those requiring precise coding of pitch information, such as musical melodies, lexical tone, and vocal emotion (Chatterjee and Peng, 2008; Hsiao and Gfeller, 2012; Luo et al., 2007; Jiam et al., 2017). Thus, music and emotion perception are often significantly poorer in CI users than in normal-hearing listeners.

Music perception ability in CI users is most commonly quantified in terms of four key structural features of music: rhythm, pitch, melody, and timbre. For adult CI patients, performance on temporal-based music tasks tends to be normal or near normal, suggesting minimal to no deficit in tempo or rhythm discrimination (Gfeller et al., 1997; Hsiao and Gfeller, 2012; Kong et al., 2004; Reynolds and Gifford, 2019). In contrast, for the reasons discussed above, pitch, melody, and timbre perception are significantly poorer (Drennan et al., 2015; Kang et al., 2009). We are greatly limited, however, if the assessment of music perception focuses only on the four perceptual elements discussed here. Data from subjective reports add great value to our understanding of music perception in the CI population, with many adult CI users being disappointed with the way music sounds. In fact, several studies report significantly lower music enjoyment ratings post-implantation compared with ratings prior to deafness (Lassaletta et al., 2007; Mirza et al., 2003). Thus, with current technology, a fulfilling sense of music appreciation remains a goal that has yet to be accomplished for many CI recipients.

An additional factor critical to our understanding in this area is the emotional element of music perception. Two primary cues are used to convey musical emotion: musical mode (the type of scale or subset of musical pitches used in the musical excerpt; e.g., major vs. minor) and musical tempo (the speed of the musical excerpt; e.g., fast vs. slow) (Eerola and Vuoskoski, 2013). Specifically, major and minor modes tend to be associated with positive and negative valence, respectively, and songs at fast tempi [i.e., ♩ = 92–196 beats per minute (bpm), Gosselin et al. (2005); ♩ = 80–255 bpm, Peretz et al. (1998)] have been associated with more positive valence compared to songs at slow tempi [i.e., ♩ = 40–60 bpm, Gosselin et al. (2005); ♩ = 20–100 bpm, Peretz et al. (1998), Balkwill and Thompson (1999), Webster and Weir (2005)].

In Western music, a finite set of 12 pitch classes (A, A#/Bb, B, C, C#/Db, D, D#/Eb, E, F, F#/Gb, G, G#/Ab) is utilized, and from these 12 notes, major or minor scales can be produced. The distinction between a major key, e.g., C major, and its parallel natural minor, C natural minor, is a lowered 3rd and 6th scale degree by a half step, or one semitone. For reference, one semitone is the difference between adjacent keys on a keyboard and is the smallest discrete interval utilized in Western music. Normal-hearing listeners can detect changes significantly smaller than one semitone, but the smallest interval detected by CI users is reportedly between 3 and 7.6 semitones, on average (7.6 semitones, Gfeller et al., 2002; 5.7 semitones, Wang et al., 2011; ~3 semitones, Drennan et al., 2015; Kang et al., 2009). Thus, for CI users, the difference between C major and C minor may be perceptually subtle or even indistinguishable.

To date, only a handful of studies have examined musical emotion perception in CI users, and even fewer have parsed out the degree to which tempo and mode cues are utilized in the CI population. Hopyan et al. (2011) studied musical emotion recognition in children with CIs and found that these individuals were significantly less accurate in their perception of musical emotion than their normal-hearing peers. A limitation of this study, however, was that tempo and mode cues were not varied independently of one another. Thus, it is unclear how the two cues were weighted by these listeners and whether one cue may have dominated their musical emotion judgments.

In order to determine how much weight listeners give to one cue over the other, researchers have begun varying mode and tempo independently of one another. Caldwell et al. (2015) presented stimuli that consisted of clips that were of positive valence (major mode at a fast tempo), of negative valence (minor mode at a slow tempo), and of ambiguous valence (major mode at a slow tempo; minor mode at a fast tempo). They showed that compared to normal-hearing listeners, CI listeners gave significantly more weight to temporal cues (tempo; fast vs. slow) than pitch cues (mode; major vs. minor) when interpreting musical emotion. Specifically, CI users' ratings of stimuli with the same tempo were similar, irrespective of mode, while normal-hearing listener ratings' differed significantly for varying mode. Similarly, Hopyan et al. (2016) altered mode, tempo, or both mode and tempo, and found that CI users relied predominantly on tempo. These findings are consistent with previous literature demonstrating that spectral cues are poorly represented for CI users, whereas temporal cues remain robust.

With the known challenges of CI listening, this raises the question of how listeners who utilize the combination of electric (via CI) and acoustic hearing in the contralateral ear (via hearing aid) may perform on tasks of musical emotion perception.

The term "bimodal hearing" is conventionally used to refer to the use of a CI in one ear and a hearing aid in the *contralateral ear.* Indeed, bimodal listeners tend to show better objective and subjective music perception outcomes compared with both unilateral and bilateral CI users (Dorman et al., 2008; El Fata et al., 2009; Gfeller et al., 2008; Sucher and McDermott, 2009). This has largely been attributed to improved access to fundamental frequency (*F*0) and low-frequency (LF) fine structure information in the non-implanted ear (e.g., Smith et al., 2002; Moore, 2003; Li et al., 2013; Dincer et al., 2018). However, much less is known about the acoustic benefits to musical emotion perception, particularly for those with significant hearing loss in the non-CI ear.

Shirvani et al. (2016) compared the musical emotion recognition abilities of children with bimodal configurations and unilateral CIs, showing that bimodal listeners performed significantly better than the unilateral CI group, yet still significantly poorer than normal-hearing listeners. However, similar to the study by Hopyan et al. (2011), they did not vary mode and tempo independently of one another. Giannantonio et al. (2015) examined musical emotion perception in 42 children with CIs, 11 of whom were bimodal listeners. These researchers systematically varied mode, tempo, and both mode and tempo cues, and found that the addition of acoustic hearing in the contralateral ear resulted in greater incorporation of the mode cue – a finding that is indicative of better access to important pitch information via acoustic hearing. Still, further research is warranted in the adult population.

The current study is a replication and extension of the previous work by Caldwell et al. (2015) to include bimodal listeners. The purpose was to examine how musical mode cues (major vs. minor) and musical tempo cues (fast vs. slow) influence the perception of musical emotion among bimodal listeners. CI-alone performance was also assessed, thereby allowing a direct comparison to the CI users' performance in the study by Caldwell et al. (2015), and also allowing for a measure of within-subject bimodal benefit. The primary hypothesis was that, unlike CI-only users, bimodal listeners would utilize both mode and tempo cues in their musical emotion judgments in a manner more similar to normal-hearing listeners. The secondary hypothesis was that LF spectral resolution in the non-implanted ear would be significantly correlated with degree of bimodal benefit for musical emotion perception. Spectral resolution in the non-implanted ear was initially quantified via psychophysical tuning curves (PTCs) (Experiment I). PTCs are considered a psychophysical analog of neural tuning curves, and measure the level of a narrowband noise masker needed to just mask a pure-tone signal fixed in level and in frequency (Moore, 1978). A smaller sample, including a portion from Experiment I, was also tested via spectral modulation detection (SMD) and neural representation of temporal fine structure via the frequency following response (FFR) for a 170-ms /da/ stimulus (Experiment II). In contrast to the within-frequency nature of PTCs, SMD provides an across-frequency measure of spectral resolution. The FFR is an auditory-evoked potential and thereby serves as an objective measure of the auditory system's spectral resolving capabilities.

EXPERIMENT I

Method

Participants

Participants included 15 adult bimodal listeners and 15 normal-hearing (NH) adult controls. Bimodal listeners ranged in age from 24 to 79 years (mean 56 years), and NH controls ranged in age from 22 to 71 years (mean 47 years). Additional demographic information for the bimodal participants is shown in **Table 1**. Normal hearing was defined as pure-tone audiometric thresholds ≤25 dB HL from 250 to 4000 Hz, bilaterally. If a hearing evaluation had not been completed within 6 months prior to the study, an audiometric evaluation was performed. A Grason Stadler GSI 61 audiometer with ER-3A insert earphones was used. Audiometric thresholds for both groups are displayed in **Figure 1**. For the NH group, the right and left ears are averaged together, and for the bimodal group, thresholds are shown for the non-implanted ear only. Although there is significant variability across participants, average hearing loss of the non-implanted ear is moderate sloping to severe. The TEN Test was used to quantify dead regions (areas with few or no functioning inner hair cells and/or auditory neurons) in the non-implanted ear of the bimodal participants (Moore et al., 2000). Dead regions were identified based on a 10-dB or greater shift criterion. Testing using the TEN test determined that 1 participant had a dead region at 500 Hz, 3 at 750 Hz, 1 at 1000 Hz, 3 at 1500 Hz, and 2 at 2000 Hz.

All procedures were explained prior to the study and informed consent was obtained. Following completion of the study, participants were compensated for their participation.

Test Environment

All testing was conducted in a single-walled sound-attenuation chamber. All music stimuli were presented at 65 dBA from a single Yamaha Model HS8 powered speaker positioned at 0° azimuth at a distance of 3 meters from the listener. Stimuli were calibrated in terms of sound pressure level at the location of the participant's head, with the participant absent. For all CI-alone testing in the soundfield, the non-CI ear was plugged with a 3M Classic foam earplug to prevent any inadvertent contribution from the acoustic hearing ear.

Cochlear Implant Programming

The CI settings used for testing were those used by the participant in everyday listening. Directional microphone settings were not activated for any of the testing, and CI-aided thresholds were between 20 and 30 dB HL from 250 to 6000 Hz for all participants.

Hearing Aid Fitting

Since the primary question of interest focused on bimodal benefit from the hearing aid ear, the authors felt it was important to fit all participants with the same device and hearing aid fitting strategy (e.g., NAL-NL2). This was done in an effort to control factors like compression schemes, signal processing, and other automatic hearing aid features. A Phonak Bolero V90 behind-the-ear (BTE) hearing aid with non-custom comply tip coupling was used for all fittings. All fittings were completed on-ear using

TABLE 1 | Bimodal participant demographics (Experiment I).

Participant	Age (years)	Gender	Manufacturer	Internal	Implant ear	Etiology	Duration of deafness	Strategy
1	72	M	AB	MidScala	R	Unknown	Longstanding, progressive	Optima-S
2	58	F	Cochlear	CI522	L	Unknown	Unknown	ACE
3	24	F	Cochlear	CI24RE (CA)	R	Unknown	Longstanding, progressive	ACE
4	64	M	AB	MidScala	R	Meniere's Disease	Longstanding, progressive	Optima-S
5	36	F	AB	MidScala	R	Unknown	Longstanding, progressive	Optima-S
6	35	F	AB	MidScala	L	Unknown	Longstanding	Optima-S
7	79	M	Cochlear	CI24RE (CA)	L	Unknown	Unknown	ACE
8	70	F	AB	MidScala	R	Unknown	Longstanding	Optima-S
9	56	F	AB	MidScala	L	Unknown	Longstanding, progressive	Optima-S
10	54	F	MED-EL	Standard	L	Unknown	Unknown	FS4-p
11	52	M	AB	MidScala	L	Sudden SNHL	Longstanding	Optima-S
12	40	F	Cochlear	CI532	L	Unknown	Unknown	ACE
13	69	M	AB	MidScala	R	Unknown	Longstanding, progressive	Optima-S
14	79	M	Cochlear	CI512	L	Sudden SNHL	5 months	ACE
15	46	F	AB	MidScala	R	Unknown	Unknown	Optima-S
Mean	56							
SD	16.87							

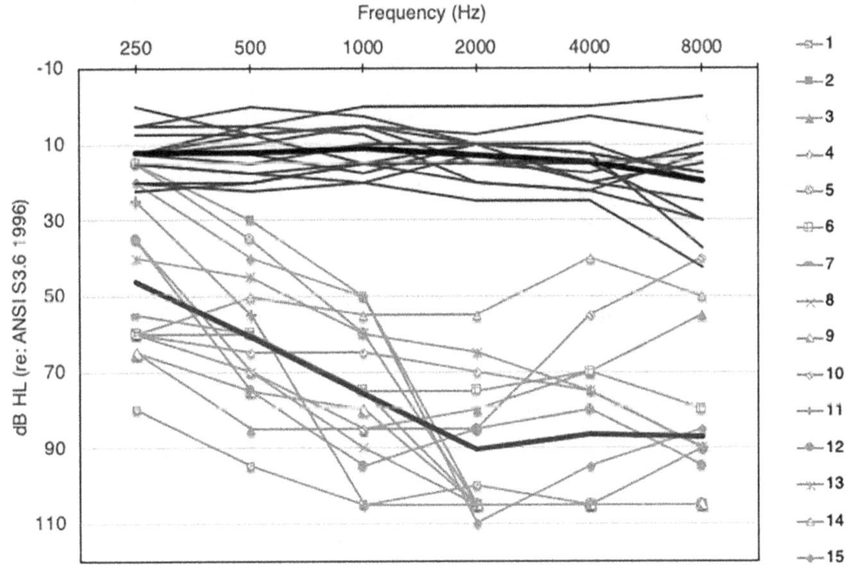

FIGURE 1 | Audiometric thresholds for NH (right and left ears averaged, solid dark gray lines) and bimodal participants (non-implanted ear only, solid light gray lines with symbols). Group means for NH and bimodal are show by the light and dark thick gray lines, respectively.

Audioscan Verifit's probe microphone system. The NAL-NL2 hearing aid prescriptive formula was used, and gain targets for 55, 65, and 75 dB SPL input levels were verified. If a match to target within ~3 dB for all input levels could not be achieved, 65 dB SPL was given priority. Features including noise reduction, acclimatization, frequency lowering, and directional microphone processing were deactivated.

Musical Emotion Perception

The musical emotion stimuli in the current study were taken from Caldwell et al. (2015), in an effort to make direct comparisons with their findings. Their stimuli were created with Finale Songwriter 2012 (MakeMusic, Inc. Eden Prairie, MN, United States), and consist of 12 four-bar melodies played on a piano with chordal accompaniment. Each melody included 10 quarter notes, 4 eighth notes, 2 half notes, and a passing chord. All clips were 20 s long. A 2 × 2 design was utilized to generate four variations of the same melody that differed in mode (major vs. minor) and tempo (fast: 180 bpm vs. slow: 60 bpm), thus resulting in either congruent or incongruent pairings of mode and tempo information. The four variations were as follows: Major/Fast (majF) – congruent, Major/Slow (majS) – incongruent, Minor/Fast (minF) – incongruent, and Minor/Slow (minS) – congruent. This resulted in 3 valence categories: positive valence (majF), negative valence (minS), and ambiguous valence (minF and majS). The ambiguous valence stimuli are considered incongruent because the mode and tempo information is conflicting. This category is particularly important because it allows one to examine how participants weight the two cues in their musical emotion perception process. If a difference exists across group/listening configurations (CI-alone vs. bimodal vs. NH) in the degree to which participants weight one cue over the other, it would be evident on the incongruent, ambiguous valence trials. During stimuli presentation, "slow" melodies were played once and "fast" melodies were repeated three times, so that both slow and fast tempo clips were the same overall duration. All four variations of the 12 melodies were presented, yielding 48 test items in total. Task instructions were delivered as follows: "You will hear several short melodies. During each melody, please focus on the emotion conveyed. After the melody is finished, you will be asked to rate it on a scale from 0 (very sad) to 10 (very happy)."

Bimodal listeners were tested in both the CI-alone and bimodal listening configurations. Order of listening configuration was alternated across participants. In order for the NH group to complete the same number of trials as the bimodal group, NH listeners were tested twice. After each 20-s stimulus was played, participants rated the stimulus on a Likert scale from + 5 (very happy) to −5 (very sad).

Musical Training and Aptitude Questionnaire

All participants completed the Ollen Musical Sophistication Index (OMSI) (Ollen, 2006) as a measure of individual musical training and aptitude. The OMSI is a 10-item, online questionnaire, which classifies individuals as "more" or "less musically sophisticated." Specifically, a score is generated which indicates the probability that a music expert would classify that individual as "more musically sophisticated." Individuals who score over 500 are considered "more musically sophisticated," and those who score less than 500 are considered "less musically sophisticated" (Ollen, 2006).

Psychophysical Tuning Curves

In Experiment I, spectral resolution in the non-implanted ear was quantified in terms of frequency selectivity at 262 Hz (C4, or "middle C") and 440 Hz (A4, or "A440"), and was measured via PTCs with narrowband noise masker. PTCs were obtained via sweeping psychophysical tuning curve (SWPTC) software (Sęk et al., 2005; Sęk and Moore, 2011). This was completed in each ear individually for participants with normal hearing and in the non-implanted ear of bimodal participants. The bandwidth for the narrowband noise masker was 20% of the signal frequency (Sęk et al., 2005) and all signal and masker parameters were selected as default by the SWPTC program (Sęk and Moore, 2011). The purpose of this measure was to quantify individual LF spectral resolution at two frequencies particularly relevant to the music domain. A440 is considered the tuning standard for music pitch (International Organization for Standardization [ISO], 1975), and both C4 (or "middle C") and A440, are within the range of the music stimuli utilized in this study. Secondarily, this was completed to examine the relationship between frequency selectivity and bimodal benefit for musical emotion perception.

With the SWPTC software, PTCs are measured using a continuous, narrowband noise masker swept in frequency. Specifically, listeners are asked to detect a pulsed sinusoidal tone in the presence of the masker with a center frequency that sweeps from high to low (reverse sweep) or from low to high (forward sweep). The tone is first presented in the absence of the noise masker to familiarize the listener with the signal of interest. The masker is then added. Instructions to the participant are to press and hold the space bar on a standard computer keyboard when the tone is heard. The masker level is increased at a rate determined by the experimenter (2 dB/sec is the default value) when the space bar is pressed. When the tone is no longer audible, the listener is instructed to release the space bar. The masker level is decreased until the space bar is pressed again, indicating that the tone is again audible. During this process, the level needed to just mask the tone is tracked. In all cases, presentation level for each frequency was determined via the threshold measurement procedure within the software. Once a threshold was determined, the presentation level was calculated to be 10 dB SL.

From this task, a measure of the Q_{10} value and tip frequency of the PTC is estimated. The Q_{10} value indicates sharpness of tuning and is calculated as the signal frequency divided by the bandwidth of the PTC 10 dB above the tip frequency. Higher values indicate sharper tuning and are associated with good frequency selectivity. Lower values indicate broader PTCs and are associated with poorer frequency selectivity, with poorest frequency selectivity approaching a Q_{10} value of 0. From the tip frequency value, tip shift can also be calculated. In this study, tip shift was determined by taking the absolute value of the difference between tip frequency and stimulus frequency. For the NH listeners, right and left ear performance was averaged together for all analyses.

DATA ANALYSIS AND RESULTS

Data analysis focused on within-subject rating differences (CI-alone vs. bimodal) and between groups rating differences (bimodal vs. NH, and CI-alone vs. NH). Bimodal benefit was defined as the difference between scores in the bimodal condition and scores in the CI-alone condition. The GraphPad Prism 7.0d (San Diego, CA, United States) and IBM SPSS Statistics Version 25 (Armonk, NY, United States) software programs were utilized for all statistical analyses. For all correlation analyses, the strength of the correlation was quantified using Cohen's (1988) classification system.

Musical Emotion Perception

There were two primary analyses of our musical emotion data – the first examined the effect of the mode cue. For this assessment, within-subject comparisons were made across the stimuli pairings for which tempo was held constant (e.g., majF vs. minF, minS vs. majS). The purpose of this analysis was to determine the extent to which listeners were able to make use of mode in their judgments. Said differently, this analysis provided

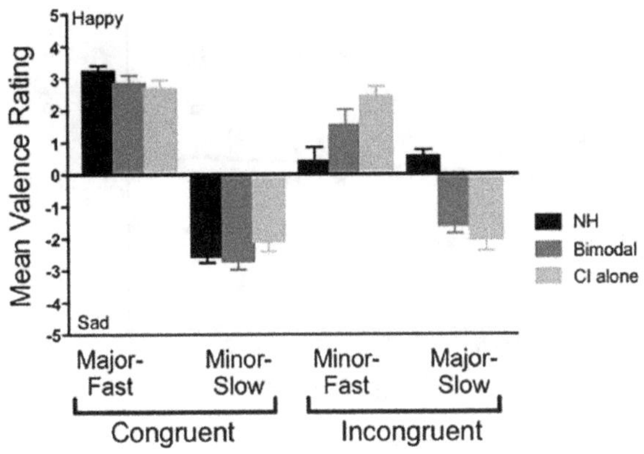

FIGURE 2 | Mean musical emotion ratings across group. Error bars represent + 1 SEM.

an examination of the extent to which ratings were dominated by the tempo cue. A Wilcoxon matched-pairs signed rank test was used for analysis with the significance level defined as $\alpha = 0.05$. For all analyses of musical emotion, non-parametric tests were used due to the ordinal nature of the data.

Figure 2 shows results from the musical emotion task for the NH listeners and the bimodal participants in both listening conditions. As discussed, the first analysis focused on the degree to which listeners utilized the mode cue. Here, valence ratings were compared across stimuli where the tempo cue was held constant (e.g., majF vs. minF, minS vs. majS). For NH listeners, results from a Wilcoxon matched-pairs signed rank test revealed significant differences in ratings for the majF vs. minF comparison ($Z = -3.408$, $p = 0.01$) and the minS vs. majS comparison ($Z = -3.408$, $p = 0.01$). Likewise, for the bimodal condition, significant differences were evident for both the majF vs. minF comparison ($Z = -2.926$, $p = 0.01$) and the minS vs. majS comparison ($Z = -3.074$, $p = 0.01$). However, for CI-alone, there were no statistically significant differences in ratings for the majF vs. minF comparison ($Z = -1.609$, $p = 0.11$) or the minS vs. majS comparison ($Z = -0.114$, $p = 0.91$). These results demonstrate that when tempo is held constant, NH and bimodal listeners make use of mode in determining the emotional valence of a piece of music, whereas CI-alone listeners do not.

The second analysis focused on the effect of group/listening condition, particularly for the incongruent stimuli pairings. For this assessment, rating differences for both minF and majS were examined, as any benefit of acoustic hearing in the bimodal condition would be evident for these stimuli. Specifically, if bimodal users perceptually combine mode information from acoustic hearing with tempo information through the CI, their emotional valence ratings of incongruent stimuli should be ambiguous, as is observed in NH listeners. A Wilcoxon matched-pairs signed rank test was used to assess differences for CI-alone vs. bimodal, and a Mann-Whitney test was used to assess differences for CI-alone vs. NH and bimodal vs. NH. Significance levels were defined as $\alpha = 0.05$.

Results from a Wilcoxon matched-pairs signed rank test showed that performance between bimodal and CI-alone listening did not differ significantly for either the minF stimulus ($Z = -1.917$, $p = 0.06$) or the majS stimulus ($Z = -1.817$, $p = 0.07$). Results from a Mann-Whitney test show that the difference in performance between bimodal and NH listeners was not significant for the minF stimulus ($U = 69$, $p = 0.07$), but was significant for the majS stimulus ($U = 7$, $p = 0.01$). The same analysis between CI-alone and NH listeners revealed a significant difference in performance for both the minF stimulus ($U = 34$, $p = 0.01$) and the majS stimulus ($U = 12$, $p = 0.01$). In other words, for the minF stimulus in particular, the addition of acoustic hearing improved CI listener performance to a level that was not significantly different from NH performance. In contrast, performance for the majS stimulus did not demonstrate this same magnitude of improvement for the bimodal listening condition.

Musical Training and Aptitude Questionnaire

Listeners achieved scores on the OMSI of 441 and 172 for the NH and bimodal groups, respectively. According to the standard OMSI scoring, both groups would be classified as "less musically sophisticated" (Ollen, 2006).

Psychophysical Tuning Curves

Frequency selectivity was evaluated at 262 and 440 Hz, and analysis focused on a comparison of sharpness of tuning, as demonstrated by the Q_{10} value for each frequency. Performance differences for the NH listeners (both ears averaged together) and the non-implanted ear of bimodal patients were compared using an independent sample t-test with the significance level defined as $\alpha = 0.05$. Of note, Q_{10} values for some of the bimodal participants (those with poorest LF thresholds) could not be calculated and were omitted from analysis (Participants 1, 3, and 14 at 262 Hz and Participants 1 and 12 at 440 Hz). Individual Q_{10} values for bimodal participants were included in **Figure 3**. For the participants for whom a Q_{10} could not be calculated, scores are represented via a hypothetical Q_{10} value of "0" and depicted as a diamond symbol.

Tables 2, 3 show the Q_{10} values and tip shift values for 262 and 440 Hz, respectively, for the NH and bimodal participants. On average, NH listeners demonstrated sharper tuning at both frequencies compared to bimodal listeners. Specifically, the difference in Q_{10} values across groups was significant for both 262 and 440 Hz using an independent sample t-test ($t_{25} = 3.04$, $p = 0.01$ and $t_{26} = 5.65$, $p = 0.01$, respectively). This finding was expected given the poorer frequency selectivity and greater variability often seen among listeners with hearing loss (Green et al., 2012). Regarding tip shift, values for NH listeners are expected to be near the test frequency (Sęk and Moore, 2011). Degree of tip shift was minimal and about equivalent for both groups for 262 Hz, and was substantially greater among bimodal listeners for 440 Hz. Our NH results for 440 Hz are consistent with Q_{10} and tip shift values reported for a similar frequency in the literature (e.g., mean Q_{10} at 500 Hz = 2.6, tip shift = 5 Hz, Shabana et al., 2014). Other studies utilizing higher

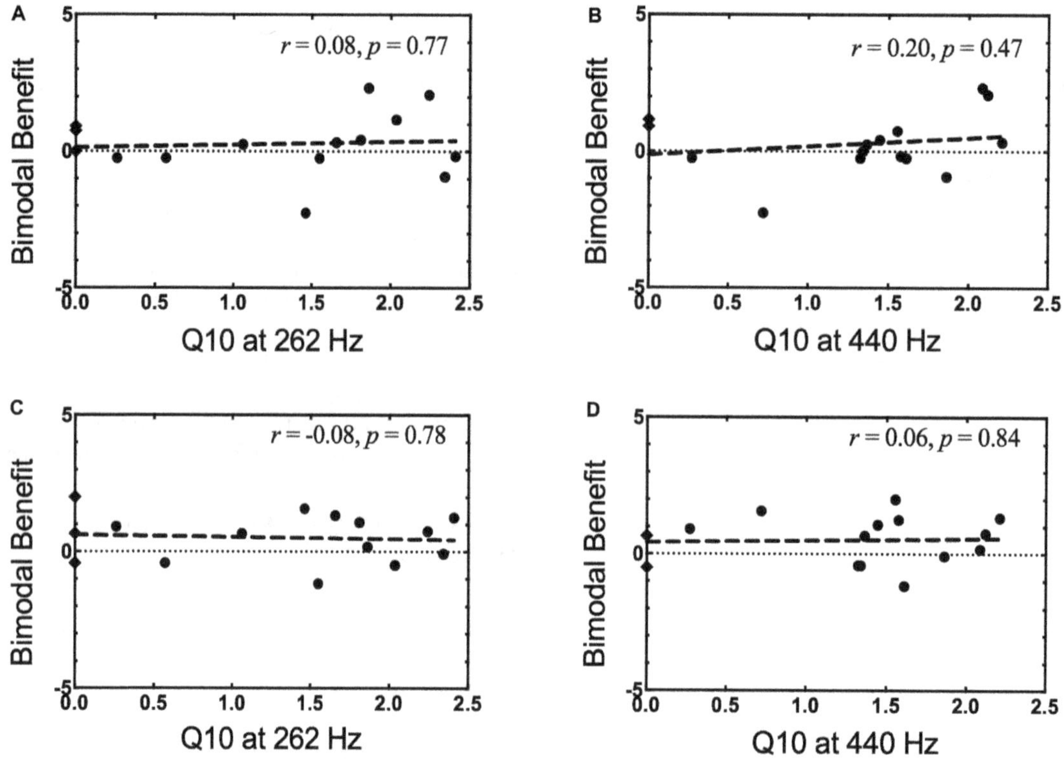

FIGURE 3 | (A–D) Bimodal benefit for musical emotion vs. Q_{10}. **(A)** minF vs. Q_{10} at 262 Hz. **(B)** minF vs. Q_{10} at 440 Hz. **(C)** majS vs. Q_{10} at 262 Hz. **(D)** majS vs. Q_{10} at 440 Hz. Q_{10} values that could not be completed were represented as a hypothetical Q_{10} value of "0" and notated by a diamond symbol.

TABLE 2 | SWPTC results for 262 Hz in NH participants (right and left ears averaged together) and bimodal participants (non-implanted ear only).

	NH		Bimodal	
	Q_{10}	Tip shift (Hz)	Q_{10}	Tip shift (Hz)
Mean	2.16	10.46	1.61	9.77
SD	0.19	7.09	0.68	11.43

TABLE 3 | SWPTC results for 440 Hz in NH participants (right and left ears averaged together) and bimodal participants (non-implanted ear only).

	NH		Bimodal	
	Q_{10}	Tip shift (Hz)	Q_{10}	Tip shift (Hz)
Mean	2.44	7.07	1.50	29.25
SD	0.33	11.72	0.55	31.69

test frequencies have found similar, albeit slightly greater results indicating sharper tuning (e.g., mean Q_{10} at 1000 Hz = ~4, mean Q_{10} at 4000 Hz = ~5, Bidelman et al., 2014).

Relationship Between Bimodal Benefit and Frequency Selectivity

In light of our second hypothesis, the relationship between spectral resolution in the non-implanted ear and bimodal benefit for musical emotion was examined. Pearson product-moment correlations between bimodal benefit for the minF stimulus and Q_{10} at 262 Hz and 440 Hz were both weak and non-significant (r = 0.08, p = 0.77 and r = 0.20, p = 0.47, respectively). This relationship is shown in **Figures 3A,B**, respectively. Pearson product-moment correlations between bimodal benefit for the majS stimulus and Q_{10} at 262 Hz and 440 Hz were also weak and non-significant (r = −0.08, p = 0.78 and r = 0.06, p = 0.84, respectively). In other words, there was no statistically significant relationship between spectral resolution – as defined via PTCs – in the non-implanted ear and bimodal benefit for musical emotion perception. This is shown in **Figures 3C,D**, respectively.

Relationship Between Bimodal Benefit and Pure Tone Average (PTA)

The relationship between bimodal benefit for musical emotion perception and LF PTA in the non-implanted ear was also examined. LF PTA was defined here as the average of thresholds at 250 and 500 Hz, and ranged from 22.5 dB HL to 87.5 dB HL. Pearson product-moment correlations between LF PTA and bimodal benefit for the minF and majS stimuli were both weak and non-significant (r = −0.10, p = 0.72 and r = −0.14, p = 0.63, respectively); thus, audiometric thresholds in the non-implanted ear were not related to bimodal benefit for musical emotion perception.

Because several participants had useable hearing above 500 Hz, both standard PTA (500, 1000, and 2000 Hz) and a high frequency (HF) PTA (4000 and 8000 Hz) were also examined. The Pearson product-moment correlation between bimodal benefit for the minF stimulus and PTA was weak and non-significant ($r = -0.19$, $p = 0.50$), as was the relationship with HF PTA ($r = -0.07$, $p = 0.82$). The Pearson product-moment correlation between bimodal benefit for the majS stimulus and PTA was also weak and non-significant ($r = -0.30$, $p = 0.27$), as was the relationship with HF PTA ($r = -0.28$, $p = 0.31$).

DISCUSSION

There were two primary questions of interest in Experiment I: (1) Are bimodal listeners able to utilize both mode and tempo cues in their musical emotion judgments in a manner more similar to NH listeners? (2) Is LF spectral resolution in the non-implanted ear, as quantified by PTCs at 262 and 440 Hz, correlated with bimodal benefit for musical emotion perception?

Are Bimodal Listeners Able to Utilize Both Mode and Tempo Cues in Their Musical Emotion Judgments in a Manner More Similar to NH Listeners?

Our primary question of interest was analyzed in two ways. The first analysis examined the effect of mode, by comparing valence ratings for the stimuli where tempo was held constant (e.g., majF vs. minF, and minS vs. majS). Our data show that both NH and bimodal listeners demonstrated significantly different ratings for the majF vs. minF and minS vs. majS comparisons. In other words, both groups accounted for mode in their ratings of incongruent stimuli. This finding among NH listeners was expected and is consistent with previous literature by Caldwell et al. (2015), where NH listeners provided significantly different ratings for stimuli that varied in mode. Importantly, our findings extend this earlier work to show that with the addition of LF acoustic hearing in the non-implanted ear, bimodal listeners were also able to consider both tempo and mode in their judgments of musical emotion.

In contrast, CI-alone listening relied almost exclusively on tempo cues, as there was no difference in valance ratings for the majF vs. minF and minS vs. majS comparisons. This finding was also consistent with Caldwell et al. (2015), where CI users provided similar ratings to stimuli with the same tempo irrespective of mode. Further, this finding was consistent with existing literature demonstrating that spectral cues are represented poorly among CI users, whereas temporal cues remain robust (Limb and Roy, 2014).

The second analysis focused on the effect of group/listening condition, particularly for the incongruent stimuli pairings. The findings presented here suggest that, on average, bimodal listening yields more typical musical emotion judgments than CI-alone, particularly for the minF stimulus, where ratings in the bimodal condition did not differ significantly from NH ratings. Results for the majS stimulus were also trending similarly, although the improvement was to a lesser degree and remained significantly different from NH performance. This finding is perhaps a product of the participants' own internal weighting of "slow" vs. "fast." It is possible that for this group of listeners, a slow tempo is considered more robust with respect to conveying emotion than is a fast tempo, and thus, the slow cue dominated more so than the fast cue for the incongruent pairings. Future research in this area may consider examining and controlling for tempo as an internal weighting factor.

Taken together, these findings yield support for our first hypothesis. The addition of acoustic hearing in the contralateral ear allowed for significantly greater use of the mode cue, and thus, ratings shifted in the direction of NH performance. Further, for the minF stimulus in particular, performance shifted to a degree that was not significantly different from NH performance.

Is Low-Frequency Spectral Resolution in the Non-implanted Ear Correlated With Bimodal Benefit for Musical Emotion Perception?

Our second question sought to determine whether improvement in the bimodal condition was related to spectral resolution in the non-implanted ear as quantified by frequency selectivity at two frequencies germane to the music domain – 262 Hz and 440 Hz. In contrast to our second hypothesis, mean tuning "sharpness" at 262 and 440 Hz did not appear to be related to bimodal benefit for musical emotion perception, as there was no correlation between bimodal benefit for either minF or majS and frequency selectivity at either frequency.

One interpretation of this finding is that the two frequencies chosen for testing may not have been particularly relevant or generalizable to the specific stimuli utilized in this study. While both frequencies are included in our chordal and melodic stimuli, they account for a relatively small portion of the total notes utilized in these tasks. Alternatively, these frequencies may be partially relevant, but perhaps an analysis of spectral resolution over a broader frequency range would yield better predictive value. SMD was examined in a portion of this sample as a means of quantifying spectral resolution over a broader spectrum and will be discussed as part of Experiment II.

Relationship Between Bimodal Benefit and PTA

Pure tone average was also not predictive of bimodal benefit for musical emotion perception. This finding carries important clinical significance, as some of the participants with the poorest thresholds received the greatest benefit for musical emotion. It is possible that interpretation of the musical mode cue may rely more heavily upon robust spectral resolution than the mere ability to detect pure tones at a low-level (or even the presence of sharp tuning at two distinct low frequencies). The clinical relevance of this finding is that we likely cannot use the audiogram as a means to determine whether a listener will derive significant musical emotion perception. Clearly, there are contributing factors that have not yet been accounted for.

Limitations

The authors recognize that there are inherent limitations to using a unidimensional rating scale for the musical emotion judgments. Further, the authors recognize that not all major mode, fast tempo music is perceived as "happy," and not all minor mode, slow tempo music is perceived as "sad." There are several additional cues that convey emotion which were not examined in this study, including dynamics, articulation, timing, timbre, consonance/dissonance, and melodic, harmonic, and rhythmic complexity (Balkwill and Thompson, 1999; Gabrielsson and Juslin, 1996). For NH listeners, all of these cues may be utilized for the perception of musical emotion (Bachorowski, 1999; Eerola and Vuoskoski, 2013; Scherer, 2003), whereas for CI users, additional cues involving changes in pitch may be distorted. The stimuli used in this study controlled for most of these additional cues while attempting to isolate the two that are most dominant – mode and tempo. However, in doing so, we may be underestimating CI users' perception of emotion in more realistic musical pieces. Cues such as dynamics, articulation, timing, and rhythmic complexity can be well-preserved with current signal processing strategies and may be significant contributors to the perception of emotion in real-world music among CI recipients.

EXPERIMENT II

Spectral resolution as measured in Experiment I focused on a within-frequency estimate provided by PTCs. However, as mentioned, spectral resolution at discrete frequencies was likely insufficient for explaining bimodal stimulation relevance for musically complex stimuli as investigated here. Thus in Experiment II, we investigated across-frequency spectral resolution using a SMD task for a broadband carrier (125–8000 Hz). In addition to SMD, we also sought to define the neural representation of periodicity and temporal fine structure via the FFR for a 170-ms /da/ stimulus. The primary question of interest in Experiment II was whether these two measures of spectral resolution may better explain bimodal benefit for musical emotion perception, as compared to the PTC data from Experiment I.

Method

Participants included 11 NH adult controls and 8 adult bimodal listeners from Experiment I, plus 1 additional bimodal participant who was not included in Experiment I analysis. Bimodal listeners ranged in age from 24 to 79 years (mean 52 years), and NH controls ranged in age from 22 to 71 years (mean 51 years). There were 5 Advanced Bionics users, 3 Cochlear users, and 1 MED-EL user in this sample. Additional demographic information for the bimodal participants is shown in **Table 4**.

Measures of Spectral Resolution

Spectral modulation detection

Spectral modulation detection was measured using the quick SMD task developed by Gifford et al. (2014). A three-interval, forced choice paradigm was used based on a modified method of constant stimuli, with two intervals consisting of a flat spectrum noise and the remaining interval consisting of a frequency modulated noise. Unlike the task described previously by Gifford et al. (2014), this version of the task used a constant modulation rate of 1.0 cyc/oct with 10 modulation depths ranging from 4 to 22 dB, in 2-dB steps (Holder et al., 2018). Sixty trials were completed (6 at each modulation depth). A percent correct score for each modulation depth was provided. Stimuli were presented to the non-implanted ear of the bimodal participants at the participant's most comfortable loudness level (levels ranged from 88–108 dB SPL; mean = 101.79 dB SPL, *SD* = 6). Presentation level across trials was roved ± 5 dB to help avoid level-based cues. NH participants did not complete the SMD task. This measure was added after the study had commenced, and thus, efforts to bring back previously enrolled participants were aimed at bimodal listeners, for whom the relationship between performance and bimodal benefit could be examined.

Frequency following response

Frequency following responses were measured using a 170-ms /da/ stimulus (fundamental frequency ($F0$) = 100 Hz, first formant ($F1$) = 700 Hz). Stimuli were delivered at a rate of 4.35 Hz using magnetically shielded Etymotic ER-3A insert earphones in a single-walled sound treated test booth. For the bimodal

TABLE 4 | Bimodal participant demographics (Experiment II).

Participant	Age (years)	Gender	Manufacturer	Internal	Implant ear	Etiology	Duration of deafness	Strategy
1	24	F	Cochlear	CI24RE (CA)	R	Unknown	Longstanding, progressive	ACE
2	64	M	AB	MidScala	R	Meniere's Disease	Longstanding, progressive	Optima-S
3	36	F	AB	MidScala	R	Unknown	Longstanding, progressive	Optima-S
4	79	M	Cochlear	CI24RE (CA)	L	Unknown	Unknown	ACE
5	70	F	AB	MidScala	R	Unknown	Longstanding	Optima-S
6	54	F	MED-EL	Standard	L	Unknown	Unknown	FS4-p
7	40	F	Cochlear	CI532	L	Unknown	Unknown	ACE
8	46	F	AB	MidScala	R	Unknown	Unknown	Optima-S
9*	55	F	AB	MidScala	R	Unknown	Unknown	Optima-S
Mean	52							
SD	17.43							

**Participant was not part of Experiment 1 dataset.*

participants, stimuli were presented at 90 dB SPL to the non-implanted ear. For the NH listeners, stimuli were presented at 80 dB SPL to either the right or left ear (counterbalanced between participants).

Each FFR was taken as the average of 3000 stimulus repetitions, with an artifact rejection of +35 μV. Low-pass and high-pass filters were set to 5000 Hz and 1 Hz, respectively, to permit *post hoc* filtering. Stimulus polarity was set as alternating, and thus allowed for analysis of envelope and temporal fine structure cues by either adding or subtracting responses to each polarity, respectively. An Intelligent Hearing System (IHS) Duet System (Smart EP, Miami FL, United States) was used for stimulus generation and presentation. All participants were positioned in a reclining chair during data collection and were instructed to remain as relaxed as possible, while still remaining awake. A vertical electrode montage with a three Ag-AgCl electrode array (Cz active, Fpz ground, earlobe reference) was utilized. The CI processor was removed during all recordings, and two runs were completed for each participant.

DATA ANALYSIS AND RESULTS

Spectral Modulation Detection

Each participant's percent correct score for each modulation depth was plotted, and a general linear model was used to create a psychometric function. More specifically, the MATLAB statistics toolbox function glmfit was used to generate a logit link function. A threshold (to the nearest dB) was determined for the modulation depth representing the 70% correct point on the psychometric function. Thus, spectral resolution was described as a threshold representing the modulation depth, in dB, yielding 70% correct. Lower thresholds indicate better spectral resolution. On average, acoustic SMD threshold for the non-implanted ear of bimodal listeners was 9.72 dB with a range of 4.56 to 17.43 dB. Individual psychometric functions are plotted in **Figure 4**.

Frequency Following Response

The two FFR recordings obtained from each participant were averaged and bandpass filtered between 70 and 3000 Hz. Spectral analysis of the averaged recording was completed using a fast fourier transform (FFT) applied over the 60–180 ms interval of the epoch, which corresponds to the steady state vowel portion of the /da/ stimulus. The envelope of the FFR is unaffected by polarity change, and thus, the FFRs obtained via stimuli of alternating polarities were added in an effort to enhance the *F*0 envelope, while simultaneously reducing the spectral components (e.g., *F*1, *F*2, etc.). The envelope amplitude spectrum at the *F*0 of the /da/ stimulus (100 Hz), in μV, was determined for each participant. *F*0 responses were considered "present" if they were above the estimated noise floor at 100 Hz calculated from the prestimulus interval from −20 to 0 ms. Based on this criterion, energy was present at the *F*0 for all participants in control and bimodal groups.

Figures 5A,B show the grand average waveform and envelope spectra for the NH group. **Figures 6A,B** show the grand average waveform and envelope spectra for the bimodal group. On average, NH listeners demonstrated larger *F*0 amplitudes compared to bimodal listeners (0.17 μV vs. 0.08 μV, respectively); however, the difference between groups was not statistically significant using an independent sample *t*-test ($t_{11 \cdot 12} = 1.542, p = 0.15$).

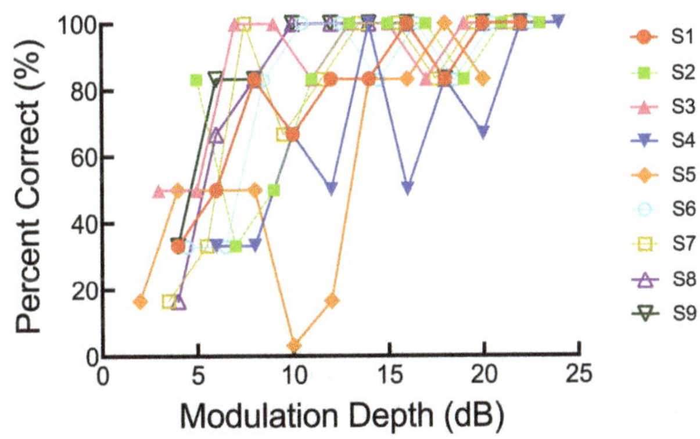

FIGURE 4 | Individual psychometric functions for the SMD task.

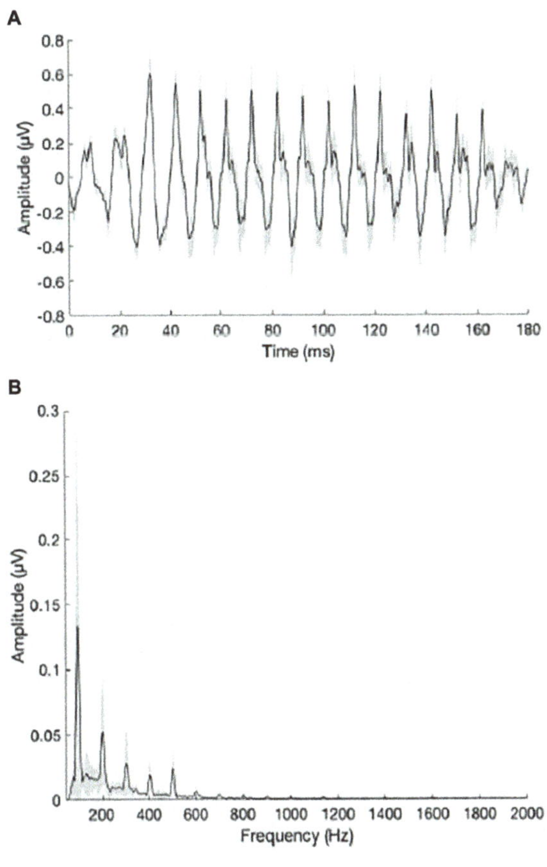

FIGURE 5 | (A) Grand average waveform for the NH group. **(B)** Grand average envelope spectrum for the NH group. The peak in the envelope spectrum at 100 Hz reflects neural phase-locking to the *F*0 of the /da/ stimulus. Shading = SEM.

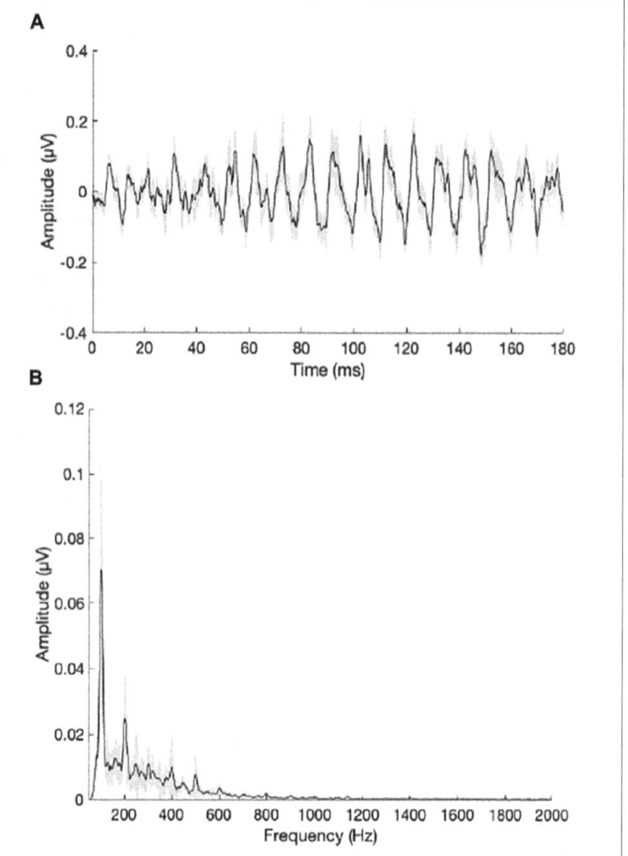

FIGURE 6 | (A) Grand average waveform for the bimodal group. **(B)** Grand average envelope spectrum for the bimodal group. The peak in the envelope spectrum at 100 Hz reflects neural phase-locking to the *F*0 of the /da/ stimulus. Shading = SEM.

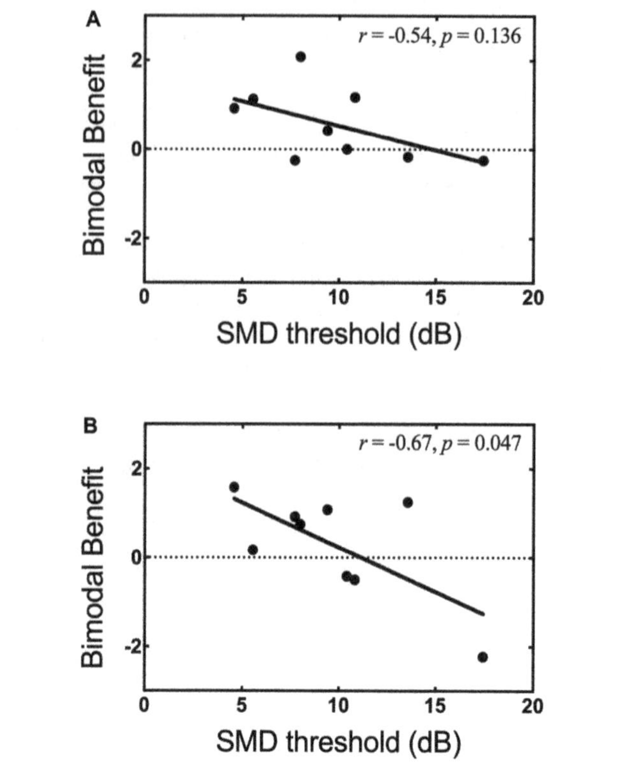

FIGURE 7 | Bimodal benefit for musical emotion vs. SMD threshold. **(A)** minF vs. SMD threshold. **(B)** majS vs. SMD threshold.

Relationship Between Bimodal Benefit and Spectral Modulation Detection

In light of our second hypothesis, the relationship between SMD threshold in the non-implanted ear and bimodal benefit for musical emotion was examined. The Pearson product-moment correlation between bimodal benefit for the minF stimulus and SMD threshold was moderate, but not statistically significant ($r = -0.54$, $p = 0.14$). There was a strong correlation between bimodal benefit for the majS stimulus and SMD threshold ($r = -0.67$, $p = 0.05$). These relationships are shown in **Figures 7A,B**, respectively. Because of the possibility that the majS correlation was driven by a single data point, the relationship with SMD threshold was re-analyzed after removing the participant with bimodal benefit of −2.22 for the majS stimulus. Upon re-analysis, the correlation between bimodal benefit for the majS stimulus vs. SMD threshold was weak and no longer statistically significant ($r = -0.233$, $p = 0.59$).

Relationship Between Bimodal Benefit and FFR

The relationship between *F*0 amplitude in the non-implanted ear and bimodal benefit for musical emotion was also examined. Of note, the bimodal listeners did not exhibit evidence for neural representation of *F*1 (700 Hz), likely due to the severity of hearing loss; thus, all analysis was focused on *F*0. The Pearson product-moment correlation between bimodal benefit for the minF stimulus and *F*0 amplitude was moderate, but not statistically significant ($r = 0.60$, $p = 0.09$). In contrast, there was a strong and statistically significant correlation between bimodal benefit for the majS stimulus and *F*0 amplitude ($r = 0.67$, $p = 0.05$). These data suggest that neural representation of *F*0 in the non-implanted ear is related, at least in part, to bimodal benefit for music emotion perception. These relationships are shown in **Figures 8A,B**, respectively. For the same reasons as discussed in the preceding paragraph, the participant with bimodal benefit of −2.22 for the majS stimulus was removed and the relationship with *F*0 amplitude was re-analyzed. Upon re-analysis, the correlation between bimodal benefit for the majS stimulus vs. *F*0 amplitude was moderate and no longer statistically significant ($r = 0.524$, $p = 0.18$).

DISCUSSION

For Experiment II, our primary research question was in relation to our secondary hypothesis: Is LF spectral resolution in the non-implanted ear correlated with bimodal benefit for musical emotion perception? Importantly, our results must be interpreted cautiously within the context of the reduced sample size in

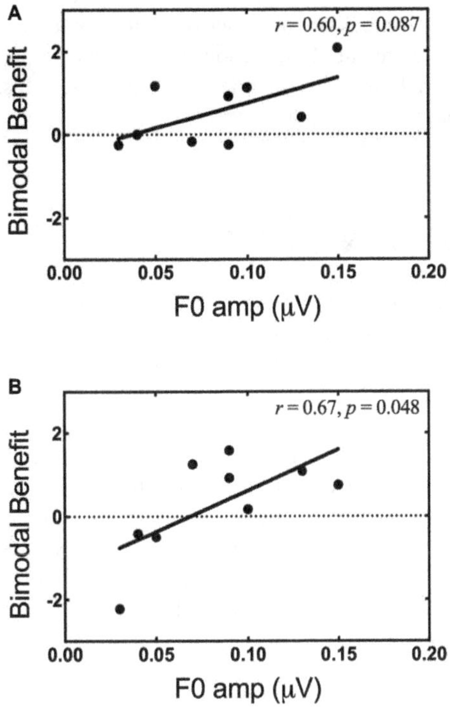

FIGURE 8 | Bimodal benefit for musical emotion vs. *F0* amplitude. **(A)** minF vs. *F0* amplitude. **(B)** majS vs. *F0* amplitude.

Experiment II. Future study in this area is warranted. Secondly, Experiment I analyses were rerun with this limited sample, and it is noteworthy that all musical emotion perception results were consistent with the original analyses, with the exception of one comparison. Results from a Wilcoxon matched-pairs signed rank test showed that performance between bimodal and CI-alone listening differed significantly for the minF stimulus ($Z = -2.193$, $p = 0.03$). In other words, this suggests that the addition of acoustic hearing improved performance with minF stimuli to a level that was significantly better than CI-alone. This is the only finding from this smaller sample that differed from Experiment I.

In Experiment II, spectral resolution was quantified behaviorally via SMD and objectively via FFR using a 170-ms /da/ stimulus ($F0 = 100$ Hz). While the FFR is not a conventional measure of spectral resolution, *per se*, it does provide information about the spectral resolving capabilities of the auditory system, as it is a neurophonic response. Our data suggest that both SMD and neural representation of *F0* amplitude may be correlated with bimodal benefit for musical emotion perception – though further study with a larger sample size is still warranted. Additionally, we should note here that the relationship between SMD thresholds and bimodal benefit for the majS stimulus must be interpreted with caution given that some of the participants exhibited non-monotonic psychometric functions (**Figure 5**). Still, both SMD and FFR yielded better predictive value than did an examination of within-channel frequency selectivity at 262 and 440 Hz, as discussed in Experiment I.

The results of Experiment II are promising. With respect to the FFR specifically, this measure holds potential for the *objective* assessment of auditory system integrity. Given its objective nature, this is particularly relevant in cases where behavioral responses are unobtainable (e.g., the pediatric population, patients with multiple disabilities, etc.). Furthermore, the FFR may serve as a useful tool in helping to guide clinical recommendation for retention of bimodal hearing or pursuit of a second CI. Indeed, the utility of the FFR as it relates to bimodal benefit extends beyond musical emotion perception, as Kessler et al. (2020) showed a significant relationship between FFR *F0* amplitude (170-ms /da/) and bimodal benefit for speech recognition. Thus, the FFR appears to hold predictive utility for bimodal benefit in both the speech and music domains. Further investigation is warranted to understand how different features of acoustic speech are neurally encoded in listeners with low frequency residual hearing.

While SMD was also correlated with bimodal benefit for musical emotion perception, Kessler et al. (2020) found no relationship between SMD and bimodal benefit for speech recognition. Therefore, the FFR may be an advantageous measure due to its predictive value with respect to bimodal benefit for both music and speech stimuli. The ability of the FFR to predict speech recognition in noise has been demonstrated across the lifespan in NH listeners and listeners with some hearing loss (Anderson et al., 2010, 2011, 2013; Song et al., 2011; Thompson et al., 2017). Further, an additional advantage is its utility for difficult-to-test populations.

Limitations

There are important limitations to note for Experiment II. First, as previously discussed, the sample size was small as only a portion of our total sample completed Experiment II. Thus, it is possible that the correlations were driven by a single data point. Indeed, when the participant with bimodal benefit of −2.22 for the majS stimulus was removed from analysis, the correlations between bimodal benefit for the majS stimulus vs. SMD threshold and *F0* amplitude were weak to moderate and were no longer statistically significant. Further study with a larger sample size is warranted to determine if this data point is truly an outlier, and if the relationships hold for larger groups. Second, hearing loss in the non-CI ear of bimodal participants was variable across participants, and additionally, our approach for determining presentation level for the SMD stimulus was based on the participant's most comfortable loudness level. Thus, given the variability in hearing sensitivity and the self-selected presentation levels, bandwidth audibility inevitably varied across participants. The individual differences in bandwidth audibility may have differentially affected performance. To better control for variability in audibility, we have interest in future investigations applying frequency-specific amplification for the FFR-stimuli as has been done by Anderson et al. (2013). Finally, while our results show significant promise, an even stronger relationship between bimodal benefit for musical emotion perception and neural representation of periodicity – and also perhaps temporal fine structure – may be shown if a "music" stimulus was used for the FFR recordings (i.e., piano stimulus), as opposed to a "speech" stimulus, as in the /da/ stimulus used here. Future studies may consider examining the same relationship using a musical stimulus for FFR.

CONCLUSION

On average, bimodal listeners receive significant benefit from acoustic hearing for musical emotion judgments. Thus, bimodal listening may not only facilitate better music perception, it may also improve musical emotion perception. Two measures of spectral resolution, SMD and FFR *F*0 amplitude for a /da/ stimulus, were significantly correlated with degree of bimodal benefit. Further study is needed with a larger sample size, though both measures may be useful in helping to guide clinical decision-making regarding retention of bimodal hearing or pursuit of a second CI. Conversely, factors such as frequency selectivity at 262 and 440 Hz, musical aptitude and training, and PTA do not appear to be strongly related to bimodal benefit for musical emotion perception. This last point is of significant clinical importance: *benefit does not appear to be related to unaided audiometric thresholds*. Thus, a severe-to-profound hearing loss does not necessarily preclude the possibility of acoustic benefit for music perception and musical emotion perception. Future investigation into the FFR via use of a "music" stimulus should be considered to further examine the relationship with bimodal benefit for musical emotion perception.

ETHICS STATEMENT

This study was carried out in accordance with the recommendations of the Vanderbilt University Institutional Review Board with written informed consent from all subjects. All subjects gave written informed consent in accordance with the Declaration of Helsinki. The protocol was approved by the Vanderbilt University Institutional Review Board.

AUTHOR CONTRIBUTIONS

In collaboration with the other co-authors, KD'O was primarily responsible for study development, recruiting participants, collecting and analyzing data, and writing the manuscript. MC and CL developed the musical emotion perception task. SS was a consultant and invaluable resource for all FFR-related methodology, data collection, and data analysis. DK recruited the participants and collected the data. RG is the first author's Ph.D. mentor, and thus, was an integral part of this project at every stage of this study. MC, CL, SS, DK, and RG all gave input prior to beginning data collection and reviewed and edited the manuscript prior to submission.

ACKNOWLEDGMENTS

The authors would like to extend thanks to Drs. Daniel Ashmead and Reyna Gordon for their helpful comments on earlier drafts of this manuscript. Portions of these data were presented at the 2018 Music and Cochlear Implant Symposium in Montreal, QC, Canada and 2019 Conference on Implantable Auditory Prostheses.

REFERENCES

Anderson, S., Parbery-Clark, A., White-schwoch, T., Drehobl, S., and Kraus, N. (2013). Effects of hearing loss on the subcortical representation of speech cues. *J. Acoust. Soc. Am.* 133, 3030–3038. doi: 10.1121/1.4799804

Anderson, S., Parbery-Clark, A., Yi, H. G., and Kraus, N. (2011). A neural basis of speech-in-noise perception in older adults. *Ear Hear.* 32, 750–757. doi: 10.1097/AUD.0b013e31822229d3

Anderson, S., Skoe, E., Chandrasekaran, B., and Kraus, N. (2010). Neural timing is linked to speech perception in noise. *J. Neurosci.* 30, 4922–4926. doi: 10.1523/JNEUROSCI.0107-10.2010

Bachorowski, J. A. (1999). Vocal expression and perception of emotion. *Curr. Dir. Psychol. Sci.* 8, 53–57. doi: 10.1111/1467-8721.00013

Balkwill, L. L., and Thompson, W. F. (1999). A cross-cultural investigation of the perception of emotion in music: psychophysical and cultural cues. *Music Percept.* 17, 43–64. doi: 10.2307/40285811

Bidelman, G. M., Schug, J. M., Jennings, S. G., and Bhagat, S. P. (2014). Psychophysical auditory filter estimates reveal sharper cochlear tuning in musicians. *J. Acoust. Soc. Am.* 136, EL33–EL39. doi: 10.1121/1.4885484

Caldwell, M., Rankin, S. K., Jiradejvong, P., Carver, C., and Limb, C. J. (2015). Cochlear implant users rely on tempo rather than on pitch information during perception of musical emotion. *Cochlear Implants Int.* 16, S114–S120. doi: 10.1179/1467010015Z.000000000265

Chatterjee, M., and Peng, S. C. (2008). Processing F0 with cochlear implants: modulation frequency discrimination and speech intonation recognition. *Hear. Res.* 235, 143–156. doi: 10.1016/j.heares.2007.11.004

Cohen, J. (1988). *Statistical Power Analysis for the Behavioural Sciences*. Cambridge MA: Academic Press.

Dincer, D., Alessandro, H., Ballantyne, D., Boyle, P., De Seta, E., DeVincentiis, M., et al. (2018). Temporal fine structure processing, pitch, and speech perception in adult cochlear implant recipients. *Ear Hear.* 39, 679–686. doi: 10.1097/AUD.0000000000000525

Dorman, M. F., Gifford, R. H., Spahr, A. J., and McKarns, S. A. (2008). The benefits of combining acoustic and electric stimulation for the recognition of speech, voice and melodies. *Audiol. Neurotol.* 13, 105–112. doi: 10.1159/000111782

Drennan, W. R., Oleson, J. J., Gfeller, K., Crosson, J., Driscoll, V. D., Won, J. H., et al. (2015). Clinical evaluation of music perception, appraisal and experience in cochlear implant users. *Int. J. Audiol.* 54, 114–123. doi: 10.3109/14992027.2014.948219

Eerola, T., and Vuoskoski, J. K. (2013). A review of music and emotion studies: approaches, emotion models, and stimuli. *Music Percept.* 30, 307–340. doi: 10.1525/mp.2012.30.3.307

El Fata, F., James, C. J., Laborde, M. L., and Fraysse, B. (2009). How much residual hearing is 'useful' for music perception with cochlear implants? *Audiol. Neurotol.gy* 14(Suppl. 1), 14–21. doi: 10.1159/000206491

Gabrielsson, A., and Juslin, P. N. (1996). Emotional expression in music performance: between the performer's intention and the listener's experience. *Psychol. Music* 24, 68–91. doi: 10.1177/0305735696241007

Gfeller, K., Oleson, J., Knutson, J. F., Breheny, P., Driscoll, V., and Olszewski, C. (2008). Multivariate predictors of music perception and appraisal by adult cochlear implant users. *J. Am. Acad. Audiol.* 19, 120–134. doi: 10.3766/jaaa.19.2.3

Gfeller, K., Turner, C., Mehr, M., Woodworth, G., Fearn, R., Knutson, J. F., et al. (2002). Recognition of familiar melodies by adult cochlear implant recipients and normal-hearing adults. *Cochlear Implants Int.* 3, 29–53. doi: 10.1179/cim.2002.3.1.29

Gfeller, K., Woodworth, G., Robin, D. A., Witt, S., and Knutson, J. F. (1997). Perception of rhythmic and sequential pitch patterns by normal hearing adults and adult cochlear implant users. *Ear and Hear.* 18, 252–260. doi: 10.1097/00003446-199706000-00008

Giannantonio, S., Polonenko, M. J., Papsin, B. C., Paludetti, G., and Gordon, K. A. (2015). Experience changes how emotion in music is judged: evidence from children listening with bilateral cochlear implants, bimodal devices, and normal hearing. *PloS One* 10:e0136685. doi: 10.1371/journal.pone.0136685

Gifford, R. H., and Dorman, M. F. (2018). Bimodal Hearing or Bilateral Cochlear Implants? Ask the Patient. *Ear Hear.* 40, 501–516. doi: 10.1097/aud.0000000000000657

Gifford, R. H., Hedley-Williams, A., and Spahr, A. J. (2014). Clinical assessment of spectral modulation detection for adult cochlear implant recipients: a non-language based measure of performance outcomes. *Int. J. Audiol.* 53, 159–164. doi: 10.3109/14992027.2013.851800

Gifford, R. H., Noble, J. H., Camarata, S. M., Sunderhaus, L. W., Dwyer, R. T., Dawant, B. M., et al. (2018). The relationship between spectral modulation detection and speech recognition: adult versus pediatric cochlear implant recipients. *Trends Hear.* 22, 2331216518771176. doi: 10.1177/2331216518771176

Gosselin, N., Peretz, I., Noulhiane, M., Hasboun, D., Beckett, C., Baulac, M., et al. (2005). Impaired recognition of scary music following unilateral temporal lobe excision. *Brain* 128, 628–640. doi: 10.1093/brain/awh420

Green, T., Faulkner, A., and Rosen, S. (2012). Frequency selectivity of contralateral residual acoustic hearing in bimodal cochlear implant users, and limitations on the ability to match the pitch of electric and acoustic stimuli. *Int. J. Audiol.* 51, 389–398. doi: 10.3109/14992027.2011.642010

Holder, J. T., Levin, L. M., and Gifford, R. H. (2018). Speech recognition in noise for adults with normal hearing: age-normative performance for AzBio, BKB-SIN, and QuickSIN. *Otol. Neurotol.* 39, e972–e978. doi: 10.1097/MAO.0000000000002003

Hopyan, T., Gordon, K. A., and Papsin, B. C. (2011). Identifying emotions in music through electrical hearing in deaf children using cochlear implants. *Cochlear Implants Int.* 12, 21–26. doi: 10.1179/146701010X12677899497399

Hopyan, T., Manno, F. A. III, Papsin, B. C., and Gordon, K. A. (2016). Sad and happy emotion discrimination in music by children with cochlear implants. *Child Neuropsychol.* 22, 366–380. doi: 10.1080/09297049.2014.992400

Hsiao, F., and Gfeller, K. (2012). Music perception of cochlear implant recipients with implications for music instruction: a review of literature. *Update Univ. S. C. Dep. Music* 30, 5–10. doi: 10.1177/8755123312437050

International Organization for Standardization (1975). *Acoustics – Standard tuning frequency (Standard musical pitch).* Available at: https://www.iso.org/standard/3601.html

Jiam, N. T., Caldwell, M., Deroche, M. L., Chatterjee, M., and Limb, C. J. (2017). Voice emotion perception and production in cochlear implant users. *Hear. Res.* 352, 30–39. doi: 10.1016/j.heares.2017.01.006

Kang, R., Nimmons, G. L., Drennan, W., Longnion, J., Ruffin, C., Nie, K., et al. (2009). Development and validation of the university of washington clinical assessment of music perception test. *Ear Hear.* 30, 411–418. doi: 10.1097/AUD.0b013e3181a61bc0

Kessler, D. M., Ananthakrishnan, S., Smith, S. B., D'Onofrio, K., and Gifford, R. H. (2020). Frequency following response and speech recognition benefit for combining a cochlear implant and contralateral hearing aid. *Trends Hear.* 24:2331216520902001. doi: 10.1177/2331216520902001

Kong, Y.-Y., Cruz, R., Jones, J. A., and Zeng, F.-G. (2004). Music perception with temporal cues in acoustic and electric hearing. *Ear Hear.* 25, 173–185. doi: 10.1097/01.aud.0000120365.97792.2f

Lassaletta, L., Castro, A., Bastarrica, M., Pérez-Mora, R., Madero, R., De Sarriá, J., et al. (2007). Does music perception have an impact on quality of life following cochlear implantation? *Acta Otolaryngol.* 127, 682–686. doi: 10.1080/00016480601002112

Li, X., Nie, K., Imennov, N. S., and Rubinstein, J. T. (2013). Improved perception of music with a harmonic based algorithm for cochlear implants. *IEEE Trans. Neural. Syst. Rehabil. Eng.* 21, 684–694. doi: 10.1109/TNSRE.2013.2257853

Limb, C. J., and Roy, A. T. (2014). Technological, biological, and acoustical constraints to music perception in cochlear implant users. *Hear. Res.* 308, 13–26. doi: 10.1016/j.heares.2013.04.009

Luo, X., Fu, Q.-J., and Galvin, J. (2007). Vocal emotion recognition by normal-hearing listeners and cochlear-implant users. *Trends Amplif.* 11, 301–315. doi: 10.1177/1084713807305301

Mirza, S., Douglas, S. A., Lindsey, P., Hildreth, T., and Hawthorne, M. (2003). Appreciation of music in adult patients with cochlear implants: a patient questionnaire. *Cochlear Implants Int.* 4, 85–89. doi: 10.1179/cim.2003.4.2.85

Moore, B. C. J. (1978). Psychophysical tuning curves measured in simultaneous and forward masking. *J. Acoust. Soc. Am.* 63, 524–532. doi: 10.1121/1.381752

Moore, B. C. J. (2003). Coding of sounds in the auditory system and its relevance to signal processing and coding in cochlear implants. *Otol. Neurotol.* 24, 243–254. doi: 10.1097/00129492-200303000-00019

Moore, B. C. J., Huss, M., Vickers, D. A., Glasberg, B. R., and Alcántara, J. I. (2000). A test for the diagnosis of dead regions in the cochlea. *Br. J. Audiol.* 34, 205–224. doi: 10.3109/03005364000000131

Ollen, J. E. (2006). *A Criterion-Related Validity Test of Selected Indicators of Musical Sophistication using Expert Ratings [Electronic Resource].* Available at: http://marcs-survey.uws.edu.au/OMSI/

Peretz, I., Gagnon, L., and Bouchard, B. (1998). Music and emotion: perceptual determinants, immediacy, and isolation after brain damage. *Cognition* 68, 111–141. doi: 10.1016/s0010-0277(98)00043-2

Reynolds, S. M., and Gifford, R. H. (2019). Effect of signal processing strategy and stimulation type on speech and auditory perception in adult cochlear implant users. *Intl. J. Audiol.* 58, 363–372. doi: 10.1080/14992027.2019.1580390

Scherer, K. R. (2003). Vocal communication of emotion: a review of research paradigms. *Speech Commun.* 40, 227–256. doi: 10.1016/s0167-6393(02)00084-5

Sęk, A., Alcántara, J., Moore, B. C., Kluk, K., and Wicher, A. (2005). Development of a fast method for determining psychophysical tuning curves. *Int. J. Audiol.* 44, 408–420. doi: 10.1080/14992020500060800

Sęk, A., and Moore, B. C. J. (2011). Implementation of a fast method for measuring psychophysical tuning curves. *Intl. J. Audiol.* 50, 237–242. doi: 10.3109/14992027.2010.550636

Shabana, M., Moore, B. C., El-Khosht, M., Selim, M. H., and Dokla, M. (2014). Fast psychophysical tuning curves of the cochlea in normal hearing individuals. *Adv. Arab. Acad. Audio Vestibul. J.* 1, 12. doi: 10.4103/2314-8667.137559

Shirvani, S., Jafari, Z., Motasaddi Zarandi, M., Jalaie, S., Mohagheghi, H., and Tale, M. R. (2016). Emotional perception of music in children with bimodal fitting and unilateral cochlear implant. *Ann. Otol. Rhinol. Laryngol.* 125, 470–477. doi: 10.1177/0003489415619943

Sladen, D. P., Carlson, M. L., Dowling, B. P., Olund, A. P., DeJong, M. D., Breneman, A., et al. (2018). Cochlear implantation in adults with asymmetric hearing loss: speech recognition in quiet and in noise, and health related quality of life. *Otol. Neurotol.* 39, 576–581. doi: 10.1097/MAO.0000000000001763

Smith, Z. M., Delgutte, B., and Oxenham, A. J. (2002). Chimaeric sounds reveal dichotomies in auditory perception. *Nature* 416, 87–90. doi: 10.1038/416087a

Song, J. H., Skoe, E., Banai, K., and Kraus, N. (2011). Perception of speech in noise: neural correlates. *J. Cogn. Neurosci.* 23, 2268–2279. doi: 10.1162/jocn.2010.21556

Sucher, C. M., and McDermott, H. J. (2009). Bimodal stimulation: benefits for music perception and sound quality. *Cochlear Implants Int.* 10, 96–99. doi: 10.1002/cii.398

Thompson, E. C., Carr, K. W., White-Schwoch, T., Otto-Meyer, S., and Kraus, N. (2017). Individual differences in speech-in-noise perception parallel neural speech processing and attention in preschoolers. *Hear. Res.* 344, 148–157. doi: 10.1016/j.heares.2016.11.007

Wang, W., Zhou, N., and Xu, L. (2011). Musical pitch and lexical tone perception with cochlear implants. *Int. J. Audiol.* 50, 270–278. doi: 10.3109/14992027.2010.542490

Webster, G. D., and Weir, C. G. (2005). Emotional responses to music: interactive effects of mode, texture, and tempo. *Motiv. Emot.* 29, 19–39. doi: 10.1007/s11031-005-4414-0

13

Pitch Matching in Cochlear Implant Users with Single-Sided Deafness: Effects of Electrode Position and Acoustic Stimulus Type

Youssef Adel[1*†], Sharon Nagel[1], Tobias Weissgerber[1], Uwe Baumann[1] and Olivier Macherey[2]

[1] Audiological Acoustics, Department of Otorhinolaryngology, University Hospital Frankfurt, Frankfurt, Germany,
[2] Aix-Marseille University, CNRS, Centrale Marseille, LMA, Marseille, France

***Correspondence:**
Youssef Adel
youssef.adel@uni-tuebingen.de

†Present address:
Youssef Adel,
Department of Otorhinolaryngology, Head and Neck Surgery, Tübingen Hearing Research Center, University of Tübingen Medical Center, Tübingen, Germany

Previous studies in patients with single-sided deafness (SSD) have reported results of pitch comparisons between electric stimulation of their cochlear implant (CI) and acoustic stimulation presented to their near-normal hearing contralateral ear. These comparisons typically used sinusoids, although the percept elicited by electric stimulation may be closer to a wideband stimulus. Furthermore, it has been shown that pitch comparisons between sounds with different timbres is a difficult task and subjected to various types of range biases. The present study aims to introduce a method to minimize non-sensory biases, and to investigate the effect of different acoustic stimulus types on the frequency and variability of the electric-acoustic pitch matches. Pitch matches were collected from 13 CI users with SSD using the binary search procedure. Electric stimulation was presented at either an apical or a middle electrode position, at a rate of 800 pps. Acoustic stimulus types were sinusoids (SINE), 1/3-octave wide narrow bands of Gaussian noises (NBN), or 1/3-octave wide pulse spreading harmonic complexes (PSHC). On the one hand, NBN and PSHC are presumed to better mimic the spread of excitation produced by a single-electrode stimulation than SINE. On the other hand, SINE and PSHC contain less inherent fluctuations than NBN and may therefore provide a temporal pattern closer to that produced by a constant-amplitude electric pulse train. Analysis of mean pitch match variance showed no differences between stimulus types. However, mean pitch matches showed effects of electrode position and stimulus type, with the middle electrode always matched to a higher frequency than the apical one ($p < 0.001$), and significantly higher across-subject pitch matches for PSHC compared with SINE ($p = 0.017$). Mean pitch matches for all stimulus types were better predicted by place-dependent characteristic frequencies (CFs) based on an organ of Corti map compared with a spiral ganglion map. CF predictions were closest to pitch matches with SINE for the apical electrode position, and conversely with NBN or PSHC for the middle electrode position. These results provide evidence that the choice of acoustic stimulus type can have a significant effect on electric-acoustic pitch matching.

Keywords: cochlear implant, pitch perception, single-sided deafness, simulation, pulse-spreading harmonic complex, binary search procedure, non-sensory bias

INTRODUCTION

Over the last two decades, the population of hearing-impaired people undergoing cochlear implantation has greatly evolved. While this treatment originally targeted patients with bilateral profound deafness, there are now increasingly more cochlear implant (CI) users with significant residual acoustic hearing in their ipsilateral or, more frequently, contralateral ear. Although this residual hearing is usually restricted to low frequencies, there exists a population of CI users with single-sided deafness (SSD) and normal or near-normal hearing (nNH) in their contralateral ear (Van Zon et al., 2015; Zeitler and Dorman, 2019). In order to enable fusion across the ears of these patients, it may be necessary to deliver to each electrode the frequency information that corresponds to its intracochlear location (Oxenham et al., 2004; Deeks et al., 2013), so that auditory nerve fibers with the same characteristic frequencies (CFs) receive the same information across ears. One way to achieve this is to perform electric-acoustic pitch matching experiments where subjects compare the pitch of a CI electrode with that evoked by acoustic stimuli differing in their spectral content. Previous pitch matching studies have shown that such measurements are difficult to conduct and usually produce very variable data (Carlyon et al., 2010; Goupell et al., 2019). This variability may have several causes, including methodological limitations as well as the choice of the acoustic stimulus type.

Methods of Electric-Acoustic Pitch Matching

A wide range of methods have been used in the literature to compare the pitches of electric and acoustic stimuli. These include magnitude estimation (Vermeire et al., 2008; Plant et al., 2014), the method of constant stimuli (Boex et al., 2006; Reiss et al., 2007, 2015; Goupell et al., 2019), the method of adjustment (Green et al., 2012; Rader et al., 2016; Maarefvand et al., 2017; Tan et al., 2017) and various kinds of adaptive forced-choice procedures (Reiss et al., 2007; Schatzer et al., 2014; Vermeire et al., 2015; Peters et al., 2016). Carlyon et al. (2010) tested several of these methods and showed they could all be potentially contaminated by different kinds of non-sensory biases. Both magnitude estimation and the method of constant stimuli require the experimenter to predefine a fixed number of acoustic stimuli with which the electrical stimulus will be compared. Carlyon et al. (2010) showed that the choice of this acoustic frequency range could have a large influence on the results. For example, in one subject, the same electrode could be matched to frequencies separated by more than two thirds of an octave for two different acoustic ranges, suggesting that the subjects were not performing real pitch comparisons but rather, and perhaps unconsciously, were basing their judgments on the frequency of the acoustic stimuli only: when the acoustic frequency was high relative to the range, they decided to judge it as "higher" than the electric stimulus, whereas when it was low relative to the range, they judged it as "lower" than the electric stimulus (see also Goupell et al., 2019). This range bias may be very problematic because the range of acoustic frequencies is usually dictated either by the amount of residual hearing of the subjects or by *a priori* estimation of the electric pitch by the experimenter, inferred from radiological findings or from preliminary pitch matches obtained *before* the experiment. An alternative to these procedures that use a fixed range of acoustic frequencies is to perform adjustment or adaptive tasks where the acoustic frequency presented on a given trial depends on the subject's response to the preceding trial. However, for these tasks, it has been shown that the pitch match can sometimes be strongly correlated with the starting frequency of the procedure, again suggesting that the subjects may not perform pitch comparisons but rather give responses converging near the acoustic stimulus they heard first (Carlyon et al., 2010; Schatzer et al., 2014). Another limitation of adjustment or adaptive tasks is that the pitch of the acoustic stimulus may not vary a lot between consecutive trials, which could distract the subjects from the task itself, especially if the stimuli vary across other dimensions (e.g., loudness or timbre), which may be more salient than the pitch dimension.

The first aim of the present study is to introduce a pitch matching method inspired from the midpoint comparison procedure (Long et al., 2005) and the binary search algorithm used in computer science. The method is relatively time-efficient and attempts to minimize the effects of non-sensory biases: it does not require *a priori* assumption on the frequency range that the electrode should be matched to and it presents acoustic stimuli whose frequency can vary considerably from trial to trial.

Choice of Acoustic Stimulus Type

Another important concern in electric-acoustic pitch matching experiments is the choice of acoustic stimulus type. While most previous studies have used sinusoids, there is evidence that the percept evoked by electric stimulation via a CI may be very different than that of a pure tone (Lazard et al., 2012). The resulting timbre differences may make pitch comparisons difficult to perform and, therefore, even more prone to non-sensory biases (Carlyon et al., 2010). To our knowledge, only three studies have used stimuli different than sinusoids; Carlyon et al. (2010) used low-rate (12 pps) electric pulse trains and matched them to bandpass-filtered acoustic pulse trains at the same rate. The advantage was that the percepts elicited by these two types of stimuli would be qualitatively similar. It is, however, unclear whether the results of these matches can be extrapolated to higher rates and lower current levels, which are typically used in clinical processors (approximately 1,000 pps). This is because different rates and/or current levels may induce shifts in the spread of excitation and thus influence the "place" pitch percept (e.g., Arnoldner et al., 2006). Green et al. (2012) tested a group of subjects with residual low-frequency hearing and measured pitch matches for different acoustic stimuli, including sinusoids, noise bands and low-rate acoustic pulse trains. Their results were very variable, but they found in one subject that the matched frequency was significantly different when using acoustic pulse trains than for sinusoids and noise bands. Maarefvand et al. (2017) have used sinusoids as well as harmonic complex tones and found that the pitch-matched frequency for each electrode was always higher when using a pure tone than the harmonic complex tone. Thus far, there is only limited evidence that the choice of acoustic stimulus type can have an effect on the electric-acoustic pitch matching results. Recently, pulse-spreading harmonic complexes (PSHCs) have been proposed as an alternative to simulate electric pulse stimulation via a CI (Hilkhuysen and Macherey, 2014). The design of PSHC addresses some of the limitations of sinusoidal or noise carriers commonly used for CI simulations, i.e., that sinusoids cannot simulate the broad spread of excitation produced by an electric current pulse and that noise bands contain intrinsic modulations which are absent in pulse trains with a constant current amplitude. PSHCs are pulsatile broadband stimuli that can simulate the broad spread of excitation and their pulse rate can be adjusted to minimize intrinsic modulations after auditory filtering (Mesnildrey et al., 2016). Furthermore, a recent evaluation in SSD subjects showed that speech processed by a vocoder using PSHC carriers was judged more similar to speech processed by the clinical CI processor than sine- or noise-vocoded speech (Karoui et al., 2019).

The second aim of the present study is to test the hypothesis that PSHCs can yield less variable pitch matches compared with sinusoids (SINE) and narrow-band noises (NBN, see **Figure 1**). Pitch was matched for an apical and a middle electrode position (E1 and E6, respectively) and compared with place-dependent CFs predicted by empirical models. Our underlying assumption was that a signal perceptually more similar to the CI should yield less variable electric-acoustic pitch matches.

MATERIALS AND METHODS

Subjects

Thirteen subjects (3 female, 10 male) with late-onset SSD and nNH in the contralateral ear participated in the study. Pure-tone air conduction thresholds were less than or equal to 20 dB HL in the frequency range from 125 to 2 kHz for all subjects, and up to 60 dB HL in the frequency range 3–8 kHz. Mean and standard deviation air conduction thresholds for the non-implanted and implanted (i.e., aided thresholds) ear, respectively, are shown in **Figure 2**. All subjects were experienced CI users (range 11 months – 7 years after implantation) with Concerto or Synchrony devices (MED-EL, Innsbruck, Austria) and either the 28-mm Flex28 electrode array (n = 10) or the 31.5-mm FlexSoft electrode array (n = 3). Subject demographics are provided in **Table 1**. Electrode migration occurred in one subject (S13, denoted by *) 5 years prior to the study and consequently, the two most basal electrodes were turned off. Tinnitus was reported in the implanted ear by 8 subjects (denoted by $^+$), one of whom also reported it in the non-implanted ear (S07). All subjects received financial compensation and reimbursement of their traveling costs. This study was carried out in accordance with the ethical standards of the institutional review board at the Goethe University Frankfurt, which approved the study protocol (IRB approval number 209/13). All subjects gave written informed consent in accordance with the Declaration of Helsinki.

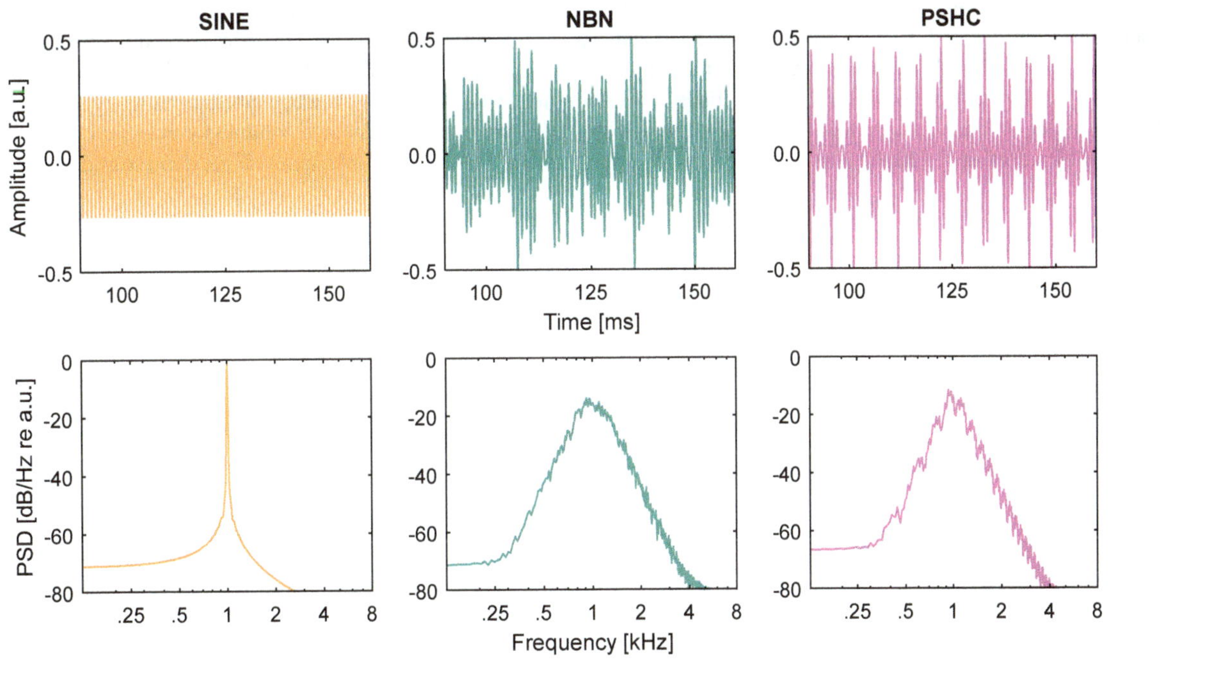

FIGURE 1 | Stimulus waveforms **(upper panels)** and power spectrum densities (PSD, **lower panels**) are shown for each acoustic stimulus type: sinusoid (SINE), narrow-band noise (NBN), and pulse spreading harmonic complex (PSHC), all centered at 1 kHz.

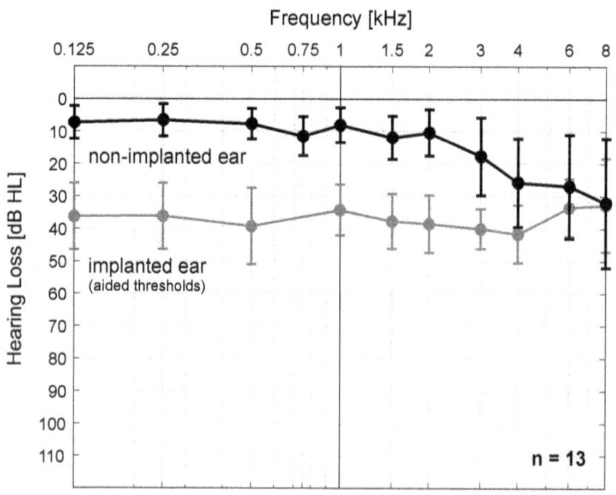

FIGURE 2 | Mean and standard deviation air conduction thresholds for the non-implanted ear, i.e., near-normal hearing (nNH, black) and implanted ear, i.e., cochlear-implant aided thresholds (gray) for all subjects (*n* = 13).

Stimuli

Electric stimuli were 400-ms biphasic cathodic-first pulse trains presented in monopolar mode. The two phases were symmetric and rectangular, had durations of 45 μs each, and were separated by a 2.1-μs inter-phase gap. All electric pulse trains were presented at a rate of 800 pps.

Acoustic stimuli were either sinusoids (SINE), 1/3-octave wide narrow bands of Gaussian noises (NBN), or 1/3-octave wide pulse spreading harmonic complexes (PSHC; Hilkhuysen and Macherey, 2014). They had a duration of 400 ms and 20-ms raised cosine onset and offset ramps. They were presented at (center) frequencies ranging between 125 and 4 kHz. NBN and PSHC were spectrally limited outside the 1/3-octave passband using 6th order Butterworth low-pass and high-pass filters, i.e., they had 36 dB per octave spectral slopes. PSHCs were presented at center frequency-dependent optimal pulse rates according to Mesnildrey et al. (2016). **Figure 1** shows waveform excerpts, i.e., amplitude over time (upper panels), and power spectrum densities (PSD, lower panels) for each stimulus type centered at 1 kHz.

Procedures

Prior to the experiment, pure-tone air conduction thresholds of the nNH ear were measured and CI electrode impedances of the implanted ear were checked. As described in detail below, the experiment started by determining electric (CI) and acoustic (nNH) loudness profiles to establish electric current and sound pressure levels at comfortable loudness. This was followed by balancing the loudness between the two stimulation modalities. After an enforced break and a short acoustic pitch demonstration, an electric pitch ranking task was conducted to verify that the subjects had no pitch reversals for the relevant electrodes. Thereafter, acoustic-acoustic pitch matching was conducted as a control measure of subjects' ability to perform pitch comparisons. Finally, electric-acoustic pitch matching procedures were carried out using the binary search procedure.

Electric and Acoustic Loudness Profiles

Electric current or sound pressure levels were initially adjusted to most-comfortable loudness (MCL), defined as rating 6 on a 10-point rating scale. Electric loudness profiles were determined by presenting pulse trains to a single CI electrode at a time, while monitoring subjects' loudness perception on a 10-point rating scale. Current level was increased from 94.5 CU (current units, 1 CU $\approx$ 1 μA) in steps of 1, 2, or 4 times 9.45 CU from rating 0 ("no percept") up to rating 7 ("loud but comfortable"), then decreased back in steps of 9.45 CU to the final rating 6 ("most comfortable"). MCL current levels were determined for electrodes E1 (apical) to E8 (basal) in ascending order. Hereafter, electric stimuli were always presented at these MCL levels.

Acoustic loudness profiles were determined for each stimulus type, i.e., SINE, NBN, or PSHC, in random order. Analogous to the electric loudness profile, a given stimulus type was presented while monitoring subjects' loudness perception on the 10-point rating scale. Initial frequency-dependent sound pressure levels

TABLE 1 | Subject demographics.

Subject	Implanted Ear	Age at Implantation [years]	Duration of CI use [years]	Age at Onset of Hearing Loss [years]	Etiology
S01	R	49	6	45	Sudden hearing loss
S02+	L	68	4	58	Sudden hearing loss
S03	R	70	5	66	Sudden hearing loss
S04+	L	53	5	40	Progressive hearing loss
S05+	R	45	5	43	Sudden hearing loss
S06	R	67	1	59	Toxic otitis
S07+	L	47	4	41	Sudden hearing loss
S08+	L	62	2	40	Head trauma
S09	R	69	7	65	Sudden hearing loss
S10+	L	37	1	36	Meningitis
S11+	L	60	3	57	Sudden hearing loss
S12+	R	53	<1	51	Sudden hearing loss
S13*	L	68	6	64	Sudden hearing loss

*L, left; R, right. *Two most basal electrodes were turned off. +Tinnitus was reported in the implanted ear.*

were based on pilot loudness-adjustment tests in NH subjects ($n = 4$, data not shown here) using the same acoustic stimuli and anchored on a 1-kHz pure tone at 65 dB SPL. Sound pressure levels were increased in steps of 1, 2, or 4 dB up to rating 7 and then decreased back in steps of 1 dB to the final rating 6. MCL sound pressure levels were determined for a given stimulus type starting at a (center) frequency of 1 kHz up to 4 kHz in half-octave steps, and then from 1 kHz down to 125 Hz in half-octave steps.

Electric-Acoustic Loudness Balancing

After having determined electric and acoustic loudness profiles, an adjustment paradigm adopted from Macherey and Carlyon (2010) was used to balance loudness between the two stimulation modalities. Each loudness-balancing trial consisted of an electric pulse train presented to the CI ear followed by an acoustic stimulus presented to the nNH ear after a 400-ms inter-stimulus gap. The electric pulse train was the reference and its level was fixed at MCL throughout a given adjustment task. The acoustic stimulus had an initial level of MCL $\pm$ 6 dB and was adjustable in steps of 0, 1, 2, or 4 dB using a graphical user interface provided to the subjects. They were asked to balance the loudness of the acoustic stimulus to that of the electric stimulus and were encouraged to make over- and undershoots before deciding on the final level. A minimum of 10 level adjustments was enforced before subjects could indicate that loudness was balanced and terminate a given adjustment task.

This procedure was carried out once for each combination of electrode (E3 or E4) and acoustic stimulus type (SINE, NBN, or PSHC) presented at different initial levels (MCL $\pm$ 6 dB), i.e., 12 possible combinations, in random order. Each acoustic stimulus was presented at a (center) frequency selected randomly without replacement from the set of frequencies ranging between 125 and 4 kHz in half-octave steps. Loudness was finally balanced for each acoustic stimulus by applying the mean adjustment of two electrodes (E3 and E4) and two different initial levels (MCL $\pm$ 6 dB), i.e., from 4 conditions, to the respective acoustic loudness profile. Each profile was then linearly interpolated by a factor of 12 to obtain a quarter-tone (i.e., 50 cents) frequency spacing. Hereafter, acoustic stimuli were always presented at these loudness-balanced MCL levels.

Note that the electrodes used for electric-acoustic loudness balancing (E3 and E4) were different than those used for electric-acoustic pitch matching (E1 and E6, see below) in order to prevent having subjects compare in loudness the same electric stimuli they would later compare in pitch, thereby avoiding such loudness comparisons from providing an additional source of bias (McDermott et al., 2008).

Acoustic Pitch Demonstration

After an enforced break at the end of the loudness balancing tasks, a short acoustic pitch demonstration was presented to accustom the subjects to the new tasks concerning pitch perception. Each demonstration trial consisted of two acoustic stimuli presented to the nNH ear, separated by a 400-ms inter-stimulus gap. Each combination of acoustic stimulus (SINE, NBN, or PSHC) and frequency order (ascending or descending) was presented three times, in random order. For each trial, a pair of (center) frequencies was selected randomly without replacement from the set of frequencies ranging between 125 and 4 kHz in half-octave steps. Each stimulus playback was visually cued and feedback was provided to indicate which stimulus was higher in pitch. Subjects were asked to listen and compare their judgment to the provided feedback.

Electric Pitch Ranking

In order to verify that the subjects had no pitch reversals for the relevant electrodes in the CI ear, the midpoint comparison procedure was used to rank electrodes according to their pitch. This procedure was adopted from Long et al. (2005), who originally developed it to optimize the fitting of auditory brainstem implants, and its implementation in CI users has been previously described in Macherey and Carlyon (2010). The procedure starts by randomly selecting a pair of electrodes without replacement from the set of electrodes to be ranked. Electric pulse trains were presented to each electrode, separated by a 400-ms inter-stimulus gap. The subjects' task was to indicate which electrode was higher in pitch, with the order of presentation randomized between trials. The procedure continues by randomly selecting additional electrodes in order to gradually rank the set of electrodes according to their pitch. To briefly illustrate this, assume that at one point of the procedure the provisional ranking of the electrodes was [E1, E3, E2, E7, E8]. The randomly selected electrode to be ranked next is E4, and is first compared to the middle-ranked electrode E2. Given an electrode pair, in this case E4 and E2, each trial consisted of an electric pulse train presented to one electrode and then to the other, with the order of electrodes randomized between trials. Each stimulus playback was visually cued without feedback. If the subject ranked one electrode higher two times in a row, then it was defined as their response. Otherwise, a third trial was presented and its result defined as their response. This best-of-three format was added to the original procedure of Long et al. (2005) to minimize confounding factors, such as lack of concentration (Levitt and Rabiner, 1967). In this illustration, if E4 was finally ranked higher in pitch than E2, then the list would be bisected and E4 compared to the consequently middle-ranked stimulus E7. If it was thereupon ranked lower in pitch than E7, then the probed electrode E4 would be added to a new provisional ranking between E2 and E7, i.e., [E1, E3, E2, E4, E7, E8]. Subsequently, the next electrode to be ranked would be randomly selected and the procedure repeated until all electrodes are ranked.

The procedure was carried out 3 times for electrodes E1 to E8 with the requirement of no pitch reversals for electrode pairs [E1, E4], [E3, E6], and [E1, E6] in at least 2 out of the 3 repetitions. These pairs were later used for catch trials and electric-acoustic pitch matching.

Acoustic-Acoustic Pitch Matching

As a control measure of subjects' ability to perform the final procedure, they were asked to match the pitch between two acoustic stimuli presented to the nNH ear, separated by a 400-ms inter-stimulus gap. Each trial consisted of a standard stimulus fixed in (center) frequency throughout a given pitch matching

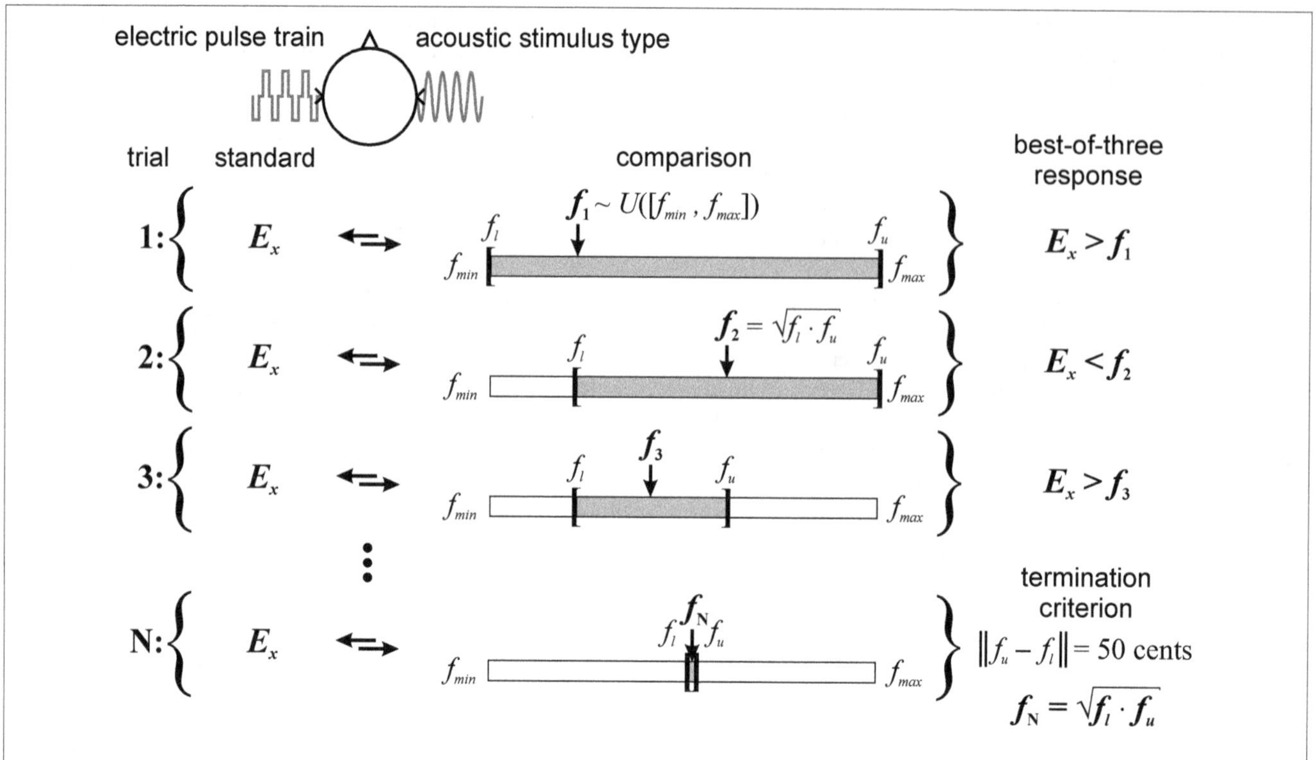

FIGURE 3 | Illustration of the *binary search procedure*: each trial consists of a standard electric pulse train fixed in electrode position (E_X) throughout a given pitch matching run (trials 1 to N), and an acoustic stimulus type. Subjects are asked to indicate whether the standard or comparison is higher in pitch, with the order of presentation randomized between trials. The (center) frequency (f_x, $x \in \{1, 2, 3, \ldots, N\}$) of the acoustic stimulus is adaptively changed according to their response, which is evaluated in a best-of-three format for each trial. The starting frequency is randomly drawn from a uniform distribution, i.e., $f_1 \sim U([f_{min}, f_{max}])$. The pitch matching range $[f_l, f_u]$ initially has the same lower and upper boundaries. In this illustration, the electric stimulus is perceived higher in pitch than the acoustic stimulus at the starting frequency (trial 1), i.e., $E_X > f_1$. Consequently, the lower boundary is set to that frequency and the next frequency (trial 2) set to the geometric mean of the current lower and upper boundaries, i.e., $f_2 = \sqrt{f_l \cdot f_u}$. The electric stimulus is then perceived lower in pitch than the acoustic stimulus, i.e., $E_X < f_2$, and the upper boundary is set to that frequency. The next frequency (trial 3) is again set to the geometric mean of the current boundaries. This iterative process is terminated (trial N) when the difference between lower and upper boundaries is a quarter-tone (i.e., 50 cents). The final pitch match f_N is defined as the geometric mean of the final boundaries.

run, and a comparison stimulus whose frequency was adaptively changed according to the binary search procedure described below (see **Figure 3**). Each stimulus playback was visually cued without feedback. This procedure was carried out 3 times for each combination of standard frequency (250 Hz or 1 kHz) and acoustic stimulus (SINE, NBN, or PSHC), in random order.

Between-subject pitch matching variability was compared with data acquired from pilot pitch matching tests in NH subjects ($n = 10$, data not shown here) using the same procedure and acoustic stimuli (NBN and PSHC) to test the effect of spectral slope on matching accuracy, with the standard fixed at 36 dB per octave and the comparison at 24, 36, or 48 dB per octave. Key differences in the NH experiment were that (i) standard and comparison stimuli were presented to contralateral ears, with the order randomized between subjects, (ii) the pitch matching range was up to 8 kHz compared with 4 kHz for SSD subjects, and (iii) NH subjects were also tested using the standard frequency of 4 kHz.

Electric-Acoustic Pitch Matching

The main and final task was to compare the pitch of an electric pulse train presented to the CI ear to that of an acoustic stimulus presented to the nNH ear as illustrated in **Figure 3**. Each pitch matching trial consisted of a standard electric stimulus fixed in electrode position (E_X) throughout a given pitch matching run (trials 1 to N), and an acoustic stimulus type, separated by a 400-ms inter-stimulus gap. The subjects' task was to indicate whether the standard or comparison was higher in pitch, with the order of presentation randomized between trials. Each stimulus playback was visually cued without feedback. The (center) frequency (f_x, $x \in \{1, 2, 3, \ldots, N\}$) of the acoustic stimulus was adaptively changed according to the *binary search procedure*: The starting frequency was randomly drawn from a uniform distribution ranging from 125 Hz (f_{min}) to 4 kHz (f_{max}), i.e., $f_1 \sim U([f_{min}, f_{max}])$. And the pitch matching range $[f_l, f_u]$ initially had the same lower and upper boundaries, i.e., 125 Hz and 4 kHz, respectively. Subjects' response was evaluated in the best-of-three format as described above. In the illustration shown in **Figure 3**, the electric stimulus was perceived higher in pitch than the acoustic stimulus at the starting frequency (trial 1), i.e., $E_X > f_1$. Consequently, the lower boundary was set to that frequency and the next frequency (trial 2) set to the geometric mean of the current lower and upper boundaries, i.e., $f_2 = \sqrt{f_l \cdot f_u}$. The electric stimulus was then perceived lower in pitch than the acoustic stimulus, i.e., $E_x < f_2$. In this case, the upper boundary was set to that frequency and the next frequency (trial 3) was again set to the geometric mean of the current boundaries. This iterative process was terminated (trial N) when the difference between the lower and upper boundaries was a quarter-tone (i.e., 50 cents). The pitch match f_N was then defined as the geometric mean of the final boundaries.

This procedure was repeated five times for each combination of electrode (E1 or E6) and acoustic stimulus type (SINE, NBN, or PSHC) in random order. A short break was enforced in the middle of the entire procedure to minimize the effect of fatigue. A given pitch matching run could be interrupted by two types of catch trials, electric or acoustic, each with 15% probability of occurrence. Electric catch trials randomly selected an electrode pair, [E1, E4] or [E3, E6], and presented an electric pulse train to each electrode in random order. Acoustic catch trials randomly selected a pair of (center) frequencies without replacement from the set of frequencies ranging between 125 Hz and 4 kHz in half-octave steps. The stimulus type tested in the current pitch matching run was presented at each frequency in random order. The subjects' task was still to indicate which stimulus was higher in pitch. Each stimulus playback was visually cued with feedback. If the response was correct, then the pitch matching run was immediately resumed. Otherwise, the catch trial was repeated twice. These catch trials aimed to impel subjects to focus on the pitch dimension by restricting these trials to a single modality, and to give them positive reinforcement on relatively easy trials.

Materials

Electric stimuli were directly transmitted to the CI using the Research Interface Box II (RIB, University of Innsbruck, Innsbruck, Austria). Acoustic stimuli were presented using a D/A converter and amplifier (24 bit, 48 kHz sampling rate, RME Fireface UC, Haimhausen, Germany), and audiometric headphones (Sennheiser HDA 200, Wedemark, Germany). All experimental procedures and graphical user interfaces were programmed in MATLAB (MathWorks, Natick, MA, United States) using the RIB library and Psychophysics Toolbox extensions (Brainard, 1997) to respectively drive the electric and acoustic stimulation hardware.

Analysis

Data are generally presented as geometric mean, or plotted as boxplots with mean values included as circles. Within-subject comparisons were calculated using repeated-measures analyses of variance (ANOVA) and Tukey's LSD post-hoc test. Linear correlation between measures was tested using Pearson's r. A p-value of less than 0.05 was considered statistically significant. Statistical analysis was performed using SPSS Statistics (IBM Corporation, Endicott, NY, United States).

In addition to analyzing electrode positions using their order on the electrode carrier, angles of insertion were estimated using postoperative X-ray images acquired with the modified Stenvers' projection (cochlear view, Xu et al., 2000), which has been described and illustrated in previous studies (Verbist et al., 2010; Rader et al., 2016).

RESULTS

Control Procedures

Electric pitch ranking using the midpoint comparison procedure was conducted to verify that the subjects had no pitch reversals for the relevant electrode pairs, which were [E1, E4] and [E3, E6] for the catch trials, and [E1, E6] for the electric-acoustic pitch matching. Only 2 subjects (S09 and S11) had pitch reversals for the pair [E3, E6] and 1 subject (S09) for the pair [E1, E6], each of which only occurred in 1 out of the 3 repetitions. Median rank differences for all subjects were 3 ranks between [E1, E4] (range 1 – 5), 3 ranks between [E3, E6] (range 2 – 5), and 5 ranks between [E1, E6] (range 4 – 6). If evaluated using the best-of-three format, 4 subjects (31%) had a "perfect" ranking, i.e., they ranked the electrodes in ascending order from E1 to E8 without any pitch reversals. If divided into the 4 apical (E1 to E4) and 4 basal (E5 to E8) electrodes, 5 subjects (38%) had perfect ranking for the apical electrodes and 8 subjects (62%) had perfect ranking for the basal electrodes.

Acoustic-acoustic pitch matching was conducted as a control measure of subjects' ability to perform pitch comparisons prior to collecting electric-acoustic pitch matching data. Pitch match distributions were comparable between conditions, which was confirmed using a two-way repeated-measures ANOVA with the factors standard frequency (250 Hz or 1 kHz) and stimulus type (SINE, NBN, or PSHC), which showed neither within-subject effects nor interaction effects. Mean absolute deviation from either standard (250 Hz or 1 kHz) was 2 semitones or lower for NBN and PSHC, which was comparable with the NH results. SINE showed the highest variance and had a mean absolute deviation of over 3 semitones from the 250-Hz standard, which could be due to octave confusions (Lockhead and Byrd, 1981). For the 4-kHz standard tested in NH subjects, mean absolute deviation was 10 semitones (minor seventh) for NBN and 8 semitones (minor sixth) for PSHC. This finding showed that pitch matching accuracy for NBN and PSHC substantially decreased at high frequencies and was thus not included in the testing of SSD subjects.

Electric and acoustic catch trials were carried out during the electric-acoustic pitch matching procedure to verify and if necessary impel subjects to focus on pitch. Mean percent correct responses were 93% for electric catch trials, 97% for SINE, 94% for NBN, and 97% for PSHC. These relatively high scores strongly suggest that the positive reinforcement of the subjects to focus on the pitch dimension was achieved.

Finally, no systematic correlations were found between starting frequency and final pitch matches, which suggests that the binary search procedure was not contaminated by this limitation previously observed for other adaptive methods (Carlyon et al., 2010). A possible explanation is that the change in frequency during the first trials is very large due to the fundamental approach of the binary search algorithm, which progressively bisects the frequency range. Therefore, it would

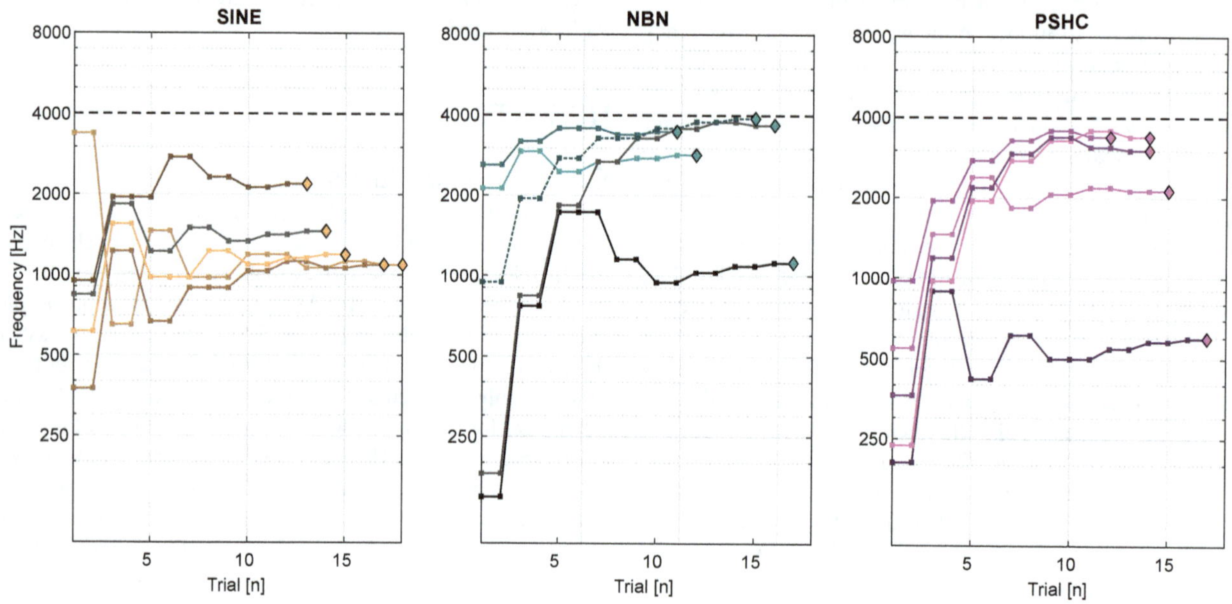

FIGURE 4 | Example of pitch matching runs for each stimulus type (SINE, NBN, or PSHC), for a given subject (S11) and electrode position (E6). The dashed horizontal gridline shows the maximum frequency at 4 kHz. For each trial, comparison (center) frequency is shown as squares. And the final pitch matches are shown as diamonds. In one pitch matching run of NBN (dashed line), the subject appears to have perceived the pitch very close to (or possibly above) the maximum frequency, but was hindered by the procedure's parameters.

TABLE 2 | Individual MLE pitch match [Hz].

Subject	E1			E6		
	SINE	**NBN**	**PSHC**	**SINE**	**NBN**	**PSHC**
S01	240.5	408.3	417.9	1233.2	–	3639.4
S02	200.0	257.6	246.1	399.1	935.5	2349.8*
S03	331.9	302.7	427.6	1124.7	1663.5	1663.5
S04	647.2	2046.6	1702.3	935.5	3027.1*	2296.3
S05	339.6	538.3	709.6	853.2	4688.5*	2958.2*
S06	363.9	155.2	186.7	502.4	709.6	1415.9
S07	339.6	576.8	427.6	1049.6	1517.2	1205.1
S08	200.0	381.1	632.5	1824.0	–	–
S09	324.4	3724.2*	1049.6	381.1	–	1910.0
S10	257.6	1482.6	853.2	760.4	–	3243.6*
S11	195.4	276.1	347.6	1352.2	2958.2*	2094.3
S12	662.3	576.8	490.9	2296.3	1663.5	1625.7
S13	246.1	295.8	381.1	1702.3	1074.1	1866.5
Mean	308.7	537.4	509.5	967.5	1711.0	2078.2

**, up to 2 matches were capped by maximum frequency at 4 kHz; –, excluded conditions because all matches were capped; MLE, maximum-likelihood estimated.*

require the subject an active effort to return to the starting frequency during the procedure in case they were not in fact comparing each matching trial independently.

Pitch Match Mean and Variance

Figure 4 shows an example of pitch matching runs for each stimulus type (SINE, NBN, or PSHC), for a given subject (S11) and electrode position (E6). The dashed horizontal gridline shows the maximum frequency at 4 kHz (f_{max}, see **Figure 3**). In one pitch matching run of NBN (dashed line), the subject appears to have perceived the pitch very close to (or possibly above) the maximum frequency, but was hindered by the procedure's parameters. This cap occurred in up to 2 pitch matching runs in 4 conditions using NBN, and in 3 conditions using PSHC (see **Table 2**, denoted by *), which were all at E6 except for once at E1. In order to take these capped trials into account, maximum-likelihood estimations (MLE) of pitch match mean and variance were calculated; for each subject and each condition, the likelihood of obtaining the collected data was computed for a wide range of means and standard deviations. The probability

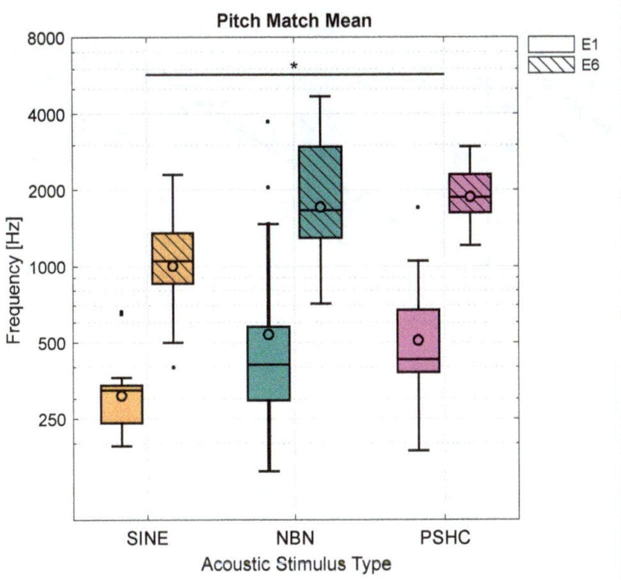

FIGURE 5 | Pitch match means for each stimulus type (SINE, NBN, or PSHC) and for each electrode position (E1 or E6) as boxplots with grand geometric means indicated as circles. Two-way repeated-measures ANOVA showed a significant effect of electrode position [$F(1,8) = 74.1$, $p < 0.001$] and acoustic stimulus type [$F(2,16) = 5.50$, $p = 0.015$]. Pairwise comparisons showed significant differences between electrode positions E1 and E6 ($p < 0.001$, not shown here) and between stimulus types SINE and PSHC (*$p = 0.017$), whereas the difference between SINE and NBN was marginally not significant ($p = 0.07$).

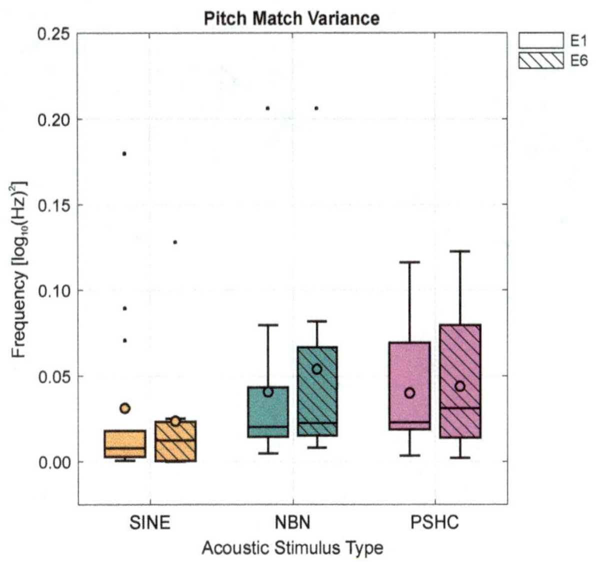

FIGURE 6 | Pitch match variances for each stimulus type (SINE, NBN, or PSHC) and for each electrode position (E1 or E6) as boxplots with mean variances indicated as circles. Two-way repeated-measures ANOVA showed neither within-subject effects nor interaction effects.

of obtaining a data point below 4 kHz was based on the normal probability density function, while the probability of obtaining a data point above 4 kHz, i.e., a capped trial, was based on the upper tail probability of the normal distribution. Hereafter, all pitch match means and variances are MLE values unless otherwise stated. In some cases, all pitch matching runs were capped and the respective condition was thus excluded from the analysis (see **Table 2**).

Figure 5 shows pitch match means for each stimulus type (SINE, NBN, or PSHC) and for each electrode position (E1 or E6) as boxplots with grand geometric means indicated as circles. **Table 2** shows grand geometric means for all conditions. A two-way repeated-measures ANOVA was performed with the factors electrode position and stimulus type ($n = 9$ due to exclusions). Mauchly's test indicated that the assumption of sphericity was not violated for any of the model effects. Both within-subject effects were significant, with $F(1,8) = 74.1$, $p < 0.001$ for the electrode position effect, and $F(2,16) = 5.50$, $p = 0.015$ for the stimulus type effect. No interaction effect was observed. Pairwise comparisons showed significant differences between electrode positions E1 and E6 ($p < 0.001$) and between stimulus types SINE and PSHC ($p = 0.017$), whereas the difference between SINE and NBN was marginally not significant ($p = 0.07$). The two-way repeated-measures ANOVA was repeated with 'actual' instead of MLE values and yielded equivalent results.

Figure 6 shows pitch match variances for each stimulus type and electrode position as boxplots with mean variances indicated as circles. SINE generally showed lower mean or median variances. And while SINE and NBN showed a few outliers, the distributions were generally comparable between electrode positions and stimulus types. This was confirmed by a two-way repeated-measures ANOVA showing neither within-subject effects nor interaction effects. Consequently, we were not able to reject the null hypothesis regarding the effect of stimulus type on the variability of pitch matches.

Pitch Match as a Function of Angle of Insertion

Figure 7 shows pitch match means for each stimulus type (SINE, NBN, or PSHC) and for each electrode position (E1 or E6) as a function of angle of insertion, which was estimated from postoperative X-ray images. Based on a histological study (Stakhovskaya et al., 2007), angles of insertion were transformed to percentage distances (or lengths) of the organ of Corti (OC) or the spiral ganglion (SG). These were then mapped to place-dependent characteristic frequencies (CFs) according to the empirically modeled Greenwood function (Greenwood, 1990). The OC frequency map $\pm$ 1 octave (solid black and gray curves, respectively) and the SG frequency map (dashed black curve) are repeated in each panel.

Residual sum of squares (SS_{res}) was calculated for each combination of stimulus type and electrode position as a measure of deviation of pitch match means from predicted CFs according to the OC or SG map. For the SG map, SINE had generally the smallest deviation for both electrode positions. However, the OC map reduced deviations for all stimulus types and electrode positions by at least a factor of 3 (up to 8) compared with the SG map, except for SINE at E6 with an increase of 47%. This

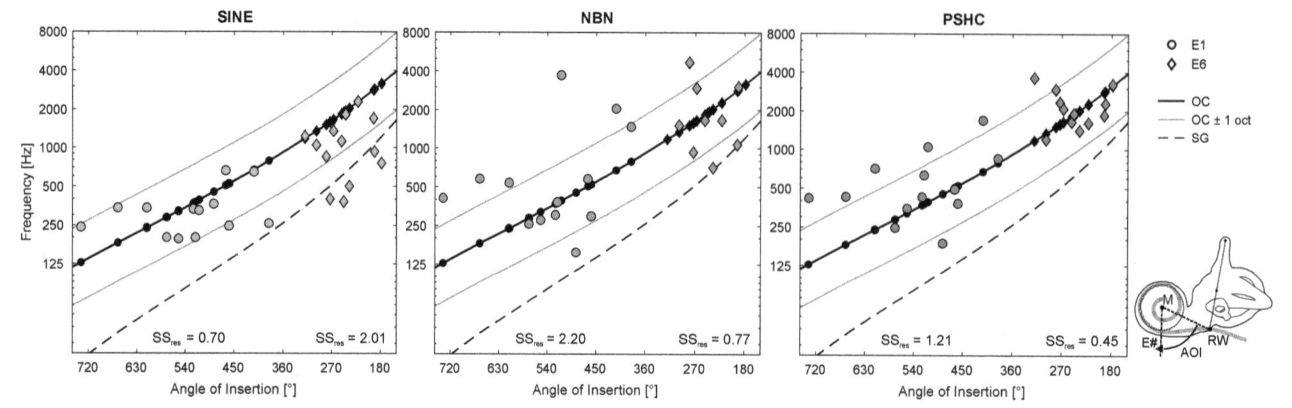

FIGURE 7 | Pitch match means for each stimulus type (SINE, NBN, or PSHC) and for each electrode position (E1 as circles, and E6 as diamonds) as a function of angle of insertion (AOI) estimated using the modified Stenvers' projection (Verbist et al., 2010). The schematic of a left cochlea shows how the AOI was measured for a given electrode (E#) by clockwise rotation at the geometric zero reference, which was defined as the line between the crossing point of the electrode array (gray) with the round window (RW), and the modiolus (M). The organ of Corti (OC) frequency map ± 1 octave (solid black and gray curves, respectively) and the spiral ganglion (SG) frequency map (dashed black curve) are repeated in each panel. Predicted characteristic frequencies according to the OC map (black filled circles or diamonds) are shown in each panel along the OC map's curve. Residual sum of squares [SS_{res}, expressed in $\log_{10}$(Hz)] for the OC map is shown for each combination of acoustic stimulus type and electrode position.

suggests that the OC map was generally a better model for our results, which is consistent with the fact that the implanted Flex28 or FlexSoft electrodes are typically placed homogenously along the lateral wall (Dhanasingh and Jolly, 2017). In **Figure 7**, SS_{res} expressed in $\log_{10}$(Hz) are shown for the OC map, for each condition. For E1, SINE had the smallest deviation, followed by PSHC, and then NBN. And for E6, PSHC had the smallest deviation, followed by NBN, and then SINE, which was generally matched lower than the predicted CFs.

These data suggest an inverse relation between electrode position and the deviation of SINE versus NBN or PSHC, which was largely confirmed by one-way repeated-measures ANOVA with the factor stimulus type for each electrode position: For E1, there was a significant within-subject effect of stimulus type, with $F(2,24) = 5.8$, $p < 0.01$. Pairwise comparisons showed that SINE pitch match means were significantly closer to CFs predicted by the OC map than either NBN or PSHC ($p = 0.035$ and $p < 0.01$, respectively). For E6, within-subject effect of stimulus type was also significant, with $F(2,16) = 5.4$, $p = 0.016$. But contrary to E1, pairwise comparisons for E6 showed that NBN and PSHC were closer to predicted CFs than SINE ($p = 0.046$ and $p = 0.021$, respectively). In both analyses, no significant differences were found between NBN and PSHC. Note, however, that the differences and by extension the inverse relation appear to be larger between SINE and PSHC than between SINE and NBN.

DISCUSSION

In this study, we minimized the effect of sensory and non-sensory biases on electric-acoustic pitch matches in CI users with SSD by controlling for loudness profiles, balancing between the two modalities, accounting for possible reversals in electric pitch perception, and implementing the binary search procedure to match pitch between electric and acoustic stimuli. While the mean pitch match variance showed no differences between acoustic stimulus types, mean pitch matches showed effects of electrode position and stimulus type, with the middle electrode always matched to a higher frequency than the apical one, and significantly higher across-subject pitch matches for PSHC compared with SINE. Mean pitch matches for all stimulus types were better predicted by CFs according to the OC map than the SG map. CF predictions were closest to pitch matches with SINE for the apical electrode position, and conversely with NBN or PSHC for the middle electrode position. In the following, we consider methodological limitations of the study design and then discuss the observed effects of acoustic stimulus type and electrode position on electric-acoustic pitch matches.

Binary Search Procedure

Although the binary search procedure has not been directly compared with other pitch matching methods, 9 of the subjects who participated in the present study were also subjects in a previous study by Rader et al. (2016) which used the method of adjustment. The acoustic stimulus type was SINE, and was matched with electric stimuli in two different conditions: pulse trains either had a fixed rate of 800 pps or they had a rate corresponding to predicted CF for the intracochlear electrode location, i.e., place-dependent rates. For each condition, 6 repetitions were obtained for electrodes E1– E6. **Figure 8** shows the variance of the pitch matches obtained for E1 and E6 using the binary search procedure (adaptive) at a fixed rate of 800 pps, and for the two adjustment procedures (adjustable) of Rader et al. (2016) at a fixed rate of 800 pps or at the place-dependent rate. While these data were not all collected on the same day and are, therefore, not directly comparable, it is worth noting that the binary search procedure could yield a much smaller variance than the adjustment procedure. This was confirmed by a two-way repeated-measures ANOVA with

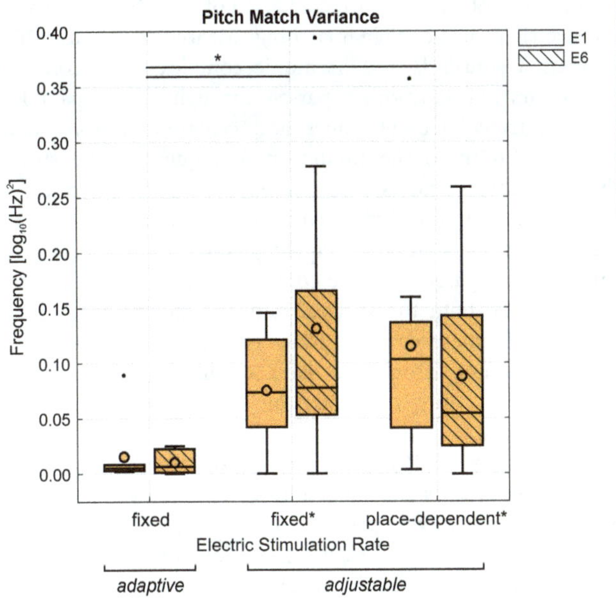

FIGURE 8 | Pitch match variances for each electrode position (E1 or E6) are compared in a subset of subjects previously tested using SINE (*n* = 9, Rader et al., 2016). Pitch matches were collected using either the binary search procedure (adaptive, from the current study) at a fixed rate of 800 pps, or the method of adjustment (adjustable, from the previous study as denoted by *) at a fixed rate of 800 pps or at the place-dependent rate. Two-way repeated-measures ANOVA showed a significant effect of matching method, with the binary search procedure significantly lower than the method of adjustment at either rate.

the factors electrode position (E1 or E6) and pitch matching method (adaptive with fixed rate, adjustable with fixed or place-dependent rate). Results showed no effect of electrode position but a significant effect of method, $F(2,14) = 7.25$, $p = 0.007$, with lower variance of the adaptive method, i.e., binary search procedure, than either adjustable methods. If this observation was confirmed in a direct comparison of pitch matching methods, it could mean that the binary search procedure is easier to perform than an adjustment task. Comparing electric-acoustic pitch matching methods, however, will remain a difficult endeavor, because there is currently no outcome measure that can be used for validation.

Although the binary search procedure does not require *a priori* assumptions on the frequency range of the acoustic stimuli, in the present study, this was not strictly the case since the acoustic frequency range was purposely limited to values ranging from 125 Hz to 4 kHz. The maximum frequency limit of 4 kHz was imposed because a pilot experiment with normal-hearing (NH) subjects showed that when using a 4-kHz standard, pitch matching accuracy for NBN and PSHC was substantially decreased. In addition, we did not anticipate that stimulation of the middle electrode (E6), which was the most basal electrode tested, would elicit pitch sensations higher than 4 kHz. Based on the results from the previous study using sinusoids (Rader et al., 2016) and on CF estimations using X-ray images, we expected E6 to be matched in the range 1–2 kHz, which was generally true for our results using SINE (see **Figure 5** and **Table 2**).

Methodological Considerations

The present study involved several methodological features with respect to the loudness-balancing procedure, the preliminary unilateral pitch comparisons, and the addition of catch trials to the main pitch matching task.

First, electric-acoustic pitch matching studies require that the acoustic and electric stimuli are equated in loudness before the subjects compare them in pitch. In most previous studies, the procedure was to first perform a *rough* pitch match between the acoustic and electric stimuli and then conduct loudness comparisons for these approximately pitch-matched stimuli (e.g., Schatzer et al., 2014). This approach may introduce an additional bias in that the subject could learn to associate a given electrode to a certain acoustic stimulus before starting the main pitch matching experiment. To avoid this potential problem, the electrodes used in this study for the loudness balancing (E3 and E4) were different than those used for the pitch matching (E1 and E6). In an earlier study, Vermeire et al. (2008) also limited the amount of loudness comparisons between the electrodes and the acoustic stimuli by only balancing one middle electrode (E6) to the acoustic sounds and then balancing all other electrodes to this middle electrode.

Second, prior to collecting electric-acoustic pitch data, each subject performed unilateral pitch comparisons separately in each modality. The electric-electric comparisons were used to verify that the two electrodes used in the main procedure (E1 and E6) were tonotopically ordered in the 'electric' pitch dimension such that subjects did not show pitch reversals. Despite the relatively large distance between neighboring electrodes of the MED-EL Flex28 electrode array (2.1 mm), only 4 out of 13 subjects could perfectly pitch rank electrodes E1 to E8. Furthermore, the variability in the ranks was larger for the 4 apical than for the 4 basal electrodes tested, consistent with previous studies in subjects with deep electrode insertions (Gani et al., 2007; Kenway et al., 2015). This suggests that the place pitch percept produced by different electrodes may not be very salient and could further depend on relative changes in the quality of sound, or timbre, as shown in a previous study using multi-dimensional scaling (Vermeire et al., 2013). The acoustic-acoustic pitch matching allowed the subjects to get accustomed to the procedure and was also used to compare their ability to match the pitch of acoustic sounds to that of NH listeners, which was largely comparable between groups for the 250-Hz and 1-kHz standards.

Effect of Acoustic Stimulus Type

Comparing the pitch of sounds with different timbres is known to be a difficult task (Micheyl and Oxenham, 2004; Carlyon et al., 2010). Carlyon et al. (2010) presented results from NH subjects tested with two procedures that used sinusoids in one ear and noise bands in the other ear and showed that, while the subjects could correctly pitch rank each type of sounds separately, their pitch match across ears were strongly influenced by range biases. It therefore appears essential to perform pitch comparisons between sounds that are relatively similar.

In the present study, we have investigated two types of broadband stimuli (NBN and PSHC), which were 1/3-octave wide and had 36-dB per octave spectral slopes. These slopes are broadly consistent with previous vocoder studies that aimed to simulate the sound of CI (reviewed in Mesnildrey and Macherey, 2015; Karoui et al., 2019). However, it is likely that the spectral slope corresponding to that of the excitation spread of a CI electrode will vary across electrodes and across subjects. In order to evaluate the impact of such variations, NH subjects (n = 10) were tested in a pilot pitch matching test. For each stimulus type (NBN or PSHC), they were asked to match a standard stimulus presented in one ear at a fixed center frequency (250 Hz, 1, or 4 kHz) with a comparison stimulus presented to the other ear with different spectral slopes (24, 36, or 48 dB per octave) and adaptively changed in frequency using the binary search procedure. For each stimulus type and standard frequency, results showed no significant differences between comparison spectral slopes. Therefore, we assume that the specific spectral slope used in the present study (i.e., 36 dB per octave) did not have a significant effect on the collected data.

The underlying hypothesis of our study was that PSHC would be perceptually closer to the sound of a CI electrode than NBN or SINE, and that pitch matches would consequently be less variable. This hypothesis could not be supported by the present data, which may be due to several reasons; first, the rate of PSHCs is defined based on the outputs of Gammatone filters which may not be valid for all SSD subjects who sometimes show hearing loss at high frequencies (Hilkhuysen and Macherey, 2014). Second, PSHCs do not simulate pulse-to-pulse interactions within a given pulse train, which are present in electrical hearing (Boulet et al., 2015). Third, PSHC can produce distortion products, particularly at a frequency corresponding to their rate (Hilkhuysen and Macherey, 2014), which are absent in direct electric stimulation of the auditory nerve via a CI electrode. The significantly higher across-subject pitch matches for PSHC compared with SINE may relate to this third point, because the temporal cue provided by the PSHC rate together with distortion products may have provided an additional pitch cue lower than the 'spectral' pitch cue corresponding to the center frequency of the stimulus. Therefore, it cannot be excluded that subjects adjusted the center frequency of the PSHC at a frequency higher than that of SINE to *compensate* for this additional pitch cue. However, the similarity between mean pitch matches obtained for NBN and PSHC is inconsistent with this explanation since this additional pitch cue is not present in NBN.

The finding that pitch matches corresponding to a given electrode depended on the type of acoustic stimulus warrants some caution when interpreting the results of electric-acoustic pitch matching studies because there is currently no scientifically based justification for using one type of sound over another. In the present study, for example, if one only considered pitch matches using SINE (see **Figure 5** and **Table 2**), then one would conclude that the subjects were adapted to their speech processor's center frequency at E6 of approximately 1.3 kHz despite the tonotopic mismatch (Reiss et al., 2007; Reiss et al., 2014) but not for E1. This conclusion, however, is not supported by the pitch matches using NBN or PSHC. Another recent study reported an effect of acoustic stimulus type on electric-acoustic pitch matching; Maarefvand et al. (2017) have used sinusoids and harmonic complex tones consisting of the first 11 harmonics passed through a bandpass filter with relatively shallow slopes and centered at a frequency equal to 1.6 times the fundamental frequency. The spectral shape of this stimulus was chosen based on the results of a study on timbre by Lazard et al. (2012). They found that the pitch-matched frequency was always higher for sinusoids compared with the complex tone. It is worth noting, however, that both the spectral centroid and the fundamental frequency of these complex tones co-varied, which may have made the comparison with electric pulses difficult since – presumably – only the place of excitation varied for the electric stimuli.

Goupell et al. (2019) raised another concern when comparing pitch between ears and modalities; they showed that range biases were strongly present in bilateral CI users when comparing the pitch of electrodes in different ears, although these same subjects could reliably pitch rank electrodes in each ear. They further suggested that differences in stimulation modalities (acoustic vs. electric) may not be the only problem associated with electric-acoustic pitch matching but that other yet unknown processes may make inter-aural pitch comparisons difficult.

Effect of Electrode Position

The tonotopic organization of the cochlea is one of the main prerequisites for the functioning of a CI. Speech processing strategies utilize this physiological property by presenting different frequency information to discrete locations along the length of the electrode array (Macherey and Carlyon, 2014). However, different CI electrode arrays generally do not reach the apex of the cochlea and thus a mismatch between frequency allocations of the speech processors and the physiological tonotopy of the auditory nerve is presently inevitable (Landsberger et al., 2015). A histological study by Stakhovskaya et al. (2007) provided relative location maps for the organ of Corti (OC) and the spiral ganglion (SG). Using the angle of insertion for each electrode position, which is estimated from postoperative X-ray images, these maps are used to calculate place-dependent characteristic frequencies (CFs) according to the empirically modeled Greenwood function (Greenwood, 1990). Recent studies investigated manipulations of these frequency maps to improve pitch perception in CI users, but have thus far shown inconsistent results.

While this individualized approach could partly account for morphological variations of the cochlea (Rask-Andersen et al., 2012; Pietsch et al., 2017), some limitations need to be taken into account; first, there is an inherent error margin in estimations based on X-ray images due to, for example, a poor resolution of electrode contacts, or if the round window is not easily identifiable since it provides the 0° reference for the frequency maps (Stakhovskaya et al., 2007; Verbist et al., 2010; Koch et al., 2017). Second, some studies based their assumptions or compared their results with the SG map, which is presumed to be the locus of neural excitation via CI (Landsberger et al., 2015; Peters et al., 2016), while other studies including the present one found their results to be better approximated by the OC map, especially when using lateral-wall electrode designs (Vermeire et al., 2008; Schatzer et al., 2014). These discrepancies underline the fact that these models are based on assumptions which cannot always be held true and should be reconsidered depending on the study approach. Third, there is a growing body of literature regarding peripheral degeneration or dead regions of spiral ganglion cells and their effect on CI function (Pfingst et al., 2015), which could further have an effect on variability between subjects.

The present study showed an effect of discrete electrode position independent of acoustic stimulus type, which is in line with an underlying tonotopic organization. However, SG and OC maps showed different results depending on stimulus type (see **Figure 7**) such that no consistent conclusions could be drawn. These results together with the aforementioned limitations raise the question whether relative distances rather than absolute place-dependent frequency estimations are more important for pitch comparisons between electric and acoustic stimulation. As mentioned above, Vermeire et al. (2013) conducted a multi-dimensional scaling study and suggested that a change in place of stimulation, i.e., electrode position, results in a perceptual change concurrent with acoustic frequency. Still, they also found another dimension showing concurrent change, which can be attributed to a change in sound quality or timbre. It is assumed that this dimension can be dependent on other factors, such as neural survival or pulse-to-pulse interactions (Boulet et al., 2015; Pfingst et al., 2015), which is in turn dependent on the electrode position *per se*, but not necessarily based on empirical models. For example, Carlyon et al. (2010) tested a subject at two different time points who showed a substantial change in matched frequency, which was later found out to be consistent with electrode migration.

Since mean pitch matches were better predicted by CFs according to the OC map for all stimulus types, we can assume it as a model of place-dependent variations in our subject group. Given this premise, we speculate that the present data may shed light on the type of acoustic stimulus that best mimics the sound of a CI electrode. For the apical position (E1), SINE pitch matches were significantly closer to predicted CFs than either NBN or PSHC. And for the more basal position (E6), NBN and PSHC were closer to predicted CFs than SINE. This supports the notion that a change in place of stimulation could lead to a change in sound quality, with pure tones better mimicking the percept elicited by electric stimulation in the apical region and wideband stimuli in the basal region. Thereby providing a possible explanation for the high variability observed in previous studies attempting to match electric with acoustic pitch in SSD subjects, since the choice of acoustic stimulus may have been optimal only for a part of their data.

CONCLUSION

Different acoustic stimulus types were used to match the pitch of electric stimulation with the underlying assumption that a signal perceptually more similar to how electric stimulation sounds should yield less variable pitch matches. While it was not possible to reject the null hypothesis regarding this effect, our data provide evidence that the choice of acoustic stimulus type can have a significant effect on electric-acoustic pitch matching results. Our results further confirm a stimulus-independent effect of electrode position which, however, is not necessarily predicted by absolute frequency mapping. This suggests that changes in place of electric stimulation are attributed to relative changes in pitch or timbre. Place-dependent characteristic frequencies predicted by an organ of Corti map suggest sinusoidal sound quality in the apex and one closer to wideband stimuli in the base. Further research is still needed to find an acoustic stimulus that better mimics the percept elicited by electric stimulation in order to investigate how cochlear implant users process pitch information.

ETHICS STATEMENT

This study was carried out in accordance with the ethical standards of the institutional review board at the Goethe University Frankfurt, which approved the study protocol (IRB approval number 209/13). All subjects gave written informed consent in accordance with the Declaration of Helsinki.

AUTHOR CONTRIBUTIONS

YA, TW, UB, and OM contributed to the conception and design of the study. YA and SN organized and conducted the experiments. YA and OM performed the statistical analysis. YA, TW, UB, and OM contributed to the interpretation of the data. YA and OM wrote the first draft of the manuscript. All authors contributed to manuscript revision, read and approved the submitted version.

ACKNOWLEDGMENTS

We are indebted to our cochlear-implant and normal-hearing subjects for their patience and effort during the experiments.

REFERENCES

Arnoldner, C., Kaider, A., and Hamzavi, J. (2006). The role of intensity upon pitch perception in cochlear implant recipients. *Laryngoscope* 116, 1760–1765. doi: 10.1097/01.mlg.0000228214.02606.42

Boex, C., Baud, L., Cosendai, G., Sigrist, A., Kos, M. I., and Pelizzone, M. (2006). Acoustic to electric pitch comparisons in cochlear implant subjects with residual hearing. *J. Assoc. Res. Otolaryngol.* 7, 110–124. doi: 10.1007/s10162-005-0027-2

Boulet, J., White, M., and Bruce, I. C. (2015). Temporal considerations for stimulating spiral ganglion neurons with cochlear implants. *J. Assoc. Res. Otolaryngol.* 17, 1–17. doi: 10.1007/s10162-015-0545-5

Brainard, D. H. (1997). The psychophysics toolbox. *Spat. Vis.* 10, 433–436. doi: 10.1163/156856897x00357

Carlyon, R. P., Macherey, O., Frijns, J. H., Axon, P. R., Kalkman, R. K., Boyle, P., et al. (2010). Pitch comparisons between electrical stimulation of a cochlear implant and acoustic stimuli presented to a normal-hearing contralateral ear. *J. Assoc. Res. Otolaryngol.* 11, 625–640. doi: 10.1007/s10162-010-0222-7

Deeks, J. M., Gockel, H. E., and Carlyon, R. P. (2013). Further examination of complex pitch perception in the absence of a place-rate match. *J. Acoust. Soc. Am.* 133, 377–388. doi: 10.1121/1.4770254

Dhanasingh, A., and Jolly, C. (2017). An overview of cochlear implant electrode array designs. *Hear. Res.* 356, 93–103. doi: 10.1016/j.heares.2017.10.005

Gani, M., Valentini, G., Sigrist, A., Kos, M. I., and Boex, C. (2007). Implications of deep electrode insertion on cochlear implant fitting. *J. Assoc. Res. Otolaryngol.* 8, 69–83. doi: 10.1007/s10162-006-0065-4

Goupell, M. J., Cosentino, S., Stakhovskaya, O. A., and Bernstein, J. G. W. (2019). Interaural pitch-discrimination range effects for bilateral and single-sided-deafness cochlear-implant users. *J. Assoc. Res. Otolaryngol.* 20, 187–203. doi: 10.1007/s10162-018-00707-x

Green, T., Faulkner, A., and Rosen, S. (2012). Frequency selectivity of contralateral residual acoustic hearing in bimodal cochlear implant users, and limitations on the ability to match the pitch of electric and acoustic stimuli. *Int. J. Audiol.* 51, 389–398. doi: 10.3109/14992027.2011.642010

Greenwood, D. D. (1990). A cochlear frequency-position function for several species - 29 years later. *J. Acoust. Soc. Am.* 87, 2592–2605. doi: 10.1121/1.399052

Hilkhuysen, G., and Macherey, O. (2014). Optimizing pulse-spreading harmonic complexes to minimize intrinsic modulations after auditory filtering. *J. Acoust. Soc. Am.* 136, 1281–1294. doi: 10.1121/1.4890642

Karoui, C., James, C., Barone, P., Bakhos, D., Marx, M., and Macherey, O. (2019). Searching for the sound of a cochlear implant: evaluation of different vocoder parameters by CI users with single-sided deafness. *Trends Hear.* 23:2331216519866029. doi: 10.1177/2331216519866029

Kenway, B., Tam, Y. C., Vanat, Z., Harris, F., Gray, R., Birchall, J., et al. (2015). Pitch discrimination: an independent factor in cochlear implant performance outcomes. *Otol. Neurotol.* 36, 1472–1479. doi: 10.1097/MAO.0000000000000845

Koch, R. W., Ladak, H. M., Elfarnawany, M., and Agrawal, S. K. (2017). Measuring cochlear duct length - a historical analysis of methods and results. *J. Otolaryngol. Head Neck Surg.* 46, 19. doi: 10.1186/s40463-017-0194-2

Landsberger, D. M., Svrakic, M., Roland, J. T., and Svirsky, M. (2015). The relationship between insertion angles, default frequency allocations, and spiral ganglion place pitch in cochlear implants. *Ear. Hear.* 36, E207–E213. doi: 10.1097/AUD.0000000000000163

Lazard, D. S., Marozeau, J., and Mcdermott, H. J. (2012). The sound sensation of apical electric stimulation in cochlear implant recipients with contralateral residual hearing. *PLoS One* 7:e38687. doi: 10.1371/journal.pone.0038687

Levitt, H., and Rabiner, L. R. (1967). Use of a sequential strategy in intelligibility testing. *J. Acoust. Soc. Am.* 42, 609–612. doi: 10.1121/1.1910630

Lockhead, G. R., and Byrd, R. (1981). Practically perfect pitch. *J. Acoust. Soc. Am.* 70, 387–389. doi: 10.1121/1.386773

Long, C. J., Nimmo-Smith, I., Baguley, D. M., O'driscoll, M., Ramsden, R., Otto, S. R., et al. (2005). Optimizing the clinical fit of auditory brain stem implants. *Ear. Hear.* 26, 251–262. doi: 10.1097/00003446-200506000-00002

Maarefvand, M., Blamey, P. J., and Marozeau, J. (2017). Pitch matching in bimodal cochlear implant patients: effects of frequency, spectral envelope, and level. *J. Acoust. Soc. Am.* 142:2854. doi: 10.1121/1.5009443

Macherey, O., and Carlyon, R. P. (2010). Temporal pitch percepts elicited by dual-channel stimulation of a cochlear implant. *J. Acoust. Soc. Am.* 127, 339–349. doi: 10.1121/1.3269042

Macherey, O., and Carlyon, R. P. (2014). Cochlear implants. *Curr. Biol.* 24, R878–R884. doi: 10.1016/j.cub.2014.06.053

McDermott, J. H., Lehr, A. J., and Oxenham, A. J. (2008). Is relative pitch specific to pitch? *Psychol. Sci.* 19, 1263–1271. doi: 10.1111/j.1467-9280.2008.02235.x

Mesnildrey, Q., Hilkhuysen, G., and Macherey, O. (2016). Pulse-spreading harmonic complex as an alternative carrier for vocoder simulations of cochlear implants. *J. Acoust. Soc. Am.* 139, 986–991. doi: 10.1121/1.4941451

Mesnildrey, Q., and Macherey, O. (2015). Simulating the dual-peak excitation pattern produced by bipolar stimulation of a cochlear implant: effects on speech intelligibility. *Hear. Res.* 319, 32–47. doi: 10.1016/j.heares.2014.11.001

Micheyl, C., and Oxenham, A. J. (2004). Sequential F0 comparisons between resolved and unresolved harmonics: no evidence for translation noise between two pitch mechanisms. *J. Acoust. Soc. Am.* 116, 3038–3050. doi: 10.1121/1.1806825

Oxenham, A. J., Bernstein, J. G. W., and Penagos, H. (2004). Correct tonotopic representation is necessary for complex pitch perception. *Proc. Natl. Acad. Sci. U.S.A.* 101, 1421–1425. doi: 10.1073/pnas.0306958101

Peters, J. P. M., Bennink, E., Grolman, W., and Van Zanten, G. A. (2016). Electro-acoustic pitch matching experiments in patients with single-sided deafness and a cochlear implant: is there a need for adjustment of the default frequency allocation tables? *Hear. Res.* 342, 124–133. doi: 10.1016/j.heares.2016.10.009

Pfingst, B. E., Zhou, N., Colesa, D. J., Watts, M. M., Strahl, S. B., Garadat, S. N., et al. (2015). Importance of cochlear health for implant function. *Hear. Res.* 322, 77–88. doi: 10.1016/j.heares.2014.09.009

Pietsch, M., Aguirre Davila, L., Erfurt, P., Avci, E., Lenarz, T., and Kral, A. (2017). Spiral form of the human cochlea results from spatial constraints. *Sci. Rep.* 7:7500. doi: 10.1038/s41598-017-07795-4

Plant, K. L., Mcdermott, H. J., Van Hoesel, R. J., Dawson, P. W., and Cowan, R. S. (2014). Factors influencing electrical place pitch perception in bimodal listeners. *J. Acoust. Soc. Am.* 136:1199. doi: 10.1121/1.4892790

Rader, T., Doge, J., Adel, Y., Weissgerber, T., and Baumann, U. (2016). Place dependent stimulation rates improve pitch perception in cochlear implantees with single-sided deafness. *Hear. Res.* 339, 94–103. doi: 10.1016/j.heares.2016.06.013

Rask-Andersen, H., Liu, W., Erixon, E., Kinnefors, A., Pfaller, K., Schrott-Fischer, A., et al. (2012). Human cochlea: anatomical characteristics and their relevance for cochlear implantation. *Anat. Rec.* 295, 1791–1811. doi: 10.1002/ar.22599

Reiss, L. A., Ito, R. A., Eggleston, J. L., Liao, S., Becker, J. J., Lakin, C. E., et al. (2015). Pitch adaptation patterns in bimodal cochlear implant users: over time and after experience. *Ear. Hear.* 36, e23–e34. doi: 10.1097/AUD.0000000000b000114

Reiss, L. A., Turner, C. W., Erenberg, S. R., and Gantz, B. J. (2007). Changes in pitch with a cochlear implant over time. *J. Assoc. Res. Otolaryngol.* 8, 241–257. doi: 10.1007/s10162-007-0077-8

Reiss, L. A., Turner, C. W., Karsten, S. A., and Gantz, B. J. (2014). Plasticity in human pitch perception induced by tonotopically mismatched electro-acoustic stimulation. *Neuroscience* 256, 43–52. doi: 10.1016/j.neuroscience.2013.10.024

Schatzer, R., Vermeire, K., Visser, D., Krenmayr, A., Kals, M., Voormolen, M., et al. (2014). Electric-acoustic pitch comparisons in single-sided-deaf cochlear implant users: frequency-place functions and rate pitch. *Hear. Res.* 309, 26–35. doi: 10.1016/j.heares.2013.11.003

Stakhovskaya, O., Sridhar, D., Bonham, B. H., and Leake, P. A. (2007). Frequency map for the human cochlear spiral ganglion: implications for cochlear implants. *J. Assoc. Res. Otolaryngol.* 8, 220–233. doi: 10.1007/s10162-007-0076-9

Tan, C. T., Martin, B., and Svirsky, M. A. (2017). Pitch matching between electrical stimulation of a cochlear implant and acoustic stimuli presented to a contralateral ear with residual hearing. *J. Am. Acad. Audiol.* 28, 187–199. doi: 10.3766/jaaa.15063

Van Zon, A., Peters, J. P., Stegeman, I., Smit, A. L., and Grolman, W. (2015). Cochlear implantation for patients with single-sided deafness or asymmetrical hearing loss: a systematic review of the evidence. *Otol. Neurotol.* 36, 209–219. doi: 10.1097/MAO.0000000000000681

Verbist, B. M., Skinner, M. W., Cohen, L. T., Leake, P. A., James, C., Boex, C., et al. (2010). Consensus panel on a cochlear coordinate system applicable in histologic, physiologic, and radiologic studies of the human cochlea. *Otol. Neurotol.* 31, 722–730. doi: 10.1097/MAO.0b013e3181d279e0

Vermeire, K., Landsberger, D. M., Schleich, P., and Van De Heyning, P. H. (2013). Multidimensional scaling between acoustic and electric stimuli in cochlear implant users with contralateral hearing. *Hear. Res.* 306, 29–36. doi: 10.1016/j.heares.2013.09.004

Vermeire, K., Landsberger, D. M., Van De Heyning, P. H., Voormolen, M., Kleine Punte, A., Schatzer, R., et al. (2015). Frequency-place map for electrical stimulation in cochlear implants: change over time. *Hear. Res.* 326, 8–14. doi: 10.1016/j.heares.2015.03.011

Vermeire, K., Nobbe, A., Schleich, P., Nopp, P., Voormolen, M. H., and Van De Heyning, P. H. (2008). Neural tonotopy in cochlear implants: an evaluation in unilateral cochlear implant patients with unilateral deafness and tinnitus. *Hear. Res.* 245, 98–106. doi: 10.1016/j.heares.2008.09.003

Xu, J., Xu, S. A., Cohen, L. T., and Clark, G. M. (2000). Cochlear view: postoperative radiography for cochlear implantation. *Am. J. Otol.* 21, 49–56. doi: 10.1016/s0196-0709(00)80075-7

Zeitler, D. M., and Dorman, M. F. (2019). Cochlear implantation for single-sided deafness: a new treatment paradigm. *J. Neurol. Surg. B Skull Base* 80, 178–186. doi: 10.1055/s-0038-1677482

14

The Role of Music in Families of Children with Hearing Loss and Normal Hearing in Australia, Finland and the UK

Valerie Looi[1,2], *Ritva Torppa*[3*], *Tania Prvan*[4] *and Debi Vickers*[5]

[1] *SCIC – An RIDBC Service, Sydney, NSW, Australia,* [2] *Advanced Bionics (Asia Pacific), Sydney, NSW, Australia,*
[3] *Logopedics and Cognitive Brain Research Unit, Department of Psychology and Logopedics, Faculty of Medicine, University of Helsinki, Helsinki, Finland,* [4] *Department of Mathematics and Statistics, Macquarie University, Sydney, NSW, Australia,*
[5] *Department of Clinical Neurosciences, The University of Cambridge, Cambridge, United Kingdom*

Correspondence:
Ritva Torppa
ritva.torppa@helsinki.fi

The primary aim of this current study was to compare the role, importance and value placed on music by families with normally hearing (NH) children, to those who had a child with a hearing loss (HL) who wore either hearing aids and/or cochlear implants. A secondary aim was to see whether this differed between the countries. Parents of children aged 2–6 years living in Australia, Finland, and the United Kingdom were invited to complete the Role of Music in Families Questionnaire (RMFQ). Two groups of participants were recruited from each country: (i) parents of NH children, and (ii) parents of children with a HL. The RMFQ had seven subsections covering topics such as music participation, attitudes to music, importance of music in the family, and future perspectives on music. Three hundred and twenty-two families of NH children, and 56 families of children with HL completed the questionnaire (Australia: 50 NH, 25 HL; Finland: 242 NH, 21 HL; United Kingdom: 30 NH, 10 HL). Analyses compared between NH and HL groups within each country, and between the three countries for the NH group, and the HL group, independently. Overall, there were few significant differences between the participation levels, role, or importance of music in families with NH children compared to those with a child who had a HL, regardless of whether the families lived in Australia, Finland or the United Kingdom. Children first started to respond to music at similar ages, and overall music participation frequency, and music enjoyment were relatively similar. The importance of music in the family was also similar between the NH and HL groups. In comparing between the countries, Finnish children had a tendency to have higher participation rates in musical activities, with few other differences noted. Overall, the results of this study indicate that children, regardless of hearing levels or country of residence, have similar levels of music engagement and enjoyment, and HL is not seen as a contraindication to music participation and involvement by the parents involved in this study.

Keywords: music, children, home environment, upbringing, hearing loss, family, culture

INTRODUCTION

Music is pervasive, transcends cultures and spoken language, and plays a multitude of different roles across the life span. For a baby or infant, singing can soothe, comfort, calm or entertain (Custodero, 2006; Ilari et al., 2011). As the baby progresses through infancy to becoming a toddler, music can also enhance language development, parental and social bonding, and musical development (Trehub, 2001; Costa-Giomi and Ilari, 2014; Virtala and Partanen, 2018). Parent–child musical activities include not only joint singing of songs, but also playing instruments, dancing, listening to music, and spontaneously making up new music or songs (Barrett, 2011). Williams et al. (2015) showed that higher regularity of these shared home musical activities was associated with children having better vocabulary, numeracy, attentional and emotional regulation, and prosocial skills.

This contribution of music to a child's upbringing and to family life seems to transcend culture and country. Ilari (2013) describes a qualitative study where unstructured interviews were conducted with 13 families of 7-year old children in nine countries (Greece, Netherlands, Denmark, England, Spain, Kenya, Taiwan, Israel, and the United States). These interviews comprised of 1–2 h home visits, where parents and children were asked to talk about their child's music participation and experiences, used in collation with photographic and text descriptions of the home, location, and musical resources in the household. Thematic analyses were conducted. Although there was no between-country comparisons made, the authors reported that all 13 families had stated that music was important in their children's lives, and that participation in organized music activities provided their child with an opportunity to discover, enjoy, and hopefully love music.

In another qualitative, natural observation study, Young and Gillen (2007) videoed a single day of home-care for seven children, aged 2.5 years, each one from a different country (Canada, Italy, Peru, Thailand, Turkey, United Kingdom, and United States). The videos were then analyzed to look for music-related activities that occurred during the day such as singing as part of the caregiver–child interaction, music that was turned on (e.g., CD) during the day, dancing, to name just a few. The authors provide a qualitative description of the musical activities observed for each child in each country, and speculate as to the potential socio-cultural factors that might have impacted on this, and how music participation is influenced by local social and cultural considerations.

There is a growing body of evidence on the associations between participation in more musical activities and improved speech perception and language skills for normally hearing (NH) listeners. Trained musicians have an increased ability to selectively engage and sustain their auditory attention, a finding referred to by some as the 'musician's advantage' (Moreno and Bidelman, 2014). This cognitive advantage may subsequently transfer from music specific skills to other categories of perception and executive functions (Schellenberg, 2004). A recent systematic review of the literature by Coffey et al. (2017) investigated the notion that music training could improve speech in noise perception for NH adults. The review reported little consistency amongst the studies in determining one mechanism behind the musician advantage, yet 18 of the 20 studies reviewed did support the existence of an advantage for musicians in speech in noise perception.

To shift the focus to children, a longitudinal study measuring children's speech in noise perception ability with music training was conducted by Slater et al. (2015). Forty six NH children (mean age of 8 years, $SD = 0.72$) were involved in the 3 years study, where they were randomly assigned to one of two groups. The first group commenced 2 years of music training (2–4 h a week) straight away, whilst the second group waited a year, and subsequently received 1 year of training. There were 38 children included in the final analyses, 19 per group, with a significant improvement for speech in noise perception being seen for the group who received 2 years of music training ($p = 0.001$). Slater et al. (2015) attributed the observed improvement to a 'musician's advantage' resulting from specific training programs, not prior musical experiences. Musical training is associated with better pre-attentive processing of speech sounds of a foreign language (Intartaglia et al., 2017) and better word learning (Dittinger et al., 2017). There are several randomized controlled trials for children with NH, and these have shown that when compared to other training, music training (especially when including singing) enhances non-musical skills including reading skills, phonological awareness (Dege and Schwarzer, 2011; Flaugnacco et al., 2015; Gordon et al., 2015; Patscheke et al., 2018), speech segmentation (Francois et al., 2013), executive function (Jaschke et al., 2018), and verbal intelligence (Jaschke et al., 2018; Linnavalli et al., 2018). The possible benefits of music training have also been shown in brain imaging studies. For example, gray matter volume in areas involved in auditory processing increases with more musical training (e.g., Schneider et al., 2002; Gaser and Schlaug, 2003), as does connectivity between frontal and auditory areas (Halwani et al., 2011; Dittinger et al., 2018; Oechslin et al., 2018).

Adolescents and adults with NH regulate their mood with music, and music has emotional, social, and psychological roles in our lives (Saarikallio and Erkkilä, 2007; Saarikallio, 2011). Hence, as music is important and beneficial through the lifespan, it is important to introduce it early into a child's life. Denac (2008) reports that early positive experiences with music will influence the child's formation of their general attitude toward musical culture and engagement, and subsequently their interest and participation in musical activities. The rate of development of a child's musical abilities is strongly linked to their early experiences of music before entering school, in which parents/caregivers and early childhood educators play a significant role (Denac, 2008).

Although the above studies have focused on NH listeners, there is no reason to believe that the benefits of music do not extend to individuals with a hearing loss (HL). The possible benefits of music and musical activities have already been recognized in the habilitation of children with HL. Playing musical instruments and singing is often used in speech and language therapy to engage them into the world of sounds, keep them attentive, and enhance their auditory perception (Estabrooks, 1994; Ronkainen, 2011). A longitudinal study by

Good et al. (2017) compared music to art lessons for 25 CI recipients (aged 6–15 years; mean = 10 years), for music and emotional prosody perception. Music training consisted of piano lessons, music theory and singing songs. The music lesson group showed significant improvements in music perception and emotional prosody discrimination at both the mid-point (3 months) and end-point (6 months), with no improvements for the children receiving art lessons. Torppa et al. (2014a) found that children with CIs who were reported to sing more at home post-implantation were more sensitive to changes in musical pitch and timbre as assessed with attention-related brain responses. Furthermore, Torppa et al. (2014b) administered a questionnaire to children with CIs, divided into two groups: (i) those having more involvement in formal and informal musical activities (active music engagement at home and outside of the home), (ii) and those having less music engagement, and assessed their performance twice (follow-up period approximately 16 months). Greater levels of active music engagement was strongly linked to better perception of the fundamental frequency (pitch), intensity, and prosodic stress in the speech stimuli, along with better development of auditory working memory. Additionally, better pitch and intensity perception was associated with better perception of speech stress. At the end of follow-up period, musically active children with CIs were better in word finding, verbal intelligence and phonological awareness, than less musically active children, with higher levels of parental singing being associated with better word finding and verbal intelligence (Torppa et al., 2019).

Gfeller et al. (2019) recently published retrospective data on a cohort of 76 pediatric CI users where they extracted pitch perception (pitch ranking of piano tones) test scores, as well as responses to two questionnaires – one on familial music engagement both whilst growing up, as well as 'currently' at the time of the study (providing a 'familial engagement in music score'), and the second on formal music involvement in classes and ensembles whilst growing up (providing a 'music engagement' score, as well as a sub-score on the duration of these music classes over time, quantified in years). They found that better pitch perception correlated with the overall 'music engagement' score, as well as the duration of time they were involved in these music classes. Interestingly, pitch perception was a significant predictor for the speech test scores (Gfeller et al., 2019). Musical training has also been shown to improve both music perception and music enjoyment for adult CI and HA users (Looi et al., 2012a,b). Overall, evidence indicates that for children and adults with HL, musical training is associated with improvements in not just music perception and music enjoyment, but also language and non-musical auditory perception skills.

Given the potential that music involvement offers to children, regardless of their hearing levels, it is important to ascertain whether parents of children with HL value music engagement in the same ways that parents of children with NH do. That is, do parents of children with HL de-prioritize music involvement or consider their child's HL as a contraindication to music involvement? This is important as it could potentially result in children with HL having less exposure to music, reduced opportunities to benefit from music participation, and/or lower music enjoyment levels compared to children with NH. Positively, there is some preliminary evidence showing that family values and priorities are more related to a child's music involvement and exposure than hearing-related factors. A study conducted by Driscoll et al. (2015) involved parents of 32 families who had a child with a CI, with 28 of these families also having another child who had NH. Parents were asked to complete a survey regarding their children's music participation and the impact of family values on musical engagement. Children were attending either preschool or primary school, with a mean age of 9.88 years (*SD* = 1.36). Correlations were performed between the parent's ratings of importance, the child's hearing ability, and their level of musical involvement. Results of this study revealed that CI and NH siblings from the same families had similar levels of musical involvement, with little difference in frequency of engagement or participation in formal lessons. That is, regardless of hearing status, children from the same family had music participation and enjoyment levels that reflected their parent's values. Importantly, there was no significant association between hearing status and musical involvement; it was the values of the parents that was the dominant factor determining if a child actively engaged with music, highlighting the significant impact parent attitudes play in children's music involvement (Driscoll et al., 2015). In line with this, the retrospective analyses by Gfeller et al. (2019) showed that current familial engagement in music was predictive of the Music Engagement Score, but age or time with the CI was not associated with music engagement.

One question that arises as a result of the Driscoll et al. (2015) study is whether the fact that the parents had a child with a CI impacted on their overall attitudes. In other words, did parents consciously (or subconsciously) change their attitude to music and the role of music in their children's lives, to compensate for their child with a CI; if their children all had NH, would attitudes or expectations have differed? Hence the main aim of this current study was to compare the role, importance and value placed on music by families who had only NH children, to those who had a child with a hearing impairment (HI) and wore either hearing aids (HAs) and/or CIs. That is, is there a difference in the role of music, and attitudes to music between families of children with NH compared to families who have a child with a HL. Is there a difference between the children's engagement with music, participation in music, or enjoyment of music? A secondary aim was to see whether this differed between three different countries – i.e., are there cultural considerations that need to be considered?

MATERIALS AND METHODS

This study was conducted in Australia, Finland, and the United Kingdom (UK), with appropriate institutional ethics approvals being obtained for all countries.

Participants

Parents of children aged between 2 to 6 years were invited to complete the questionnaire. There were two groups of participants for each country – families with NH children (NH group), and families who had a child with a HL (HL group). Children in the HL group could use either hearing aids (HAs) and/or CIs, fitted unilaterally, bilaterally or bimodally (CI in one ear, HA in the contralateral ear), but had to have been fitted with their first hearing device at age two or younger. Families of children with additional disabilities and families of NH children who had a sibling with a HL were excluded from the study. As this was an anonymous online survey, it was not possible to pre-screen individuals against the inclusion and exclusion criteria. Participants had to click they had read and agreed to the online Participant Information Consent Form statement before proceeding, and that they met the study criteria.

Materials

The Role of Music in Families Questionnaire (RMFQ), initially developed by Looi et al. (2018) was furthered for this study. There were three versions of this questionnaire, one for parents of children with NH, one for parents of children fitted with HA(s), and one for families of children fitted with CI(s). It had seven subsections, which covered the topics of: A-General Information, B-Childhood Music Participation and Experiences, C-Attitudes and Reactions to Music, D-Music Resources, E-Overall Importance of Music in the Household and Family, F-Music Listening Preferences and G-Future Perspectives. The survey comprised both closed- and open-ended questions, taking an estimated 30–45 min to complete. For Finland, an extra section H was added covering questions related to speech production, singing, and factors that encourage singing, however, these will not be covered in this paper. The RMFQ was broadly adapted from the Music Engagement Questionnaire: preschool and elementary (MEQ-P/E) used by Driscoll et al. (2015), with several major changes. Firstly, the RMFQ extended beyond the MEQ-P/E by having three separate surveys for the three sub-groups of families, and included children with HAs. The MEQ-P/E had a total of 26 questions, while the RMFQ had a total of 82 questions covering a broader range of topics. The target age group for the RMFQ was children aged 2–6 years, as opposed to the MEQ-P/E which included children up to 12 years of age. Finally, the MEQ-P/E was designed for families who had one child with a CI, and one child with NH. That is, comparisons were intra-family, rather than between-families as in the current study.

Procedure

The three versions of the RMFQ were initially pilot tested with five families in Australia to ensure it was clear, response options were valid, and questions were interpreted as expected. The questionnaires were then translated for Finland, with country-specific adaptations and pilot testing being conducted in Finland and the UK. The adaptations were predominantly in the first section, with response categories to demographic questions being changed to suit the country (e.g., the income ranges, education categories etc.). The RMFQ was then uploaded onto an online survey portal. In Australia and Finland, Qualtrics[1] was utilized. In the UK, University College of London web-based, secure survey tool "Opinio" was used (UCL, 2019)[2]. The questionnaire could be completed on a computer, tablet and/or smart phone, and no personal identifying information was collected.

In all countries, flyers containing the study information and questionnaire links were distributed via a number of hearing-related organizations, clinics, and charities. Data collection time varied slightly between the three countries, but was approximately 3 months.

Data Analysis

Data from the HA and CI questionnaires were grouped together to form a HL group, with analyses predominantly focusing on comparing this group to the NH group. It should be noted that Section B included questions related to the frequency of participation in, and enjoyment of, various musical activities. These were scored with different scales between countries. Frequency was scored on a 7-point scale for Australia and Finland: 0 = don't know, 1 = less than monthly; 2 = once a month; 3 = 2–3 times a month; 4 = once a week; 5 = 2–3 times a week; 6 = 4–6 times a week; 7 = daily. For the UK, a 6-point scale was used: 0 = don't know, 1 = less than monthly; 2 = once a month; 3 = 2–3 times a month; 4 = once a week; 5 = 2–6 times a week; 6 = daily. Hence for analyses, a 6-point scale was used, with responses in categories '5' and '6' from Australian and Finnish respondents being combined. Enjoyment was scored on a scale from 1 to 10 (1 = Does not Enjoy; 10 = Very much enjoys). Data was analyzed to assess for differences within each country for the effect of a HL (i.e., NH vs. HL for the same country), as well as between the three countries (i.e., Australia vs. Finland vs. UK) for (i) NH families and (ii) HL families.

Based on the research questions, statistical comparisons were predominantly made: (1) between countries, separately for NH and HI children; (2) between NH and HI children, only within each of the three countries (but not between countries; i.e., for example, no comparisons were made between NH children from one country to HI children from a different country).

As the exact statistical test used varied for the different sections due to the different types of data and different comparisons made, details of the test(s) used will be provided in the Results section under the applicable subsection. In general, for most of the statistical comparisons, Mood's Median tests were used as distributions of the data did not have the same shape (an assumption required for tests such as the Mann–Whitney *U*, or Kruskal–Wallis tests). The assumptions for parametric tests such as t-tests and/or Analyses of Variance (ANOVA) were not met on most occasions. Comparisons between proportions were made using Chi-square tests, or Fisher's Exact test when the assumptions for the Chi-square test failed (i.e., if more than 20% of cells had an expected count below 5; the Chi-Square tests needs this to be no more than 20% for the results to be valid). Bonferroni corrections were made for all multiple comparisons. Correlational analyses were performed using Spearman's Rank Correlations, as the bivariate normality assumption was violated. As is inherent to questionnaires, the number of respondents

[1] www.qualtrics.com/uk/research-core/survey-software/

[2] https://www.ucl.ac.uk/isd/services/learning-teaching/e-learning-staff/e-learning-core-tools/opinio

differed for some of the questions, and where applicable, the number of respondents who answered a particular question is provided in the tables provided. Analyses were performed using either SPSS version 23.0 and/or Minitab version 17.0.

RESULTS

In total across the three countries there were 322 families of NH children, and 56 families of children with HL. For Australia, there were 50 NH children (29 Male, 21 Female) with a mean age of 4.00 years (*SD* 1.102), and 25 hearing impaired (HI) children (15 Male, 10 Female) with a mean age of 3.54 years (*SD* 0.603). The NH children were significantly older than the HI children in Australia (p = 0.022; two-sample t-test). For Finland, the mean age of the 242 NH children (109 Male, 132 Female) was 3.92 years (*SD* 1.195), with the mean age of the 21 HI children (6 Male, 15 Female) being 3.42 years (*SD* 1.257). The UK cohort comprised 30 NH children (15 Male, 14 Female, 1 no response) with a mean age of 4.17 years (*SD* 1.341), and 10 HI children (5 Male, 5 Female), mean age 3.95 years (*SD* 1.252). There was no statistically significant difference between the ages of the NH and HI children in Finland, or the UK (Mood's Median Tests). There was also no statistically significant difference between the ages of the NH children across the three countries, or the ages of the HI children across the three countries (Mood's Median Tests).

Section A – General Information

This section covered general demographic and hearing-related information. Combined across the NH and HL groups, 92% of the surveys were completed by the mother in Australia, 99% in Finland and 95% in the UK. For Australia, 91% of the respondents spoke English as their main language at home, with 99% of the children being born in Australia, and 100% brought up in Australia. Eighty percent identified their culture as 'Australian.' For Finland, 98% of respondents spoke Finnish as their main language, 99.6% were brought up in Finland, and 96% identified their culture as 'Finnish.' For the UK, 70% of the respondents spoke English as their main home language, 85% were brought up in the UK, and 65% of them identified their culture as 'British.' For Australia, the most typical maternal education level was a Bachelor degree (33%), with 4% at the highest educational level (Ph.D. or Doctorate). Finnish results were very similar to Australia, with the most typical maternal education level being a Bachelor degree (38%), and 4% at the highest educational level (Ph.D. or Doctorate). For the UK 48% of respondents had a Bachelor Degree and 7.5% were educated to Ph.D./Doctoral level.

For the children in the HL group, the mean age diagnosed with HL was in Australia 0.39 years (*SD* 0.909), 0.71 years (*SD* 1.017) in Finland, and 0.78 years (*SD* 1.57) in the UK. The UK HL cohort included two children with progressive hearing losses, hence the large standard deviation. The level of HL the child was diagnosed with was most typically moderate in the right ear (28%) and moderately severe in the left ear (24%) for Australia. In Finland, the majority of children had a profound loss (both ears) (57%), with 29% having bilateral moderate losses. In the UK, the cohort contained three children (30%) with moderate bilateral losses, one child with a bilateral moderately severe loss, five children with bilateral severe to profound losses, and one child with a slightly asymmetric losses with the poorer ear being moderately severe. For Finland and the UK, all HA users (Finland, N = 7; UK, N = 4) and all CI users (Finland, N = 14; UK, N = 6) were fitted bilaterally. In Australia, of the 17 HA users, 13 were bilaterally aided, 4 unilaterally aided. Seven of the eight CI children were bilaterally implanted, with the other using bimodal stimulation. For the CI recipients, the mean age at of implantation was 1.45 years (*SD* 0.960) in Australia, 0.85 years (*SD* 0.245) in Finland, and 2.33 years (*SD* 1.212) for the UK. For the HA users, the mean age of first HA fitting was 0.87 years (*SD* 1.263) in Australia, 1.12 years (*SD* 1.046) for Finland, and 1.18 years (*SD* 1.891) for the UK. The mean time with their respective hearing device, in years, was: Australia, CI, 2.20 (*SD* 1.336), HA, 2.42 (*SD* 0.955); Finland, CI, 2.42 (*SD* 1.318), HA, 2.11 (1.318); UK; CI, 1.92 (*SD* 1.531), HA, 2.92 (*SD* 1.215).

Section B – Childhood Music Participation and Experiences

This section asked about the child's engagement in a wide range of music-based activities. Responses to question B1, "At what age did your child first start paying attention to music?" indicated that Australian NH children first attended to music at an average age of 0.62 years (*SD* = 0.89) while the 22 HI responses indicated an average age of 0.81 years (*SD* = 0.089), with no significant difference between the two groups (Mood's Median Test).

Question B5 asked parents "How often did you sing in front of your child (face to face) during the last year?" This was followed for the NH group by the question, "How often did you sing in front of your child (face to face) during the first year of his/her life, and for the HI group (Australia and Finland only)" – "How often did you sing in front of your child (face to face) in the first year after they received their CI/HA(s)?" The scales and results are displayed in **Table 1**.

For the question related to the amount of singing in the last year (Q B5), for the NH families, Fisher's Exact Test showed there was a significant difference between the three countries, with *post hoc* comparisons showing that the distribution of scores for Finland was significantly different to the UK distribution (p = 0.004) (see **Table 2** for the crosstabs, showing the distribution of responses for both the NH and HI groups). The means and distributions indicate that parents in Finland sang more than in UK. For the families of children with HL, there was

TABLE 1 | Mean of responses to questions B5 and B6 for parental singing.

Question	Australia		Finland		UK	
	NH	HL	NH	HL	NH	HL
B5	5.1 (1.3) (n = 48)	5.3 (0.96) (n = 21)	5.4 (0.95) (n = 242)	5.4 (1.2) (n = 21)	4.9 (1.5) (n = 30)	4.6 (1.6) (n = 10)
B6	5.7 (0.57) (n = 48)	5.6 (0.59) (n = 21)	5.6 (0.66) (n = 242)	5.5 (0.51) (n = 21)	5.6 (1.1) (n = 30)	Was not asked

6 = Daily, 5 = 2–6 times a week, 4 = Once a week, 3 = 2–3 times a month, 2 = once a month, 1 = Less than once a month, 0 = Don't know.

TABLE 2 | Distribution of responses for question B5.

Response	Australia		Finland		UK		All countries	
	NH *n* (%)	HL *n* (%)	NH *n* (%)	HL *n* (%)	NH *n* (%)	HL *n* (%)	NH *n* (%)	HL *n* (%)
0	1 (2.1)	0	0	0	0	0	1 (0.3)	0 (0)
1	0	0	4 (1.7)	0	2 (6.7)	1 (10.0)	6 (1.9)	1 (1.9)
2	2 (4.2)	1 (4.8)	0	2 (9.5)	2 (6.7)	0	4 (1.3)	3 (5.8)
3	2 (4.2)	0	9 (3.7)	0	0	1 (10.0)	11 (3.4)	1 (1.9)
4	2 (4.2)	1 (4.8)	12 (5.0)	0	4 (13.3)	2 (20.0)	18 (5.6)	3 (5.8)
5	20 (41.7)	9 (42.9)	76 (31.4)	5 (23.8)	7 (23.3)	2 (20.0)	103 (32.2)	16 (30.8)
6	21 (43.8)	10 (47.6)	141 (58.3)	14 (66.7)	15 (50.0)	4 (40.0)	177 (55.3)	28 (53.8)

6 = Daily, 5 = 2–6 times a week, 4 = Once a week, 3 = 2–3 times a month, 2 = once a month, 1 = Less than once a month, 0 = Don't know. n, number of responses.

no difference between the countries. Within each country, a statistically significant difference in the distribution of parental singing of NH children compared to HI children was found for Finland only. Compared to Finnish NH families, it can be observed that more Finnish parents of children with HI sang 'daily' or 'once a month' for their child, while less of them sang 'less than once a week,' '2–3 times in month,' or '2–6 times a week.'[3] No other statistically significant differences were found.

Questions B7 - B23 covered a range of different music activities as listed in **Table 3**. Respondents were asked whether their child participated in each of these activities. Parents were first asked, "Has your child ever participated in this activity?" (Yes/No). The results are presented in **Figure 1**. If they answered yes, then the child's frequency of participation was scored on a scale from 0 to 6, as detailed earlier in the 'data analysis' section, with this data used to calculate the Overall Music Participation Frequency Score (OMPFS) calculation (discussed below).

When the NH data was examined as a whole (i.e., combining the participation rates for all three countries), it was observed that all of the children participated in musical activities; for example, 100% of children listened to music informally, 97% danced, and 96% created their own songs or musical performances. In comparing between the countries, for the NH group, there were significant differences for participation (yes/no) in Singing Groups, Instrumental Groups, Special Children's Music Programs, Dance Classes, Family Music Activities (e.g., singing or playing music together), Online Music Training Programs/Games, Independent Music Exploration, Creating Songs/Music Performances informally, and Music Concerts (Chi-square tests, or Fisher's Exact Tests). The Finnish cohort participated significantly more ($p < 0.005$) than both the Australian and UK cohort for Singing Groups, Instrumental Groups, and Online Music Training Programs/Games. Both the Finnish and Australian cohort participated significantly more than the UK cohort ($p < 0.005$) in Special Children's Music Programs, Independent Music Exploration, Creating/making up Music or Singing Songs informally, and Music Concerts. Finnish children participated more in Family Music Activities than UK children, but UK children participated more in Dance Classes than Finnish children ($p < 0.005$ for both). Overall for the NH children, where there was a significant difference, the Finnish children had greater participation levels, with little difference between the Australian and UK children. The UK children tended to have the lowest participation rates overall.

[3]It is important to point out that the Fisher's Exact Test compares the distribution of data, rather than the means. For example, in this case, a number was assigned to each category, so the M itself is somewhat meaningless (e.g., the M would be different if a different number was assigned to the categories. Due to the data being categorical, looking at the number of responses to each category (i.e., the distribution of the data) provides more meaningful comparisons. Hence the reason the M is the same in this case, but the results are still statistically different.

TABLE 3 | Section B question/instrument association.

Question	Activity	Classification
B7	Music Lessons (formal lessons – instrument or voice)	Formal activities
B8	Singing Groups (e.g., choir)	
B9	Instrumental Groups (e.g., orchestra or band)	
B10	Special children's music programs (e.g., Kindermusik, Yamaha, Suzuki music groups)	
B11	Dance classes (formal lessons – e.g., ballet, tap, jazz)	
B12	Other music programs or activities (e.g., those organized and run by the school, community, religious organizations etc.)	
B13	Music classes (at preschool/kindergarten/childcare)	
B15	Listening to music informally (e.g., in the car, bedtime, playtime etc.)	Informal activities
B16	Social music activities (informal, not organized activities – e.g., playing with friends)	
B17	Musical videos (TV, online, Youtube etc.)	
B18	Family music activities	
B19	Online music training or music games	
B20	Independent music exploration (e.g., playing homemade music instruments etc.)	
B21	Creating/making up songs or music performances for play or fun	
B22	Dancing informally	
B23	Live music concerts (e.g., children's music bands, Hi-5, The Wiggles, etc.)	

B14 asked parents, if their child was not typically involved with music, to select the applicable reasons.

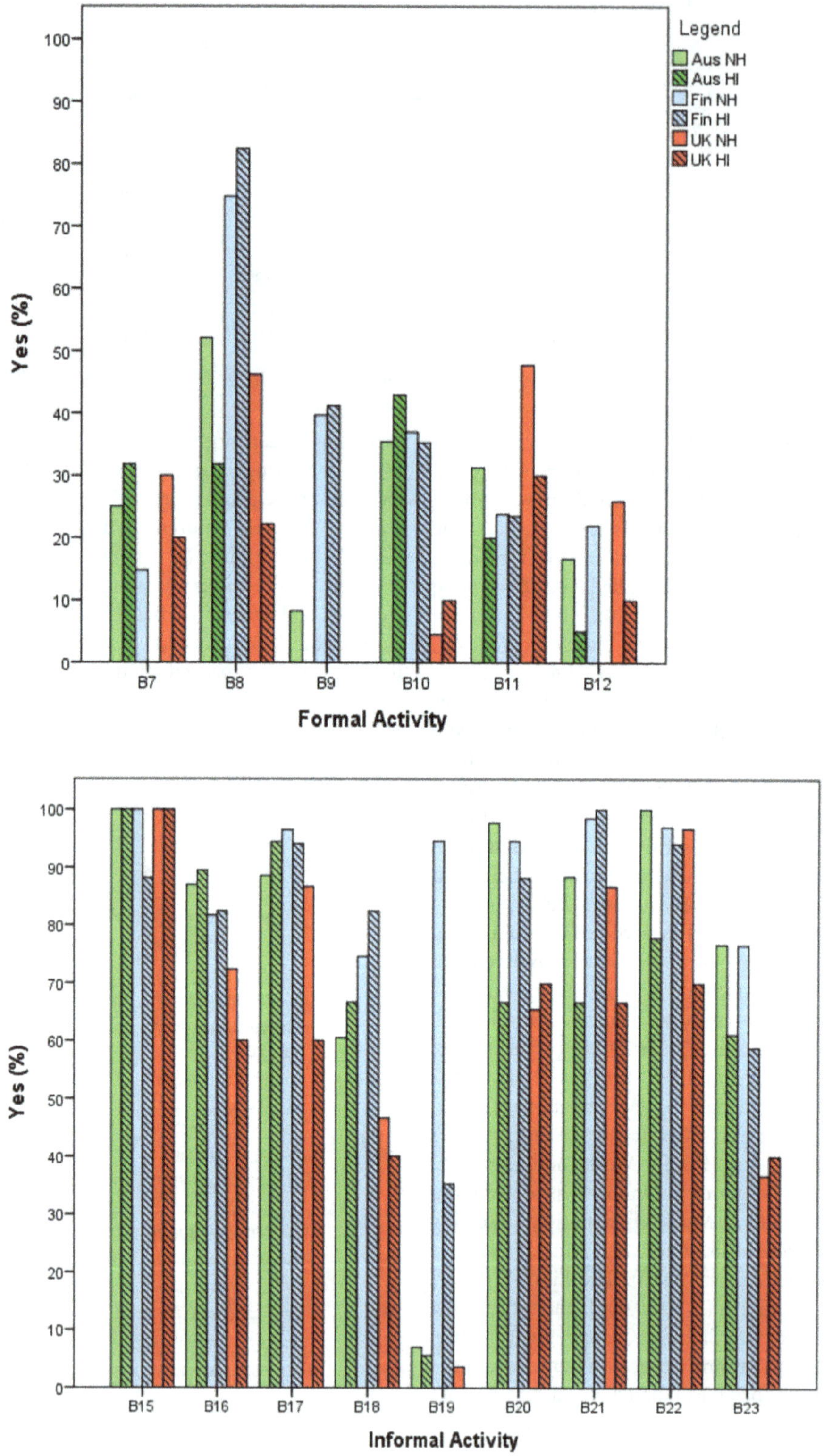

FIGURE 1 | Percentage of children who had participated in each activity, for the 6 participant groups. The top panel displays the formal activities, the bottom panel displays the informal activities. Formal: B7, Music Lessons; B8, Singing Groups; B9, Instrumental Groups; B10, Special children's music programs; B11, Dance classes; B12, Other organized music programs or activities; B13, Music classes at preschool/kindergarten/childcare; Informal: B15, Listening to music informally; B16, Social music activities; B17, Musical videos; B18, Family music activities; B19, Online music training or music games; B20, Independent music exploration; B21, Creating/making up songs or music performances for play or fun; B22, Dancing informally; B23, Live music concerts. B13's response scale was different in Finland, and therefore is not presented in this figure.

For the HI group, the Finnish cohort participated in Singing Groups as well as in Creating Music or Songs informally more than both the Australian and UK children. Their greater participation rates in online music training programs than the UK children was approaching significance ($p = 0.057$). Australian children had significantly higher rates of Formal Music Lessons than the Finnish children ($p = 0.012$). There were no other statistically significant differences. Overall for the HI children, less significant differences were observed than for the NH group. The within-country comparisons for participation in specific activities between NH and HI children were conducted using Fisher's Exact Test. The only significant differences were, for Australia, for Independent Music Exploration ($p = 0.002$) and Dancing Informally ($p = 0.005$), for Finland, for Other Music Programs/Activities ($p = 0.027$) and Listening to Music Informally ($p = 0.005$), and for the UK, Dancing Informally ($p = 0.042$). In all cases, NH participation rates were higher.

Overall Music Participation Frequency (OMPFS)

To get an overview of the average frequency of participation in music activities, an 'Overall Music Participation Frequency' score (OMPFS) was calculated for each participant by averaging their frequency of participation scores from questions B7–B23, with frequency being classified on a scale from 0 to 6, as described earlier. These mean of these scores are shown in **Table 4**. As only activities that the child participated in were included in the calculation, the number of activities averaged differed for each child. When comparing between countries, one-way ANOVAs showed that the Finnish HI children had higher participation scores than the UK HI children ($p = 0.011$). Within each of the three countries, there was no difference between the NH and HI children.

Overall Music Enjoyment Score (OMES)

In addition to the OMPFS, an Overall Music Enjoyment Score (OMES) was calculated for each child, by averaging the ratings for the activities that the child participated in; again, the number of activities included in this calculation differed between the individual participants. The mean of these scores are shown in **Table 4**. Mood's Median Tests showed that scores from the NH children in the UK were significantly higher than the NH Australian children ($p = 0.016$), and also higher than the NH Finnish children ($p = 0.030$), with no other differences. There were also no differences between any of the countries for the HI children, nor any differences between the NH and HI within each of the three countries That is, overall, NH and HI children from the same country had similar music enjoyment and participation scores.

TABLE 4 | Mean and SD for OMPFS and OMES scores.

Mean (*SD*)	Australia		Finland		UK	
	NH (*n* = 37)	HL (*n* = 16)	NH (*n* = 219)	HL (*n* = 19)	NH (*n* = 30)	HL (*n* = 10)
OMPFS (/6)	2.4 (0.63)	2.1 (0.63)	2.4 (0.83)	2.7 (0.84)	2.3 (0.74)	1.8 (0.82)
OMES (/10)	8.8 (0.91)	8.8 (1.17)	8.8 (0.95)	8.7 (1.08)	9.2 (1.21)	9.2 (1.25)

OMPFS: 6 = Daily, 5 = 2–6 times a week, 4 = Once a week, 3 = 2–3 times a month, 2 = once a month, 1 = Less than once a month, 0 = Don't know. n = number of responses. OMES: Scale from 1 to 10 (1 = "did not enjoy," and 10 = "very much enjoyed").

Section C – Childhood Music Participation and Experiences

This section asked about the child's participation in, and reactions to, music, and was slightly different for the UK than for Australia and Finland. In Australia and Finland, the first question was only for the HI children, and asked parents whether their child's reaction to music has changed over time since receiving their HA and/or CI. There were 36 responses in total for both countries, of which 18/36 (50%) said their child immediately became more interested in music, 4/36 (11%) said it was a gradual increase in interest in music, with 12/36 (33%) saying there was no change in their reaction. There were two 'other' responses. For the UK, parents of HI children were asked to rate on a scale from 1 (does not enjoy at all) to 10 (very much enjoys), whether their child enjoyed music overall. Of the 10 parents that responded, seven gave the maximum rating of '10,' and there was one rating of '7,' and one rating of '4.'

For all three countries, and all groups (including the NH group), this was followed by the question "Which of the following best describes your child's response to music generally, in the last 6 months" with a 5-point rating scale: 1 = very much enjoys music; 2 = enjoys some aspects of music; 3 = neither enjoys nor dislikes; 4 = somewhat negative; and 5 = dislikes music. None of the NH parents selected 'somewhat negative' or 'dislikes music' and only 1 parent from the HL group rating 'somewhat negative,' with no ratings of 'dislikes music.' Statistical analyses showed no differences between the three countries nor between the NH and HI groups for the proportions who selected each option. The Australian and Finnish questionnaire for HI families then asked about factors that may make music listening more, and less enjoyable for their child with a HA or CI. Eleven different factors were listed, with respondents asked to mark all the factors that made music more enjoyable, and subsequently in the next question, all the factors that made music less enjoyable. There were also two additional options: "I am not aware of any situations that. . .(makes music more/less enjoyable)," and "Other (please specify)." Results are presented in **Figures 2, 3**. Across countries, having visual input with the music, followed by a quiet listening environment, were the two most commonly selected factors that helped to make music more enjoyable, with a noisy listening environment overwhelmingly selected as the factor that made music less enjoyable.

Section D – Music Resources for Child

The questions in this section asked parents if they had discussed their child's music participation with teachers, therapists or other professionals, if they had utilized music information from any of the HA or CI companies, and if they had purchased musical instruments or music resources for their child. For the NH group, only 17% of respondents said they had discussed their child's music participation with professionals, compared to 55% for

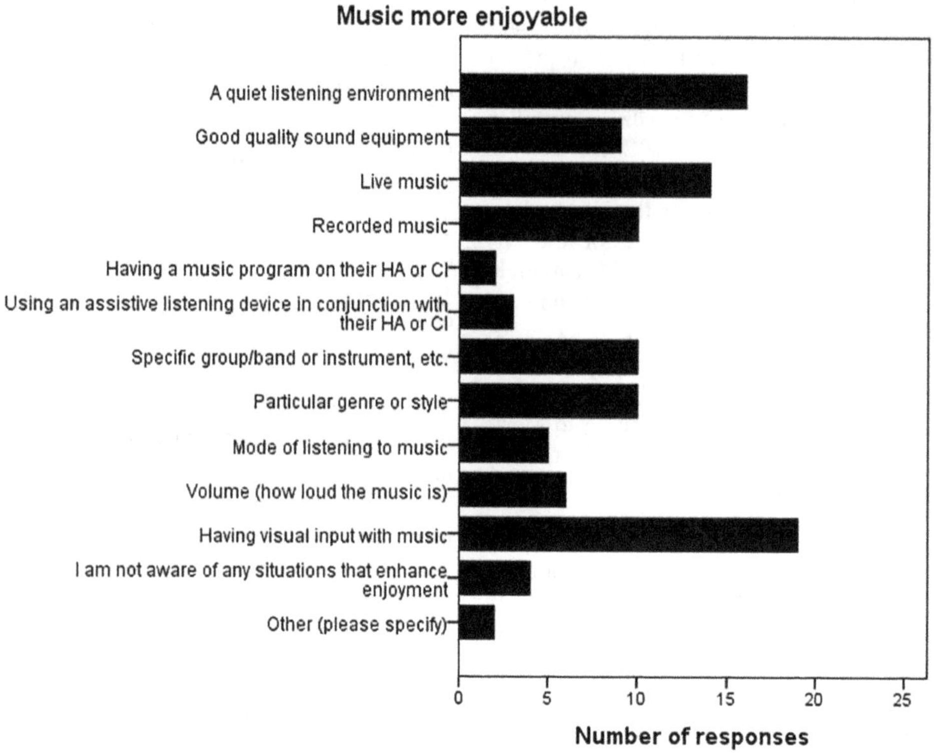

FIGURE 2 | Factors that make music listening more enjoyable. Parents could select more than one factor, and the bars represent the number of time that factor was selected (Australia and Finland only; $n = 45$).

the HL group. Statistical analyses (performed with Chi-Squared Tests or Fisher's Exact Tests) showed that for each country, the difference between the NH and HL groups was statistically significant (or approaching significance) ($p = 0.09$ for Australia; $p < 0.001$ for Finland; $p = 0.055$ for UK), with no country difference within each of these two groups.

With regard to purchasing musical instruments, 67% of the NH group and 72% of the HL group said they had purchased (or were renting, or in the process of purchasing) musical instruments for their child, with no differences within or between the countries. Ninety-two percent of the NH group and 80% of the HL group had purchased physical music resources (e.g., music books, music toys, DVD/Video, CDs) for their child. For the NH group, more Finnish parents had purchased resources than Australian ($p = 0.011$) or UK parents ($p = 0.005$). For the HL group, there was no significant country differences noted. Within each country, the difference between the NH and HL groups was only significant for the Finnish cohort ($p = 0.007$; NH higher).

Section E – Overall Importance of Music in Your Household and Family

This section aimed to evaluate how important music was in the family and child's life. All statistical analyses were conducted with Mood's Median tests, with *post hoc* Chi square tests conducted where applicable. Parents were firstly asked to rate 'music is important to our family's life' on a scale from 1 to 10 (1 = not at all important; 10 = very important). Results are shown in **Table 5**.

Between-country comparisons for the NH group were statistically significant ($p = 0.0004$), with this difference being the UK parents rating music as significantly more important in their family's life than the Finnish parents ($p = 0.002$). There were no other significant differences. Within each country, there was no difference between the NH and HL group.

When asked to rate how important music was in their child's life (same scale as for 'family life'), similar results were found with the UK parents of NH children rating music as significantly more important than Finnish parents of NH children ($p = 0.001$), with no significant country difference for the HI children, nor any significant difference between the two groups within each of the three countries individually (**Table 5**).

The third key question asked parents to rate the importance of music in their other children's life (see **Table 5**). For the NH children, the UK parents' ratings were significantly higher than both the Australian and Finnish parents' ratings (Australia: $p = 0.001$; Finland: $p = 0.010$), with no country differences for the HI group. Again there were no differences between the NH and HL groups for any of the three countries.

Section F – Child's Music Listening Preferences

The first question of this section asked parents 'How much music would your child actively listen to, or be involved with each week'

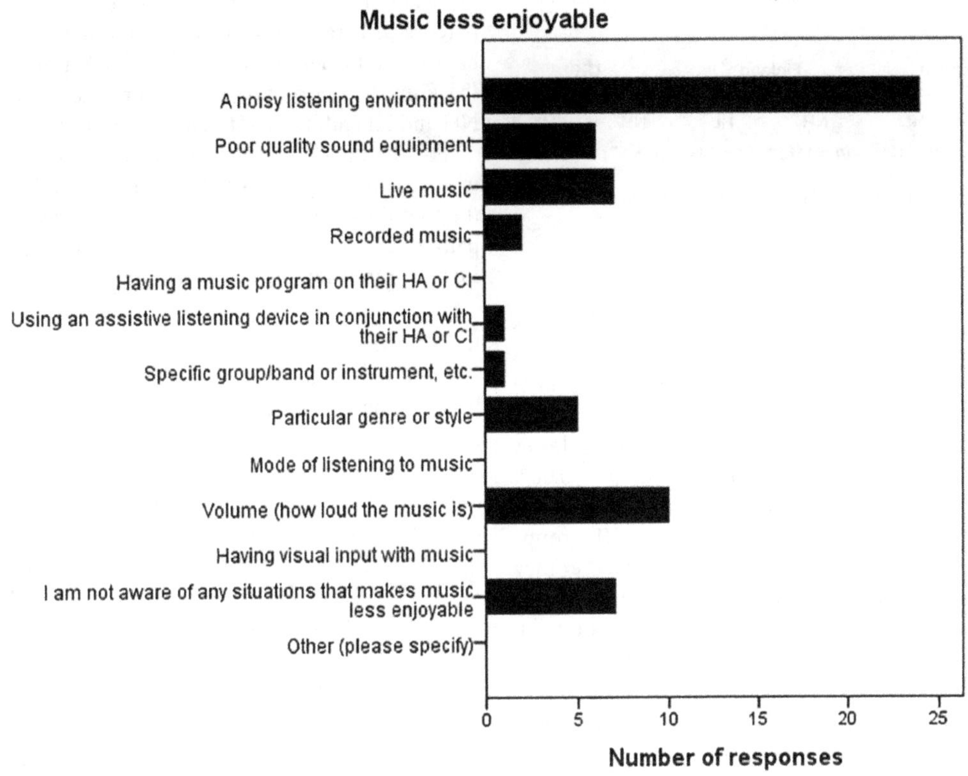

FIGURE 3 | Factors that make music listening less enjoyable. Parents could select more than one factor, and the bars represent the number of time that factor was selected (Australia and Finland only; *n* = 45).

TABLE 5 | Mean and SD (and 'n') for Section E, Section F and Section G.

Question	Australia		Finland		UK	
	NH	**HL**	**NH**	**HL**	**NH**	**HL**
Music is important in our family's life	8.3 (1.54)	7.5 (2.28)	7.4 (1.63)	7.3 (1.41)	8.9 (1.47)	7.9 (3.09)
	n = 40	*n* = 16	*n* = 184	*n* = 19	*n* = 25	*n* = 8
Music is important in the child's life	8.5 (1.60)	8.4 (2.02)	7.7 (1.46)	7.7 (1.53)	9.1 (1.26)	7.9 (2.71)
	n = 39	*n* = 16	*n* = 183	*n* = 19	*n* = 26	*n* = 9
Music is important in our other children's lives (if applicable)	6.7 (3.59)	4.6 (3.89)	8.0 (2.16)	8.1 (1.64)	9.2 (1.39)	6.2 (2.79)
	n = 39	*n* = 16	*n* = 126	*n* = 11	*n* = 17	*n* = 6
My child loves music	9.0 (1.45)	8.6 (1.86)	8.7 (1.45)	8.7 (1.45)	9.4 (1.01)	9.0 (1.73)
	n = 37	*n* = 16	*n* = 180	*n* = 19	*n* = 22	*n* = 7
My child is good at music	6.4 (2.04)	6.0 (2.00)	8.2 (1.68)	7.4 (1.61)	7.8 (1.80)	6.8 (3.31)
	n = 37	*n* = 16	*n* = 180	*n* = 19	*n* = 19	*n* = 6
I think my child will be actively participating in music for the next 5 years	8.2 (1.67)	8.9 (1.34)	8.4 (1.96)	8.1 (1.91)	8.7 (1.40)	9.1 (1.46)
	n = 37	*n* = 16	*n* = 180	*n* = 19	*n* = 23	*n* = 8
I think my child with be actively participating in music in high school	7.2 (2.19)	7.1 (2.54)	7.3 (2.23)	6.2 (2.24)	7.9 (1.76)	8.1 (2.48)
	n = 37	*n* = 16	*n* = 180	*n* = 19	*n* = 23	*n* = 8
If music was optional at school, do you think your child would do it?	7.8 (1.91)	7.8 (2.30)	7.5 (2.01)	5.6 (1.57)	8.3 (2.05)	9.0 (1.92)
	n = 37	*n* = 16	*n* = 180	*n* = 19	*n* = 24	*n* = 7

Mean (SD) are provided, with the 'n' being the number of families who responded to that question. All scores are from 1–10; 1 being the poorest/lowest.

(in hours)? Results are displayed in **Table 6**. Independent Samples Median Tests showed no significant differences between NH and HI children within each country, or between the countries for the NH, or HL groups.

The next two questions then asked parents to rate on a slider scale (which was subsequently converted into a number from 1 to 10 where 1 was the poorest): (i) 'My child loves music,' and (ii) 'in my opinion, my child is good at music.' As

TABLE 6 | Means for 'How much music would your child listen to or be involved in each week (hrs).'

Hours	Australia		Finland		UK	
	NH (n = 28)	HL (n = 12)	NH (n = 118)	HL (n = 11)	NH (n = 17)	HL (n = 4)
Mean (SD)	7.0 (7.6)	9.7 (12.4)	4.8 (5.4)	4.5 (3.8)	9.4 (8.6)	5.8 (4.2)
Median	4.0	5.0	3.0	3.0	7.0	6.5

can be seen from the results shown in **Table 5**, overall ratings were extremely high for the first question. Mood's Median Tests with *post hoc* Chi-Square tests (and Bonferroni corrections) were used to compare between the countries. These analyses showed that the NH Finnish ratings were significantly lower than the Australian or UK NH ratings (Australia: p = 0.007; UK: p = 0.003), with no country difference for the HL group nor any significant differences between the NH and HL groups within each country. The NH Australian ratings on whether they felt their child was good at music was significantly lower when compared to both the Finnish and UK NH children (Finland: p < 0.001; UK: p = 0.004). Again there were no differences for the HL group, or within the countries between the NH and HIL groups. There were no significant between-country differences for either the NH or HL groups in the proportion of children who would initiate age-appropriate music experiences themselves and within each country, the only difference was for Finland, with significantly more NH children doing this (Fisher's Exact Test; p = 0.031).

Section G – Future Perspectives

The first three questions of this section asked parents: (i) I think my child will be actively participating in music for the next 5 years; (ii) I think my child will be learning a musical instrument, playing in a band, or singing in a choir when they are in high school; and (iii) If music was an optional subject at primary school, do you think your child would do it? The response was made on a slider-rating scale (converted to a number between 1 and 10 where 1 was the poorer or 'less likely' score). Finally parents were asked whether they would support it if their child wanted to pursue music as a career (yes/no). Results for these three questions are presented in **Table 5**. Mood's Median Test with *post hoc* Fisher's Test with Bonferroni corrections (where applicable) were used for analyses of the first two questions, and Fisher's Exact Test used for the proportional data in the last question.

There were no between, or within country differences for the first question of this section. For the second question, responses were similar between the countries for the NH children, but for the HI children, Finnish parents had significantly lower expectations than UK parents (p = 0.033). Within the countries, the only significant difference was for Finland with parents of NH children having significantly higher expectations than parents of HI children (p = 0.022). With regard to whether they thought their child would do music if it was an optional school subject, the parents of Finnish HI children had significantly lower expectations of this happening than both the Australian and UK parents (Australia: p = 0.009; UK: p = 0.001), with no difference between countries for the NH children. Within each country, only the Finnish cohort showed a significant difference between the NH and HI children (NH higher; p = 0.001).

For the final question, the overwhelming response was 'yes,' with 95% of the parents of both the NH and HI children saying they would support their child if music was their chosen career path, with no significant between or within country differences for the proportion of parents who said 'yes.'

Correlations

Correlational analyses were conducted to look for associations between the OMPFS or OMES and both key participant variables (age for both groups, and for the hearing impaired group, age diagnosed with HL and age fitted with device), as well as the following four questions in Sections E and F: (i) importance of music in your family's life; (ii) importance of music in your child's life; (iii) my child loves music; (iv) my child is good at music. For the NH group, there was a weak negative correlation between age and the OMES (Spearman's ρ = −0.129; p = 0.029), with no significant correlation between age and the OMPFS. That is, older participants provided slightly lower enjoyment ratings for the activities they participated in. There were no other significant correlations for the HL group.

For the NH group, there were significant moderate correlations between both the OMES and OMPFS and all four questions listed above. For the HL group, there were significant moderate correlations between the OMES and the rating of the importance of music in the child's life, as well as between both the OMES and the OMPFS and the ratings of 'my child loves music' and 'my child is good at music.' There were no significant correlations for either the OMES or OMPFS and the rating of how important music is in the family's life for the HL group. These results are shown in **Table 7**.

DISCUSSION

The major aim of the current study was to compare the role of, and attitudes to, music between families of children with

TABLE 7 | Correlations between OMPFS and OMES, and questions from Section E and F, for both NH and HI groups.

Question	NH		HI	
	OMPFS	OMES	OMPFS	OMES
How important is music in your family's life?	ρ = 0.454 (p < 0.001)	ρ = 0.444 (p < 0.001)	Not significant	Not significant
How important is music in your child's life?	ρ = 0.504 (p < 0.001)	ρ = 0.512 (p < 0.001)	ρ = 0.459 (p = 0.002)	Not significant
'My child loves music'	ρ = 0.459 (p < 0.001)	ρ = 0.587 (p < 0.001)	ρ = 0.468 (p = 0.002)	ρ = 0.543 (p < 0.001)
'My child is good at music'	ρ = 0.400 (p < 0.001)	ρ = 0.399 (p < 0.001)	ρ = 0.418 (p = 0.007)	ρ = 0.423 (p = 0.006)

NH to families with children with a HL, with a secondary aim of seeing if these results differed between three countries. The overall results showed very few differences between NH and HI children, regardless of whether the families lived in Australia, Finland or the UK, suggesting that it is the family's attitude to music and the role it plays in the household, rather than a child's hearing thresholds, that determines children's involvement and engagement with music. There were few differences between the countries, either, suggesting that this finding of familial influence is fairly consistent, at least across the three countries involved in this study.

Families of NH Children vs. Families of HI Children

Children, regardless of their hearing abilities, first started attending to music at similar ages (NH: 0.62 years; HI: 0.81 years). Briggs (1991) provides a list of music development milestones for NH children from birth to age 11. Our NH findings are relatively consistent with their developmental progression proposing that an infant will first respond to being sung to with fixed attention or cessation of movement at age 2 months, and will 'calm' or quieten to quiet music at around 3 months of age. Around the age of 6–8 months, the child will start to search for, and attend to, music when it is played. There has yet to be any published research on how a HL impacts on these music developmental milestones, however, our results are consistent with the proposition that these early music attention milestones would be the similar for HI children, provided they were appropriately aided or implanted at an early age.

Driscoll et al. (2015) in their cohort of 16 preschool aged American children with CIs reported that their participants first started attending to music at a somewhat older age of 1.81 years; no results for their NH children were provided nor was the age at implantation, or experience with the CI, given for children with CIs. This delay of 1 year in attending to music may be partially due to the fact that the HI children in Driscoll's study were all CI recipients, as opposed to the mix of CI and HA users in the current study. Children with implants would have had a greater degree of HL, and would probably have received minimal auditory input during the time before they got the implant, hence the older age before they attended to music. It is also interesting to note here that in the current study, 50% of the parents in the HL group, compared to 25% of parents in Driscoll et al.'s (2015) study, reported that their child with a HL became immediately interested in music when they received their devices for hearing. The age of implantation (or initial HA fitting) was not provided by Driscoll et al. (2015), and if their cohort was implanted at a later age, it may also explain the delay in attending to music. During periods of deafness, the brain reorganizes to compensate for the lack of auditory input; once this auditory input if provided, further reorganization occurs. However, this takes time (Kral and Sharma, 2012).

To examine music engagement and participation, parents were provided with a list of 15 different music activities and asked to indicate which of these their child participated in, and the frequency of participation. Of these 15 activities, there was only a maximum of two activities where the NH cohort had a significantly higher proportion of children participating than HI children (and only one in the UK). There was no significant difference in the overall frequency of participation (as measured by the OMPFS), or enjoyment levels (as measured by the OMES), between NH and HI children. This is supported by the later question asking parents 'How much music would your child actively listen to, or be involved with each week,' where no significant difference was found between NH and HI children. Further demonstrating the overall high levels of music enjoyment reported in this study, when parents were asked about their child's response to music in the last 6 months, none of the NH parents selected 'somewhat negative' or 'dislikes music' and only one parent from the HL group rated 'somewhat negative,' with no ratings of 'dislikes music.' That is, only one parent out of 308 who answered this question (combined NH and HL groups) said their child has a negative response to music, and only four parents (three from the NH group and one from the HL group) indicated a neutral reaction of 'neither enjoys nor dislikes.'

There were no differences for any country between the proportion of NH and HI families who had procured (e.g., purchased, rented) at least one musical instrument for their child, with an overwhelming majority of parents having purchased physical music resources for their child (e.g., music books, DVDs, CDs, videos etc.). Finland was the only country where there was a significant difference between parents of NH compared to HI children; the former were significantly more likely to purchase music resources for their child.

There were also no differences between NH and HI families in rating how important music was in their family's life, in their child's life, or in the lives of their other children (where applicable). Overall for the NH and HI families, the mean ratings (out of 10) of as to how important music was in the family's life, and in their child's life were very high (NH: 7.7, 8.0; HI 8.0, 8.0, respectively out of 10), implying that music is an important part of family and upbringing, at least in these three developed Western nations. Driscoll et al. (2015), for their group of 16 children using CIs found very similar results, reporting a mean of 7.9/10, when asked to rate the importance of music in the household. No data was provided for the NH children in their study. In the current study, parents also provided similar ratings for whether their child loved music, was good at music, and if they self-initiated music, regardless of the child's hearing status. This is consistent with the assertion that having a child with a HL does not impact on the role that music plays in the family, or a parent's attitude to having their child engage and participate in music-related activities.

The final section of the questionnaire asked about the future, and their prediction of their child's future involvement with music-related activities, as well as how supportive they would be of their child's continued active engagement with music. The overwhelming response from both the NH and HL groups was that parents would support their child's future involvement with music (95% of parents from both groups saying 'yes'), and that they expected their child to be actively involved in music activities for the next 5 years (mean scores for all groups was greater than

8/10). All participant groups, except for the parents of Finnish HI children, had mean scores above 7/10 that their child would be learning a music instrument, playing in a band or singing in a choir, when the child was in high school. Given that all of the children in this study were aged 6 years or younger, this indicates that parent's believe their child will continuing to participate in formal musical activities for many years to come.

Factors That Make Music Listening More/Less Enjoyable for Children With HL

Parents were specifically asked about factors that impacted on their child's music listening experience. For the HI children, having visual input with the music, and a quiet listening environment were the highest rated factors for improving music enjoyment, with a noisy listening environment followed by an inappropriate music volume being the most frequently rated factors that detracted from music enjoyment. Looi and She (2010) and Looi et al. (2019) asked postlingually deafened adult CI and HA users, respectively, about factors that impacted on their music listening enjoyment. In line with the present results, for both adult CI and HA users, being able to watch the performer or following the musical score/words (which are visual cues), and a quiet listening environment were also highly rated factors by the majority of adults that improved music enjoyment, with music volume (e.g., too loud/soft) and an echoey/reverberant room being highly rated factors detracting from music listening ('noisy listening environment' was not specifically asked in the adult studies). Collectively the results imply that factors which make music perception more difficult also reduce music enjoyment, whilst those making perception easier increase the listener's enjoyment. Many of these factors overlap with variables that impact on speech perception, and by taking the time to proactively modify the listening environment would serve to benefit both speech, and music perception.

It is interesting to note that a special or separate music listening program was rarely selected as a factor to improve music listening for children or adults; it was selected by 2/45 parents in this study and 28/100 in the adult HA study (Looi et al., 2019). Hence it is questionable as to the extent these programs offered by device manufacturers genuinely improve music listening for the typical HI listener, or it may be that many CI or HA users are unfamiliar with the programs.

Comparisons Between the Countries

A secondary aim of this study was to see whether there were any country/cultural differences in the role music plays in families of children in Australia, Finland and UK. To the authors' knowledge, this has not yet been examined in existing research involving families with HI children.

Normally Hearing Children

Overall there were some between-country differences observed for the families with NH children in this study, particularly in the actual rates of participation in different music activities for children. However, the mean frequency of participation for the activity (as calculated with the OMPFS) between the countries was not statistically significant. Every single child listened to music, 97% danced, 96% created music performances informally. The present results fit with a Slovenian study by Denac (2008) where 176 kindergarten children (aged 5–6) were interviewed on the music activities they most preferred to participate in at home. They found that 'listening to music' (56%), dancing or moving to music (55%), and singing songs (48%) were the popular informal home music activities. Similarly in a Brazilian study by Ilari et al. (2011), all but one mother reported that they listened to music with their child, with 52% saying they also danced to this music with their child, and 43% saying they played along with the music whilst dancing. Our results are also in line with the findings from Williams et al. (2015) who reported that 42% of their Australian families engaged in music activities with their children 6–7 days a week, 32% using it 3–5 days a week, 23% for 1–2 days a week, and only 4% had not used music in the last week. It would seem that children, regardless of the country they live in, enjoy listening to music, and dancing to music.

In looking at the participation rates for individual activities, for all three countries, listening to music informally and dancing informally had the highest participation rates. There were some interesting observations made in comparing the participation data between the countries. Finnish children participated in singing groups, instrumental groups and online music training programs/games significantly more than either the UK or Australian children, and Finnish parents reported to spend significantly more time singing to their child in the last year than UK parents. In Finland, many parents participate with their children in or send them to 'music play schools,' which are common, low-cost activities, routinely provided at many daycares and usually taught by a music pedagogist (Huotilainen and Tervaniemi, 2018; Linnavalli et al., 2018). In these groups, children sing and play instruments, which may explain the high participation rates in singing and instrumental groups reported by Finnish parents.

The UK children participated significantly less in special children's music programs, independent music exploration, creating/making up music or songs, and music concerts than either the Australian or Finnish children. It is difficult to determine the reason(s) for these differences. It may be that the availability and access to these different activities may be different across the countries. For example, one could speculate that the reduced availability or access to, and/or higher costs to attend, these special music programs in the UK may make it more challenging for parents, or that the availability and access to children's singing groups or instrumental groups is higher in Finland (e.g., more groups available, closer to home, lower costs).

One other worthwhile finding to highlight was that the present results showed that parents sang, on average, 2–6 times a week to their children. Ilari et al. (2011) reported that 90% of the mothers in their study said they sang to their child, and half reported that others in the family (e.g., fathers, siblings etc.) also sang to the infant. This suggests that parental singing is an inherent part of a child's upbringing, which is important given research indicating that more parental singing potentially benefits not only parent–child bonding, but also encourages children to sing and is associated with better attention, speech perception in noise and language skills (Torppa et al., 2018, 2019).

Interestingly, although the trend in music participation rates was for the Finnish cohort to have the highest proportion of children participating in many of the activities, and the UK children the lowest proportion, the Finnish parents had significantly lower ratings than UK parents when asked to rate the importance of music in their family's life, and in their child's life. For the latter, Finnish parents ratings were also significantly lower than Australian parents. This seems somewhat contradictory; one would expect that if a parent was willing to make the time effort to enroll their child in a large number of music activities or engage them in music making opportunities, then they must see some potential benefit or value to providing those musical opportunities. This may be related to country differences in deciding what is 'important' versus 'less important' when prioritizing different factors, or language or cultural differences in interpreting the term 'important.' For example, it may be that if music is a 'routine' or 'expected' part of Finnish culture and upbringing, being integrated routinely into daily life, then it is not necessarily seen by parents to be something special or a 'priority.' Alternatively, it may simply be that Finnish parents are more conservative when providing ratings on these kind of scales. Finnish parents also provided significantly lower ratings than Australian or UK parents as to whether their child loved music, although Australian parents provided significantly lower ratings than Finnish or UK parents as to whether their child was good at music.

For the OMES, a measure of the levels of enjoyment of the activities the children participated in, overall enjoyment scores were generally high (means ranging between 8.8 and 9.2 out of 10), with ratings from the UK NH children being higher than both the Australian and Finnish children. When asked about their child's general response to music in the last 6 months, 99% of all the NH children had a positive response to music. Attitudes to music and the importance of music in the family unit were fairly similar across countries, and there were no country differences for any of the 'future perspectives' questions, for the NH children. Parents had high expectations when asked whether they thought their child would be participating in music activities for the next 5 years. When asked if they thought their child would be learning a musical instrument, playing in a band and/or singing in a choir in high school (i.e., more than 5 years from the time they were completing the questionnaire), expectations were still relatively high of this happening. An overwhelming 95% of parents said they would support their child if their child wanted to pursue music as a career. Thus, results from this cohort of NH children were similar to results from published results from other countries, suggesting that the value of music is recognized by parents globally, and children all around the world enjoy participating in, and listening to, music.

Hearing Impaired Children

There were even fewer between-country differences for the HI children. There was no differences in the age children started attending to music for the three countries, nor in the amounts parents sang to their child in the last year, or in the first year after they received their hearing device.

For the 15 music activities in Section B, similar to their NH counterparts, the Finnish HI children had significantly higher rates of participation in formal singing groups, as well as in making up or creating music/songs, than both the Australian and UK children. Further, only the Finnish children participated in instrumental groups – none of the Australian or UK HI children participated in these formal instrumental groups. Australian children had significantly higher rates of formal music lessons than the Finnish children, though. A similar trend seen in the NH data was observed in the HI data, in that Finnish children tended to have the highest proportion participating in most activities, and the UK the lowest proportion.

The OMPFS also showed that Finnish children participated in their chosen activities significantly more frequently than the UK children, with no difference between the Australian and Finnish, or Australian and UK children. The most commonly undertaken activity for Finnish children was creating or making up music/songs (100% of the children did this), followed by watching musical videos (94%). In contrast, for both the Australian and UK children, listening to music informally was the most commonly undertaken activity, followed by watching musical videos for Australia (94%) and independent music exploration as well as dancing informally for the UK children (70% for both). Several Finnish parents of children with HL reported that professionals such as speech therapists had informed them about the benefits of music participation and had recommended that they sing, and make music, with their child(ren), and therefore they made a conscious effort to integrate music into their daily family life. This may be one of the reasons for the country differences found for the Finnish HI children. It is also possible that music is an inherent part of more families' lives in Finland than other countries, regardless of whether their child has NH or a HL. Kirschner and Ilari (2014) collected information on music participation and involvement for 41 Brazilian and 36 German preschool children. Half of the children in each country participated in weekly music education classes, but there were between-country differences when it came to music in the family home. Brazilian parents spent significantly more time than the German parents each day on active music making activities such as singing, or playing instruments at home with their children. The Brazilian children were also significantly more likely to sing and dance spontaneously than the German children. The authors discuss how 'music learning' is somewhat different between the countries, with Germany tending to be more dominated by formal music lessons or participation in an organized music group (e.g., choir, band etc.), whereas Brazilian children tended to learn to sing, dance and play music informally as part of their daily life (e.g., seeing it on TV, dancing/singing in the community etc.). The authors suggested that these findings indicate a culture-specific social learning process in learning musical conventions.

In the current study, music enjoyment levels were high, and similar between the countries. This enjoyment was also demonstrated with only one of the parents in this group amongst the whole cohort rating that their child's response to music was 'somewhat negative'; that is, 96% of the HI children enjoyed music. This is consistent with findings from Gfeller et al. (1998), Trehub et al. (2009), and Rocca (2012), who all report that the majority of children with HL enjoy, and benefit from, participating in music. Although research indicates that adults using CIs (Looi et al., 2007; Looi and She, 2010; Limb and Roy, 2014), or hearing aids (Chasin and Russo, 2004; Looi et al., 2007, 2018) have lower levels of enjoyment and perceptual accuracy for music compared to both NH adults as well as to when they had better levels of hearing, it must be remembered that most children are born with their HL, and/or acquire their HL at a very young age. Therefore they do not have a 'normal hearing' auditory template for music, but rather their memory and auditory template for music is one acquired whilst listening with their HA(s) and/or CIs. They have learnt to hear music that way, and therefore do not know any different.

There were no differences between the countries in parental ratings for how important music was in their family, or HI child's lives. There were also no differences in parental ratings of how much their child loved music, how good they were at music, or whether they self-initiated music experiences for themselves. It is worthwhile highlighting here the high ratings for all six participant groups (NH and HI children in all countries) for 'My child loves music,' with all mean scores above 8.6 out of 10.

Finally, in looking toward the future, scores for whether parents thought their child would be actively participating in music for the next 5 years were high, with no difference between the countries. Finnish parents were less optimistic than UK parents as to whether their child would be participating in music in high school (i.e., learning an instrument, playing in a band or singing in a choir) and less optimistic than both UK and Australian parents as to whether their child would choose to do music at school if it was an optional subject.

Overall, there were few between-country differences for the HL cohort, and these differences were primarily in the activities the children in each country participated in. It is noted that the number of HI participants in each country was small, which would have reduced the sensitivity of the statistical testing.

Correlations

Aside from the very weak negative correlation between age and OMES for the NH group, there were no significant correlations between either the frequency of music participation (OMPFS) or music enjoyment (OMES) and age-related participant variables (age, and for HI group, age diagnosed with HL, and age fitted with device) for either the NH and HI group. This is in contrast to the findings from LeBlanc et al. (1999) who tested 2042 students, aged 8–18, from Greece, South Korea, and the United States on their music preference, using an 18 item music listening test with Likert-type response scales. The authors looked at the factors of age, gender, and country on the music preference scores, finding a significant difference in music preference ratings between the three countries, with the variables of age and gender also contributing significantly to the ratings, and the variability in the ratings. In contrast, adult studies with CI recipients have found that neither age diagnosed with a HL or length of time with the device have been significantly correlated with music perception or enjoyment scores (Gfeller et al., 2008; Looi et al., 2012a). There are very few pediatric music perception studies involving children using CI or HAs, where correlations have been calculated to outcomes. Looi and Radford (2011) found pitch ranking scores of CI and HA users were not associated with age or duration of device use (age diagnosed with HL was not investigated), and Gfeller et al. (2019) did not find that age, age diagnosed with HL, age of implantation, or time with the CI were predictive of pitch ranking scores. The current authors could not find any hearing-impaired pediatric music appreciation studies where the researchers looked at whether participant variables were associated with the music participation or enjoyment scores.

For the NH group, both the OMPFS and OMES were moderately correlated to the importance of music for the family and child, and the parent-judged ratings of their child's love of, and ability with, music. That is, the more important music was in the family and/or child's life, the more often the child participated in music activities, and the more they were rated to enjoy these activities. Similarly, if parents felt their child loved music and/or were good at it, participation frequency and enjoyment was also higher. These results support the proposition that music enjoyment and participation are related to the importance of music in the familial, and individual's life.

For the HI group, music enjoyment was higher in families who rated music as being more important in their child's life, however, music importance in the child's or family's life did not associate with the OMPFS. Both the OMPFS and OMES were higher for children whose parents rated that they loved music, and/or were good at music. These correlations inherently make sense, although as is the nature of correlations, one cannot be sure if the children participate more because they enjoy it more and/or are thought to be better at it, or if it is because they enjoy it more or are better at it, which the parents had noticed, so subsequently they are provided more opportunities to participate. It is interesting to note that the importance of music in the family's life was not significantly correlated with OMPFS, which is in contrast to the findings from Driscoll et al. (2015) for families who had a child with a CI as well as a NH sibling. This may be due to the fact that the OMPFS was a calculation of the number of times the children participated in their chosen music activities (i.e., frequency of participation), as opposed to the actual overall quantity of participation. That is, a child who participated in one activity every day would have a higher OMPFS than a child who participated in three activities once a week. Regardless, parents in this study do see music as important for their child with a HL, and provide them with regular opportunities to participate and engage with music.

Limitations

One of the major limitations of this study was the large difference in group sizes – both between the NH and HL groups, as well as between the countries, which reduced the power of the statistical analyses, with much of the data violating assumptions for parametric testing. Additionally, there were relatively fewer HL participants than NH participants, with the HL data combining both CI and HA users.

Although the study is the first to compare between three different countries, including one non-English speaking country, all three countries are considered developed, 'Western' nations, all speaking a non-tonal language. Hence the cultural differences between these countries may be less than if compared to an Eastern, Latin-American, or African country. Additionally, it is acknowledged that 'country' and culture are different, and one cannot equate culture with nationality, or even country of residence with nationality. However, as discussed in the results for Section A, parents were also asked what 'culture' they identified with, with 80% of Australians, 96% Finnish, and 65% of the UK families responding 'Australian,' 'Finnish' and 'British,' respectively.

SUMMARY AND CONCLUSION

The results of this study indicate that children, regardless of hearing levels or country of residence, have similar levels of music engagement and enjoyment. HL is not seen as a contraindication to music participation and involvement by the parents involved in this study, and families with HI children had similar attitudes and expectations of music for their child to families of NH children, with music being an important part of family life for the majority of respondents. When considered in conjunction with the findings of Driscoll et al. (2015), it could be propounded that the majority of parents do not significantly change their attitude to music or the role that music should play in a child's upbringing, regardless of the child's hearing thresholds. Overall, these findings are extremely positive, given the benefits that music training and participation offers to children across all facets of their development and upbringing.

ETHICS STATEMENT

The studies involving human participants were reviewed and approved by (1) The Macquarie University Human Sciences and Humanities Research Ethics Committee, Australia, (2) University of Helsinki Ethical Review Board in the Humanities and Social and Behavioural Sciences, Finland, (3) University College London Psychology and Language Sciences Ethics Board, UK. Written informed consent to participate in this study was provided by the participants' legal guardian/next of kin.

AUTHOR CONTRIBUTIONS

VL conceived the study and the protocol, developed the questionnaires, oversaw the study, and led the Australian data collection. RT and DV were responsible for reviewing the questionnaires, adapting them for Finland and the UK (respectively), led their respective country's data collection, and commented and reviewed the manuscript. TP analyzed the data and developed the figures. VL, RT, and TP compiled the tables. VL wrote the first version of the manuscript with the assistance of RT. RT was responsible for the modification of the manuscript to the final format, and submission, and is the corresponding author.

ACKNOWLEDGMENTS

We wish to thank Cherilee Rutherford for her work in developing the questionnaire; Jack Tuckerman and Chi Lo from Macquarie University for their role in the Australian data collection; Australian Hearing, The Shepherd Centre, RIDBC, and The Speech & Hearing Clinic at Macquarie University for assistance with recruitment in Australia; Sanna Kotkas, Reetta Viljanen, and Elisabet Kaila for their work in translating the questionnaires into Finnish; CICERO learning (Mari Tervaniemi); Elisabet Kaila, LapCI ry, Satakieliohjelma, Kuulovammaisten Lasten Vanhempien Liitto (KLVL), Kuuloliitto, Kuulo Auris, Lindfors Foundation, speech therapists, and other professionals in the clinics of university hospitals in Finland for assistance with recruitment in Finland; Lawson Falshaw who set up the online questionnaire for the UK and assisted with UK data collection; the National Deaf Children's Society and Cochlear Implanted Children's Support Group for assisting with UK data collection, and all the parents who completed the questionnaire, or were involved with pilot testing of the questionnaires.

REFERENCES

Barrett, M. S. (2011). Musical narratives: a study of a young child's identity work in and through music-making. *Psyhol. Music* 39, 403–423. doi: 10.1177/0305735610373054

Briggs, C. A. (1991). A model for understanding musical development. *Music Ther.* 10, 1–21. doi: 10.1093/mt/10.1.1

Chasin, M., and Russo, F. A. (2004). Hearing aids and music. *Trends Amplif.* 8, 35–47. doi: 10.1177/108471380400800202

Coffey, E. B. J., Mogilever, N. B., and Zatorre, R. J. (2017). Speech-in-noise perception in musicians: a review. *Hear. Res.* 352, 496–499. doi: 10.1016/j.heares.2017.02.006

Costa-Giomi, E., and Ilari, B. (2014). Infants' preferential attention to sung and spoken stimuli. *J. Res. Music Educ.* 62, 188–194. doi: 10.1177/0022429414530564

Custodero, L. A. (2006). Singing practices in 10 families with young children. *J. Res. Music Educ.* 54, 37–56. doi: 10.1177/002242940605400104

Dege, F., and Schwarzer, G. (2011). The effect of a music program on phonological awareness in preschoolers. *Front. Psychol.* 2:124. doi: 10.3389/fpsyg.2011.00124

Denac, O. (2008). A case study of preschool children's musical interests at home and at school. *Early Child. Educ. J.* 35, 439–444. doi: 10.1007/s10643-007-0205-4

Dittinger, E., Chobert, J., Ziegler, J. C., and Besson, M. (2017). Fast brain plasticity during word learning in musically-trained children. *Front. Hum. Neurosci.* 11:223. doi: 10.3389/fnhum.2017.00233

Dittinger, E., Valizadeh, S. A., Jancke, L., Besson, M., and Elmer, S. (2018). Increased functional connectivity in the ventral and dorsal streams during retrieval of novel words in professional musicians. *Hum. Brain Mapp.* 39, 722–734. doi: 10.1002/hbm.23877

Driscoll, V., Gfeller, K., Tan, X., See, R. L., Cheng, H.-Y., and Kanemitsu, M. (2015). Family involvement in music impacts participation of children with cochlear implants in music education and music activities. *Cochlear Implants Int.* 16, 137–146. doi: 10.1179/1754762814y.0000000103

Estabrooks, W. (1994). *Auditory-Verbal Therapy for Parents and Professionals.* Washington DC: Alexander Graham Bell Association for the deaf.

Flaugnacco, E., Lopez, L., Terribili, C., Montico, M., Zoia, S., and Schön, D. (2015). Music training increases phonological awareness and reading skills in developmental dyslexia: a randomized control trial. *PLoS One* 10:e0138715. doi: 10.1371/journal.pone.0138715

Francois, C., Chobert, J., Besson, M., and Schön, D. (2013). Music training for the development of speech segmentation. *Cereb. Cortex* 23, 2038–2043. doi: 10.1093/cercor/bhs180

Gaser, C., and Schlaug, G. (2003). Brain structures differ between musicians and non-musicians. *J. Neurosci.* 23, 9240–9245. doi: 10.1523/JNEUROSCI.23-27-09240.2003

Gfeller, K., Driscoll, V., and Schwalje, A. (2019). Beyond technology: the interaction of perceptual accuracy and experiential factors in pediatric music engagement. *Otol. Neurotol.* 40, e290–e297. doi: 10.1097/mao.0000000000002123

Gfeller, K., Oleson, J., Knutson, J. F., Breheny, P., Driscoll, V., and Olszewski, C. (2008). Multivariate predictors of music perception and appraisal by adult cochlear implant users. *Volta Rev.* 19, 120–134. doi: 10.3766/jaaa.19.2.3

Gfeller, K., Witt, S. A., Spencer, L. J., Stordahl, J., and Tomblin, B. (1998). Musical involvement and enjoyment of children who use cochlear implants. *Volta Rev.* 100, 213–233. doi: 10.1179/1754762814Y.0000000103

Good, A., Gordon, K. A., Papsin, B. C., Nespoli, G., Hopyan, T., Peretz, I., et al. (2017). Benefits of music training for perception of emotional speech prosody in deaf children with cochlear implants. *Ear Hear.* 38, 455–464. doi: 10.1097/aud.0000000000000402

Gordon, R. L., Fehd, H. M., and McCandliss, B. D. (2015). Does music training enhance literacy skills? A meta-analysis. *Front. Psychol.* 6:1777. doi: 10.3389/fpsyg.2015.01777

Halwani, G. F., Loui, P., Rüber, T., and Schlaug, G. (2011). Effects of practice and experience on the arcuate fasciculus: comparing singers, instrumentalists, and non-musicians. *Front. Psychol.* 2:156. doi: 10.3389/fpsyg.2011.00156

Huotilainen, M., and Tervaniemi, M. (2018). Planning music-based amelioration and training in infancy and childhood based on neural evidence. *Ann. N. Y. Acad. Sci.* 1423, 146–154. doi: 10.1111/nyas.13655

Ilari, B. (2013). Concerted cultivation and music learning: global issues and local variations. *Res. Stud. Music Educ.* 35, 179–196. doi: 10.1177/1321103x13509348

Ilari, B., Moura, A., and Bourscheidt, L. A. (2011). Between interactions and commodities: musical parenting of infants and toddlers in Brazil. *Music Educ. Res.* 13, 51–67. doi: 10.1080/14613808.2011.553277

Intartaglia, B., White-Schwoch, T., Kraus, N., and Schön, D. (2017). Music training enhances the automatic neural processing of foreign speech sounds. *Sci. Rep.* 7, 1–7. doi: 10.1038/s41598-017-12575-1

Jaschke, A. C., Honing, H., and Scherder, E. J. A. (2018). Longitudinal analysis of music education on executive functions in primary school children. *Front. Neurosci.* 12:103. doi: 10.3389/fnins.2018.00103

Kirschner, S., and Ilari, B. (2014). Joint drumming in Brazilian and German preschool children: cultural differences in rhythmic entrainment, but no prosocial effects. *J. Cross Cult. Psychol.* 45, 137–166. doi: 10.1177/0022022113493139

Kral, A., and Sharma, A. (2012). Developmental neuroplasticity after cochlear implantation. *Trends Neurosci.* 35, 111–122. doi: 10.1016/j.tins.2011.09.004

LeBlanc, A., Jin, Y. C., Stamou, L., and McCrary, J. (1999). Effect of age, country, and gender on music listening preferences. *Bull. Coun. Res. Music Ed.* 141, 72–76.

Limb, C. J., and Roy, A. T. (2014). Technological, biological, and acoustical constraints to music perception in cochlear implant users. *Hear. Res.* 308, 13–26. doi: 10.1016/j.heares.2013.04.009

Linnavalli, T., Putkinen, V., Lipsanen, J., Huotilainen, M., and Tervaniemi, M. (2018). Music playschool enhances children's linguistic skills. *Sci. Rep.* 8:8767. doi: 10.1038/s41598-018-27126-5

Looi, V., Gfeller, K., and Driscoll, V. D. (2012a). Music appreciation and training for cochlear implant recipients: a review. *Sem. Hear.* 33, 307–334. doi: 10.1055/s-0032-1329222

Looi, V., King, J., and Kelly-Campbell, R. (2012b). A music appreciation training program developed for clinical application with cochlear implant recipients and hearing aid users. *Sem. Hear.* 33, 361–380. doi: 10.1055/s-002-2 4038

Looi, V., McDermott, H., McKay, C., and Hickson, L. (2007). Comparisons of quality ratings for music by cochlear implant and hearing aid users. *Ear Hear.* 28, 59S–61S. doi: 10.1097/AUD.0b013e31803150cb

Looi, V., and Radford, C. J. (2011). A comparison of the speech recognition and pitch ranking abilities of children using a unilateral cochlear implant, bimodal stimulation or bilateral hearing aids. *Int. J. Pediatr. Otorhinolaryngol.* 74, 472–482. doi: 10.1016/j.ijporl.2010.12.023

Looi, V., Rutledge, K., and Prvan, T. (2019). Music appreciation of adult hearing aid users and the impact of different levels of hearing loss. *Ear Hear.* 40, 529–544. doi: 10.1097/aud.0000000000000632

Looi, V., and She, J. (2010). Music perception of cochlear implant users: a questionnaire, and its implications for a music training program. *Int. J. Audiol.* 49, 116–128. doi: 10.3109/14992020903405987

Looi, V., Tuckerman, J., Lo, C., Prvan, T., and Rutherford, C. (2018). The role of music in families of children with hearing loss in Australia & South Africa. *Presentation at the 34th World Congress in Audiology*, Cape Town, 28–31.

Moreno, S., and Bidelman, G. M. (2014). Examining neural plasticity and cognitive benefit through the unique lens of musical training. *Hear. Res.* 308, 84–97. doi: 10.1016/j.heares.2013.09.012

Oechslin, M. S., Gschwind, M., and James, C. E. (2018). Tracking training-related plasticity by combining fMRI and DTI: the right-hemisphere ventral stream mediates musical syntax processing. *Cerebr. Cortex* 28, 1209–1218. doi: 10. 1093/cercor/bhx033

Patscheke, H., Degé, F., and Schwarzer, G. (2018). The effects of training in rhythm and pitch on phonological awareness in four- to six-year-old children. *Psychol. Music* 47, 376–391. doi: 10.1177/0305735618756763

Rocca, C. (2012). A different musical perspective: improving outcomes in music through habilitation, education, and training for children with cochlear implants. *Sem. Hear.* 33, 425–433. doi: 10.1055/s-0032-132 9229

Ronkainen, R. (2011). Enhancing listening and imitation skills in children with cochlear implants: the use of multimodal resources in speech and language therapy. *J. Interact. Res. Commun. Disord.* 2, 245–269. doi: 10.1558/jircd. v2i2.245

Saarikallio, S. (2011). Music as emotional self-regulation throughout adulthood. *Psychol. Music* 39, 307–327. doi: 10.1177/0305735610374894

Saarikallio, S., and Erkkilä, J. (2007). The role of music in adolescents' mood regulation. *Psychol. Music* 35, 88–109. doi: 10.1177/030573560706 8889

Schellenberg, E. G. (2004). Music lessons enhance IQ. *Psychol. Sci.* 15, 511–514. doi: 10.1111/j.0956-7976.2004.00711.x

Schneider, P., Scherg, M., Dosch, H. G., Specht, H. J., Gutschalk, A., and Rupp, A. (2002). Morphology of Heschl's gyrus reflects enhanced activation in the auditory cortex of musicians. *Nat. Neurosci.* 5, 688–694. doi: 10.1038/nn871

Slater, J., Skoe, E., Strait, D. L., O'Connell, S., Thompson, E., and Kraus, N. (2015). Music training improves speech-in-noise perception: longitudinal evidence from a community-based music program. *Behav. Brain Res.* 291, 244–252. doi: 10.1016/j.bbr.2015.05.026

Torppa, R., Faulkner, A., Huotilainen, M., Järvikivi, J., Lipsanen, J., Laasonen, M., et al. (2014a). The perception of prosody and associated auditory cues in early-implanted children: the role of auditory working memory and musical activities. *Int. J. Audiol.* 53, 182–191. doi: 10.3109/14992027.2013.87 2302

Torppa, R., Huotilainen, M., Leminen, M., Lipsanen, J., and Tervaniemi, M. (2014b). Interplay between singing and cortical processing of music: a longitudinal study in children with cochlear implants. *Front. Psychol.* 5:1389. doi: 10.3389/fpsyg.2014.01389

Torppa, R., Faulkner, A., Kujala, T., Huotilainen, M., and Lipsanen, J. (2018). Developmental links between speech perception in noise, singing, and cortical processing of music in children with cochlear implants. *Music Percept.* 36, 156–174. doi: 10.1525/MP.2018.36.2.156

Torppa, R., Faulkner, A., Laasonen, M., Lipsanen, J., and Sammler, D. (2019). Links of prosodic stress perception and musical activities to language skills of children with CIs and normal hearing. *Ear Hear.* doi: 10.1097/AUD.0000000000000763 [Epub ahead of print].

Trehub, S. E. (2001). Musical predispositions in infancy. *Ann. N. Y Acad. Sci.* 930, 1–16. doi: 10.1111/j.1749-6632.2001.tb05721.x

Trehub, S. E., Vongpaisal, T., and Nakata, T. (2009). Music in the lives of deaf children with cochlear implants. *Ann. N. Y. Acad. Sci.* 1169, 534–542. doi: 10.1111/j.1749-6632.2009.04554.x

Virtala, P., and Partanen, E. (2018). Can very early music interventions promote at-risk infants' development? *Ann. N. Y. Acad. Sci.* 1423, 92–101. doi: 10.1111/nyas.13646

Williams, K. E., Barrett, M. S., Welch, G. F., Abad, V., and Broughton, M. (2015). Associations between early shared music activities in the home and later child outcomes: findings from the longitudinal study of australian children. *Early Child. Res. Q.* 31, 1131–1124. doi: 10.1016/j.ecresq.2015.01.004

Young, S., and Gillen, J. (2007). Toward a revised understanding of young children's musical activities: reflections from the "Day in the Life" project. *Curr. Musicol.* 84, 79–99.

15

Effects of Low Frequency Residual Hearing on Music Perception and Psychoacoustic Abilities in Pediatric Cochlear Implant Recipients

Mustafa Yüksel[1], Margaret A. Meredith[2] and Jay T. Rubinstein[3]*

[1] Audiology and Speech Disorders Program, Institute of Health Sciences, Marmara University, Istanbul, Turkey, [2] Childhood Communication Center, Seattle Children's Hospital, Seattle, WA, United States, [3] Virginia Merrill Bloedel Hearing Research Center, Department of Otolaryngology – Head and Neck Surgery, University of Washington, Seattle, WA, United States

***Correspondence:**
Mustafa Yüksel
mustafa.yuksel@marmara.edu.tr*

Studies have demonstrated the benefits of low frequency residual hearing in music perception and for psychoacoustic abilities of adult cochlear implant (CI) users, but less is known about these effects in the pediatric group. Understanding the contribution of combined electric and acoustic stimulation in this group can help to gain a better perspective on decisions regarding bilateral implantation. We evaluated the performance of six unilaterally implanted children between 9 and 13 years of age with contralateral residual hearing using the Clinical Assessment of Music Perception (CAMP), spectral ripple discrimination (SRD), and temporal modulation transfer function (TMTF) tests and compared findings with previous research. Our study sample performed similarly to normal hearing subjects in pitch direction discrimination (0.81 semitones) and performed well above typical CI users in melody recognition (43.37%). The performance difference was less in timbre recognition (48.61%), SRD (1.47 ripple/octave), and TMTF for four modulation frequencies. These findings suggest that the combination of low frequency acoustic hearing with the broader frequency range of electric hearing can help to increase clinical CI benefit in pediatric users and decisions regarding second-side implantation should consider these factors.

Keywords: cochlear implant, residual hearing, hearing preservation, music perception, psychoacoustics

INTRODUCTION

Profoundly deaf patients can receive cochlear implants (CIs) and the advantages of electrical stimulation in restoring hearing capacity and speech understanding are well known. However, music perception and speech perception in noise are still generally poor in CI recipients without residual acoustic hearing, due to spectrotemporal limitations of electrical stimulation (Gfeller et al., 2002b, 2007; Nimmons et al., 2008; Won et al., 2010, 2011; Drennan et al., 2015). Combining acoustic hearing with electric stimulation, if available, can be advantageous and CI users who have residual low frequency hearing in the non-implanted ear or in the implanted ear can perform better on such tasks (Gantz and Turner, 2004; Gantz et al., 2006; Golub et al., 2012; Roland et al., 2016). There are different ways to achieve combined acoustic and electric hearing. CI users can use the residual hearing in the implanted ear when residual hearing is preserved, so called

Hybrid (Cochlear Ltd., Sydney) or EAS (MED-EL, Innsbruck, Austria) hearing, or benefit from the residual hearing in the contralateral non-implanted ear, so-called bimodal hearing, with or without a hearing aid. The aim of both methods is to combine the high frequency information of electrical stimuli with the low frequency information of acoustic hearing to provide better spectral and temporal information via the combination than a CI can provide alone.

The benefits of combined acoustic and electric hearing are especially significant in music perception (Gfeller et al., 2006; Golub et al., 2012; Driscoll et al., 2016; Kelsall et al., 2017; Cheng et al., 2018; Parkinson et al., 2019). Gfeller et al. (2006) conducted two different experiments. In the first, authors compared 4 Hybrid CI users implanted with shorter electrode arrays with 39 CI users implanted with standard length electrodes and 17 normal hearing adults using an open-set melody recognition test. In the second, authors compared 14 Hybrid CI users implanted with shorter electrode arrays with 174 standard CI users implanted with standard length electrodes and 21 normal hearing adults using a closed set test of musical instrument identification. Hybrid CI users performed significantly better than standard CI users on both tests and similar to normal hearing subjects in melody recognition with lyrics. Dorman et al. (2008) evaluated and compared the melody recognition abilities of 15 CI users with and without a hearing aid in the non-implanted ear. Acoustic only (70.6%) and EAS (71.2%) modes were similar but the electric only mode (52%) was significantly poorer than the other two conditions. More recently, Kelsall et al. (2017) demonstrated that Hybrid CI users (N = 50) implanted with shorter electrode arrays performed similarly to normal hearing subjects in a pitch perception task using complex tones and the average score was 1.1 semitones. Conventional CI users tested in related studies have scores around three semitones. Melody perception was 65.9% and almost three times better than in conventional CI users. Timbre recognition was also better, but the difference was limited with Hybrid users scoring 56.6% and conventional CI users scoring 42.5%. The authors concluded that Hybrid CI users maintain music perception abilities postoperatively better than typically observed with conventional CIs.

To determine whether the preserved acoustic cues contribute to superior performance, Parkinson et al. (2019) examined the music perception of normal hearing subjects with acoustic simulations of Hybrid implants and compared electric only, acoustic only, and electro-acoustic conditions. Results showed better performance with the electric-acoustic condition (67.9%) in melody recognition scores compared to the electric-only condition (39.1%), but there was no effect of stimulation condition on timbre recognition scores. Researchers also compared the findings with the Hybrid L24 US clinical trial (Roland et al., 2016) and the results showed a similar pattern. The authors attributed the better melody recognition performance to the availability of low frequency spectral cues in the acoustic domain. In general, low frequency residual hearing appears highly beneficial for pitch and melody perception but less so for timbre perception.

Speech and musical sounds contain multiple frequency and timing cues that vary in a complex manner. Both normal hearing and CI systems need a detailed representation of acoustic signals in spectral and temporal domains to fully perceive such complex signals, but spectral and temporal sensitivity is limited in current implants as a result of biological and technological constraints. Won et al. (2010) evaluated the spectral and temporal sensitivity and music perception abilities of 42 adult CI recipients. Spectral sensitivity was shown to correlate with the three subtests of the Clinical Assessment of Music Perception (CAMP) test (Kang et al., 2009), but there was no correlation between temporal sensitivity and music perception. A similar study was performed with pediatric CI recipients (8–16 years of age) and the authors suggested that the spectral sensitivity might be decisive in the children's performance (Jung et al., 2012). Heng et al. (2011) and Kong et al. (2011) both evaluated the relationship between timbre perception and temporal sensitivity in CI recipients and both studies emphasized the importance of temporal sensitivity in the perception of timbre. Recently Choi et al. (2018) evaluated the spectrotemporal modulation sensitivity and music perception of normal hearing listeners, hearing aid users, and CI recipients, and there was a significant correlation between music perception abilities and spectrotemporal modulation sensitivity, but there was no correlation between music perception and spectral or temporal modulation sensitivities alone. Golub et al. (2012) compared Hybrid CI recipients with standard CI recipients and pitch perception and spectral ripple discrimination (SRD) performance were significantly better in the Hybrid group and there was no advantage of residual acoustic hearing for temporal sensitivity.

Since there is no US FDA approval for the Hybrid or EAS systems for individuals younger than 18 years of age, reported outcomes in this age group with preserved residual hearing after implantation are limited. Benefit of combined acoustic and electric hearing on music emotion judgment (Giannantonio et al., 2015) and perception (Shirvani et al., 2016) and faster reaction time on music perception tests (Polonenko et al., 2017) were shown in bimodal CI users with a contralateral hearing aid. While these studies emphasize the benefit of combined electric and contralateral acoustic hearing, it is also possible to electro-acoustically stimulate the same ear and even the same single neuron (Tillein et al., 2015; Sato et al., 2017) with Hybrid and EAS systems. But there are only two studies directly evaluated the Hybrid or EAS system using subjects under 18 years of age. Driscoll et al. (2016) evaluated the music perception of five adolescents using Hybrid implants (13–18 years of age) with complex pitch ranking (PR-C), melodic error detection, and melody recognition. The performance of the Hybrid implant users on the three tests was significantly better than the traditional implant users and very similar to normal hearing peers. Recently Cheng et al. (2018) assessed the speech perception and melody contour identification of 35 children in unilateral (CI only) and bimodal (with hearing aid on the contralateral ear) conditions. Subjects performed significantly better in the bimodal condition on the melody contour identification and Mandarin tone recognition tests and results suggested that combined electric and acoustic hearing can improve both music and tonal speech perception in CI users.

Given the apparent benefits of bimodal hearing, there is an ongoing debate over when bimodal hearing may have benefits over bilateral CIs (Cullington and Zeng, 2011; Looi and Radford, 2011; Bartov and Most, 2014; Giannantonio et al., 2015; Polonenko et al., 2017; Gifford and Dorman, 2018). Studies reported that bimodal benefit is highly dependent on the degree of hearing loss, amount of pre-operative acoustic experience, and CI benefit (Looi and Radford, 2011; Illg et al., 2014; Dorman et al., 2015) and also the testing material used to evaluate the benefit. Standard clinical measures of speech perception alone are probably not reliable to determine second-side CI candidacy (Gifford and Dorman, 2018). Therefore, this study was intended to assess spectral and temporal sensitivity and music perception in older children with progressive hearing loss who have residual hearing in the contralateral ear to determine if, as expected, their outcomes were adult-like. We also intended to evaluate the benefits of residual acoustic hearing on music perception and spectral and temporal sensitivity in this age group. It is hoped that such measures can improve candidacy selection for second-side cochlear implantation in children with residual hearing in the unimplanted ear.

MATERIALS AND METHODS

Subjects

Six unilaterally implanted children between 9 and 13 years (M = 10.6 years) of age participated in this study. Subjects spoke English as their native language and had limited formal music training. **Table 1** describes the demographics and etiology of hearing loss if known. All subjects passed newborn hearing screening bilaterally, have normal cochlear anatomy and early speech, and language development was normal by parent report. All subjects except S6 were deafened progressively while S6 had stable hearing thresholds through all of childhood. Mean age at diagnosis was 3.9 years and all subjects started to use hearing aids not later than 6 months after the diagnosis (mean age 4.1 years). Mean age at implantation was 5.2 years and all of the participants were using their implants for 4–8 years at the time of the study. All subjects received Cochlear Ltd. Devices using the Advanced Combination Encoder strategy at 900 Hz stimulation rate per channel. During the testing only one subject (S6) was wearing her hearing aid since she was the only one using a hearing aid in the unimplanted ear regularly. The other five subjects were not using an aid in the contralateral ear by the time of the study though some had earlier in their lives. Audiograms for the contralateral ear are shown for five subjects (**Figure 1A**). S6 has a significantly different audiometric configuration from the rest of the group, therefore we presented her audiogram separately (**Figure 1B**). The protocol was approved by the Seattle Children's Hospital and University of Washington Institutional Review Boards and all subjects and their parents gave written informed consent.

All tests were conducted in a sound-treated double walled room (IAC) with custom MATLAB programs and a sound field presentation level of 65 dB A. All stimuli were presented via a loudspeaker that was positioned at 0° azimuth and 0° elevation at a 1-m distance from the subjects.

TABLE 1 | Demographics, etiology of hearing loss, and speech perception scores.

	Participant demographics										
	Demographics					Cochlear implant			Speech perception scores		
No.	Age	Age at diagnosis (months)	Age at hearing aid (months)	Age at first CI (months)	Etiology	Device	Processor	Surgical approach	CNC (words) (%)	AzBio quiet (%)	AzBio + 5 SNR (%)
1.	10	50	51	58	TMPRSS33 mutation	CI422	Nucleus 6	Round window	84	98	65
2.	12	25	28	46	TMPRSS33 mutation	CI512	Nucleus 6	Cochleostomy	80	95	42
3.	9	27	27	38	TMPRSS33 mutation	CI422	Nucleus 5	Round window	56	86	59
4.	11	75	76	84	Unknown	CI422	Nucleus 6	Round window	88	99	47
5.	11	75	76	84	Unknown	CI422	Nucleus 6	Round window	100	98	52
6.	13	51	53	60	Connexin26	CI422	Nucleus 5	Round window	80	90	66
Mean	11	50.5	51.83	61.67							

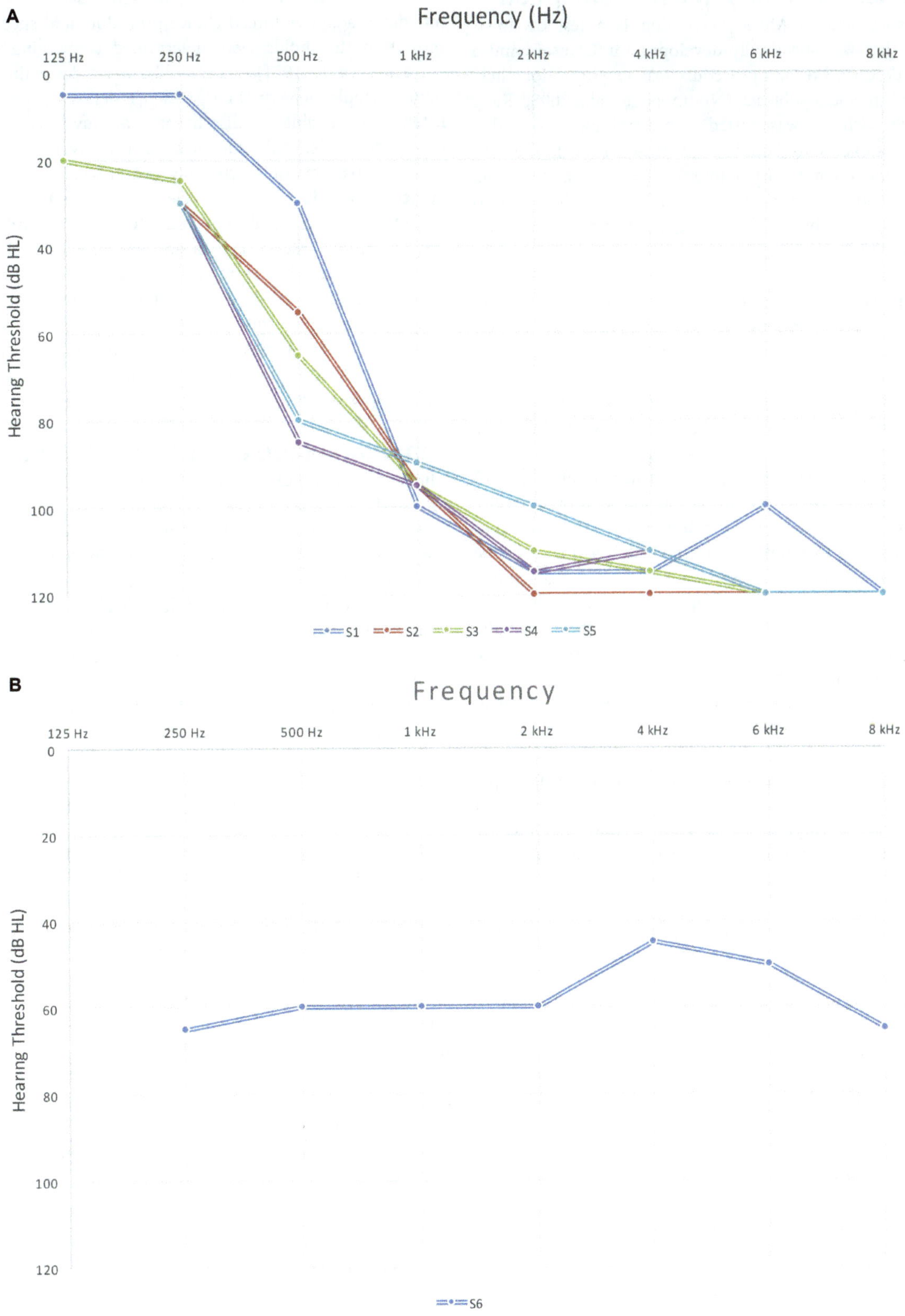

FIGURE 1 | Audiometric configuration for unimplanted ears of study subjects: **(A)** five study subjects and **(B)** S6 with different configuration.

Clinical Assessment of Music Perception

Clinical Assessment of Music Perception is a test of music perception that was specifically developed for CI users and a previously described testing procedure was employed for pitch, timbre, and melody subtests (Nimmons et al., 2008; Kang et al., 2009). Each test was started with a training session that allowed the subjects to familiarize themselves with the task which allowing them to listen four different pitch pairs and 12 melodies and 8 instruments twice. During training sessions feedback was given, but in the actual testing no feedback was given to the subjects.

The complex pitch direction discrimination (PDD) test was a two alternative forced choice procedure in which the subject identifies the synthesized tone with a higher pitch. Two buttons (1 and 2) were presented on a computer screen and subjects were instructed to select the button corresponding to the tone with the higher pitch. Three base frequencies (262, 330, and 392 Hz) were used as a reference stimulus and in each tone pair the comparison stimulus interval was changed by the step size of one semitone. The initial pitch pair has an interval of 12 semitones and each correct response was followed by a smaller interval with incorrect responses followed by larger intervals. The discrimination threshold in semitones was estimated as the mean interval size for three base frequencies, each determined from the mean of the final six of eight reversals. A reversal at zero was automatically added by the test algorithm when the subjects answered correctly at a one semitone interval to create an accurate psychometric function.

Twelve well-known melody clips were played three times in random order in the melody recognition subtest. Rhythmic cues were removed from the melodies and each note of each melody has the same length and time signature with identical tempo. All melodies played in notes with a duration of 500 ms in an 8 note pattern at a tempo of 60 beats per minute. Each melody was prerecorded as five versions with different intensities per note (±4 dB) and each time a different version was played randomly to avoid intensity cues. After listening to the melody, subjects were asked to identify the melody by selecting the title of the song from the closed set of names. Measured outcome was a total percent correct score calculated after 36 melody presentations.

In timbre recognition, subjects were asked to identify a musical instrument from a closed set of names with the picture of the corresponding instrument. Eight instruments playing an identical five-note sequence were used and all instruments were recorded live with attempted identical phrasing. A total percent of instruments correctly identified was calculated after 24 presentations.

Spectral Ripple Discrimination

The SRD test is an adaptive task and previously described stimuli and procedures were used (Won et al., 2007). The stimuli were generated by summing 200 pure tone frequency components with a duration of 500 ms and a rise/fall time of 150 ms. Each stimulus was either a standard (reference) or inverted ripple (ripple phase – reversed). The stimuli had a bandwidth of 100–5000 Hz and the ripple densities differed by ratios of 1.411. The test paradigm used a two up and one down adaptive forced-choice procedure and spectral ripple resolution thresholds were determined converging on 70.7% correct (Levitt, 1971). Thresholds were determined as the highest ripple density (in ripples per octave – rpo) at which listeners were able to discriminate an inverted signal from two standard stimuli, identical to the inverted one except that the positions of spectral peaks and valleys were reversed. Subjects were instructed to select the respective number of different/inverted signal from computer screen. Testing included three adaptive tracks. The mean threshold of a single track was determined by averaging the final 8 of 13 reversals. The final SRD thresholds were determined by averaging three adaptive tracks. A few examples were shown to subjects prior to the actual test until the examiner is confident the subject understood the task and as the actual testing began no feedback was given.

Temporal Modulation Transfer Function

The temporal modulation transfer function (TMTF) test used in this study was adapted from Bacon and Viemeister (1985) and modified by Won et al. (2011). Stimuli consisted of two intervals, one with unmodulated and one with sinusoidally amplitude modulated (SAM) wide-band noise and subjects were instructed to choose the interval with the modulation. Total duration of the stimuli was 2 s and each interval was 1 s. Modulation frequencies of 10, 50, 100, and 300 Hz were used to keep the attention of the subjects since three tests were taking approximately 90 min and this also allowed analysis of the high pass characteristic of the TMTF. Modulated stimuli were created with the following equation:

$$y(t) = [f(t)]\, x[1 + m_i \sin(2\pi f_m t)]$$

In this equation, t indicates time and x indicates multiplication, $f(t)$ is the wideband Gaussian noise carrier, m_i is the modulation index (modulation depth), f_m is the modulation frequency, and $y(t)$ is the resulting signal. To compensate the intensity increment for the SAM stimuli the modulated waveform was divided by a factor of $1 + (m_i^2/2)$. A two interval two alternative forced-choice test with two down one up adaptive procedure was used. Measured outcome was the modulation depth (m_i) threshold (MDT) for each modulation frequency, converging on 70.7% (Levitt, 1971). The starting modulation depth was 100% and decreasing in steps of 4 dB for the first four reversals and 2 dB for the next 10 reversals. MDT for each modulation frequency was obtained from the average of the final 10 reversals. Reported values are in dB relative to 100% modulation depth.

RESULTS

Since our study sample was small, results from previous studies conducted with the same testing material in the same research center were used as a reference and values are shown in the respective figures.

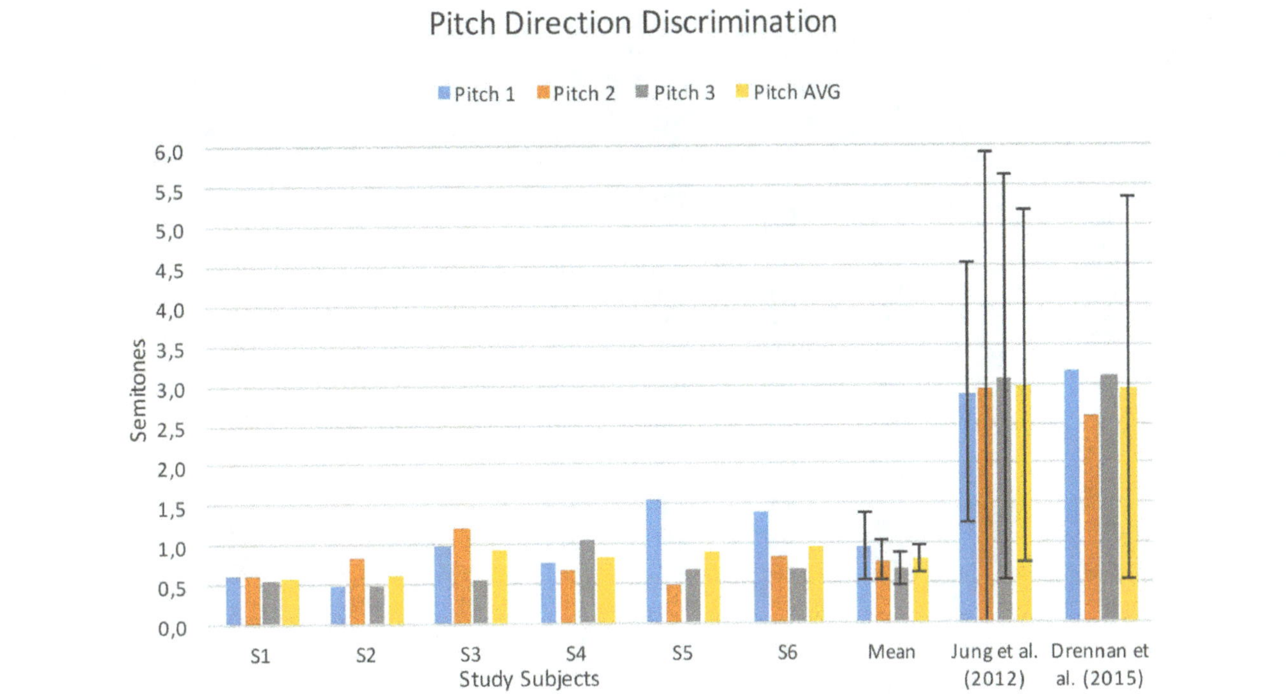

FIGURE 2 | Individual and mean pitch direction discrimination scores for study subjects and mean scores from previous studies. Error bars indicate ±1 standard deviation. AVG, average. Data adopted from Jung et al. (2012) and Drennan et al. (2015).

CAMP

Pitch direction discrimination, timbre recognition, and melody recognition scores of six study subjects and mean values from previous studies conducted with normal hearing subjects and standard length electrode CI users (Kang et al., 2009; Jung et al., 2012; Drennan et al., 2015) for reference are shown in **Figures 2, 3**.

Mean PDD thresholds for the study sample were 0.97 (±0.43) for 262 Hz; 0.78 (±0.25) for 330 Hz; 0.67 (±0.20) for 391 Hz; and 0.81 (±0.16) semitones on average. Jung et al. (2012) assessed 11 prelingually deafened pediatric CI users with standard length electrodes and no residual hearing and subjects scored 2.98 (±2.23) semitones on average and 145 postlingually deafened adult CI users in the Drennan et al. (2015) study scored 2.95 (±2.40) semitones on average (**Figure 2**). Mean PDD threshold of normal hearing subjects in Kang et al. (2009) study was 1.0 (±0.03).

The timbre recognition score of the subjects was 48.61% (±8.06) on average. Pediatric users of CIs without residual hearing in a previous study scored 34.09% (±13.15) on average (Jung et al., 2012). Adult CI recipients in the Drennan et al. (2015) study and adults with Hybrid devices in electro-acoustic mode in Parkinson et al. (2019) study scored 43.2 (±22%) and 40.7 (±19.7%), respectively (**Figure 3A**). Mean timbre recognition of normal hearing subjects in Kang et al. (2009) study was 94.2 (±4.0%).

On the melody recognition subtest the subjects scored 43.37% (±19.49) on average and with that score our study sample performed almost four times better than the children from a previous study without residual hearing (Jung et al., 2012). In reference studies adult CI users scored 26.20% (±19.90) on average (Drennan et al., 2015) and adult Hybrid users in the electric-acoustic condition in the Parkinson et al. (2019) study scored 67.90% (±21.10) on average (**Figure 3B**). Mean melody recognition of normal hearing subjects in Kang et al. (2009) study was 87.5% (±8.3%).

Spectral Ripple Discrimination

Mean spectral ripple threshold of study subjects was 1.47 (±0.85) rpo. Pediatric and adult CI recipients and adult Hybrid CI recipients in previous studies have mean spectral ripple thresholds at 2.08 (±1.6), 2.10 (0.40) and 4.60 (±0.60) rpo, respectively (**Figure 4A**).

Temporal Modulation Transfer Function

Temporal modulation detection thresholds in four modulation frequency are shown in **Figure 4B**. Two previous reference studies were conducted with adult CI recipients (Won et al., 2011; Golub et al., 2012) but the values were quite similar. The low pass shape of the present study's TMTFs is similar to TMTFs measured in previous studies.

DISCUSSION

This study demonstrates the benefit of low frequency residual hearing on music perception measurements in CI recipients. Such benefit was shown in previous studies with bimodal users

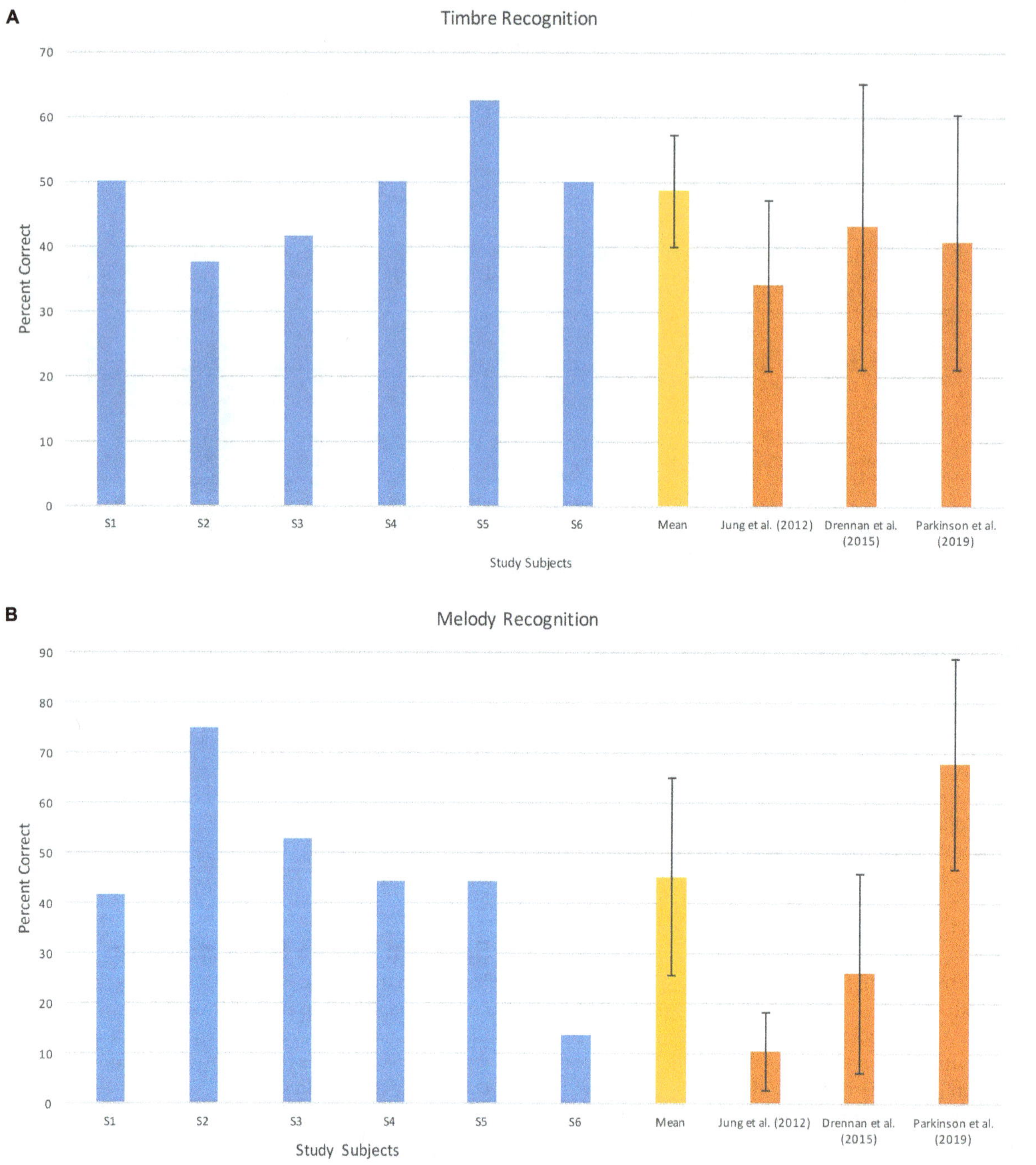

FIGURE 3 | Individual and mean timbre **(A)** and melody **(B)** recognition scores for study subjects and mean scores from previous studies. Error bars indicate ±1 standard deviation. Data adopted from Jung et al. (2012), Drennan et al. (2015), and Parkinson et al. (2019).

(Bartov and Most, 2014; Cheng et al., 2018), Hybrid CI recipients (Driscoll et al., 2016), and acoustic simulations of the electric-acoustic condition (Parkinson et al., 2019).

The complex PDD performance of our study sample was very close to normal hearing subjects in previous studies (Gfeller et al., 2002a; Kang et al., 2009) with values ranging between 0.59 and 0.96 semitones. Adolescent Hybrid CI users in the Driscoll et al. (2016) study performed between 1 and 6 semitones but the PR-C Test was used in that study and the best score in PR-C is 1 semitone while the best score in PDD of CAMP is 0.50 semitones. Also the participants in our study had progressive hearing losses but there was no comparable information given in the Driscoll et al. (2016) study. Adult Hybrid CI users in the Kelsall et al. (2017) study performed the same pre (with hearing aids) and post operatively (mean = 1.1 semitones) in the PDD test and this observation is an important evidence for

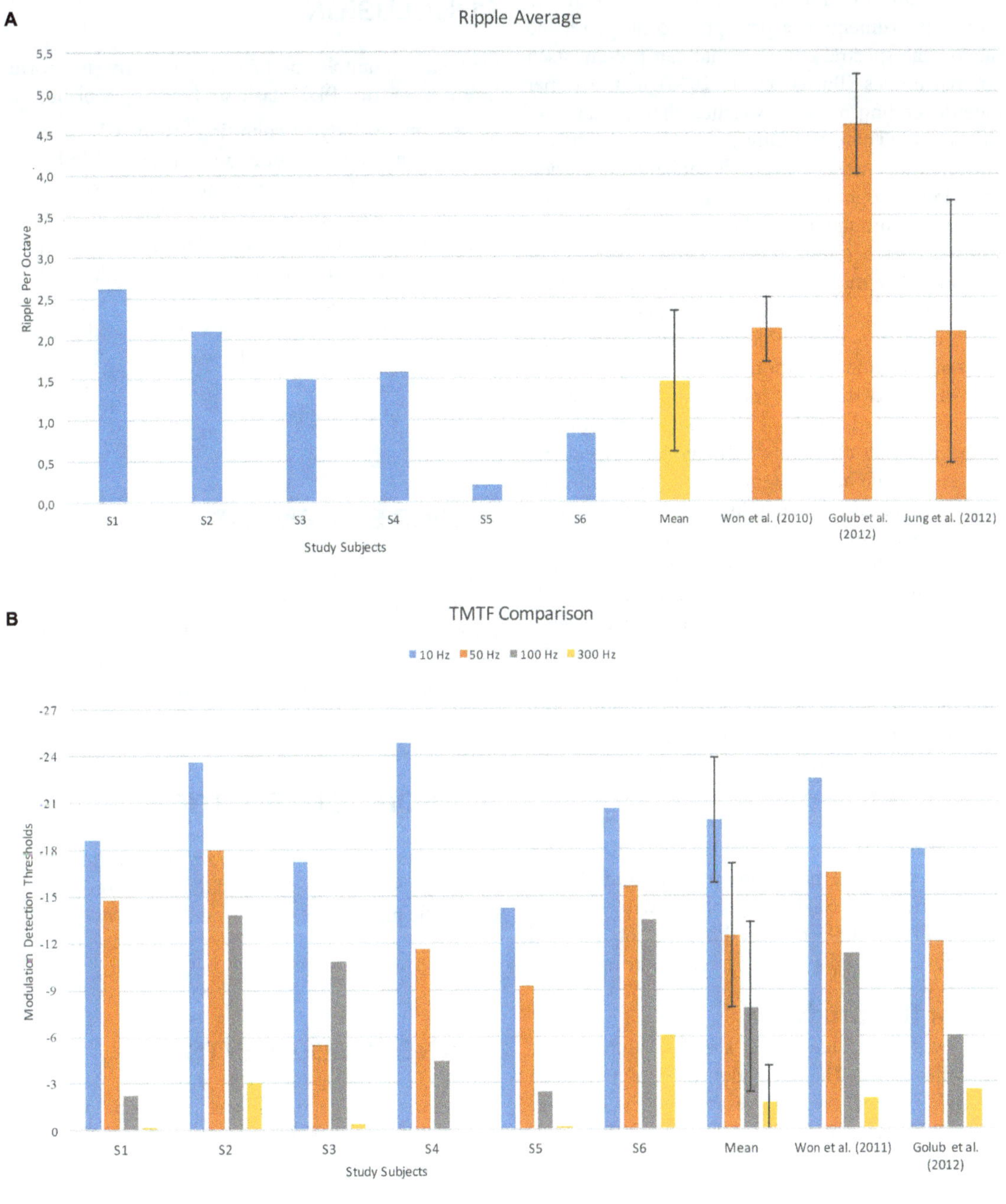

FIGURE 4 | Spectral ripple discrimination **(A)** and TMTF **(B)** performance of study subjects and mean scores from previous studies. Error bars indicate ±1 standard deviation. Data adopted from Won et al. (2010), Golub et al. (2012), and Jung et al. (2012).

the benefit of low frequency hearing on pitch perception. This benefit is especially significant, since the pitch range evaluated in CAMP is a direct reflection of western musical instruments and melody intervals that mainly focused on octaves around middle C (262 Hz). In the other two measurements of music perception, the study sample performed better than CI recipients without any acoustic hearing, particularly for melody recognition. We believe that the superior performance in the melody recognition can be related to the PDD, since the melodies were sequential tones with changing pitches in an isochronous manner and as mentioned earlier, these pitches are well within the residual hearing range of subjects 1–5. Unlike the PDD test, the participants did not reach the normal range in the melody recognition test. This finding is consistent with Jung et al. (2012) study where child CI users with standard length electrode arrays performed similarly to adults in the PDD test but performed below chance level on the melody recognition test. It should be considered that perception of melodies requires more attention and memory-related performance compared to the PDD test and this requirement might be dominant for children. Performance was significantly worse than normal hearing in timbre recognition. Timbre of musical instruments is a perceptual concept related to salient peaks on the spectral envelope that can present itself as formants or harmonics (Burred et al., 2006) in the upper frequency range depending on the resonance characteristics of respective instruments (Toole and Olive, 1988). Therefore, the timbre recognition task is more related to broadband perception than pitch and melody recognition tasks and hence dependent on the well-known spectral limitations of CIs.

The superior performance seen in music perception was not evident in SRD and TMTF measurements. The SRD test stimulus has a frequency range of 100–5000 Hz and the perception of high frequency information above 1000 Hz is critical for ripple detection. Effects of age and maturation were studied previously and it has been suggested that SRD matures at 7 years of age in CI recipients (Horn et al., 2017). This is based not only on chronological age but also on CI age (DiNino and Arenberg, 2018) for congenitally deaf children. Our study sample consisted of children with progressive hearing loss who may develop normal central auditory function regardless of implantation age (Sharma and Dorman, 2006). Also, Jung et al. (2012) found no difference between adult and pediatric CI recipients in SRD testing. Therefore, we can speculate that the absence of difference can be expected due to the hearing loss above 1 kHz. In the same study by Jung et al. (2012) the difference between Schroeder-phase discrimination scores at 50 and 200 Hz of adult and pediatric CI groups was statistically significant and it is known that temporal auditory processing can be influenced by age (Brennan et al., 2018), become adult like at age of 11 years in normal hearing individuals (Buss et al., 2017) and development of temporal modulation sensitivity is delayed in pediatric CI users (Park et al., 2015). The precise maturation process in implanted children, and the effects of residual hearing and progressive hearing loss are still not known, but the effect of age and maturation must be considered when interpreting our results.

Limitations of the Study

Our sample size was small due to the specific nature of the CI recipients in this study. This limitation precludes detailed statistical analysis. It is believed, however, that the findings present valuable information to assist decisions on when to perform second-side implantation in older children with residual hearing.

CONCLUSION

Our study sample performed similarly to normal hearing listeners in the PDD task and also performed substantially better on melody recognition than CI recipients without residual hearing in previous studies. Timbre recognition, SRD, and TMTF performances were similar to previous studies of implant recipients. These findings must have taken into account when deciding whether to proceed with second-side implants in children with residual hearing. CI recipients who perform similarly to normal hearing individuals in any behavioral measure is an important and atypical outcome measurement post implantation, hence preserving this ability should be a priority for clinicians.

ETHICS STATEMENT

This study was carried out in accordance with the recommendations of the Declaration of Helsinki with written informed consent from all subjects. The protocol was approved by the Seattle Children's Hospital and the University of Washington Institutional Review Boards.

AUTHOR CONTRIBUTIONS

MY conducted the tests and wrote the manuscript. MM evaluated the subjects. JR conceptualized the study, reviewed the data, and edited the manuscript.

ACKNOWLEDGMENTS

A portion of this paper was accepted for presentation at the 16th Symposium on CIs in Children in Hollywood, FL, United States, 10–13 July 2019.

REFERENCES

Bacon, S. P., and Viemeister, N. F. (1985). Temporal modulation transfer functions in normal-hearing and hearing-impaired listeners. *Audiology* 24, 117–134. doi: 10.3109/00206098509081545

Bartov, T., and Most, T. (2014). Song recognition by young children with cochlear implants: comparison between unilateral, bilateral, and bimodal users. *J. Speech Lang. Hear. Res.* 57, 1929–1941. doi: 10.1044/2014_JSLHR-H-13-0190

Brennan, M. A., Mccreery, R. W., Buss, E., and Jesteadt, W. (2018). The influence of hearing aid gain on gap-detection thresholds for children and adults with hearing loss. *Ear Hear.* 39, 969–979. doi: 10.1097/AUD.0000000000000558

Burred, J., Röbel, A., and Rodet, X. (2006). "An accurate timbre model for musical instruments and its application to classification," in *Proceedings of the Workshop on Learning the Semantics of Audio Signals*, (Athens).

Buss, E., Porter, H. L., Hall, J. W. III, and Grose, J. H. (2017). Gap detection in school-age children and adults: center frequency and ramp duration. *J. Speech Lang Hear. Res.* 60, 172–181. doi: 10.1044/2016_JSLHR-H-16-0010

Cheng, X., Liu, Y., Wang, B., Yuan, Y., Galvin, J. J. III, Fu, Q. J., et al. (2018). The benefits of residual hair cell function for speech and music perception in pediatric bimodal cochlear implant listeners. *Neural Plast.* 2018:4610592. doi: 10.1155/2018/4610592

Choi, J. E., Won, J. H., Kim, C. H., Cho, Y.-S., Hong, S. H., and Moon, I. J. (2018). Relationship between spectrotemporal modulation detection and music perception in normal-hearing, hearing-impaired, and cochlear implant listeners. *Sci. Rep.* 8:800. doi: 10.1038/s41598-017-17350-w

Cullington, H. E., and Zeng, F. G. (2011). Comparison of bimodal and bilateral cochlear implant users on speech recognition with competing talker, music perception, affective prosody discrimination, and talker identification. *Ear Hear.* 32, 16–30. doi: 10.1097/AUD.0b013e3181edfbd2

DiNino, M., and Arenberg, J. G. (2018). Age-related performance on vowel identification and the spectral-temporally modulated ripple test in children with normal hearing and with cochlear implants. *Trends Hear.* 22:2331216518770959. doi: 10.1177/2331216518770959

Dorman, M. F., Cook, S., Spahr, A., Zhang, T., Loiselle, L., Schramm, D., et al. (2015). Factors constraining the benefit to speech understanding of combining information from low-frequency hearing and a cochlear implant. *Hear. Res.* 322, 107–111. doi: 10.1016/j.heares.2014.09.010

Dorman, M. F., Gifford, R. H., Spahr, A. J., and Mckarns, S. A. (2008). The benefits of combining acoustic and electric stimulation for the recognition of speech, voice and melodies. *Audiol. Neurootol.* 13, 105–112. doi: 10.1159/000111782

Drennan, W. R., Oleson, J. J., Gfeller, K., Crosson, J., Driscoll, V. D., Won, J. H., et al. (2015). Clinical evaluation of music perception, appraisal and experience in cochlear implant users. *Int. J. Audiol.* 54, 114–123. doi: 10.3109/14992027.2014.948219

Driscoll, V. D., Welhaven, A. E., Gfeller, K., Oleson, J., and Olszewski, C. P. (2016). Music perception of adolescents using electroacoustic hearing. *Otol. Neurotol.* 37, e141–e147. doi: 10.1097/MAO.0000000000000945

Gantz, B. J., and Turner, C. (2004). Combining acoustic and electrical speech processing: Iowa/Nucleus hybrid implant. *Acta Otolaryngol.* 124, 344–347. doi: 10.1080/00016480410016423

Gantz, B. J., Turner, C., and Gfeller, K. E. (2006). Acoustic plus electric speech processing: preliminary results of a multicenter clinical trial of the Iowa/Nucleus Hybrid implant. *Audiol. Neurotol.* 11, 63–68. doi: 10.1159/000095616

Gfeller, K., Olszewski, C., Turner, C., Gantz, B., and Oleson, J. (2006). Music perception with cochlear implants and residual hearing. *Audiol. Neurootol.* 11(Suppl. 1), 12–15. doi: 10.1159/000095608

Gfeller, K., Turner, C., Mehr, M., Woodworth, G., Fearn, R., Knutson, J. F., et al. (2002a). Recognition of familiar melodies by adult cochlear implant recipients and normal-hearing adults. *Cochlear Implants Int.* 3, 29–53. doi: 10.1002/cii.50

Gfeller, K., Witt, S., Woodworth, G., Mehr, M. A., and Knutson, J. (2002b). Effects of frequency, instrumental family, and cochlear implant type on timbre recognition and appraisal. *Ann. Otol. Rhinol. Laryngol.* 111, 349–356. doi: 10.1177/000348940211100412

Gfeller, K., Turner, C., Oleson, J., Zhang, X., Gantz, B., Froman, R., et al. (2007). Accuracy of cochlear implant recipients on pitch perception, melody recognition, and speech reception in noise. *Ear Hear.* 28, 412–423. doi: 10.1097/aud.0b013e3180479318

Giannantonio, S., Polonenko, M. J., Papsin, B. C., Paludetti, G., and Gordon, K. A. (2015). Experience changes how emotion in music is judged: evidence from children listening with bilateral cochlear implants, bimodal devices, and normal hearing. *PLoS One* 10:e0136685. doi: 10.1371/journal.pone.0136685

Gifford, R. H., and Dorman, M. F. (2018). Bimodal Hearing or Bilateral Cochlear Implants? Ask the Patient. *Ear Hear.* 40, 501–516. doi: 10.1097/aud.0000000000000657

Golub, J. S., Won, J. H., Drennan, W. R., Worman, T. D., and Rubinstein, J. T. (2012). Spectral and temporal measures in hybrid cochlear implant users: on the mechanism of electroacoustic hearing benefits. *Otol. Neurotol.* 33, 147–153. doi: 10.1097/MAO.0b013e318241b6d3

Heng, J., Cantarero, G., Elhilali, M., and Limb, C. J. (2011). Impaired perception of temporal fine structure and musical timbre in cochlear implant users. *Hear. Res.* 280, 192–200. doi: 10.1016/j.heares.2011.05.017

Horn, D. L., Dudley, D. J., Dedhia, K., Nie, K., Drennan, W. R., Won, J. H., et al. (2017). Effects of age and hearing mechanism on spectral resolution in normal hearing and cochlear-implanted listeners. *J. Acoust. Soc. Am.* 141, 613–613. doi: 10.1121/1.4974203

Illg, A., Bojanowicz, M., Lesinski-Schiedat, A., Lenarz, T., and Buchner, A. (2014). Evaluation of the bimodal benefit in a large cohort of cochlear implant subjects using a contralateral hearing aid. *Otol. Neurotol.* 35, e240–e244. doi: 10.1097/MAO.0000000000000529

Jung, K. H., Won, J. H., Drennan, W. R., Jameyson, E., Miyasaki, G., Norton, S. J., et al. (2012). Psychoacoustic performance and music and speech perception in prelingually deafened children with cochlear implants. *Audiol. Neurotol.* 17, 189–197. doi: 10.1159/000336407

Kang, R., Nimmons, G. L., Drennan, W., Longnion, J., Ruffin, C., Nie, K., et al. (2009). Development and validation of the university of washington clinical assessment of music perception test. *Ear Hear.* 30, 411–418. doi: 10.1097/AUD.0b013e3181a61bc0

Kelsall, D. C., Arnold, R. J. G., and Lionnet, L. (2017). Patient-reported outcomes from the united states clinical trial for a hybrid cochlear implant. *Otol. Neurotol.* 38, 1251–1261. doi: 10.1097/MAO.0000000000001517

Kong, Y., Mullangi, A., Marozeau, J., and Epstein, M. (2011). Temporal and spectral cues for musical timbre perception in electric hearing. *J. Speech Lang. Hear. Res.* 54, 981–994. doi: 10.1044/1092-4388(2010/10-0196)

Levitt, H. (1971). Transformed up-down methods in psychoacoustic. *J. Acoust. Soc. Am.* 2:467. doi: 10.1121/1.1912375

Looi, V., and Radford, C. J. (2011). A comparison of the speech recognition and pitch ranking abilities of children using a unilateral cochlear implant, bimodal stimulation or bilateral hearing aids. *Int. J. Pediatr. Otorhinolaryngol.* 75, 472–482. doi: 10.1016/j.ijporl.2010.12.023

Nimmons, G. L., Kang, R. S., Drennan, W. R., Longnion, J., Ruffin, C., Worman, T., et al. (2008). Clinical assessment of music perception in cochlear implant listeners. *Otol. Neurotol.* 29, 149–155. doi: 10.1097/mao.0b013e31812f7244

Park, M.-H., Won, J. H., Horn, D. L., and Rubinstein, J. T. (2015). Acoustic temporal modulation detection in normal-hearing and cochlear implanted listeners: effects of hearing mechanism and development. *J. Assoc. Res. Otolaryngol.* 16, 389–399. doi: 10.1007/s10162-014-0499-z

Parkinson, A. J., Rubinstein, J., Drennan, W., Dodson, C., and Nie, K. (2019). Hybrid music perception outcomes: implications for melody and timbre recognition in cochlear implant recipients. *Otol. Neurotol.* 40, e283–e289. doi: 10.1097/MAO.0000000000002126

Polonenko, M. J., Giannantonio, S., Papsin, B. C., Marsella, P., and Gordon, K. A. (2017). Music perception improves in children with bilateral cochlear implants or bimodal devices. *J. Acoust. Soc. Am.* 141, 4494–4507. doi: 10.1121/1.4985123

Roland, J. T. Jr., Gantz, B. J., Waltzman, S. B., Parkinson, A. J., and Group, M. C. T. (2016). United States multicenter clinical trial of the cochlear nucleus hybrid implant system. *Laryngoscope* 126, 175–181. doi: 10.1002/lary.25451

Sato, M., Baumhoff, P., Tillein, J., and Kral, A. (2017). Physiological mechanisms in combined electric-acoustic stimulation. *Otol. Neurotol.* 38, e215–e223. doi: 10.1097/MAO.0000000000001428

Sharma, A., and Dorman, M. F. (2006). Central auditory development in children with cochlear implants: clinical implications. *Adv. Otorhinolaryngol.* 64, 66–88. doi: 10.1159/000094646

Shirvani, S., Jafari, Z., Motasaddi Zarandi, M., Jalaie, S., Mohagheghi, H., and Tale, M. R. (2016). Emotional perception of music in children with bimodal fitting and unilateral cochlear implant. *Ann. Otol. Rhinol. Laryngol.* 125, 470–477. doi: 10.1177/0003489415619943

Tillein, J., Hartmann, R., and Kral, A. (2015). Electric-acoustic interactions in the hearing cochlea: single fiber recordings. *Hear. Res.* 322, 112–126. doi: 10.1016/j.heares.2014.09.011

Toole, F. E., and Olive, S. E. (1988). The modification of timbre by resonances: perception and measurement. *J. Audio Eng. Soc.* 36, 122–142.

Won, J. H., Drennan, W. R., Kang, R. S., and Rubinstein, J. T. (2010). Psychoacoustic abilities associated with music perception in cochlear implant users. *Ear Hear.* 31, 796–805. doi: 10.1097/AUD.0b013e3181e8b7bd

Won, J. H., Drennan, W. R., Nie, K., Jameyson, E. M., and Rubinstein, J. T. (2011). Acoustic temporal modulation detection and speech perception in cochlear implant listeners. *J. Acoust. Soc. Am.* 130, 376–388. doi: 10.1121/1.3592521

Won, J. H., Drennan, W. R., and Rubinstein, J. T. (2007). Spectral-ripple resolution correlates with speech reception in noise in cochlear implant users. *J. Assoc. Res. Otolaryngol.* 8, 384–392. doi: 10.1007/s10162-007-0085-8

16

Place and Temporal Cues in Cochlear Implant Pitch and Melody Perception

Brett A. Swanson[1], Vijay M. R. Marimuthu[2] and Robert H. Mannell[2]*

[1] Cochlear Ltd., Sydney, NSW, Australia, [2] Department of Linguistics, Faculty of Human Sciences, Macquarie University, Sydney, NSW, Australia

Correspondence:
Brett A. Swanson
bswanson@cochlear.com

The present study compared pitch and melody perception using cochlear place of excitation and temporal cues in six adult nucleus cochlear implant (CI) recipients. The stimuli were synthesized tones presented through a loudspeaker, and recipients used the Advanced Combinational Encoder (ACE) sound coding strategy on their own sound processors. Three types of tones were used, denoted H3, H4, and P5. H3 tones were harmonic tones with fundamental frequencies in the range C3–C4 (131–262 Hz), providing temporal pitch cues alone. H4 tones were harmonic tones with fundamental frequencies in the range C4–C5 (262–523 Hz), providing a mixture of temporal and place cues. P5 tones were pure tones with fundamental frequencies in the range C5–C6 (523–1046 Hz), providing place pitch cues alone. Four experimental procedures were used: pitch discrimination, pitch ranking, backward modified melodies, and warped modified melodies. In each trial of the modified melodies tests, subjects heard a familiar melody and a version with modified pitch (in randomized order), and had to select the unmodified melody. In all four procedures, many scores were much lower than would be expected for normal hearing listeners, implying that the strength of the perceived pitch was weak. Discrimination and ranking with H3 and P5 tones was poor for two-semitone intervals, but near perfect for intervals of five semitones and larger. H4 tones provided the lowest group mean scores in all four procedures, with some pitch reversals observed in pitch ranking. Group mean scores for P5 tones (place cues alone) were at least as high as those for H3 tones (temporal cues alone). The relatively good scores on the melody tasks with P5 tones were surprising, given the lack of temporal cues, raising the possibility of musical pitch using place cues alone. However, the alternative possibility that the CI recipients perceived the place cues as brightness, rather than musical pitch *per se*, cannot be excluded. These findings show that pitch perception models need to incorporate neural place representations alongside temporal cues if they are to predict pitch and melody perception in the absence of temporal cues.

Keywords: cochlear implant, pitch, melody, discrimination, sound coding

INTRODUCTION

Normal Hearing

For a pure tone in normal hearing, a place cue to pitch is provided by the location of the peak response on the basilar membrane, and a temporal cue to pitch is provided by neural phase locking, i.e., the neurons tend to fire in phase with the basilar membrane vibration (Moore, 1997; Oxenham, 2013). For a harmonic tone, the perceived pitch is equal to the fundamental frequency

(F0), regardless of the amplitudes of the harmonics, even if there is no energy at F0 (a "missing fundamental"). The resolved harmonics are those lower harmonics which produce distinct peaks in the basilar membrane response. Each resolved harmonic provides a distinct place and temporal cue. The remaining (i.e., unresolved) harmonics do not provide a clear place cue (because a broad region of the cochlea is excited), but do provide a temporal cue (because the basilar membrane response is amplitude modulated at F0) (Plack and Oxenham, 2005).

Place cues to pitch in normal hearing are not very reliable: as the amplitude of a pure tone increases, the peak of basilar membrane excitation shifts basally, and the neural firing rate saturates over a region near the peak, yet the perceived pitch is relatively stable (Moore, 1997). Further evidence of the importance of temporal cues is that tones containing only unresolved harmonics do provide pitch percepts, albeit not as strong as that produced by resolved harmonics (Moore and Rosen, 1979; Houtsma and Smurzynski, 1990).

Timbre is the perceptual quality that allows two tones that have the same pitch, loudness, and duration to be distinguished. One aspect of timbre is brightness. Increasing the amplitudes of the high harmonics relative to the low harmonics increases the perceived brightness of a tone. Brightness can be ordered on a low-to-high scale, and the results of brightness ranking experiments can be predicted by the spectral centroid ("center of gravity") of the tones (Plomp, 1976; Schubert and Wolfe, 2006). Multi-dimensional scaling experiments suggest that pitch and brightness are independent perceptual dimensions (Plomp, 1976).

A melody can be defined as a sequence of notes, typically varying in pitch and duration. To transpose a melody means to shift the entire melody up or down in pitch, adding (or subtracting) a constant number of semitones to each note. Transposing a melody does not change its identity; only the intervals (the differences in pitch from one note to the next) are important (Attneave and Olson, 1971). The contour of a melody is defined as the sequence of up or down changes in pitch, i.e., the direction of the steps, ignoring their size. Dowling and Fujitani (1971) showed that listeners have a good memory for the precise interval sizes of familiar melodies. However, distorted versions of familiar melodies that preserved the contour but changed the interval sizes could still be recognized reasonably well.

Cochlear Implants

Cochlear implant (CI) temporal pitch cues can be investigated by stimulating a single electrode with a varying pulse rate. For pulse rates in the range of about 50–300 pulses per second, CI recipients can recognize melodies (Eddington et al., 1978; Pijl and Schwarz, 1995b), judge the size of presented musical intervals (Pijl and Schwarz, 1995b; McDermott and McKay, 1997; Pijl, 1997), and adjust pulse rates to produce a specified interval from either a fixed or randomized reference pulse rate, demonstrating an ability to transpose intervals (Pijl and Schwarz, 1995a; McDermott and McKay, 1997; Pijl, 1997). At these pulse rates, the neural firing is entrained to the stimulation pulses, i.e., the timing of neural firing is the same as the pulse timing (McKay et al., 1994). Similar pitch percepts are produced by varying the modulation frequency of an amplitude-modulated high rate pulse train (McKay et al., 1994; McDermott and McKay, 1997; Kong et al., 2009). The pitch is stronger for deeper modulation depths, and for shallow depths, the pitch may be higher than the modulation frequency (Vandali et al., 2013).

Cochlear implant place pitch cues can be investigated by varying the electrodes that are stimulated (Nelson et al., 1995). Several studies suggest that CI place pitch and temporal pitch are independent perceptual dimensions (Tong et al., 1983; McKay et al., 2000). The single CI recipient in McDermott and McKay (1997) could estimate a musical interval when two electrodes were stimulated in succession, but with little knowledge of the electrode placement, there was no objective way of determining the "correct" interval, and his estimates were more variable than those created when varying pulse rate on one electrode. McDermott and McKay (1994) found that sequential stimulation on two nearby electrodes evoked a place pitch percept that was intermediate to that of either electrode when stimulated by itself, and suggested that the percept depended on the centroid of the neural excitation pattern. Laneau et al. (2004) conducted a study in which four CI recipients pitch-ranked harmonic tones processed by the ACE strategy, using standard and alternative filter banks. In one condition, the filter envelopes were low-pass filtered to remove the amplitude modulation (temporal cues), leaving only place cues, and the results were predicted well by the centroid model.

There is an intriguing resemblance between the spectral centroid model for brightness in normal hearing and for place pitch in CI. The perceptual independence of temporal and place percepts in CI is also reminiscent of the independence of pitch and brightness in normal hearing. If CI place percepts were more akin to brightness than to musical pitch, then it would be expected that good scores could be obtained using CI place cues alone on discrimination and ranking tasks, but not on tasks that involve melodies (Moore and Carlyon, 2005). The present study investigated this hypothesis by comparing CI recipient performance on discrimination, ranking, and melody tasks, with stimuli that provided place cues alone or temporal cues alone.

In CI experiments that aim to independently manipulate temporal and place pitch cues, stimulus pulses are customarily delivered to a CI recipient under the control of a research interface. The present study also aims to demonstrate that CI temporal and place pitch cues can be studied by applying judiciously chosen audio signals to a recipient's own sound processor. To this end, the results will be compared to those of our previous study (Marimuthu et al., 2016) investigating pulse rate cues to pitch in the same set of subjects, with stimuli delivered via a research interface. The present study also builds upon an earlier study (Swanson et al., 2009) in which melodies were presented by playing pure tones to the recipients' processors.

MATERIALS AND METHODS

Subjects

Six post-lingually-deafened adult CI recipients, with at least 1 year of implant usage, participated in the study. These were the

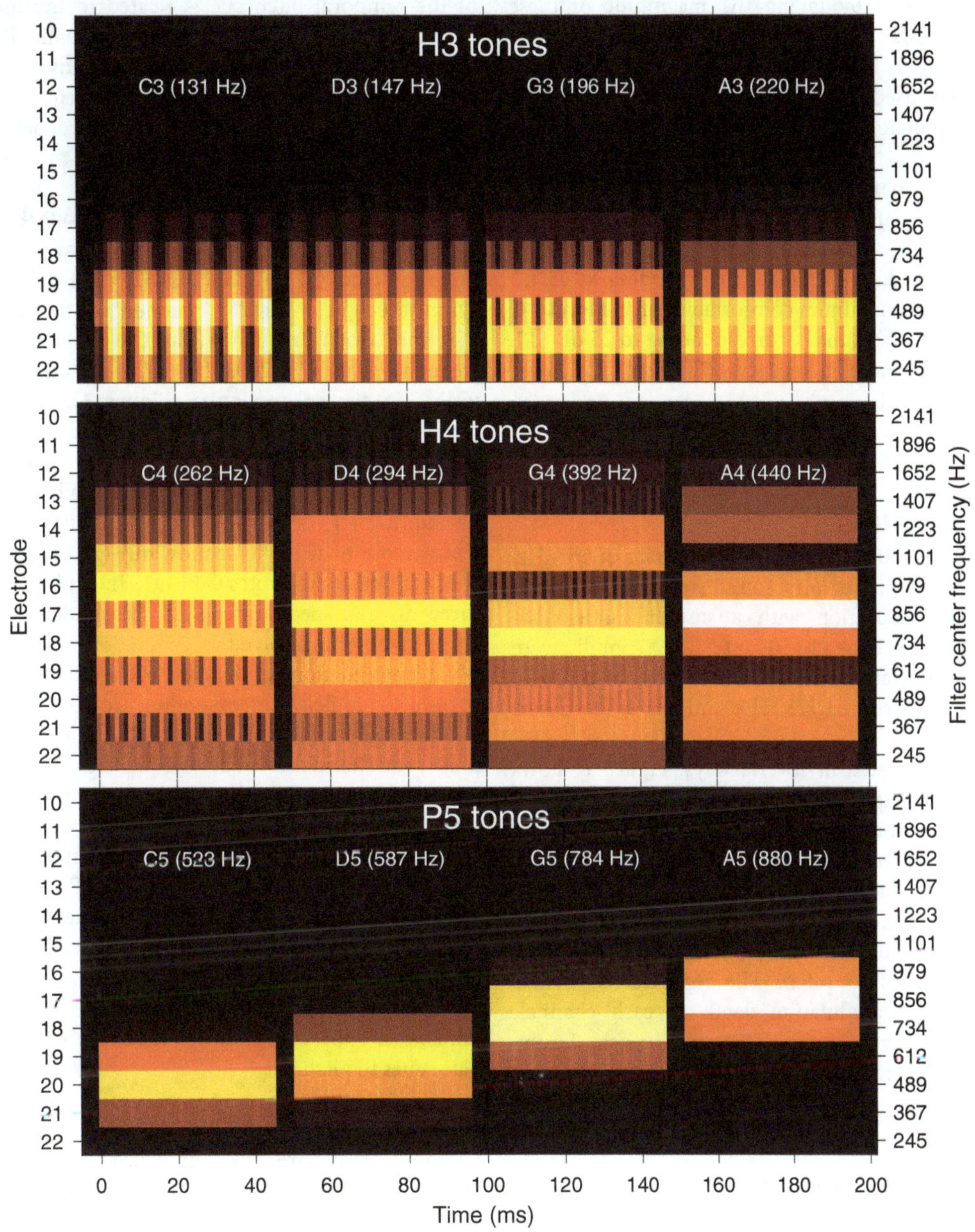

FIGURE 1 | Filter bank envelopes (spectrograms) for each note. Amplitude is indicated by the color (black: zero, white: full scale). Electrodes in the Nucleus® CI system are labeled from E22 (most apical) to E1 (most basal). E1–E9 had negligible energy for these tones and are not shown. The **center** frequencies of the corresponding filters are indicated on the **right** axis. A 45 ms excerpt of each of the four notes C, D, G, and A is shown (each note was 300 ms in duration with 50 ms rise and fall). Each note is also labeled with its fundamental frequency in hertz. **Top**: H3 tones (temporal cues only). **Middle**: H4 tones (temporal and place cues). **Bottom**: P5 tones (place cues only).

same subjects as in our previous study on rate-pitch perception (Marimuthu et al., 2016).

Cochlear Implant Signal Processing

During the testing, all subjects used their own sound processor which implemented the Advanced Combinational Encoder (ACE) processing strategy (Vandali et al., 2000; Swanson et al., 2007). The ACE filter bank was based on a 128-point fast Fourier transform (FFT) with a Hann window. The audio sampling rate was 15,659 Hz, thus the FFT provided a bank of 64 filters with center frequencies spaced linearly at multiples of 122 Hz (Harris, 1982), and a 6 dB bandwidth of 245 Hz (two bins) (Harris, 1978). The FFT filters with center frequencies from 245 to 1101 Hz were allocated to the eight lowest frequency (most apical) electrodes (**Figure 1**). Wider filters for the more basal electrodes were formed by summing adjacent FFT bins. Each filter output sample was a complex number, and the envelope of each filter was calculated by taking the magnitude of these complex numbers; this is known as quadrature envelope detection (Swanson et al., 2007). All subjects used 22 electrodes, except for S4, who used 20 electrodes (E4 and E13 were deactivated). The eight lowest frequency filters were identical in all subjects.

After each FFT, a maxima-selection block examined each set of filter envelopes, and selected the eight channels with the largest amplitude for stimulation. Instantaneous non-linear compression was applied. Amplitudes corresponding to 65 dB SPL were mapped to the maximum comfortable current level ("C level") of that channel. Amplitudes corresponding to 25 dB SPL were mapped to the threshold current level ("T level'), and lower amplitudes were discarded.

Subject S2 used a channel stimulation rate of 500 Hz, and the remaining subjects used 900 Hz.

Stimulus Description

All the stimuli were synthesized at a sampling rate of 16 kHz, and presented via loudspeaker in a sound-treated room. Each note was 300 ms in duration with a smooth (sinusoidal-shaped) rise and fall time of 50 ms. The stimuli were presented at a comfortable loudness level. Three types of tones were used, here denoted H3, H4, and P5, as described in detail below.

The stimuli are illustrated in several ways. **Figure 1** shows the envelopes at the output of the ACE filter bank, plotted as 22-channel spectrograms. **Figure 2** contains alternative representations of these envelopes to better visualize the place and temporal cues. The left set of panels in **Figure 2** shows the spectral profiles (i.e., each corresponding to a vertical slice through the spectrograms of **Figure 1**), indicating the availability of place cues to pitch. The right set of panels in **Figure 2** shows the modulation depth in each channel, indicating the availability of temporal cues to pitch. Lastly, **Figure 3** shows the corresponding pulse sequences resulting from the ACE strategy with eight maxima and a channel stimulation rate of 900 Hz.

H3 Tones: Harmonic Tones in Octave 3

H3 tones were harmonic tones in octave 3, i.e., having F0s in the range from C3 to C4 (131–262 Hz). In synthesizing the H3 tones, harmonics were summed with zero phase, and with unity amplitude up to a corner frequency of C5 (523 Hz), and then with amplitude decreasing at -36 dB per octave up to an upper frequency of C6 (1046 Hz). This spectral shaping is visible in the spectrograms (**Figure 1**). The individual harmonics were not resolved by the ACE filter bank. As a result, the four notes (C3, D3, G3, A3) had the same spectral profile (**Figure 2**), and the resulting pulse sequences (**Figure 3**) activated the same set of electrodes (E14–E22), with the same peak amplitudes, and hence there were negligible place pitch cues.

Multiple harmonics fell into each ACE filter, resulting in envelopes with amplitude modulation at the fundamental frequency, clearly visible in the spectrograms (**Figure 1**). The corresponding pulse sequences (**Figure 3**) had current level modulation at F0, providing a temporal pitch cue. The salience of the temporal pitch cue is related to the modulation depth (Vandali et al., 2013). The modulation depth (**Figure 2**) differed across channels within one note, depending on the alignment of the harmonics to the filter center frequencies. The average modulation depth reduced as F0 increased, being deepest for C3 and shallowest for A3.

H4 Tones: Harmonic Tones in Octave 4

H4 tones were harmonic tones in octave 4, i.e., having F0s ranging from C4 to C5 (262–523 Hz). The H4 tones were synthesized in a similar manner to the H3 tones, except that the corner frequency was C6 (1046 Hz) and the upper frequency was C7 (2093 Hz). This spectral shaping is again visible in the spectrograms (**Figure 1**). As the fundamental frequency increased, the ACE filter bank progressively resolved the harmonics. For example, referring to **Figure 2**, the spectral profile of the note C4 reflected the overall spectral shaping; the harmonics were not resolved because their spacing (262 Hz) was comparable to the filter bandwidth (245 Hz). In contrast, the spectral profiles for notes G4 (392 Hz) and A4 (440 Hz) showed three distinct spectral peaks, corresponding to the first three harmonics being resolved.

The modulation depth (**Figure 2**) exhibited a complementary pattern: channels corresponding to peaks in the spectral profile had the least modulation. In the note C4, the first four harmonics had frequencies close to the center frequencies of the filters driving electrodes E22, E20, E18, and E16. Thus, those channels were dominated by a single harmonic and had negligible amplitude modulation. Conversely, electrodes E21, E19, and E17 responded to two harmonics, and were deeply modulated. As F0 increased, there were fewer channels that responded to two harmonics, and the modulation depth decreased. Note A4 had very little modulation. **Figure 3** shows the corresponding pulse sequences. Thus, the H4 tones offered a mixture of temporal and place cues to pitch.

P5 Tones: Pure Tones in Octave 5

P5 tones were pure tones in octave 5, i.e., in the frequency range from C5 to C6 (523–1046 Hz). These tones were the same as those used by Swanson et al. (2009). As shown in **Figures 1**, **2**, the spectral profiles of the four notes (C5, D5, G5, A5) had peaks on successive electrodes (E20, E19, E18, E17, respectively). Because the ACE filters have broad, bell-shaped frequency responses, each of these pure tones activated multiple electrodes. A large change in fundamental frequency (e.g., C5 to A5) resulted in the activation of a different set of electrodes. A smaller change in fundamental frequency (e.g., C5 to D5) resulted in an overlapping set of electrodes being activated, with changes in the relative amplitude of the pulses on those electrodes, providing an intermediate place-pitch cue (McDermott, 2004).

As explained earlier, because ACE incorporates quadrature envelope detection (Swanson et al., 2007), the filter envelopes (**Figure 1**) and resulting pulse sequences (**Figure 3**) had no amplitude modulation, and thus provided no temporal pitch cues (**Figure 2**).

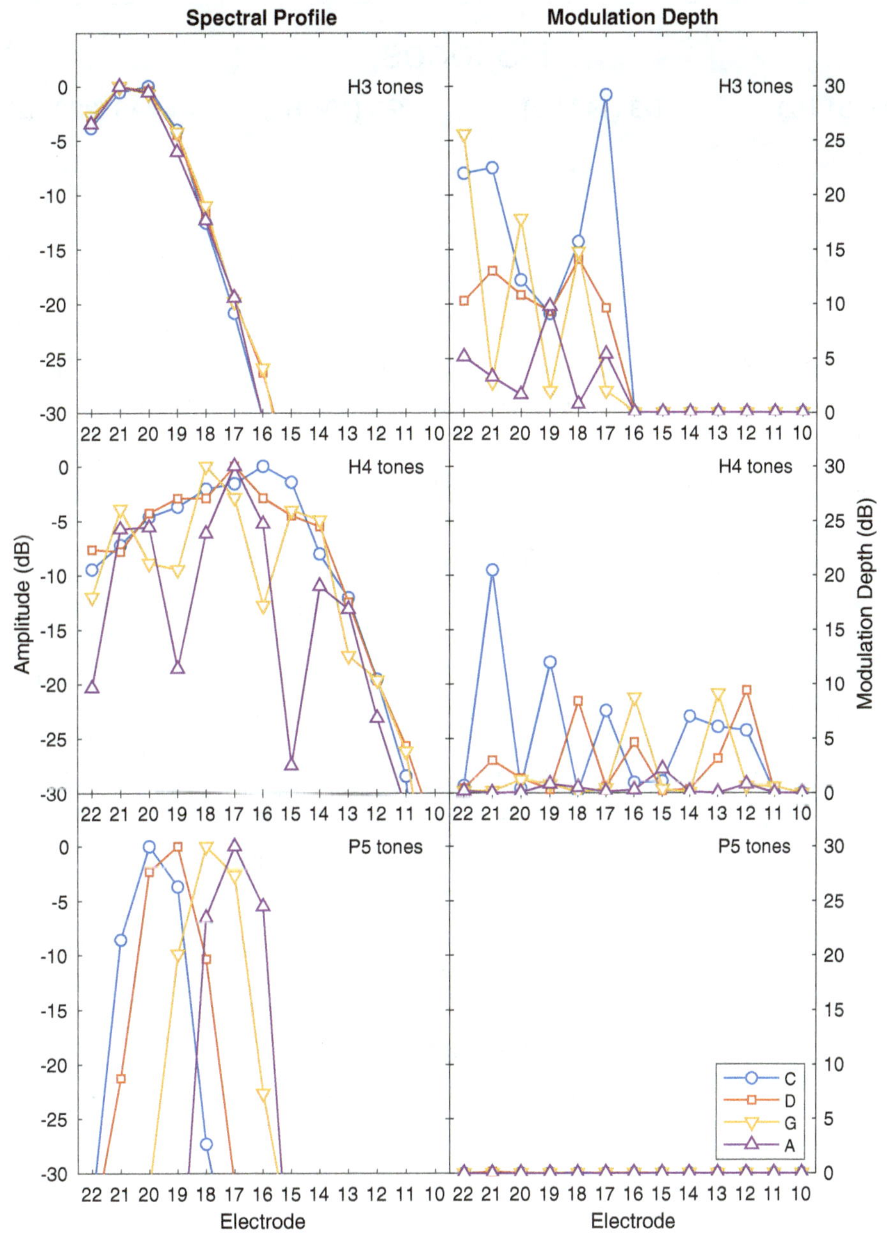

FIGURE 2 | Representation of place and temporal cues in the ACE filter bank envelopes. The **left** set of panels shows the spectral profiles for each note, indicating the availability of place pitch cues. Each panel shows the peak amplitude in dB in each channel, corresponding to a vertical slice through the spectrograms in **Figure 1**. The **right** set of panels shows the amplitude modulation depth for each note, indicating the availability of temporal pitch cues. Each panel shows the modulation depth in dB in each channel. For those notes that had modulation, the modulation frequency was equal to the fundamental frequency of the note, as shown in the labels of **Figure 1**. The abscissa indicates the electrode number allocated to each filter; E1–E9 had negligible amplitude for these notes and are not shown. **Top panels**: H3 tones, where no harmonics were resolved, showing negligible differences in the spectral profile between notes, and deep modulation. **Middle panels**: H4 tones, spanning the range of fundamental frequencies from unresolved (C4) to resolved (A4) harmonics, with shallower modulation. **Bottom panels**: P5 tones, where each note produced a single peak in the spectral envelope, with no modulation.

Psychophysical Experimental Procedures

Four experimental procedures were used: discrimination, ranking, and two variants of the modified melodies test: backward melodies and warped melodies. These procedures (except for discrimination) were also used by Marimuthu et al. (2016).

Discrimination and Ranking

For both the discrimination and ranking procedures, a set of four notes in the same octave were used: {C, D, G, A}. There are six possible pairings of these notes: {CD (2), GA (2), DG (5), CG (7), DA (7), CA (9)}, where the interval in semitones between the notes is given in parentheses. In each trial of the

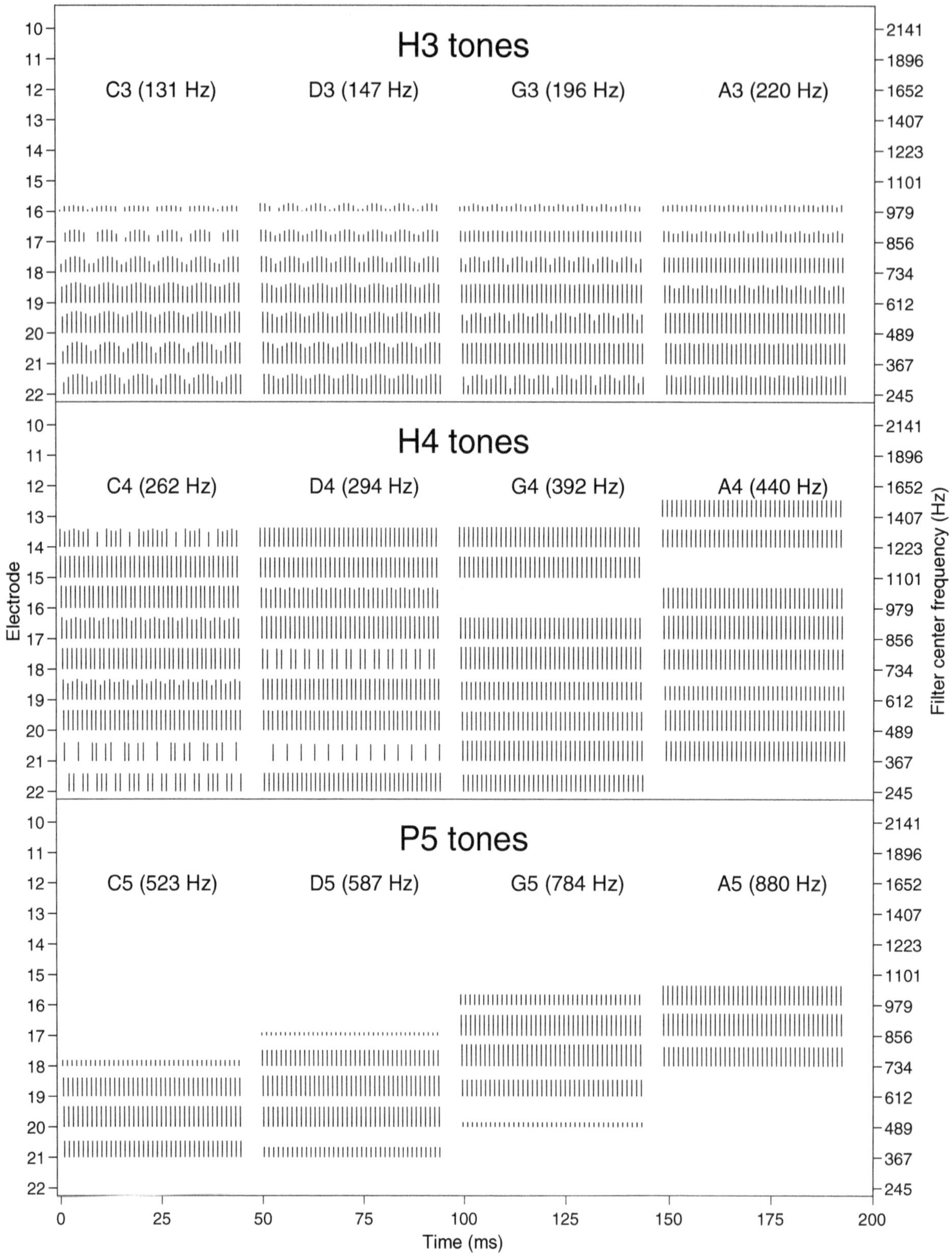

FIGURE 3 | Pulse sequences (electrodograms) for each note. Each pulse is represented by a vertical line, with the horizontal position indicating the start time (onset) of the pulse, the vertical position indicating the electrode number (indicated on the **left** axis), and the height of the line representing the current level. E1–E9 had no pulses for these notes and are not shown. The **center** frequencies of the corresponding filters are indicated on the **right** axis. A 45 ms excerpt of each of the four notes is shown, as in **Figure 1**. **Top**: H3 tones (temporal cues only). **Middle**: H4 tones (temporal and place cues). **Bottom**: P5 tones (place cues only).

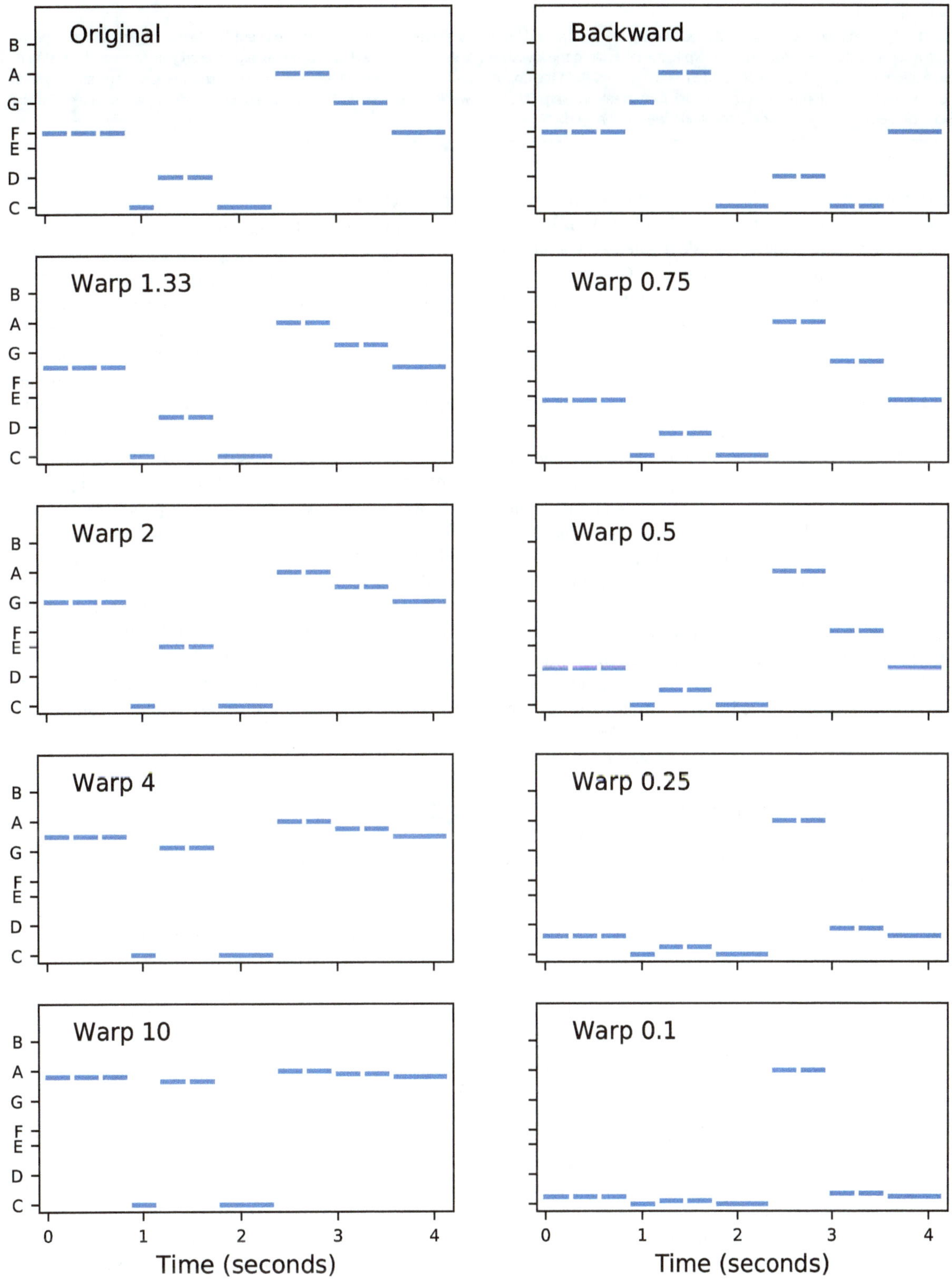

FIGURE 4 | Melodies used in the modified melodies test. Each note is represented by a horizontal line, with length indicating duration and vertical location indicating fundamental frequency. The vertical axis is logarithmic in frequency (i.e., linear in semitones), with note names indicated. Each single note was 300 ms in duration. The **top left panel** shows the original (i.e., correct) melody "Old MacDonald." The **top right panel** shows the backward melody, which has the same rhythm as the original, but a completely different contour (e.g., the first step in the original is down, from F to C, but the first step in backward is up, from F to G). The remaining *(Continued)*

FIGURE 4 | Continued
panels show the warped melodies. In each warped melody, the highest and lowest notes were unchanged, but the intermediate notes were shifted in pitch according to a "warp factor." For example, in Warp 2, the intervals in the lower part of the range were doubled in size (e.g., the original two-semitone step up from C to D became a four-semitone step up from C to E), and the intervals in the upper part of the range were halved (e.g., the original two-semitone step down from A to G became a one-semitone step down from A to G#). Conversely, in Warp 0.5, the lower intervals were halved and the upper intervals were doubled. The contour of the warped melodies (i.e., the directions of the steps) was unchanged.

discrimination procedure, the subject was asked to select the note that was different out of four alternatives (e.g., CCAC). In each trial of pitch ranking, the subject was asked whether a sequence of three notes with the first note repeated (e.g., CCA) was either rising or falling in pitch. In both discrimination and ranking, an experimental block comprised 48 trials (six pairings × two orders × four repetitions).

Modified Melodies

In each trial of the modified melodies test (Swanson, 2008; Swanson et al., 2009), the name of a familiar melody was displayed to the subject, and its opening phrase was presented twice (in randomized order): once correctly and once with modified pitch. The rhythm was unchanged. The subject was asked to select either the first presentation or the second as the correct version. Trials alternated between two melodies: "Old MacDonald had a farm" and "Twinkle twinkle little star," which each had a range of nine semitones. The set of interval sizes in the two melodies was {1, 2, 5, 7, 9} semitones; thus, all the intervals larger than one semitone were common to the discrimination and ranking procedures. On each trial, both the correct and modified melodies were transposed by either 0, 1, 2, or 3 semitones, so the total range of notes in a block of trials was an octave.

There were two types of pitch modification: backward and warped. **Figure 4** displays the original melody of "Old MacDonald" and each of the modified versions used in the study. In backward melodies, the contour of the melody was changed, without changing the set of notes in the melody, by playing the notes in reverse order. Each block comprised 16 trials (two melodies × four transpositions × two repetitions).

In warped melodies, the contour of the melody was maintained, but the sizes of the musical intervals were modified by a "warp factor." The warp factor determined the amount of expansion or compression of the intervals (refer to **Figure 4** for details). A warp factor of 1.0 would leave the intervals unchanged, and hence warp factors further away from 1.0 (either above or below 1.0) had more distorted intervals. A block of warped melodies trials always contained a reciprocal pair of warp factors (in randomized order). All subjects were first tested with the block labeled "W10| 0.1," in which half the trials were original vs. warp 10, and the other half were original vs. warp 0.1. Subjects were subsequently tested with blocks of trials which progressively increased in difficulty: W4| 0.25, W2| 0.5, and W1.33| 0.75. An informal adaptive rule was applied for each tone type, so that if a subject scored at chance levels, the remaining more difficult blocks were not always tested. Each block comprised 16 trials (two melodies × two warp factors × four transpositions).

Objectives

The H3 tones were designed to provide temporal cues to pitch, but no place cues. Conversely, the P5 tones were designed to provide place cues to pitch, but no temporal cues. The primary objective of the study was to compare performance between H3 and P5 tones. Many studies have examined CI pitch perception with temporal cues, but few studies have explored musical pitch with place cues. If performance on the discrimination and ranking tasks was comparable between H3 and P5 tones, but performance on the modified melodies test was better with H3 than P5 tones, then it would imply that place cues had more in common with brightness than with true musical pitch.

A secondary objective was to compare performance between H3 and H4 tones. This was of interest because octave 4 (starting at middle C) is very common in music, and normal hearing listeners would be expected to have similar pitch ranking ability for H3 and H4 tones. In contrast, it was hypothesized that CI recipients would have worse performance with H4 than H3 tones, because the upper limit of temporal pitch is typically around 300 Hz, and furthermore the H4 tones exhibited a transition from unresolved to resolved harmonics (**Figure 1**), yielding a complex mixture of temporal and place cues.

RESULTS

It was apparent from an initial examination of the results that subject S2 had the lowest scores of any subject for the H3 tones. It was hypothesized that this was because S2 used an ACE map with a channel stimulation rate of 500 Hz in the present study, in contrast to 900 Hz for the other subjects. McKay et al. (1994) recommended that the channel stimulation rate should be at least three to four times the modulation frequency to adequately sample the amplitude modulation waveform. As the primary objective was to compare H3 tones (temporal cues) and P5 tones (place cues), it was decided that the results of S2 should be excluded from any analysis involving temporal cues.

The results were analyzed in several ways. The first analysis applied a Monte Carlo simulation (bootstrap) approach using the binomial distribution (Simon, 1997; Swanson, 2008) to compare scores for H3 and P5 tones (primary objective) and for H3 and H4 tones (secondary objective). As a concrete example, subject S1 had CG discrimination scores of 10 correct out of 16 trials for H3 tones and 15 correct out of 16 trials for P5 tones. The null hypothesis was that the probability of success was the same for H3 and P5 tones. The simulation estimated the probability of observing scores differing by 5 or more if the null hypothesis was true. The best estimate of the null-hypothesis probability (denoted p_0) is the mean score across the two tone types, i.e.,

$p_0 = 25/32 = 0.78$. In each simulation run, two random numbers were generated from the binomial distribution, with $n = 16$ (the number of trials), and $p = p_0 = 0.78$. The run was classified as an extreme event if the absolute difference between the two simulated scores was greater than or equal to the difference in the subject's actual scores (5); this was a two-sided test. The p-value for the comparison was estimated as the proportion of extreme events in one million simulation runs, in this case $p = 0.0526$, just missing significance. This approach was extended to examine the scores for a subject across all note pairs. The null hypothesis was that the probability of success varied across the six note pairs, but that at each note pair, it was the same for H3 and P5 tones, yielding a vector of six p_0 values. In each simulation run, six pairs of random numbers were generated using the corresponding p_0 values. The run was classified as an extreme event if the absolute value of the mean difference between the six pairs of simulated scores was greater than or equal to the mean difference in the subject's actual scores (in this case, 16.7 percentage points). As before, the p-value was estimated as the proportion of extreme events in one million simulation runs (in this case, $p = 0.002$). Finally, to examine the group results across the five subjects, the mean scores across tone types yielded a vector of $5 \times 6 = 30$ p_0 values. Each simulation run generated 30 pairs of simulated scores, and was classified as extreme if the absolute value of the mean difference across the 30 simulated scores was greater than or equal to the mean difference in the 30 actual scores. The per-subject and group results are listed in **Table 1**.

The second analysis was a more traditional ANOVA, but as the results followed a binomial distribution and included many instances of 100% scores, an ANOVA on the percent-correct scores was not considered appropriate. Instead, the scores were first converted into d' sensitivity values (Macmillan and Creelman, 2004). A third analysis applied the non-parametric Friedman test, using the MATLAB Statistics Toolbox (The MathWorks, Inc.). The results for each type of procedure were analyzed separately. The Friedman test is less sensitive than the other tests because it does not consider the size of the differences. For the ANOVA and Friedman analyses, pair-wise differences were subsequently examined with Tukey's honestly significant difference criterion (using multcompare in MATLAB). The means and comparison intervals were plotted (**Figure 8**) such that two means differed significantly ($p < 0.05$) if their comparison intervals did not overlap.

TABLE 1 | Results of binomial paired comparisons of scores for H3 vs. P5 tones and H3 vs. H4 tones (excluding subject S2).

Comparison	Procedure	Subject	Mean difference (%)	p-value
P5 – H3	Discrimination	S1	16.7	2e-03**
		S3	2.1	0.68
		S4	6.2	0.12
		S5	2.1	0.84
		S6	−2.1	0.77
		Group	5.0	0.02*
	Ranking	S1	11.5	1e-02**
		S3	5.2	0.13
		S4	5.2	0.20
		S5	10.4	0.11
		S6	−2.1	0.72
		Group	6.0	2e-03**
	Modified melodies	S1	−9.4	0.30
		S3	11.9	9e-03**
		S4	2.3	0.60
		S5	−0.8	0.91
		S6	−2.1	0.71
		Group	2.0	0.33
H4 – H3	Discrimination	S1	5.2	0.43
		S3	−9.4	0.12
		S4	−15.6	7e-03**
		S5	0.0	1.00
		S6	−12.5	0.045*
		Group	−6.5	0.013*
	Ranking	S1	−9.4	0.13
		S3	−25.0	7e-05**
		S4	−15.6	6e-03**
		S5	4.2	0.61
		S6	−17.7	8e-04**
		Group	−12.7	5e-06**
	Modified melodies	S1	−14.1	0.12
		S3	−40.6	1e-05**
		S4	−56.2	3e-07**
		S5	−10.9	0.015*
		S6	−2.3	0.72
		Group	−19.6	2e-06**

The fourth column shows the mean difference between percent-correct scores, and the fifth column shows whether this difference was significant (under a two-sided test), with an asterisk denoting $p < 0.05$ and two asterisks denoting $p < 0.01$.

Discrimination and Ranking

Subjects completed two blocks of trials for each tone type; except that only one block was performed by S3 for H4 tones and by S5 for all tone types. **Figure 5** shows the percent-correct discrimination scores, for each pair of notes, for the three tone types. Similarly, **Figure 6** shows the corresponding pitch ranking scores. Scores for subject S2 are shown, but were excluded from the group mean and the statistical analysis. As expected, the overall trend in both procedures was for scores to increase as the interval size increased from two to nine semitones. In our previous study of rate pitch (Marimuthu et al., 2016), the scores were aggregated based on the interval size; however, here the scores for each note pair are reported, because the scores often differed significantly for note pairs that had the same interval (e.g., CG vs. DA 7-semitone ranking scores for H4 tones).

Regarding the primary objective (**Table 1**), the group mean score was 5 percentage points better with P5 tones than with H3 tones ($p = 0.02$) for discrimination and 6 percentage points better for ranking ($p = 0.002$). For both procedures, the individual subject comparisons only reached significance for one subject (S1). Given that most scores at the larger intervals were near ceiling for both P5 and H3 tones, these mean differences were mainly due to instances such as S3, S4, and S5 scoring 100% for ranking GA for P5 tones, but substantially lower for H3 tones.

Regarding the secondary objective (**Table 1**), the group mean score was 6.5 percentage points lower with H4 tones than with

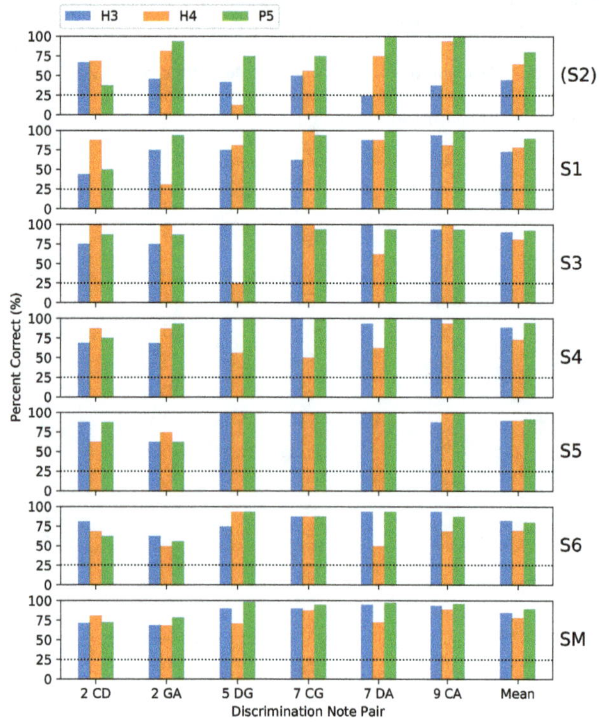

FIGURE 5 | Percent-correct discrimination scores for the three tone types. Each of the **upper panels** shows the scores for a single subject (S1–S6). The **lower panel** (labeled "SM") shows the group mean scores, excluding subject S2 (who used a 500 pps stimulation rate, unlike the other subjects who used 900 pps). The abscissa labels indicate the note pair, with the interval in semitones preceding the note names, and the right-most set of bars (labeled "Mean") showing the score averaged across note pairs. The chance score of 25% is indicated by a dotted line.

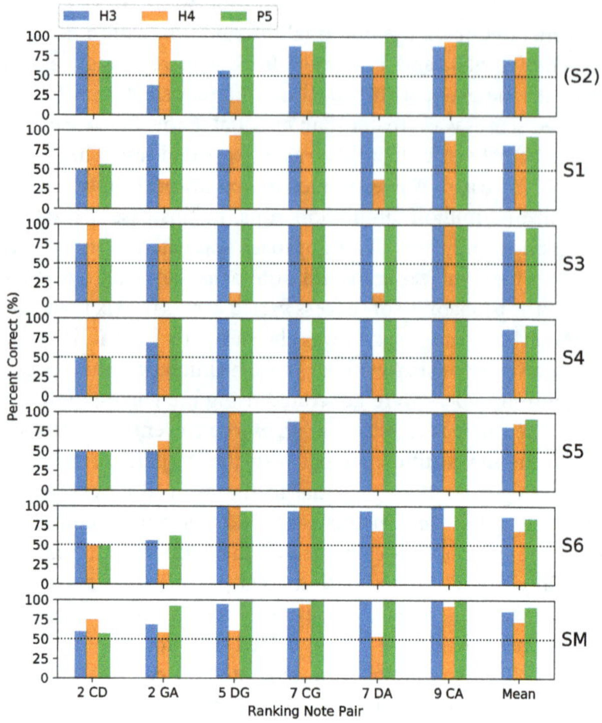

FIGURE 6 | Percent-correct pitch ranking scores, in the same format as **Figure 5**, except that the chance score is 50%. S2 was again excluded from the group mean.

H3 tones (p = 0.01) for discrimination and 12.7 percentage points lower for ranking ($p < 0.001$). Subjects S4 and S6 showed significant differences for discrimination, and subjects S3, S4, and S6 for ranking. The larger difference for ranking (compared to discrimination) was driven by the occurrence of pitch reversals for the H4 tones (**Figure 6**), i.e., scores significantly worse than chance (50%). Pitch reversals are listed in **Table 2** and did not occur for the other tone types.

Because discrimination was a four-alternative forced-choice (4AFC) task, whereas ranking was a 2AFC task, the percent-correct scores for the two procedures should not be directly compared. Instead, the percent-correct scores were converted to d' sensitivity, and a repeated-measures (within subject) ANOVA was performed with factors of procedure (discrimination and ranking), tone type, and note pair (**Table 3**). There were significant main effects of procedure (p = 0.04), tone type (p = 0.008), and note pair (p = 0.0001). All the interactions of these factors were also significant ($p < 0.05$).

According to the Friedman test, discrimination scores for the three tone types were not significantly different (p = 0.20). The Friedman test showed that ranking scores for the three tone types were significantly different (p = 0.017), and pairwise comparisons showed P5 significantly better than H4 (**Figure 8**).

Modified Melodies

All of the subjects confirmed that they were familiar with the two melodies from earlier in their life when they had better hearing, but often remarked that neither of the two alternatives in a trial sounded as they remembered the specified melody. Subjects were asked informally to identify the instruments that had played the melodies, and their responses are shown in **Table 4**. Subjects generally reported that the different tone types sounded like different instruments. Given that the tones were not intended to mimic any specific instrument, there was no "correct"

TABLE 2 | Pitch ranking reversal scores, and corresponding discrimination scores.

			Ranking			Discrimination		
Subject	**Tone type**	**Note pair**	**Score**	**%**	***p***	**Score**	**%**	***p***
S2	H4	5 DG	3/16	19	0.011*	2/16	12	0.94
S3	H4	5 DG	1/8	12	0.035*	2/8	25	0.63
S3	H4	7 DA	1/8	12	0.035*	5/8	62	0.027*
S4	H4	5 DG	0/16	0	1.5e-05**	9/16	56	0.0075**
S6	H4	2 GA	3/16	19	0.011*	8/16	50	0.027*

Scores are given as "number of correct responses/number of trials," and also as percent correct (%). For ranking, p is the probability of obtaining a score as low or lower if the null hypothesis of no perceived pitch difference (p_0 = 0.5) was true. Conversely, p for discrimination is the probability of obtaining a score as high or higher if the null hypothesis of no perceived pitch difference (p_0 = 0.25) was true. An asterisk denotes $p < 0.05$ and two asterisks denote $p < 0.01$.

TABLE 3 | Results of ANOVA analyses of *d'* sensitivity (excluding subject S2).

Analysis	Factor	*F*-value	Prob > *F*
Repeated measures ANOVA for discrimination and ranking	Procedure	8.4261	0.0440
	Tone_type	9.2606	0.0083
	Note_pair	9.8448	0.0001
	Procedure:tone_type	5.7226	0.0286
	Procedure:note_pair	3.1347	0.0300
	Tone_type:note_pair	2.2808	0.0318
	Procedure:tone_type:note_pair	2.4175	0.0234
Repeated measures ANOVA for modified melodies backward and W10| 0.1	Procedure	6.5584	0.0626
	Tone_type	5.9651	0.0260
	Procedure:tone_type	1.6113	0.2582
Repeated measures ANOVA for H3 tones and rate-pitch	Procedure	21.5707	0.0000
	Tone_type	5.0933	0.0870
	Procedure:tone_type	0.8502	0.5564
ANOVA on group mean for all procedures	Procedure	9.61	0.0104
	Tone_type	21.08	0.0019

TABLE 4 | Subjects' responses when asked to identify the instrument that played the melodies in the modified melodies procedures.

Subject	H3 tones	H4 tones	P5 tones
S1	Oboe	Trumpet or oboe	Penny whistle or flute
S2	Saxophone	Clarinet	(Could not say)
S3	Wind instrument: trumpet	Wind instrument	Flute
S4	Oboe	Wind instrument: trumpet	Flute or oboe or clarinet
S5	Oboe	Violin	Flute or clarinet
S6	Bassoon	Clarinet	Woodwind: clarinet

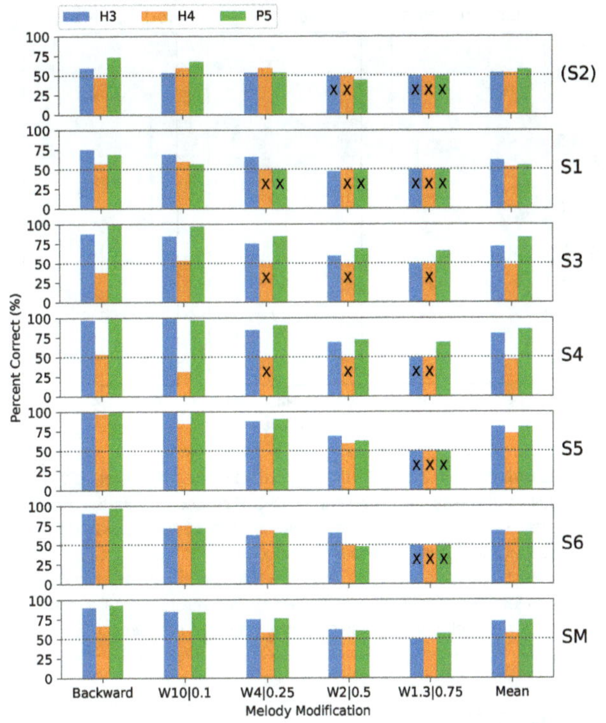

FIGURE 7 | Percent-correct backward melodies scores and warped melodies scores for each subject, and the group mean scores. The format is similar to **Figure 6**. S2 was again excluded from the group mean. Missing scores for the more difficult warp factors are plotted as chance level (50%) but marked with an "X."

answer, but many responses were common to several subjects, and the responses were generally consistent with the octave range. Interestingly, the most common response for P5 tones was a flute, which has relatively weak higher harmonics compared to other instruments (Schubert and Wolfe, 2006). Almost all responses were wind instruments, most likely due to the temporal envelope of each note, which had a gradual (50 ms) attack and release.

Subjects completed two blocks of trials for each condition; except that only one block was performed by S3 for H4 backward melodies and by S4 for H3 warped melodies. **Figure 7** shows the percent-correct discrimination scores, for backward and warped melodies, for the three tone types. Scores for subject S2 are shown, but were excluded from the group mean and the statistical analysis. Because of the adaptive rule, there were many missing scores for the more difficult warp factors. The missing scores were given an imputed value of 50% (chance level) for visualization purposes (including calculating the mean scores in **Figure 7**), but are marked with an "X."

A wider range of performance across subjects was exhibited than with discrimination or ranking, with subjects S1 and S2 rarely scoring above chance, while each remaining subject had some scores at or near ceiling. Scores were similar for backward and W10| 0.1, and the warped melodies scores decreased progressively as the warp factor approached 1.0. Scores for H3 and P5 tones were similar, with lower scores for H4 tones.

The binomial analysis for each subject utilized the backward scores and all the warp scores for that subject that were common to the pair of tone types under comparison. Regarding the primary objective, the group mean scores for P5 tones were 2 percentage points higher than with H3 tones, but the difference was not significant (**Table 1**). Subject S3 had significantly better scores with P5 tones, by 11.9 percentage points ($p = 0.009$).

Regarding the secondary objective, the group mean score was 19.6 percentage points lower with H4 tones than with H3 tones ($p < 0.001$) (**Table 1**). All subjects had lower scores with H4 tones, by very large and significant margins for S3, S4, and S5.

The ANOVA statistical analysis only included the scores for the backward and W10| 0.1 modifications, which had no missing data. A repeated-measures (within subject) ANOVA on *d'* sensitivity was performed with factors of modification type (backward and W10| 0.1) and tone type (**Table 3**). There was a significant effect of tone type ($p = 0.026$), while the effect of modification type just missed significance ($p = 0.063$). According to the Friedman test, modified melodies scores for the three tone types were significantly different ($p = 0.019$), and pairwise comparisons showed that H4 was significantly worse than both H3 and P5 (**Figure 8**).

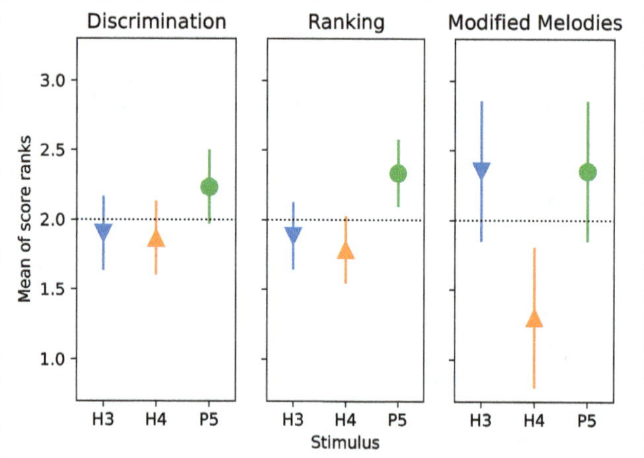

FIGURE 8 | Mean of score ranks (Friedman test) for discrimination, ranking, and modified melodies (backward and W10| 0.1) procedures, for the three tone types. S2 was excluded from the analysis. The dashed horizontal line indicates that if there was no difference between conditions, all would have a mean rank of 2 (mean of {1, 2, 3}). Pair-wise differences were examined with Tukey's honestly significant difference criterion: two means differ significantly ($p < 0.05$) if their comparison intervals ("error bars") do not overlap.

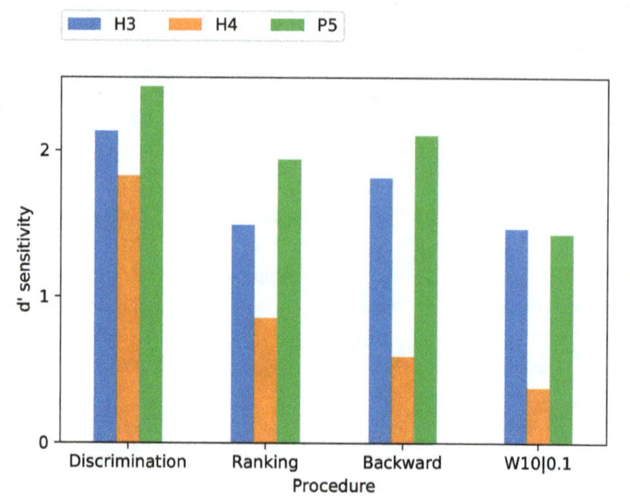

FIGURE 9 | Comparison of group mean *d'* sensitivity scores for the three tone types across the four procedures. Subject S2 was excluded from the analysis.

All Procedures

To allow an analysis across all procedures, the modified melodies backward and W10| 0.1 percent correct scores were averaged across subjects, and the discrimination and ranking percent correct scores were averaged across both subjects and note pairs. The *d'* sensitivity scores calculated from these group mean percent-correct scores for each tone type and procedure are shown in **Figure 9**. The group means were lowest for H4 tones in all four procedures, and highest for P5 tones in three procedures (the exception being W10| 0.1, where P5 and H3 tones had almost equal group means). A two-way ANOVA on *d'* (**Table 3**) revealed very significant effects of tone type ($p = 0.002$). Pair-wise comparisons showed that *d'* was significantly lower for H4 tones than both H3 tones ($p = 0.008$) and P5 tones ($p = 0.002$), with H3 and P5 not differing significantly.

The discrimination task yielded a higher *d'* sensitivity than the other procedures for all three tone types. The previously mentioned two-way ANOVA on group mean *d'* (**Table 3**) also revealed a significant effect of procedure ($p = 0.01$). Pair-wise comparisons showed that *d'* was significantly greater for discrimination than for ranking ($p = 0.045$) and modified melodies backward ($p = 0.008$), while the comparison between discrimination and W10| 0.1 just missed significance ($p = 0.07$).

DISCUSSION

The Centroid Model for Place Cues

Laneau et al. (2004) modeled the place pitch of a CI stimulation pulse sequence by the centroid c, calculated as:

$$c = \frac{\sum_k k\, a(k)}{\sum_k a(k)} \quad (1)$$

where k is the channel number and $a(k)$ is the amplitude of the corresponding filter envelope. However, this fails to consider the mapping from amplitude to stimulus current. In the ACE strategy, amplitude values that are below a base level are discarded and do not produce a stimulation pulse. These discarded low amplitudes cannot affect the perceived pitch, so they were excluded from the centroid calculation.

The ability to rank or discriminate two stimuli based on place pitch should depend on the difference between the two centroids. **Figure 10** shows the centroids of the four notes (C, D, G, A), for the three tone types, together with the corresponding centroid differences for the six note pairs. Centroids are given in units of channel numbers, e.g., a centroid of 3.5 would mean that the stimulation pattern was centered midway between the third channel (E20) and the fourth channel (E19). The centroids of the four H3 notes were practically identical (just below channel 3, E20), and the centroid differences were negligible, consistent with our earlier claim that there were no place pitch cues for H3 tones.

The horizontal axis of **Figure 10** (upper panel) is linear in semitones, with notes C, D, G, and A being located at 0, 2, 7, and 9 semitones, respectively. The centroids of the P5 notes were reasonably close to lying on a straight line, i.e., the centroid was approximately linearly related to the fundamental frequency. Referring to **Figure 10** (lower panel), the centroid difference clearly increased with the interval size. If the relationship had been perfectly linear, then the centroid differences for the P5 note pairs CD and GA (both two-semitone intervals) would have been equal, as would those for CG and DA (seven semitones). Instead, the centroid difference for GA was larger than that for CD; and the centroid difference for DA was larger than that for CG. A Monte Carlo binomial analysis (including S2, because only place cues were involved) showed GA group mean scores 14.6 percentage points higher than CD scores for discrimination ($p = 0.035$), and 29.2 percentage points higher for ranking ($p < 0.001$). Thus, the centroid model correctly predicted that

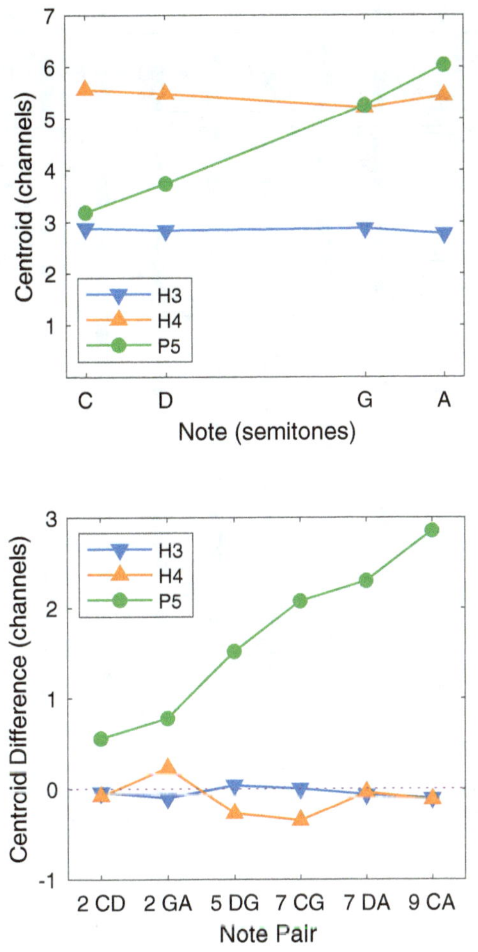

FIGURE 10 | Upper panel: Spectral centroid for the four notes C, D, G, and A for each tone type. **Lower panel**: Spectral centroid difference for each note pair, for each tone type. In the abscissa labels, the note names are preceded by the corresponding interval in semitones.

the P5 scores for GA would be higher than those for CD, despite both having a two-semitone interval. The centroid model also predicted that the P5 scores for DA would be higher than that for CG, but the differences were not significant because both were near ceiling.

The scores for H4 tones exhibited large variations both between subjects and also between note pairs for the same subject. Scores for the note pairs DG and DA were particularly inconsistent, with subject S5 scoring 100% for both in discrimination and ranking, while the remaining subjects each had instances of low scores. The erratic performance with H4 tones may have been caused by the transition from unresolved to resolved harmonics. Examining the H4 stimuli in **Figures 1, 3**, it appears that notes C4 and D4 provided primarily temporal cues to pitch, while notes G4 and A4 provided primarily place cues. With the six note pairs delivered in random order in one block of trials, it may have been difficult for subjects to switch attention between place and temporal cues, or confusing to compare a "temporal cue" note with a "place cue" note, such as in the pairs DG and DA.

Furthermore, the place cues for H4 tones were misleading in some cases. The spectral peak of D4 was on E17, while the peak of G4 was more apical, on E18 (**Figures 1, 2**). Consequently, the centroid of G4 was slightly lower than that of D4 (**Figure 10**). Thus, although the fundamental frequency increased by five semitones from D4 to G4, the place pitch apparently decreased. In the pair DA, both D4 and A4 had their spectral peak on E17, and had negligible difference in the spectral centroid, and so had much the same place pitch. Referring to **Table 2**, note pairs DG and DA produced significant pitch reversals for three subjects: S2, S3, and S4. Presumably these subjects were giving more weight to place cues than temporal cues in their ranking judgments. Pitch reversals by CI recipients have also been observed with more natural stimuli such as sung vowels (Sucher and McDermott, 2007; Swanson, 2008; Vandali and van Hoesel, 2012).

Comparison of Procedures

There are several factors that could contribute to discrimination scores being higher than ranking scores. The ranking task required the subject to order the stimuli along a perceptual scale from low to high, while in the discrimination task, the subject merely had to detect a difference between stimuli, without having to apply any ordering to them. Thus, it is possible that judging the direction of a pitch change was more difficult than detecting a difference in pitch, as has been reported with normal hearing listeners (Moore and Peters, 1992).

Although it was intended that the notes differed only in pitch, it is also possible that there were other unintended differences between the notes. Despite the stimuli having the same acoustic amplitude, it is possible that the loudness of the pulse sequences that were delivered varied between stimuli, as no loudness balancing of the stimuli was conducted. The 4AFC discrimination task has the inherent problem that the researcher cannot be sure that the subject is using pitch to distinguish the stimuli.

A final factor is the presence of pitch reversals. A subject experiencing a pitch reversal is consistently ranking the notes in the wrong order, but can clearly tell the notes apart, and so a high score on the discrimination task for that note pair would be expected. Referring to **Table 2**, three out of the five pitch reversals had corresponding discrimination scores significantly higher than chance. The decrement in performance of the H4 tones relative to the other tone types was smallest for the discrimination procedure. On balance, it is recommended that the 4AFC discrimination task used here should be avoided in future CI pitch studies, primarily because pitch reversals are not apparent.

The modified melodies test required subjects to decide which of two alternatives best matched their memory of a named familiar melody. Compared to discrimination or ranking, the modified melodies test is more cognitively demanding, so it is not surprising that its scores were lower. Both the contour and the exact interval sizes of familiar melodies are stored in long-term memory (Dowling and Fujitani, 1971). The backward modification required subjects to detect a mismatch in the contour between their memory and each presentation (e.g., a pitch step down instead of up), which in principle only required the ability to rank the pitch of consecutive notes. As might be expected, subjects S2, S3, and S4, who experienced a pitch ranking reversal for the five-semitone DG pair of H4 tones, scored at chance levels for all modified melody conditions with H4 tones.

The warp modification was designed to preserve the melodic contour and change the interval sizes. However, it could be argued that warp factors as extreme as W10| 0.1 did effectively change the contour, as many intervals were compressed into imperceptibly small steps, so that the warped melody was likely perceived to contain long sequences of repeated notes (**Figure 4**). Therefore, the important question of whether place cues alone can support judgments of musical interval size is best addressed by the scores on the more difficult warp factors. The best performing subjects provided evidence supporting this proposition, with scores on P5 tones significantly above chance by subject S3 for W2| 0.5 (22/32, $p = 0.025$), and by subject S4 for both W2| 0.5 (23/32, $p = 0.01$) and W1.3| 0.75 (22/32, $p = 0.025$).

Comparison With Previous CI Studies

In our previous study (Marimuthu et al., 2016), the same six subjects performed the procedures of ranking, backward modified melodies, and warped modified melodies as per the present study, but with different stimuli. Each note was a synthetic pulse sequence with a pulse rate equal to the fundamental frequency, so that only rate pitch cues were available. Four spatial stimulation patterns were used, denoted Apex (a single apical electrode), Mid (a single mid electrode), Dual (two electrodes, apical and mid), and Scan (eleven electrodes, from apical to mid). No significant differences were found between scores for the four spatial patterns for pulse rates in the range C3–C4, implying that the strength of the rate pitch percept was independent of electrode place, and of the number of electrodes.

Figure 11 compares the present results for H3 tones with the previous rate pitch results, averaged over the four spatial patterns. The fundamental frequencies of the H3 tones were the same as the pulse rates of the rate pitch stimuli (C3–C4), and the pattern of results was very similar, consistent with other studies that have compared amplitude modulation and pulse rate cues (McKay et al., 1994; Kong et al., 2009).

Subject S2 had the lowest scores of any subject on the H3 tones, and the largest difference (10.5 percentage points) between the H3 and rate pitch mean scores. As mentioned previously, this was most likely because subject S2 used a 500 Hz channel stimulation rate, and so S2 was excluded from the subject mean in **Figure 11**, and from the following analysis. When converted to d', a repeated-measures (within subject) ANOVA showed no significant effect of stimulus type ($p = 0.087$, **Table 1**). Thus, the performance with pulse sequences that were amplitude-modulated at F0 was similar to that with pulse sequences with the pulse rate equal to F0. The H3 tones provided temporal cues on nine electrodes, and consistent with Marimuthu et al. (2016), there was no apparent benefit over having temporal cues on a single electrode.

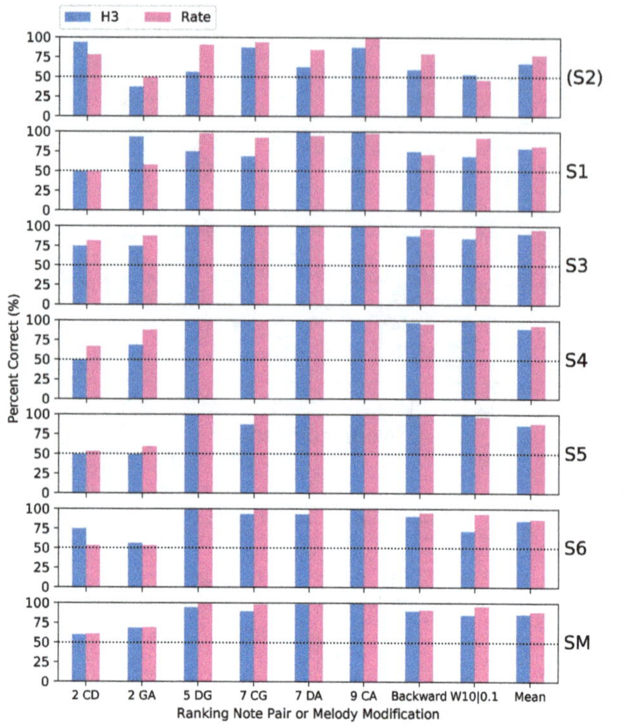

FIGURE 11 | Percent-correct ranking and modified melodies scores for H3 tones, together with corresponding scores for rate-pitch stimuli from a previous study with the same subjects and procedures (Marimuthu et al., 2016). The format is the same as **Figure 6**. S2 was again excluded from the group mean.

The present results can also be compared to those in another previous study that used the same P5 tones. Results for six CI recipients were reported in Swanson et al. (2009), and one additional subject was reported in Swanson (2008). An earlier version of the modified melodies test was utilized, which included only a single familiar melody ("Old MacDonald"). Four pitch modifications were tested: "Backward" (as in the present study) and "Exchange" altered the melodic contour; while the "Nudge" type preserved the contour, and changed an interval size by either two ("Nudge2") or five ("Nudge5") semitones. Scores significantly above chance were obtained by all seven subjects for Backward; by six subjects for Exchange, by four subjects for Nudge5; and by one subject for Nudge2. This is consistent with the results using P5 tones in the present study, where most subjects scored highly for backward, and a small subset of subjects were sensitive to interval size changes in the more difficult warp factors.

Implications for Cochlear Implant Music Perception

The present study investigated CI pitch perception using the recipients' own sound processors, with audio signals presented via loudspeaker. This method provides a bridge between real-world listening conditions and psychophysics experiments that deliver synthetic pulse sequences via a research interface.

In Singh et al. (2009), CI recipients used their own sound processors to perform a closed-set melody identification task, with melodies comprised either pure tones or harmonic tones in three F0 ranges: low (104–262 Hz), middle (207–523 Hz), and high (414–1046 Hz). Their upper F0s were identical to that of the three F0 ranges of the present study, although their lower F0s were four semitones lower. In experiment 1, they found better scores with harmonic tones for the middle F0 range than the low F0 range, contrary to the present study, where H4 tones produced worse scores than H3 tones on all procedures. Their harmonic tones had spectral profiles extending up to 4 kHz, so that more higher harmonics would have been resolved, possibly providing more reliable place cues and explaining the difference in results. Alternatively, it may have been due to their recipients using a variety of implant devices and sound processing strategies. Regardless, it appears that tone parameters that would have little impact on pitch scores for normal hearing listeners can have a large impact for CI recipients.

In experiment 2 of Singh et al. (2009), pure tones in the high F0 range produced better scores than harmonic tones in any F0 range, which is consistent with the present study. Singh et al. (2009) labored under the misconception that pure tones would provide good temporal cues, but two of the four recipients in experiment 2 used the Nucleus 24 implant with the ACE strategy, for which the pure tones would have provided no temporal cues. Thus, Singh et al. (2009) inadvertently provided evidence that place cues can support melody identification. One lesson is that knowledge of the algorithms implemented on the sound processor is necessary if it is desired to manipulate or even understand the cues that will be available to a CI recipient.

For some subjects in the present study, performance with pulse rate cues was no worse at octave 4 than at octave 3 (Marimuthu et al., 2016). This suggests that their lower scores with H4 tones, compared to H3 tones, were due to the sound processor failing to provide adequate temporal cues (**Figure 2**), rather than the temporal cues exceeding the recipient's upper limit for temporal pitch. This implies that pitch perception for the H4 tones would be improved by a sound coding strategy such as OPAL (Vandali and van Hoesel, 2011, 2012; Vandali et al., 2017, 2018), which enhances temporal cues by providing deeper amplitude modulation over a wider range of F0s.

Finally, it should be remembered that the melodies in the present study consisted of a single note at a time. Even under these ideal conditions, CI recipients' perception of contour and interval size was worse than that of normal hearing listeners. Real-world music typically comprises multiple instruments playing together, with each instrument often playing chords comprising multiple simultaneous notes. Unsurprisingly, this additional complexity generally results in poor music perception (McDermott, 2004).

Comparison With Normal Hearing Performance

An informal comparison can be made with normal hearing performance. Frequency discrimination thresholds for pure tones (such as the P5 tones), expressed as a percentage of reference frequency, are less than 1% for listeners with normal hearing (Moore, 1997). F0 discrimination thresholds for harmonic tones with resolved harmonics (such as the H3 and H4 tones) are generally even better (Spiegel and Watson, 1984).

Assuming that an F0 discrimination threshold corresponds to a score of 75% correct on a 2AFC ranking task, then rough estimates of the mean thresholds for the CI recipients in the present study (excluding S2) were 12% (two semitones) for P5 tones, 19% (three semitones) for H3 tones, and 50% (seven semitones) for H4 tones, i.e., more than an order of magnitude worse than normal hearing. It can be inferred that the strength of the pitch perceived by the CI recipients in the present study was relatively weak.

It is informative to compare CI temporal pitch to the pitch of temporal cues alone in normal hearing. Houtsma and Smurzynski (1990) measured normal hearing F0 discrimination thresholds of 2.5–3% for tones containing only unresolved harmonics at F0 = 200 Hz. Kaernbach and Bering (2001) reported that F0 discrimination thresholds for high-pass filtered click trains containing only unresolved harmonics were as low as 1.2% at F0 = 100 Hz, but increased as the filter cutoff frequency increased. This was consistent with earlier results by Cullen and Long (1986), who reported F0 discrimination thresholds for high-pass filtered click trains at F0 = 100 Hz in the range 3–13% across four normal hearing listeners. The best CI recipient in the present study (S3) scored 75% correct for two-semitone intervals (12% F0 change) for H3 tones, which was just in the normal hearing performance range.

Implications for Models of Normal Hearing Pitch Perception

The relatively good performance on melody tasks using CI place cues is surprising for two reasons. The first reason is the disparities between the place cues in normal hearing and CIs. The frequencies assigned to the CI electrodes do not match the characteristic frequencies of a normal cochlea, and the intermediate place pitch cues depend on the details of sound processing, such as the amplitude roll-off of the filters. Nevertheless, it appears that some recipients can utilize the approximately linear relationship between fundamental frequency and spectral centroid (**Figure 10**) in the ACE strategy to make judgments of musical interval sizes.

The second reason is that obtaining a musical pitch sensation in the absence of temporal cues has no counterpart in normal hearing. Because neural phase locking is limited to about 5 kHz, pure tones above that frequency provide place cues without temporal cues, but they do not support melody perception (Attneave and Olson, 1971). A sound component that excites a distinct place in the apical to mid region of the cochlea is always accompanied by matching temporal cues: if it has a bandwidth narrow enough to only excite a localized region of the cochlea, then it must resemble a sinusoid, and so the neural firing times will provide a pitch cue.

The goal of a pitch perception model is to predict the pitch that a listener would perceive in response to a given sound. An important aspect to be modeled is the strength of the pitch percepts, which can be quantified by scores on pitch tests. Historically, models of pitch perception have been challenged and refined by applying esoteric sounds that do not commonly occur in the natural environment. Models that use only place cues cannot explain the pitch of a tone containing only unresolved harmonics (Moore and Rosen, 1979), or of amplitude-modulated noise (Burns and Viemeister, 1981). This can only be explained by models that analyze neural firing times (Moore, 1997). Licklider (1951) proposed that an autocorrelation analysis is performed on the neural spike trains at each cochlear place. Meddis and Hewitt (1991) implemented a computer model that summed neural autocorrelation functions across cochlear place, demonstrating accurate predictions of pitch and pitch strength for a wide variety of sounds. Cariani and Delgutte (1996) measured neural firing times in cat auditory nerves, and found that the distributions of inter-spike intervals were consistent with these models.

One issue for autocorrelation models is the absence of physiological evidence for a calibrated neural delay line of up to 30 ms at each cochlear place. Loeb et al. (1983) proposed a spatial cross-correlation model, employing the basilar membrane traveling wave delay instead of a neural delay line. The basilar membrane response to a resolved harmonic shows a large phase shift in the vicinity of the peak. Thus, comparing neural firing times across nearby places in the cochlea yields similar behavior to an autocorrelation model (Shamma, 1985; Carney et al., 2002). Shamma and Klein (2000) showed that such a model can produce a strong response to resolved harmonics, and a weaker response to unresolved harmonics.

To summarize, the most successful pitch models assign a crucial role to neural firing times. Moore and Carlyon (2005) wrote that "a demonstration that pitch can be conveyed purely by place-of-excitation cues would disprove models which propose that timing cues are essential for pitch perception." It is acknowledged that CI place pitch and CI temporal pitch are extremely impoverished compared to the strong pitch produced by resolved harmonics in normal hearing. However, the pitch of CI temporal cues resembles the pitch of unresolved harmonics in normal hearing, and although weak, both support judgments of the size of musical intervals, and the recognition of melodies, and both are widely accepted to be true musical pitch (Moore and Carlyon, 2005). The present study suggests that CI place cues provide pitch of similar strength to CI temporal cues, and support similar levels of melody recognition. Hence, the present results imply that a truly comprehensive pitch model should not only produce a weak pitch percept for temporal cues in the absence of place cues, it should also produce a weak pitch percept for place cues in the absence of temporal cues.

An alternative explanation is that the recipients in this study perceived the CI place cues as brightness, consistent with the spectral centroid model of brightness in normal hearing, but that they could utilize brightness to score well on the modified melodies test. McDermott et al. (2008) reported a set of experiments showing that normal hearing listeners were able to recognize patterns in brightness (and loudness). In each trial, subjects heard a randomly-generated five-note sequence, followed by a transposed sequence, and were asked whether the contours of the two sequences were the same or different. The notes in a sequence varied in either pitch, brightness, or loudness. Subjects performed best when both sequences were pitch sequences, but scores were still well above chance when both were brightness sequences, or when the two sequences were of different types (e.g., a pitch sequence compared to a brightness sequence). In the final experiment, subjects were presented with familiar "melodies" played as either pitch, brightness, or loudness sequences, and asked to name them. Performance with brightness and loudness sequences was well above chance, and was similar to performance with pitch sequences where all the intervals had been stretched by a factor of two. The backward melodies in the present study had an incorrect contour, so it is possible that subjects could utilize brightness cues to identify them.

In a later study (McDermott et al., 2010), subjects were presented with two pairs of notes differing in either pitch, brightness, or loudness, and asked which of the two intervals was wider. Subjects were able to make judgments of interval sizes for brightness (and loudness), although the thresholds for brightness interval size, measured in semitones, were twice as large as thresholds for pitch interval size (i.e., subjects were less accurate for brightness than pitch). However, the experiments in McDermott et al. (2010) did not provide a musical context for the intervals. The warped melodies in the present study had incorrect interval sizes, but merely being able to judge which of two isolated intervals was larger would not be sufficient to score well; subjects had to decide which melody had the musically-correct intervals. In summary, it is not clear whether brightness cues could explain the scores of the CI recipients in the present study; evaluating normal hearing listeners on the modified melodies test with brightness sequences may help to resolve the issue.

McDermott et al. (2008) did not provide much in the way of subjective reports. Although subjects could recognize that a particular loudness sequence had the same up-and-down pattern as the pitch changes in a familiar melody, this could simply reflect general pattern-matching cognitive abilities, and it seems unlikely that anyone would claim that they could "hear a melody" in a pattern of loudness changes (Moore and Rosen, 1979). Because brightness scores were similar to loudness scores in McDermott et al. (2008), the same may be true of brightness contours. Ultimately, we must rely on the CI recipients to tell us whether they could hear a melody in the P5 tone sequences. Based on their subjective reports (**Table 4**), it seems that they did. Subjects readily described the P5 melodies as being played by wind instruments, just as they did with the H3 and H4 melodies; indeed, the labels of oboe and clarinet were applied to all three tone types. There was no indication that the P5 tones provided a different type of perceptual experience to the H3 tones.

CONCLUSION

Cochlear implant pitch perception was measured using discrimination, ranking, and the modified melodies test. Group mean scores for H4 tones were significantly poorer than H3 tones, most likely because of inadequate temporal cues and misleading place cues. Some subjects experienced pitch reversals with H4 tones, eliminating any ability to perceive melodies. Group mean scores for P5 tones (place cues alone) were at least as high as those for H3 tones (temporal cues alone).

The scores with P5 tones were qualitatively consistent with a centroid model of place pitch perception. Despite the similarity to the centroid model for brightness in normal hearing, the results suggest that CI place cues can provide a sense of musical pitch, albeit much weaker than that provided by pure tones in normal hearing.

ETHICS STATEMENT

The studies involving human participants were reviewed and approved by the Macquarie University and Sydney South West Area Health Service Human Research Ethics Committees. The patients/participants provided their written informed consent to participate in this study.

AUTHOR CONTRIBUTIONS

All authors contributed to the conception and design of the study. BS wrote the experimental software and the first draft of the manuscript. VM tested the subjects. BS and VM performed the statistical analysis, contributed to manuscript revision, and read and approved the submitted version.

ACKNOWLEDGMENTS

We wish to thank the cochlear implant recipients for their contribution and PC for his detailed review.

REFERENCES

Attneave, F., and Olson, R. K. (1971). Pitch as a medium: a new approach to psychophysical scaling. *Am. J. Psychol.* 84, 147–166.

Burns, E. M., and Viemeister, N. F. (1981). Played-again SAM: further observations on the pitch of amplitude-modulated noise. *J. Acoust. Soc. Am.* 70, 1655–1660. doi: 10.1121/1.387220

Cariani, P. A., and Delgutte, B. (1996). Neural correlates of the pitch of complex tones. I. Pitch and pitch salience. *J. Neurophysiol.* 76, 1698–1716. doi: 10.1152/jn.1996.76.3.1698

Carney, L., Heinz, M., Evilsizer, M., Gilkey, R., and Colburn, H. (2002). Auditory phase opponency: a temporal model for masked detection at low frequencies. *Acta Acust. United Acust.* 88, 334–347.

Cullen, J. K. Jr., and Long, G. R. (1986). Rate discrimination of high-pass-filtered pulse trains. *J. Acoust. Soc. Am.* 79, 114–119. doi: 10.1121/1.393762

Dowling, W. J., and Fujitani, D. S. (1971). Contour, interval, and pitch recognition in memory for melodies. *J. Acoust. Soc. Am.* 49, 524–531. doi: 10.1121/1.1912382

Eddington, D. K., Dobelle, W. H., Brackmann, D. E., Mladejovsky, M. G., and Parkin, J. (1978). Place and periodicity pitch by stimulation of multiple scala tympani electrodes in deaf volunteeers. *ASAIO J.* 24, 1–5.

Harris, F. J. (1978). On the use of windows for harmonic analysis with the discrete Fourier transform. *Proc. IEEE* 66, 51–83. doi: 10.1109/proc.1978.10837

Harris, F. J. (1982). The discrete fourier transform applied to time domain signal processing. *IEEE Commun. Mag.* 20, 13–22. doi: 10.1109/MCOM.1982.1091013

Houtsma, A. J. M., and Smurzynski, J. (1990). Pitch identification and discrimination for complex tones with many harmonics. *J. Acoust. Soc. Am.* 87, 304–310. doi: 10.1121/1.399297

Kaernbach, C., and Bering, C. (2001). Exploring the temporal mechanism involved in the pitch of unresolved harmonics. *J. Acoust. Soc. Am.* 110, 1039–1048. doi: 10.1121/1.1381535

Kong, Y.-Y., Deeks, J. M., Axon, P. R., and Carlyon, R. P. (2009). Limits of temporal pitch in cochlear implants. *J. Acoust. Soc. Am.* 125, 1649–1657. doi: 10.1121/1.3068457

Laneau, J., Wouters, J., and Moonen, M. (2004). Relative contributions of temporal and place pitch cues to fundamental frequency discrimination in cochlear implantees. *J. Acoust. Soc. Am.* 116, 3606–3619. doi: 10.1121/1.1823311

Licklider, J. C. R. (1951). A duplex theory of pitch perception. *Experientia* 7, 128–134. doi: 10.1007/bf02156143

Loeb, G. E., White, M. W., and Merzenich, M. M. (1983). Spatial cross-correlation. *Biol. Cybern.* 47, 149–163.

Macmillan, N. A., and Creelman, C. D. (2004). *Detection Theory: A User's Guide.* London: Psychology Press.

Marimuthu, V., Swanson, B. A., and Mannell, R. (2016). Cochlear implant rate pitch and melody perception as a function of place and number of electrodes. *Trends Hear.* 20:2331216516643085. doi: 10.1177/2331216516643085

McDermott, H. J. (2004). Music perception with cochlear implants: a review. *Trends Amplif.* 8, 49–82. doi: 10.1177/108471380400800203

McDermott, H. J., and McKay, C. M. (1994). Pitch ranking with nonsimultaneous dual-electrode electrical stimulation of the cochlea. *J. Acoust. Soc. Am.* 96, 155–162. doi: 10.1121/1.410475

McDermott, H. J., and McKay, C. M. (1997). Musical pitch perception with electrical stimulation of the cochlea. *J. Acoust. Soc. Am.* 101, 1622–1631. doi: 10.1121/1.418177

McDermott, J. H., Keebler, M. V., Micheyl, C., and Oxenham, A. J. (2010). Musical intervals and relative pitch: frequency resolution, not interval resolution, is special. *J. Acoust. Soc. Am.* 128, 1943–1951. doi: 10.1121/1.3478785

McDermott, J. H., Lehr, A. J., and Oxenham, A. J. (2008). Is relative pitch specific to pitch? *Psychol. Sci.* 19, 1263–1271. doi: 10.1111/j.1467-9280.2008.02235.x

McKay, C. M., McDermott, H. J., and Carlyon, R. P. (2000). Place and temporal cues in pitch perception: are they truly independent? *Acoust. Res. Lett. Online* 1, 25–30. doi: 10.1121/1.1318742

McKay, C. M., McDermott, H. J., and Clark, G. M. (1994). Pitch percepts associated with amplitude-modulated current pulse trains in cochlear implantees. *J. Acoust. Soc. Am.* 96, 2664–2673. doi: 10.1121/1.411377

Meddis, R., and Hewitt, M. J. (1991). Virtual pitch and phase sensitivity of a computer model of the auditory periphery. I: pitch identification. *J. Acoust. Soc. Am.* 89, 2866–2882. doi: 10.1121/1.400725

Moore, B. C. J. (1997). *An Introduction To The Psychology Of Hearing*, 3rd Edn. London: Academic Press.

Moore, B. C. J., and Carlyon, R. P. (2005). "Perception of pitch by people with cochlear hearing loss and by cochlear implant users," in *Pitch: Neural Coding and Perception Springer Handbook of Auditory Research*, eds C. J. Plack, A. J. Oxenham, R. R. Fay, and A. N. Popper, (New York: Springer), 234–277. doi: 10.1007/0-387-28958-5_7

Moore, B. C. J., and Peters, R. W. (1992). Pitch discrimination and phase sensitivity in young and elderly subjects and its relationship to frequency selectivity. *J. Acoust. Soc. Am.* 91, 2881–2893. doi: 10.1121/1.402925

Moore, B. C. J., and Rosen, S. M. (1979). Tune recognition with reduced pitch and interval information. *Q. J. Exp. Psychol.* 31, 229–249.

Nelson, D. A., Van Tasell, D. J., Schroder, A. C., Soli, S., and Levine, S. (1995). Electrode ranking of "place pitch" and speech recognition in electrical hearing. *J. Acoust. Soc. Am.* 98, 1987–1999. doi: 10.1121/1.413317

Oxenham, A. J. (2013). Revisiting place and temporal theories of pitch. *Acoust. Sci. Technol. Ed. Acoust. Soc. JPN* 34, 388–396. doi: 10.1250/ast.34.388

Pijl, S. (1997). Labeling of musical interval size by cochlear implant patients and normally hearing subjects. *Ear Hear.* 18, 364–372. doi: 10.1097/00003446-199710000-00002

Pijl, S., and Schwarz, D. W. F. (1995a). Intonation of musical intervals by deaf subjects stimulated with single bipolar cochlear implant electrodes. *Hear. Res.* 89, 203–211. doi: 10.1016/0378-5955(95)00138-139

Pijl, S., and Schwarz, D. W. F. (1995b). Melody recognition and musical interval perception by deaf subjects stimulated with electrical pulse trains through single cochlear implant electrodes. *J. Acoust. Soc. Am.* 98, 886–895. doi: 10.1121/1.413514

Plack, C. J., and Oxenham, A. J. (2005). "The psychophysics of pitch," in *Pitch: Neural Coding and Perception Springer Handbook of Auditory Research*, eds C. J. Plack, A. J. Oxenham, R. R. Fay, and A. N. Popper, (New York: Springer), 1–6.

Plomp, R. (1976). *Aspects of Tone Sensation*. London: Academic Press.

Schubert, E., and Wolfe, J. (2006). Does timbral brightness scale with frequency and spectral centroid? *Acta Acust. United Acust.* 92, 820–825.

Shamma, S., and Klein, D. (2000). The case of the missing pitch templates: How harmonic templates emerge in the early auditory system. *J. Acoust. Soc. Am.* 107, 2631–2644. doi: 10.1121/1.428649

Shamma, S. A. (1985). Speech processing in the auditory system II: lateral inhibition and the central processing of speech evoked activity in the auditory nerve. *J. Acoust. Soc. Am.* 78, 1622–1632. doi: 10.1121/1.392800

Simon, J. L. (1997). *Resampling: The New Statistics*. Available at: http://www.resample.com/content/text (accessed November 13, 2019).

Singh, S., Kong, Y.-Y., and Zeng, F.-G. (2009). Cochlear implant melody recognition as a function of melody frequency range, harmonicity, and number of electrodes. *Ear Hear.* 30, 160–168. doi: 10.1097/AUD.0b013e31819342b9

Spiegel, M. F., and Watson, C. S. (1984). Performance on frequency-discrimination tasks by musicians and nonmusicians. *J. Acoust. Soc. Am.* 76, 1690–1695. doi: 10.1371/journal.pone.0187881

Sucher, C. M., and McDermott, H. J. (2007). Pitch ranking of complex tones by normally hearing subjects and cochlear implant users. *Hear. Res.* 230, 80–87. doi: 10.1016/j.heares.2007.05.002

Swanson, B. A. (2008). *Pitch Perception With Cochlear Implants*. Ph.D. thesis, University of Melbourne, Parkville, MO. Available at: http://hdl.handle.net/11343/39587 (accessed November 13, 2019).

Swanson, B. A., Dawson, P., and McDermott, H. (2009). investigating cochlear implant place-pitch perception with the modified melodies test. *Cochlear Implants Int.* 10, 100–104. doi: 10.1179/cim.2009.10.Supplement-1.100

Swanson, B. A., Van Baelen, E., Janssens, M., Goorevich, M., Nygard, T., and Van Herck, K. (2007). "Cochlear implant signal processing ICs," in *Proceedings of the IEEE 2007 Custom Integrated Circuits Conference*, (San Jose: IEEE), 437–442.

Tong, Y. C., Blamey, P. J., Dowell, R. C., and Clark, G. M. (1983). Psychophysical studies evaluating the feasibility of a speech processing strategy for a multiple-channel cochlear implant. *J. Acoust. Soc. Am.* 74, 73–80. doi: 10.1121/1.389620

Vandali, A., Dawson, P., Au, A., Yu, Y., Brown, M., Goorevich, M., et al. (2018). Evaluation of the optimized pitch and language strategy in cochlear implant recipients. *Ear Hear.* 40, 555–567. doi: 10.1097/AUD.0000000000000627

Vandali, A. E., Dawson, P. W., and Arora, K. (2017). Results using the OPAL strategy in mandarin speaking cochlear implant recipients. *Int. J. Audiol.* 56, S74–S85. doi: 10.1080/14992027.2016.1190872

Vandali, A. E., Sly, D., Cowan, R., and van Hoesel, R. J. M. (2013). Pitch and loudness matching of unmodulated and modulated stimuli in cochlear implantees. *Hear. Res.* 302, 32–49. doi: 10.1016/j.heares.2013.05.004

Vandali, A. E., and van Hoesel, R. J. M. (2011). Development of a temporal fundamental frequency coding strategy for cochlear implants. *J. Acoust. Soc. Am.* 129, 4023–4036. doi: 10.1121/1.3573988

Vandali, A. E., and van Hoesel, R. J. M. (2012). Enhancement of temporal cues to pitch in cochlear implants: Effects on pitch ranking. *J. Acoust. Soc. Am.* 132, 392–402. doi: 10.1121/1.4718452

Vandali, A. E., Whitford, L. A., Plant, K. L., and Clark, G. M. (2000). Speech perception as a function of electrical stimulation rate: using the Nucleus 24 cochlear implant system. *Ear Hear.* 21, 608–624. doi: 10.1097/00003446-200012000-00008

Permissions

All chapters in this book were first published by Frontiers; hereby published with permission under the Creative Commons Attribution License or equivalent. Every chapter published in this book has been scrutinized by our experts. Their significance has been extensively debated. The topics covered herein carry significant findings which will fuel the growth of the discipline. They may even be implemented as practical applications or may be referred to as a beginning point for another development.

The contributors of this book come from diverse backgrounds, making this book a truly international effort. This book will bring forth new frontiers with its revolutionizing research information and detailed analysis of the nascent developments around the world.

We would like to thank all the contributing authors for lending their expertise to make the book truly unique. They have played a crucial role in the development of this book. Without their invaluable contributions this book wouldn't have been possible. They have made vital efforts to compile up to date information on the varied aspects of this subject to make this book a valuable addition to the collection of many professionals and students.

This book was conceptualized with the vision of imparting up-to-date information and advanced data in this field. To ensure the same, a matchless editorial board was set up. Every individual on the board went through rigorous rounds of assessment to prove their worth. After which they invested a large part of their time researching and compiling the most relevant data for our readers.

The editorial board has been involved in producing this book since its inception. They have spent rigorous hours researching and exploring the diverse topics which have resulted in the successful publishing of this book. They have passed on their knowledge of decades through this book. To expedite this challenging task, the publisher supported the team at every step. A small team of assistant editors was also appointed to further simplify the editing procedure and attain best results for the readers.

Apart from the editorial board, the designing team has also invested a significant amount of their time in understanding the subject and creating the most relevant covers. They scrutinized every image to scout for the most suitable representation of the subject and create an appropriate cover for the book.

The publishing team has been an ardent support to the editorial, designing and production team. Their endless efforts to recruit the best for this project, has resulted in the accomplishment of this book. They are a veteran in the field of academics and their pool of knowledge is as vast as their experience in printing. Their expertise and guidance has proved useful at every step. Their uncompromising quality standards have made this book an exceptional effort. Their encouragement from time to time has been an inspiration for everyone.

The publisher and the editorial board hope that this book will prove to be a valuable piece of knowledge for researchers, students, practitioners and scholars across the globe.

List of Contributors

Morrison M. Steel, Melissa J. Polonenko, Sara Giannantonio and Talar Hopyan
Archie's Cochlear Implant Laboratory, The Hospital for Sick Children, Toronto, ON, Canada

Blake C. Papsin and Karen A. Gordon
Archie's Cochlear Implant Laboratory, The Hospital for Sick Children, Toronto, ON, Canada
Department of Otolaryngology-Head and Neck Surgery, University of Toronto, Toronto, ON, Canada

Barbara Tillmann
CNRS UMR5292, INSERM U1028, Auditory Cognition and Psychoacoustics Team, Lyon Neuroscience Research Center, Lyon, France
University of Lyon, Lyon, France Université Claude Bernard Lyon 1, Villeurbanne, France

Bénédicte Poulin-Charronnat and Charles Delbé
CNRS UMR5292, INSERM U1028, Auditory Cognition and Psychoacoustics Team, Lyon Neuroscience Research Center, Lyon, France
University of Lyon, Lyon, France
Université Claude Bernard Lyon 1, Villeurbanne, France
LEAD-CNRS, UMR5022, Université Bourgogne Franche-Comté, Dijon, France

Etienne Gaudrain
CNRS UMR5292, INSERM U1028, Auditory Cognition and Psychoacoustics Team, Lyon Neuroscience Research Center, Lyon, France
University of Lyon, Lyon, France
Université Claude Bernard Lyon 1, Villeurbanne, France
University Medical Center Groningen, University of Groningen, Groningen, Netherlands

Idrick Akhoun
School of Psychological Sciences, The University of Manchester, Manchester, United Kingdom

Eric Truy
University of Lyon, Lyon, France
Université Claude Bernard Lyon 1, Villeurbanne, France
CNRS UMR5292, INSERM U1028, Brain Dynamics and Cognition Team, Lyon Neuroscience Research Center, Lyon, France

Lionel Collet
University of Lyon, Lyon, France
Université Claude Bernard Lyon 1, Villeurbanne, France

Sina Tahmasebi, Tom Gajęcki and Waldo Nogueira
Department of Otolaryngology, Medical University Hannover and Cluster of Excellence "Hearing4all", Hanover, Germany

Kate Gfeller
School of Music, College of Liberal Arts and Sciences, The University of Iowa, Iowa City, IA, United States
Department of Communication Sciences and Disorders, College of Liberal Arts and Sciences, The University of Iowa, Iowa City, IA, United States
Iowa Cochlear Implant Clinical Research Center, Department of Otolaryngology, The University of Iowa Hospitals and Clinics, Iowa City, IA, United States

Virginia Driscoll
School of Music, College of Liberal Arts and Sciences, The University of Iowa, Iowa City, IA, United States
Iowa Cochlear Implant Clinical Research Center, Department of Otolaryngology, The University of Iowa Hospitals and Clinics, Iowa City, IA, United States

Adam Schwalje
Iowa Cochlear Implant Clinical Research Center, Department of Otolaryngology, The University of Iowa Hospitals and Clinics, Iowa City, IA, United States

Christina Fuller
Department of Otorhinolaryngology, Head and Neck Surgery, University Medical Center Groningen, University of Groningen, Groningen, Netherlands
Research School of Behavioral and Cognitive Neurosciences, Graduate School of Medical Sciences, University of Groningen, Groningen, Netherlands
Department of Otorhinolaryngology, Treant Zorggroep, Emmen, Netherlands

Deniz Başkent and Rolien Free
Department of Otorhinolaryngology, Head and Neck Surgery, University Medical Center Groningen, University of Groningen, Groningen, Netherlands
Research School of Behavioral and Cognitive Neurosciences, Graduate School of Medical Sciences, University of Groningen, Groningen, Netherlands

Molly L. Erickson, Katie Faulkner, Patti M. Johnstone, Mark S. Hedrick and Taylor Stone
Department of Audiology and Speech Pathology, University of Tennessee Health Science Center, Knoxville, TN, United States

Ruth MacMullen Mallalieu
University Library, The University of Sheffield, Sheffield, United Kingdom

Aleksander Mansouri
Independent Scholar, Brighton, MA, United States

Gaelen McCormick
Eastman School of Music, University of Rochester, Rochester, NY, United States

Renee Blue O'Connell
Independent Scholar, Charlottesville, VA, United States

Jake Spinowitz
Independent Scholar, San Francisco, CA, United States

Bettina Gellinek Turner
Independent Scholar, Newburyport, MA, United States

Steffen Spangmose, Jens Hjortkjær and Jeremy Marozeau
Hearing Systems Group, Department of Health Technology, Technical University of Denmark, Lyngby, Denmark

Bjørn Petersen, Anne Sofie Friis Andersen, Niels Trusbak Haumann, Elvira Brattico and Peter Vuust
Center for Music in the Brain, Department of Clinical Medicine, Aarhus University and The Royal Academy of Music, Aarhus/Aalborg, Aarhus, Denmark

Andreas Højlund and Martin J. Dietz
Center of Functionally Integrative Neuroscience, Aarhus University, Aarhus, Denmark

Franck Michel
Audiological Clinic, Department of Otorhinolaryngology, Head and Neck Surgery, Aarhus University Hospital, Aarhus, Denmark

Søren Kamaric Riis
Oticon Medical, Smørum, Denmark
Iowa Cochlear Implant Clinical Research Center, Department of Otolaryngology–Head and Neck Surgery, Carver College of Medicine, University of Iowa, Iowa City, IA, United States

Emily R. Spitzer, David M. Landsberger and David R. Friedmann
Department of Otolaryngology–Head and Neck Surgery, New York University School of Medicine, New York, NY, United States

John J. Galvin III
House Ear Institute, Los Angeles, CA, United States

Katelyn Berg and Robert Dwyer
Department of Hearing and Speech Sciences, Vanderbilt University Medical Center, Nashville, TN, United States

Jack Noble
Department of Hearing and Speech Sciences, Vanderbilt University Medical Center, Nashville, TN, United States
Department of Electrical Engineering and Computer Science, Vanderbilt University, Nashville, TN, United States
Department of Otolaryngology, Vanderbilt University Medical Center, Nashville, TN, United States

Benoit Dawant and Robert Labadie
Department of Electrical Engineering and Computer Science, Vanderbilt University, Nashville, TN, United States
Department of Otolaryngology, Vanderbilt University Medical Center, Nashville, TN, United States

Virginia Richards
Department of Cognitive Science, University of California, Irvine, Irvine, CA, United States

René Gifford
Department of Hearing and Speech Sciences, Vanderbilt University Medical Center, Nashville, TN, United States
Department of Otolaryngology, Vanderbilt University Medical Center, Nashville, TN, United States

Kristen L. D'Onofrio, David M. Kessler and René H. Gifford
Cochlear Implant Research Laboratory, Department of Hearing and Speech Sciences, Vanderbilt University, Nashville, TN, United States

Meredith Caldwell
Vanderbilt University Medical Center, Nashville, TN, United States

Charles Limb
Department of Otolaryngology–Head and Neck Surgery, University of California, San Francisco, San Francisco, CA, United States

Spencer Smith
Department of Communication Sciences and Disorders, The University of Texas at Austin, Austin, TX, United States

Youssef Adel, Sharon Nagel, Tobias Weissgerber and Uwe Baumann
Audiological Acoustics, Department of Otorhinolaryngology, University Hospital Frankfurt, Frankfurt, Germany

Olivier Macherey
Aix-Marseille University, CNRS, Centrale Marseille, LMA, Marseille, France

Valerie Looi
SCIC - An RIDBC Service, Sydney, NSW, Australia
Advanced Bionics (Asia Pacific), Sydney, NSW, Australia

Ritva Torppa
Logopedics and Cognitive Brain Research Unit, Department of Psychology and Logopedics, Faculty of Medicine, University of Helsinki, Helsinki, Finland

Tania Prvan
Department of Mathematics and Statistics, Macquarie University, Sydney, NSW, Australia

Debi Vickers
Department of Clinical Neurosciences, The University of Cambridge, Cambridge, United Kingdom

Mustafa Yüksel
Audiology and Speech Disorders Program, Institute of Health Sciences, Marmara University, Istanbul, Turkey

Margaret A. Meredith
Childhood Communication Center, Seattle Children's Hospital, Seattle, WA, United States

Jay T. Rubinstein
Virginia Merrill Bloedel Hearing Research Center, Department of Otolaryngology - Head and Neck Surgery, University of Washington, Seattle, WA, United States

Brett A. Swanson
Cochlear Ltd., Sydney, NSW, Australia

Vijay M. R. Marimuthu and Robert H. Mannell
Department of Linguistics, Faculty of Human Sciences, Macquarie University, Sydney, NSW, Australia

Index